INTERDISCIPLINARY REHABILITATION OF LOW BACK PAIN

INTERDISCIPLINARY REHABILITATION OF LOW BACK PAIN

Edited by

C. DAVID TOLLISON, PhD
Pain Therapy Centers
Greenville Hospital System
Greenville, South Carolina

Associate Clinical Professor
Department of Anesthesiology
Medical College of Georgia
Augusta, Georgia

MICHAEL L. KRIEGEL, PhD
Pain Therapy Centers
Greenville Hospital System
Greenville, South Carolina

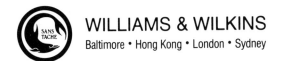

WILLIAMS & WILKINS
Baltimore • Hong Kong • London • Sydney

Editor: Michael G. Fisher
Associate Editor: Carol Eckhart
Copy Editor: Megan Westerfeld
Design: Ray Lowman
Illustration Planning: Bets Ltd.
Production: Barbara J. Felton

Copyright· © 1989
Williams & Wilkins
428 East Preston Street
Baltimore, Maryland 21202, USA

Accurate indications, adverse reactions, and dosage schedules for drugs are provided in this book, but it is possible that they may change. The reader is urged to review the package information data of the manufacturers of the medications mentioned.

Printed in the United States of America

Library of Congress Cataloging in Publication Data

Interdisciplinary rehabilitation of low back pain.
  Includes index.
  1. Backache—Patients—Rehabilitation. 2. Backache—
Treatment. I. Tollison, C. David, 1949–
II. Kriegel, Michael L. [DNLM: 1. Backache—therapy.
WE 755 I598]
RD771.B217I57 1989   617'.56   88-36281
ISBN 0-683-08336-8

89 90 91 92 93
1 2 3 4 5 6 7 8 9 10

To my mother, Louise J. Tollison

C.D.T.

To my wife, Linda H. Kriegel, and daughter, Ashley

M.L.K.

PREFACE

We must all die. But that I can save a person from days of torture, that is what I feel as my great and ever new privilege. Pain is a more terrible lord of mankind than even death himself.

Albert Schweitzer

Pain in the lower back is one of the most common, yet complex, disorders encountered in modern medical practice. Authorities report that over 50% of those persons surveyed complained of back pain during the preceding year, with spinal pain ranking second only to headaches as the leading cause of employee absenteeism in our country (*Nuprin Pain Report,* Louis Harris and Associates, 1986). Consider the following facts:

75 million Americans have back pain
7 million new victims suffer back pain each year
4 million back pain sufferers are unable to work
89 million workdays are lost per year because of back pain
5 billion dollars are spent annually on tests and treatments for back pain
1.9 billion dollars are lost to the gross national product because of decreased productivity of back patients
20% of all occupational injuries involve the spine
32% of all workers' compensation dollars are spent on the spine
60% of all long-term disabilities involve the spine

Despite the fact that eight of every 10 Americans will suffer an episode of low back pain during their lives, the successful treatment of this common disorder remains a perplexing challenge to clinicians.

Historically, treatment of lower back complaints has consisted of either surgical intervention or conservative care, characterized primarily by bed rest, muscle relaxant medications, and passive physical therapy modalities. While surgery remains an effective treatment of choice in carefully selected lower back diagnoses, generally the results are disappointing. Likewise, the results of conservative and traditional medical management in nonsurgical back pain are discouraging. The frustration experienced by clinicians and patients has recently served as a catalyst for the development of a more aggressive, interdisciplinary, rehabilitative approach to treatment.

Today interdisciplinary rehabilitation of low back pain is an accepted and growing part of medical practice. Thousands of physicians and health professionals of various disciplines, along with hospitals and independent treatment centers, now either specialize in back pain rehabilitation or offer services as part of a broad pain management practice. Recently a clinically effective armamentarium of treatment techniques has been developed to assist the professionals. These new techniques, in concert with the innovative delivery of time-honored modalities, have brought focus on the practice of interdisciplinary rehabilitation of low back pain as the promising direction to pursue in the treatment of spinal pain.

What is the distinguishing value of an interdisciplinary approach? The practice of medicine has historically utilized an acute care model with solo practitioners providing direct services to patients on an individual basis. Despite advancing technical knowledge and the concomitant increase in medical specialization, the acute illness–individual provider model has remained largely unchanged. Perhaps the increased specialization within medicine has, in reality, resulted in a narrower perspective on patients and fractionalization of medical care. Although this time-honored model may be appropriate treatment for the majority of acute diseases, chronic conditions and disorders such as intractable back pain, with inherent sets of complex medical, psychological, social, and legal problems, have led to an identified need for a comprehensive team approach to treatment.

Turk and Steig (Turk DC, Steig RL: Chronic pain: the necessity of interdisciplinary communication. *Clin J Pain* 3:163–167, 1987) characterized the value of an interdisciplinary team in this manner: An interdisciplinary team ideally consists of a core group of individuals who (a) share a common conceptualization of pain patients; (b) synthesize the diverse sets of information based on their own evaluation, as well as those of outside consultants, into an intelligent differential diagnosis and treatment plan for each patient; (c) work together to formulate and implement a comprehensive rehabilitation plan based on the available data; (d) share a common philosophy of disability management; and, perhaps most importantly, (e) act as a functional unit whose members are willing to learn from each other and modify, when appropriate, their own opinions based on the combined observations and expertise of the entire group.

Addressing the unique value of an interdisciplinary, clinical, rehabilitative treatment of lower back pain, this book is designed as a comprehensive practice guide. It is written for use by practicing internists, neurologists, orthopaedic surgeons, neurosurgeons, rheumatologists, family practice physicians, psychiatrists, physiatrists, psychologists, physical therapists, chiropractors, occupational therapists, pain medicine specialists, and other interested health professionals. The content is an attempt to blend carefully all aspects of nonsurgical back treatment within a comprehensive interdisciplinary style. Organized in a logical and easy-reference "treatment modality" format, the text features the contributions of a highly distinguished panel of nationally recognized authorities who have prepared information in their respective areas of expertise while adhering to the interdisciplinary theme of the book. The underlying goal of the book is to bridge the present gap between theory and practice by providing a comprehensive reference for clinical practice that emphasizes practical information essential for evaluating and treating low back pain in an interdisciplinary, rather than a partitioned, fashion.

Section 1 of the text establishes a required foundation for understanding, diagnosing, and treating low back pain in an interdisciplinary fashion. Four chapters are devoted to an emphasis on the importance of interdisciplinary practice and a differentiation of surgical versus nonsurgical treatment. A discussion of physical and psychological examinations of the lower back pain patient reveals the multidimensional quality of low back pain.

Section 2 is a pragmatic, clinical presentation of the role of neural blockage and needle therapies in the interdisciplinary treatment of low back pain. With both diagnostic and therapeutic value, nerve blocks and trigger point injections play a critical role in comprehensive management. In addition, a practical presentation of acupuncture, an often misunderstood technique, is outlined in a traditionally anatomic and physiologic manner.

Section 3 offers a detailed presentation of physical medicine modalities and techniques in treatment. Four chapters carefully integrate physical medicine into the comprehensive evaluation and treatment of individuals suffering lower back pain and provide specific information on clinical utility.

Section 4 specifically details the value of a pharmacologic approach to treatment. This comprehensive section outlines the use of systemic analgesics, nonsteroidal anti-inflammatory agents, and psychopharmacologic medications in the treatment of low back pain and incorporates their use within an interdisciplinary approach.

Section 5 maintains the comprehensive interdisciplinary focus of the text by integrating the important role of psychological therapies into a nonsurgical, rehabilitative approach. The value and specifics of behavioral management, group therapy, and family therapy in the treatment of lower back pain are thoroughly discussed. In addition, a chapter on hypnotic analgesia provides interesting clinical information that should prove useful in treatment.

The sixth and final section of the text provides useful and practical information on a collection of topics carefully chosen because of their impact on interdisciplinary treatment of lower back pain. The benefits of comprehensive pain centers, work hardening, back schools, and work capacity evaluations are outlined along with the clinical specifics of lumbar traction in treatment. In addition, a comprehensive presentation of the interesting functional restoration approach to spinal rehabilitation is detailed.

This text is thought to represent a clinical first. While several available texts and chapters target selected aspects of physical medicine modalities, psychological rehabilitation, pharmacology, and other components of a comprehensive treatment approach, to our knowledge there is no text exclusively devoted to the detailed nonsurgical interdisciplinary management of lower back pain.

While we should remain always mindful that the term "lower back pain" describes an anatomic location of discomfort and is not technically an ac-

ceptable diagnosis, the science of nonsurgical rehabilitation is rapidly maturing into an effective treatment alternative for thousands of individuals in pain. The time has come. The need exists.

C. David Tollison, PhD
Michael L. Kriegel, PhD

ACKNOWLEDGMENTS

The publication of a book such as this is generally credited to the editors, contributing authors, and publisher. Yet anyone who has labored intently in the preparation of a text readily knows that countless other individuals contribute, both directly and indirectly, to the final product. Although recognizing the important contribution of every individual who positively influenced this project is impossible, we shall attempt to identify a limited number of persons and we hereby extend our sincere appreciation to each of these and numerous unnamed others.

First, we would like to extend our appreciation to the contributing authors. Twenty-nine authors gave their time, talents, knowledge, and considerable expertise to this book. Each is a highly regarded authority with multiple demands on his/her time and attention. Yet each cheerfully cooperated with the numerous requests inherent in such a project as this. Thank you!

We would also like to extend our appreciation to Williams & Wilkins. Nancy Collins originally championed this project during its initial stages prior to Michael Fisher, Editor, competently assuming editorial control through completion. Carol Eckhart, Associate Editor, was consistently of invaluable assistance in all aspects of coordination and development. Her expertise, enthusiasm, and personality have made our working relationship both productive and enjoyable.

We also owe a debt of personal gratitude to many other people, some of whom include: Thomas E. Hassett III, our friend and colleague; John R. Satterthwaite, M.D., Medical Director of Pain Therapy Centers; Jack A. Skarupa, President, and the Board of Directors of the Greenville Health Corporation; Mrs. Melinda Davis, Administrative Assistant, for her skilled work in coordinating all aspects of this text; and Mrs. Sharon Ellis, for all that she does for our practice.

The first editor also extends appreciation and gratitude to Joseph W. Tollison, M.D., and his family, Betty, Joey, and Julie; Walter E. and Ellen T. Hayden; Dr. Jerry C. Langley and his family, Sandy, Spencer, and Brittany; and Fred and Louise Surett. Particular appreciation is extended to my wife and children—Linda, Courtney, and David.

The second editor extends appreciation and gratitude to Thomas and Ann Kriegel, his parents, who always believed in him.

C. David Tollison, PhD
Michael L. Kriegel, PhD

CONTRIBUTORS

J. Hampton Atkinson, Jr., MD
(Chapter 15)
Department of Psychiatry
University of California at San Diego
School of Medicine
La Jolla, California

Laurence A. Bradley, PhD
(Chapter 4)
Section on Medical Psychiatry
The Bowman Gray School of Medicine
Wake Forest University
Winston-Salem, North Carolina

Thomas H. Budzynski, PhD
(Chapter 12)
Behavioral Medicine Associates
Bellevue, Washington

Jeffrey R. Cram, PhD
(Chapter 12)
Biofeedback Institute of Seattle
Seattle, Washington

W. David Crews, Jr., MS
(Chapter 17)
Psychological Associates of Lynchburg
Oakdale Circle
Lynchburg, Virginia

Daniel M. Doleys, PhD
(Chapter 16)
Adjunct Associate Professor
University of Alabama at Birmingham
and
Director, Behavioral Programs
AMI Brookwood Medical Center
Birmingham, Alabama

Frederick J. Evans, PhD
(Chapter 19)
Adjunct Professor
Department of Psychiatry
University of Medicine and Dentistry of
New Jersey
Robert Wood Johnson Medical School
Piscataway, New Jersey

Teresa Ferrer-Brechner, MD
(Chapter 5)
Adjunct Professor
Department of Anesthesiology
and
Director, UCLA Pain Management Center
University of California at Los Angeles
Los Angeles, California

Lawrence W. Friedmann, MD, FACA, FICA
(Chapter 7)
Chairman, Department of Physical Medicine and
Rehabilitation
Nassau County Medical Center
and
Professor of Rehabilitation Medicine
State University of New York
Stony Brook, New York

Robert J. Gatchel, PhD
(Chapter 25)
Research Director
Productive Rehabilitation Institute of Dallas
for Ergonomics
Dallas, Texas

W. Doyle Gentry, PhD
(Chapter 17)
Psychological Associates
of Lynchburg and
Clinical Professor of
Behavioral Medicine and
Psychiatry, University
of Virginia School of
Medicine

Kimberly S. Gochneaur, BA
(Chapter 16)
Stress Management Department
AMI Brookwood Medical Center
Birmingham, Alabama

Gary D. Goldish, MD
(Chapter 23)
Institute for Low Back Care
Minneapolis, Minnesota
and
Rehabilitation Medicine Service
Minneapolis Veterans Administration
Minneapolis, Minnesota

Harold J. Gottlieb, PhD
(Chapter 20)
Director, Comprehensive Back Services
Advanced Rehabilitation Management
Pomona, California

Hamilton Hall, MD, FRCSC
(Chapter 22)
Medical Director
The Canadian Back Institute
and
Associate Professor, Department of Surgery
Division of Orthopaedics
University of Toronto
Toronto, Ontario, Canada

Thomas G. Kantor, MD
(Chapter 14)
Professor of Clinical Medicine
New York University Medical Center
New York, New York

Barbara K. Kornblau, JD, OTR
(Chapter 21)
Occupational Therapist and Attorney at Law
Miami, Florida

Stuart C. Kozinn, MD
(Chapter 3)
Institute for Bone and Joint Disorders
Phoenix, Arizona

Michael L. Kriegel, PhD
(Chapter 1)
Pain Therapy Centers
Greenville Hospital System
Greenville, South Carolina

Jerry C. Langley, DC
(Chapter 11)
Greenville, South Carolina

Stephen J. Lipson, MD
(Chapter 3)
Associate Professor, Orthopedic Surgery
Harvard Medical School
Boston, Massachusetts

Leonard N. Matheson, PhD
(Chapter 24)
Director, Employment and Rehabilitation Institute
of California
Anaheim, California

Tom G. Mayer, MD
(Chapter 25)
Clinical Professor of Orthopedic Surgery
University of Texas Southwestern Medical Center
and
Medical Director
Productive Rehabilitation Institute of Dallas
for Ergonomics
Dallas, Texas

Russell K. Portenoy, MD
(Chapter 13)
Director, Analgesic Studies
Pain Service
and
Assistant Attending Neurologist
Department of Neurology
Memorial Sloan-Kettering Cancer Center
New York, New York
and
Assistant Professor of Neurology
Cornell University Medical Center
Ithaca, New York

John C. Rowlingson, MD
(Chapter 6)
Professor, Department of Anesthesiology
and
Director, Pain Management Center
University of Virginia Medical Center
Charlottesville, Virginia

Ranjan Roy, Adv, DipSW
(Chapter 18)
Professor, Department of Psychiatry
School of Social Work
University of Manitoba
Winnipeg, Manitoba, Canada

Mark A. Slater, PhD
(Chapter 15)
Adjunct Assistant Professor
Department of Psychiatry
University of California at San Diego
La Jolla, California
and
Psychology Service
San Diego Veterans Medical Center
San Diego, California

Rajka Soric, MD, MSc, FRCPC
(Chapters 9 and 10)
Department of Rehabilitation Medicine
Mount Sinai Hospital
Toronto, Ontario, Canada

C. David Tollison, PhD
(Chapter 1)
Pain Therapy Centers
Greenville Hospital System
Greenville, South Carolina
and
Associate Clinical Professor
Department of Anesthesiology
Medical College of Georgia
Augusta, Georgia

George A. Ulett, MD, PhD
(Chapter 8)
Psychosomatic Medicine and Psychiatry, Inc.
St. Louis, Missouri
and
Clinical Professor of Psychiatry
St. Louis University School of Medicine
and
Director, Department of Psychiatry
Deaconness Hospital
St. Louis, Missouri

Clark Watts, MD
(Chapter 2)
Professor of Surgery, Neurosurgery
Division of Neurological Surgery
University of Missouri–Columbia
School of Medicine
Columbia, Missouri

CONTENTS

Section 1
INTRODUCTION

Chapter 1

INTERDISCIPLINARY REHABILITATION:

AN OVERVIEW

C. DAVID TOLLISON, PhD
MICHAEL L. KRIEGEL, PhD

The field of nonsurgical rehabilitation of low back pain has fast become one of the most rapidly growing treatment approaches in modern health care. A wide variety of health care professionals are now engaged in the clinical practice of low back pain rehabilitation, including physicians and surgeons of various medical specialties, medical psychologists, physical therapists, nurses, occupational therapists, vocational counselors and specialists, social workers, and health educators. Trends in the training of the health care professionals, including the development of didactic and practicum experiences in nonsurgical pain management for physicians and other professionals, reflect the growing acceptance of the principles and methods of pain rehabilitation and are a tribute to their acknowledged effectiveness in clinical use.

The growth and increased sophistication of nonsurgical rehabilitation has been stimulated by a vastly increased literature in the areas of assessment/evaluation, application, and analysis of specialized clinical care. The chapters in this text summarize new developments and outline the clinical application of nonsurgical rehabilitative treatment techniques for low back pain. These chapters are intended to provide practitioners of various disciplines with a central source of clinical information on the nonsurgical practice of interdisciplinary rehabilitation of low back pain.

CURRENT ISSUES

The relatively brief history of rehabilitative treatment of low back pain has been marked by vigorous and healthy dialogues, ranging from arguments concerning differing theoretical foundations to disagreements over terminology. The issues in terminology center, in part, on the concept of multidisciplinary versus interdisciplinary treatment approaches, while theoretical differences exist as to whether chronic pain is centrally or peripherally generated.

MULTIDISCIPLINARY VERSUS INTERDISCIPLINARY TREATMENT

Although multidisciplinary team treatment approaches have been much heralded in the restorative care of low back pain, there is a need to consider what is involved when this generic term is employed. "Multidisciplinary" is generally used to connote the clinical involvement of a group of specialists, although the authors have seen the term generously employed in several marginal program marketing publications to refer to as few as two specialists. Nevertheless, while the term "multidisciplinary" initially appears as an improvement over the traditional single-provider modus operandi, the phrase "multidisciplinary team" tells nothing of the nature of team interactions, the mechanics of team operation, the delegation of responsibility, the quality of communication among team members, or even the composition of the team (1). If what occurs in practice is that clinical information is provided by diverse consulting specialists, who represent the composition of the "team," while an identified coordinator synthesizes the information and develops and delivers the treatment plan, then there is little advance beyond the solo practitioner model.

In the evaluation and nonsurgical treatment of low back pain, an alternative to the multidisciplinary model is that of an "interdisciplinary team." An interdisciplinary team ideally consists of a group of core professionals who (a) share a common conceptualization of the patient in pain; (b) synthesize the diverse sets of information based on their clinical evaluations, as well as those of outside consultants, into an intelligent differential diagnosis and treatment plan for each patient; (c) work together to formulate and implement a comprehensive rehabilitation plan based on the available data; (d) share a common philosophy of disability management; and, perhaps most importantly, (e) act as a functional unit whose members are willing to learn from each other and modify, when appropriate, their own opinions based on the combined observations and expertise of the entire team (1).

If one considers the delivery of nonsurgical rehabilitative treatment of low back pain as existing on a continuum of solo provider—multidisciplinary team—interdisciplinary team, it is the opinion of the authors, based on limited observations, that the field of low back pain rehabilitation remains primarily concentrated in the multidisciplinary model with a recent and alarming gradual shifting back toward the single-discipline or solo-provider approach. Although it has become widely recognized that persistent low back pain is a complex phenomenon that has an impact on multiple aspects of a victim's functioning, there appears a recent proliferation of unimodal treatment centers providing single-discipline or, at best, multidisciplinary treatment. One sees this regression most prominently in so-called work hardening programs as well as physical therapy treatment centers.

Work hardening programs are theoretically designed to provide specialized clinical services to occupationally disabled patients who have reached maximum medical improvement (2). The proposed goal of such programs is to assist these individuals in achieving a desired physical state required to return to employment following a lengthy period of disability and physical deterioration (2). However, with the potent influences of a competitive market and free enterprise, one must wonder how frequently physical therapy centers and work hardening programs refer patients who are inappropriate for limited-scope treatment to comprehensive interdisciplinary programs. The influence of third-party payors intent upon identifying the least expensive treatment alternative possible generates additional concern.

According to Turk and Stieg, the treatment of patients suffering intractable pain should be addressed by an interdisciplinary team consisting of members from the disciplines of medicine, psychology, physical therapy, and occupational therapy (1). Since each team member has specific areas of expertise, the contribution of each member to decision making, planning, and clinical delivery is essential and of equal importance. Yet, it is the synthesis of these disciplines into a functioning interdisciplinary team, rather than merely the participation of various disciplines, that truly represents state-of-the-art rehabilitative care of low back pain.

PERIPHERAL VERSUS CENTRAL PAIN

The continuing controversy over the peripheral versus central etiology of chronic benign pain remains an important and unresolved issue that has a great impact on the treatment of low back pain. For example, the basic peripheralist's view of pain establishes the etiology of discomfort within the nervous system and the nociceptive process. Furthermore, the peripheralist believes that if the underlying pain generator or the "organic" mechanism producing the chronic pain can be eliminated, the patient's suffering will be relieved (3). In an effort to achieve this goal, the peripheralist may choose among various concepts and treatment modalities such as injectable steroids, nerve blocks, acupuncture, medications designed to alter basic neurochemistry, and surgical interventions designed to effect structural changes. Such modalities as hot packs, ultrasound, spinal manipulation, and transcutaneous electrical nerve stimulation also follow the general principles of the peripheralist's model in their attempt to reduce or eliminate nociceptive stimulation as the pain culprit. These treatment approaches are generally the basis of a unimodal treatment approach and, in fact, are consistent with the medical "disease" model of acute pain where professionals of various disciplines share in patient care in a serial or "turn-taking" manner (4). There is little utility for an interdisciplinary approach in the peripheralist's model, and the serial consultation mode of traditional medicine tends to dominate this type of approach.

By marked contrast, the centralist's view of chronic benign pain considers an array of factors in the etiology of pain as generated within the central nervous system. Such factors may include the patient's verbalizations of discomfort, socioeconomic variables, family problems, vocational and avocational aspects, and emotional and intellectual factors, as well as the cultural context within which these variables occur (1). Consequently, the centralist views pain as much more than the "sum of its parts" and adheres to a broader and more comprehensive approach to assessment (5). By definition the molar nature of the centralist's view mandates the necessity of an interdisciplinary approach to treatment, but with a special emphasis on the broad spectrum of psychosocial treatments, including selected antidepressant medications, and a rejection of those modalities consistent with the peripheral model (6).

Central and peripheral are two opposing theories as to the cause and appropriate treatment of chronic low back pain. As is so frequently the case, both models enjoy the credibility of noted advocates and a research base of clinical substantiation. Obviously, the question becomes which model is correct, and it should be remembered that such a decision heavily influences our approach to the treatment of a large and deserving population of pain sufferers.

Sometimes far removed from the level of expansive theoretical oration is the clinical practitioner with daily responsibilities for making difficult treatment decisions that have an impact on numerous patients in pain. It is at this one-to-one, human level of practical clinical application that the bipolar clarity of central versus peripheral models often becomes clouded. As the reader will determine in subsequent chapters, a variety of treatment approaches have proven beneficial in the nonsurgical care of low back pain. Some of these approaches, such as nerve blocks and acupuncture, fall into the category of the peripheral model, whereas other approaches, such as behavioral management and group therapy, are considered consistent with the central model. However, there are other rehabilitative approaches, such as work hardening and "back school," that may be argued to be partially consistent with both the peripheral and the central models. While additional research is needed to better define the clinical effectiveness of available treatment techniques, perhaps the current state of the art is best represented by an eclectic clinical approach whereby a variety of modalities, regardless

of whether they fit the central or peripheral model, are collectively administered in an interdisciplinary fashion (7). If one adheres to a philosophy that chronic benign low back pain is a biopsychosocial phenomenon comprised of the interaction of nociceptive sensory stimulation, psychological factors (i.e., cognitive, affective, and behavioral), and socioenvironmental factors (e.g., reinforcement from significant others and the health care system), the comfort of both the practitioner and the patient may be facilitated. From a biopsychosocial perspective, pain is neither solely somatic nor exclusively psychological; it is the interaction among these factors that produces the subjective experience of pain. Consequently, a multimodal interdisciplinary approach to the rehabilitation of low back pain currently appears to be the treatment of choice.

INTERDISCIPLINARY REHABILITATION: A MODEL PROGRAM

The comprehensive nonsurgical rehabilitation of low back pain is most often delivered in so-called pain centers or clinics, although there has been a proliferation of unimodal physical therapy programs as of late. Since pain centers vary greatly in terms of scope, philosophy, comprehensiveness, staffing, modalities, and the like, our present purpose is to outline one such interdisciplinary program and to illustrate how the complex process of evaluation and nonsurgical rehabilitation of low back pain occurs in such a setting.

The Pain Therapy Center of Greenville (South Carolina) was developed in 1980 as part of a 50-bed rehabilitation division of the Greenville Hospital System. Today, the Pain Therapy Center of Greenville serves as the flagship program of Pain Therapy Centers, a growing network of over 10 hospital-based programs located in the southeastern and midwestern United States. An interdisciplinary staff of health care professionals, including medical psychologists, physicians, physical therapists, behavior therapists, occupational therapists, nurses, and vocational specialists, devote their total time and attention to pain rehabilitation. Consultants representing neurology, neurosurgery, rheumatology, internal medicine, orthopedic surgery, and family medicine are also actively involved.

Although the details of nonsurgical rehabilitative treatment are individualized for every patient, the general approach is consistent. Physician-referred patients deemed appropriate for specialized rehabilitation as a result of participation in a comprehensive preadmission evaluation are actively involved in an average 18-day inpatient or outpatient interdisciplinary program emphasizing a nonsurgical rehabilitative approach to the physical, psychological, and vocational recovery of patients suffering intractable benign pain. This effort consists of an active "sports medicine" functional restoration approach to physical therapy, characterized by objective daily measures of progress in increasing strength, stamina, endurance, and range of motion, while clinical outcome is objectively measured by means of comprehensive pre-post functional capacities evaluations. The advantage of medical interventions, including pharmacologic care, nerve blocks and injection therapies, and various physical medicine techniques, is assessed on a continual basis by physicians and other professional staff. Other components of the rehabilitative program, including various educational classes, vocational interventions, relaxation and biofeedback training, and individual and group psychotherapy, are conducted in a behavioral therapeutic setting. Active patient participation in a highly structured, intensive, graded, interdisciplinary program of comprehensive nonsurgical rehabilitation is emphasized, and treatment goals include (a) increased physical activity, (b) decreased intake or elimination of analgesic agents, (c) decreased subjective estimates of pain, (d) decreased utilization of and dependence on health care facilities and providers, and (e) return to employment and productivity.

Since 1980, the Pain Therapy Center of Greenville has conducted evaluations on and treated over 5000 patients in pain. Table 1.1 outlines descriptive characteristics from a recent sampling of 100 consecutively treated patients with a diagnosis of chronic back pain (8). Historically 60% of all patients are referred by orthopaedic and neurosurgeons, while internal medicine and family physicians collectively refer the majority of the remainder. Approximately 80% of our patients complain of low back pain and 9% of chronic headaches, and the remainder are diagnosed as suffering with a variety of pain complaints.

PREADMISSION EVALUATION

Patient selection based on a comprehensive evaluation process is the first step in an interdisciplinary rehabilitation program. Each patient referred to our program is initially scheduled for an outpatient preadmission evaluation to determine his/her potential for specialized pain management and nonsurgical restorative treatment. Admissions criteria include the following:

Table 1.1
Characteristics of 100 Patients with Chronic Back Pain[a]

	NO.	MEAN	RANGE
Men	56		
Women	44		
Workmen's compensation	72		
Age		42.6 years	19–66 years
Education		10.3 years	3–17 years
Time since onset of pain		32 months	5–96 months
Medications for pain		2.2	0–7
Major back operations		2.1	0–6
Time since last employment[b]		22 months	1–77 months

[a] From Tollison CD, Kriegel ML, Downie GR: Chronic low back pain: results of treatment at the Pain Therapy Center. *South Med J* 78:1291–1295, 1986.
[b] For housewives, months since beginning to require help with housework.

1. No clinical evidence of pain etiology that is determined likely to respond to conventional medical or surgical interventions.
2. Referral by a physician with medical records of appropriate diagnostics.
3. Patient's cooperation and participation in a variety of tests and examinations.
4. Cooperation and active participation of the patient's spouse and family.
5. Clinical staff agreement that the patient is motivated to reduce pain and disability.
6. No evidence of severe psychological/psychiatric disturbance.

During the preadmission evaluation, every patient is examined by a physician, clinical psychologist, physical therapist, and vocational specialist, and family members are interviewed by a social worker. Each staff member reviews the medical records on every patient prior to the evaluation.

The medical and physical therapy components of the preadmission evaluation include a careful review of the patients' medical and surgical records as well as all diagnostic tests and procedures, a detailed pain interview, and a thorough physical examination and functional assessment. Particular attention is given to measurement of range of motion and discrepancies between pain behavior and observed or inferred abnormality. Occasionally patients are asked to undergo electrodiagnostic studies and/or radiographic studies to upgrade and compliment the diagnostic data base where indicated. The medical and physical therapy examinations also serve to define physical limitations and to better identify specific amounts, types, and rates of physical activities indicated as medically advisable at the outset and at subsequent points throughout the restorative treatment program.

The psychological evaluation is intended to determine the general psychological and personality status of every patient and to explore for systematic relationships between pain behavior and reinforcing consequences. In addition to the detailed clinical/pain interview, psychological testing in the form of the Minnesota Multiphasic Personality Inventory (MMPI), Millon Behavioral Health Inventory (MBHI), and Beck Depression Inventory is administered, with interpretation based on standards consistent with a population of patients in pain (8, 9).

A vocational history and interview are conducted by a certified vocational evaluator in order to identify vocational experience, skills, and interests of patients who may require vocational assistance in returning to or modifying employment. Since appropriate employment and productivity is considered, within our philosophy, to be physically and psychologically therapeutic, considerable emphasis is placed on identifying and satisfying those factors that may otherwise prohibit a return to a level of employment consistent with any physical or psychological limitations.

While referred patients participate in the structured preadmission evaluation, our social worker interviews family members, who are required to accompany the patient to the initial examination. The social work interview is intended to investigate family response and reinforcement of pain behavior and to identify the impact of every patient's pain on his/her family. During the interview a determination is also made as to whether the family is agreeable to participating in required weekly family training sessions. Furthermore, it has been our experience that communications training and marital counseling are frequently necessary in facilitating new interactional patterns between spouses and family members and in aiding in the transition from the pain program to the home or work environment.

PREADMISSION STAFFING

Following the preadmission evaluation, the professional staff meets and formally presents clinical findings and opinions. With the admissions criteria as a general guide, each staff member is allowed one vote for or against an offer of program admission. Those patients judged as not meeting the admissions criteria receive particular attention, since it is our policy to forward to the referring physician a summary of formal treatment and management recommendations on all patients, including those individuals not offered program admission.

Since 1981, approximately 22% of referred patients examined in the preadmission evaluation have been rejected for program admission. It is our firm belief that as a specialized elective pain rehabilitation and restoration program, accountability to patients, referring physicians, insurance carriers, and employers with a financial and/or personal interest in treatment success is critically important. As a result, admissions criteria are relatively stringent and we attempt to offer admission only to those individuals demonstrating adequate motivation and potential for success. Of the 22% rejected for program admission, 63% have been judged as demonstrating inadequate motivation to reduce pain and disability, 28% were judged as suffering severe psychological/psychiatric disturbance requiring traditional psychological/psychiatric referral, and the remaining 9% were rejected for a variety of reasons including lack of cooperation in the preadmission evaluation or a belief on the part of our staff that further traditional medical diagnostics and/or treatment were indicated.

THERAPEUTIC MODALITIES

Programs designed for the treatment of chronic benign low back pain vary greatly in terms of scope, philosophy, intensiveness, staffing, modalities, and so on. It is our firm belief that appropriate treatment must be active and interdisciplinary, emphasizing as much objective measurement as possible and fostering patient responsibility and independence. Consequently, while rehabilitation goals represent specific and measurable outcome events, treatment is broadly comprehensive and intensive.

In the sections to follow we briefly outline some of the primary therapeutic modalities used in our center and describe some of the more salient aspects or each. However, because of the comprehensive scope of the treatment program and the limitation of this chapter, only a partial listing of therapeutic modalities is possible.

Physical Therapy

Research has indicated that a program of regular stretching, strengthening, endurance, stamina, and physical reconditioning exercises is an important part of chronic benign pain rehabilitation, particularly in cases of low back pain (8). Flexion, general conditioning, and range-of-motion exercises have been proven to be important in reducing the amount of pain that patients report (10), and when introduced as part of a multimodal behavioral program as early as within 2 days of pain onset, result in a superior clinical outcome when compared to traditional conservative medical management (11).

In our program, patients are routinely scheduled for two daily classes of physical reactivation exercises totaling more than 2½ hours each day. No passive physical therapy is offered; all components are active and intensive and utilize a work-to-quota approach to increasing strength, walking distances, sitting and standing tolerances, bicycle riding, range of motion, and physical endurance (7).

Patients are introduced to physical therapy by explaining the rationale of a graded program of physical reconditioning and through a 2-day program of establishing appropriate baseline measures on a sampling of physical exertional stations (7). During this time, an individualized program of morning and afternoon stretching exercises is also outlined for every patient from a general collection of appropriate and effective exercises designed by Center staff (7).

Following baseline measurement, a daily work-to-quota system is implemented that is maintained throughout each patient's hospitalization and follow-up (12). Increased physical activity is also encouraged outside the scheduled reactivation classes. Patients are required to walk stairs rather than use the elevator, go through the hospital cafeteria line for meals, make their own beds, and clean their rooms. Treatment is goal oriented and emphasizes each patient's responsibility for his/her own treatment program, as well as increased physical strength, stamina, endurance, and independence.

In addition to stretching and strengthening exercises, our physical therapists also use transcutaneous electrical nerve stimulation (TENS) units, electrical therapies, mobilization techniques, and a variety of physical medicine modalities (see Chapters 9 and 10) in the treatment protocol. Of particular clinical benefit has been a technique termed "myofascial release," a manipulative-motion technique designed to induce muscular relaxation in spasming muscles.

Medicine

Program physicians are responsible for detailed history and physical examinations as part of the preadmission evaluation, as well as determining the need for further diagnostic tests or medical consultations. Diagnostic and therapeutic nerve blocks, trigger point injections, and a range of physical

Table 1.2
Pain Cocktail Formulas[a]

INGREDIENT	AMOUNT
PAIN COCKTAIL A	
Theragran liquid	20 ml
Flavored diluent	316 ml
Meperidine 100 mg/ml injection 100/15-ml dose	24 ml
PAIN COCKTAIL B	
Theragran liquid	20 ml
Flavored diluent	328 ml
Meperidine 100 mg/ml injection 50/15-ml dose	12 ml
PAIN COCKTAIL C	
Theragran liquid	20 ml
Codeine soluble tablets 30 mg (48 tablets)	1.44 g
Flavored diluent qs to a total of 60/15-ml dose	360 ml
PAIN COCKTAIL D	
Theragran liquid	20 ml
Codeine soluble tablets 30 mg. (24 tablets)	720 mg
Flavored diluent qs to a total of 30/15-ml dose	360 ml
PAIN COCKTAIL E	
Theragran liquid	20 ml
Flavored diluent	340 ml

[a]*Expiration on all cocktails is 6 months.*

medicine modalities are considered on an individual basis for every patient. Medication deceleration and regulation is a primary responsibility of our physicians, who frequently utilize a "pain cocktail" formula in analgesic detoxification (Table 1.2).

References to chronic low back pain generally identify a constellation of symptoms, including depression (13). The incidence of pain in depression has been reported to average 65% and the incidence of depression in chronic pain has been reported to be as high as 87% (14). A significant majority of patients treated in our program are judged to be clinically depressed by means of psychological testing and clinical interviews (8). Therefore, depression and pain may share common pathophysiology and potentiate negative effects on patients' coping and pain tolerance. Accordingly, tricyclic antidepressants are commonly prescribed by our physicians for patients suffering the combination of depression and low back pain (15). Of the two general groupings of tricyclic antidepressants, the tertiary amines, including doxepin and amitriptyline, have received considerable attention in the pain management literature. This is primarily due to research suggesting the effectiveness of doxepin and amitriptyline in blocking the reuptake of serotonin in excess of norepinephrine blockage and to research suggesting that serotonic enhancement helps raise the pain threshold, improves sleep, and relieves depression (13).

Because most chronic low back pain patients have been repeatedly examined and treated medically, the physicians in interdisciplinary rehabilitation programs must adopt philosophies, attitudes, and behaviors that are at variance with their years of training and experience in the traditional medical model. As expected, this can potentially create a wide variety of control and clinical problems for many physicians as well as the interdisciplinary team. For example, physicians must be capable of and willing to forfeit the ultimate control of the patient's care and encourage the blending of their talents with the talents, experiences, and expertise of the other members of the rehabilitation team. They must be capable of accepting the bitterness and frustration that many chronic patients harbor toward physicians in general for their failure to cure the patients' pain. Likewise, they must recognize that there is no singular therapeutic technique, whether it be injection, surgery, or pill, that will have as great a positive impact on chronic pain symptomatology as a multimodal clinical approach. In our experience, this last criterion generally represents the most difficult hurdle for physicians, particularly surgeons, who are accustomed to time-efficient and significant structural therapeutic change through operative intervention (see Chapter 2).

Vocational and Occupational Therapy

Many patients suffering chronic benign low back pain are vocationally disabled as the result of pain intensity and the cumulative and wide-ranging ramifications and effects of any chronic disorder. Perhaps some of these individuals will be unable to return to previously performed heavy physical labor and must consider less strenuous occupations, whereas other patients require specialized treatment and assistance in returning to previous employment. Further complicating this scenario is our patients' resistance to exploring return-to-work issues because of fears of failure, increased pain, possible reinjury, and potential loss of workers' compensation, which they often see as their only source of financial security. It is our opinion that returning disabled low back pain patients to employment is an appropriate and worthy goal of any comprehensive rehabilitation program, and our experience that exemplary results in return-to-work

efforts are mandated by workers' compensation insurance companies.

In response to return-to-work and productivity issues, we established in 1987 a comprehensive interdisciplinary program for vocationally disabled patients. The Workers' Rehabilitation and Recovery Center (WRRC) is specifically designed to return persons to productive employment following injury, prolonged medical recovery, and disability. It has three primary components: functional restoration, work simulation, and vocational intervention.

Functional Restoration

Prolonged physical inactivity, often complicated by bed rest, medications, and surgery, results in a negative catabolic state of musculoskeletal and cardiopulmonary function. Treatment requires a concentrated program of physical restoration, so the individual can meet the physical demands of employment. The WRRC patients work several hours a day under the supervision of a physical therapist to build strength, stamina, and endurance in a goal-oriented quota system of physical restoration. The result is an individual with the strength, stamina, and endurance to return to employment. In addition, the specially trained physical therapist may evaluate back-injured patients using the Isometric Strength Testing Unit (ISTU). The ISTU is a sophisticated diagnostic tool that accurately measures the back strength and functional utility of the spine by assessing physical performance in a variety of work-related postures. It then uses strength-designed software to compare the patient's isometric back strength and performance against that of a normal population.

Work Simulation

The most striking feature of the WRRC is its comprehensive work simulation environment, reproducing the specific job conditions in which the patient worked prior to injury. Patients work under the supervision of an occupational therapist in a variety of comprehensively designed work stations. Goals include increasing the patient's productivity and work tolerance, improving work rate and habits, and increasing confidence and proficiency in a structured work environment. Patients start at baseline levels consistent with their limitations and build endurance until they are working a full 8-hour day. The WRRC also attempts to offer patients more realistic preparation for their return to employment. Each work environment is contained within a cubicle and features authentic equipment, specific floor and wall coverings, and full-wall photographic murals. The murals were photographed in area companies and industries to add to the authenticity of the patient's workplace. In this way the WRRC serves as a "bridge" between disability and employment.

Vocational Intervention

Between preadmission and admission, a WRRC vocational specialist visits the worker's place of employment to perform a detailed job analysis. Specific data are gathered for computerized analysis on weights lifted, distances traveled, repetitions made, and other activities constituting a job profile, in order to develop an objective assessment of what the worker did and what he/she needs to do in work simulation. Besides shaping the work simulation program, the analysis resolves discrepancies between the patient's perception of his/her job and the employer's perception by providing an objective view of the work situation. This, of course, is one of the basic aims of vocational intervention, to handle and facilitate detailed and frequent communications between workers, physicians, employers, insurance companies, and attorneys. The result is frequently the difference between "employable" and "employed."

Relaxation and Biofeedback

Formalized progressive relaxation and biofeedback training, as part of a multimodal interdisciplinary treatment program, have proven valuable in helping patients learn to modify physiologic and psychological tension associated with chronic pain (7). Our typical patient does not know which of his/her muscles are tense, cannot accurately judge whether he/she is relaxed, does not realize any connection between prolonged tension and pain, and does not know how to relax (7). Relaxation training has proven helpful in breaking the "pain-tension-pain cycle" of chronic pain and in teaching patients to gain control over both physiologic and psychological functioning. (16).

In our program, progressive muscular relaxation instruction takes place in a dimly lit, quiet room specifically designated for relaxation training. Patients are encouraged to visit the relaxation room on their own during unscheduled times, and audio recordings of the progressive relaxation technique, along with portable tape players, are available for use in every patient's room. In addition, formalized relaxation therapy is scheduled daily. Patients are instructed in a specialized relaxation technique designed by program staff based, in part, on combining imagery and muscle-tensing techniques (7).

Electromyogram (EMG) biofeedback training is also utilized with selected low back pain patients exhibiting high levels of muscular bracing and tension in an effort to reduce pain intensity through reduction of maladaptive neuromuscular behaviors. Furthermore, EMG biofeedback is occasionally utilized to instruct proper posture and gait in patients more severely impaired by back pain.

Learning to relax can be a powerful tool in combating low back pain, and is frequently cited by our patients as one of the more beneficial aspects of the total rehabilitation program (7). Furthermore, pain control, anxiety relief, and improved sleep through instruction facilitates the transfer of responsibility of pain management to the patient.

Patient Education

It is our philosophy that patient education plays a valuable and unique role in effective pain rehabilitation. We have found that an alarming number of our patients have previously consented to multiple spinal surgeries with no concept of the surgical procedure, what a disk or vertebra looks like, the function of the spine, or even what to expect after surgery (7). Consequently, patient education in the form of didactic lectures and discussions is afforded a priority position within our treatment approach. Presentations and discussions led by psychologists, physicians, nurses, physical therapists, and vocational counselors have proven helpful in explaining to patients the continuing mechanism of low back pain, the value of proper body mechanics and physical reactivation, and why surgery usually cannot simply "cut out" the cause of chronic back pain.

In our organization, all disciplines participate in the educational process; however, the nursing service assumes primary responsibility for coordination and instruction. Nurses are in the unique position of having substantial observational time with patients and frequently continue instruction and reinforcement outside of the classroom in one-to-one relationships with patients.

A daily scheduled 1-hour educational class that is a particular favorite among our patients is termed "Pain School." Pain School incorporates over 50 prepared and outlined lectures and group discussions of specific topics requested by our patients. Each of these specific topics falls under one of 11 general categories found to have a significant impact on effective pain rehabilitation. Lectures and discussions of problem areas, such as sexual functioning and physical disability and how chronic low back pain can affect an individual's behavior and personality, are empirically judged as beneficial in allowing patients to more effectively deal with their pain problems. Lectures in basic anatomy and physiology, as well as presentations and discussions of the various types of medications, are particularly popular topics.

One class each week is devoted to dealing openly and honestly with how secondary gains, such as financial compensation and avoidance of responsibility, may occasionally be associated with chronic low back pain. Problems associated with workers' compensation claims and disability determination are thoroughly discussed in a nonjudgmental, educationally oriented fashion.

Finally, involvement of the spouse and family is considered a critical aspect of rehabilitative treatment. Family members are considered "extenders" of health professionals and are recognized as being capable of providing either potent reinforcement or extinction of the treatment regimen. Regular family training sessions are held during the course of treatment. Basics of behavior modification are taught and rehearsed, and family members are held responsible for practicing these principles at home.

Psychology

The clinical psychologist in a pain rehabilitation program must have specialized training and experience in medicine, especially in the areas of neurology, neurosurgery, and orthopaedic medicine (4). He/she must be willing to listen and answer questions and concerns about traditionally defined medical areas and, obviously, to correctly respond to such queries. The psychologist who views his/her role in the traditional sense of a mental and emotional health caretaker and refuses to become highly knowledgeable of the patient's physical problems is certain to fail as an integral part of the rehabilitation team (4).

Patients who have long suffered benign low back pain are almost universally unaccepting of a psychological approach to pain management, or of any approach that directly or indirectly suggests a psychological etiology of pain. Frequently these patients have endured inference by health professionals that the pain is "all in their heads," and reject any associated approach. To accept such an approach likely threatens their perception of pain as physical or mechanical in origin and may also jeopardize their workers' compensation benefits.

The interdisciplinary pain rehabilitation approach emphasizes a therapeutic model that addresses both the nociceptive and emotional components of low back pain (4). Consequently, all components of the pain phenomenon must be addressed, including financial compensation, secondary gain, avoidance and time-out from work and responsibilities, and other operant reinforcers, as well as body mechanics, muscle strengthening, posture, and other more physiologic mechanisms of pain. Goal-directed patient education is part of the psychologist's therapeutic armamentarium, and both individual and group instruction is offered in topics such as neuroanatomy and neurophysiology of pain, spinal biomechanics, pharmacology, spinal surgery, sexual dysfunction, depression and pain, and a variety of additional topics. Furthermore, persuasion, reassurance, support, and confrontation, as well as suggestion and other behavioral techniques, are utilized by all staff members. In our program it is not uncommon too find a psychologist explaining spinal anatomy to a patient or to witness an anesthesiologist or orthopaedic surgeon discussing with a patient the role of depression in chronic low back pain symptomatology. Psychotherapy, in its broadest sense, is coordinated by the psychologist but routinely delivered by all members of the interdisciplinary rehabilitation team.

TREATMENT RESULTS

A recent clinical outcome investigation was conducted to assess multimodal interdisciplinary rehabilitation effectiveness (8). One hundred patients consecutively admitted to the Pain Therapy Center of Greenville program with a diagnosis of chronic low back pain served as subjects. All patients were adults with a mean age of 42.6 years (range of 19–66 years). Fifty-six per cent of the admissions were male and 72% of the sample were injured in occupational accidents and admitted under workers' compensation. The mean time from pain onset to program admission was, 32 months and the average length of vocational disability was 22 months. The mean number of major spinal surgeries for the group was 2.1 and the average number of medications taken for pain complaints was 2.2.

Each of the 100 patients in this sample had active and current low back pain that had not responded to multiple traditional medical interventions and treatments in the past. All patients were admitted for comprehensive program participation based on the following criteria:

1. Pain of at least 6 months' duration.
2. No significant clinical evidence of surgically or medically remediable pain.
3. Referral by a physician or service agency after appropriate medical workup.

4. Cooperation in psychological and physical examination and testing.
5. Cooperation and active involvement of the patient's spouse and family.
6. Staff agreement that the patient is motivated to reduce pain and disability.
7. No debilitating psychological/psychiatric disturbance.

The results of this clinical outcome investigation indicated that all 100 patients had increased physical strength, stamina, endurance, range of motion, and overall physical activity, with the total increase per patient averaging 356%. These measurements were recorded daily, but statistical analysis compared physical measurements recorded at the time of admission (baseline) and at discharge. At 12-month follow-up, 83 patients were evaluated to determine maintenance of treatment gains. (Because our program is a regional referral center serving a number of southern states, 17 patients could not return for 1-year follow-up owing to excessive distances.) Of the 83 patients who returned for follow-up, 74 (89%) had successfully maintained the treatment gains as measured at discharge.

Eighty-four patients (84%) were taking an average of 2.2 medications for pain (including narcotics) at the time of program admission (16 patients were taking no medication for pain). At discharge 74 patients (88%) formerly taking medications were taking no medication for pain, and the average number of medications (1.0 medications, no narcotics) taken by the remaining 10 patients showed a 55% reduction. At 12-month follow-up, 63 patients (75%) who were taking medication at the time of admission were taking no medication for pain, and the average number of medications (1.1 medications, no narcotics) taken by the remaining patients indicated a reduction of 50%.

Subjective pain intensity was rated daily by each patient on a 5-point scale of intensity, but for purposes of analysis, significant decreases in subjective pain intensity were noted at discharge and at 1-year follow-up. Utilizing the daily rating scale, 69 patients (69%) reported subjective decreases in pain intensity and increased ability to cope with residual pain. At discharge, the average decrease in pain intensity was 31%. At 12-month follow-up, 61 patients reported decreases in pain intensity averaging 40%. Furthermore, the majority of patients also reported an increased ability to relax, improved sleep, and renewed confidence in their ability to function independently.

Overuse of medical care also sharply decreased after specialized treatment. At 1-year follow-up, 15 patients continued under active medical care and 85 patients reported no additional visits to physicians or hospitalizations for pain except for appointments initiated by workers' compensation personnel. This represents an 85% reduction in use of health care and a significant reduction in health care expenditures.

At the time of admission to our program, three patients with low back pain were working daily. At the time of discharge, 37 additional patients (38%) returned to full-time employment or were attending school or vocational training. Twelve-month follow-up indicated that an additional 27 patients (28%), for a total of 67 patients, were working or attending school daily, an increase of 66% from admission. Of the remainder, 5 patients had taken early retirement and 28 had not returned to employment.

A more recent clinical outcome study was conducted to investigate the effectiveness of the comprehensive interdisciplinary rehabilitation program described in this chapter in the treatment of both acute and chronic low back pain (17). The central issues in this research addressed the clinical effectiveness of comprehensive interdisciplinary rehabilitation of pain of a recent onset, and a comparison of treatment outcomes in populations suffering either acute or chronic low back pain.

Twenty-six consecutively admitted patients (group A) with a diagnosis of acute low back pain of less than 2 months' duration and 30 consecutively admitted patients (group B) with a diagnosis of chronic low back pain of greater than 6 months' duration served as subjects in this clinical outcome investigation. Each of the subjects suffered active and constant low back pain that had not responded to medical interventions. Tables 1.3 and 1.4 characterize the acute and chronic pain groups, respectively. Patients were treated under the same general format and are considered comparable in the data reported.

The results of this investigation (17) indicated that group A increased physical strength, stamina, endurance, and overall physical activity by an average of 228%, and group B demonstrated an average increase of 244%. Objective measurements were recorded daily, but statistical analyses compared objective physical measurements recorded at the time of program admission (baseline) and at discharge. At 3-month follow-up, 24 group A patients and 25 group B patients were evaluated to determine maintenance of treatment gains. (Seven patients could not return for 3-month follow-up

Table 1.3

Characteristics of Acute Low Back Pain Patients

CHARACTERISTIC	NO.	MEAN	RANGE
Men	16		
Women	10		
Workers' compensation cases	20		
Age		44.4 years	33–52 years
Education		11 years	6–16 years
Duration of pain		43 days	2–60 days
Medication for pain		2.7	0–5
Percentage having undergone surgery	15		
Duration of vocational disability[a]		36 days	0–60 days

[a] For housewives, days since beginning to require assistance with housework.

because of excessive distances.) Of the 24 patients in group A returning for follow-up, 22 (92%) had successfully maintained treatment gains as compared to functional status measured at discharge. Of the 25 patients in group B returning for follow-up, 20 (80%) had successfully maintained the level of increased physical activity (Table 1.5).

In a comparison of medication intake, 21 patients (81%) in group A were taking an average of 2.7 medications for pain (including narcotics) at the time of program admission, and 20 patients (67%) in group B were taking an average of 2.2 analgesic

Table 1.4

Characteristics of Chronic Low Back Pain Patients

CHARACTERISTIC	NO.	MEAN	RANGE
Men	17		
Women	13		
Workers' compensation cases	22		
Age		42.9 years	33–60 years
Education		10.4 years	5–17 years
Duration of pain		409 days	199–793 days
Medications for pain		2.2	0–6
Percentage having undergone back surgery	20		
Duration of vocational disability[a]		283 days	0–651 days

[a] For housewives, days since beginning to require assistance with housework.

Table 1.5

Average Treatment Outcome of Acute (Group A) and Chronic (Group B) Low Back Pain Patients

	DISCHARGE	FOLLOW-UP
Increase in physical activity		
Group A	228% increase	92% maintenance
Group B	244% increase	80% maintenance
Elimination of medication intake		
Group A	76% elimination	86% maintenance
Group B	85% elimination	79% maintenance
Reduction in subjective pain intensity		
Group A	44% reduction	72% reduction
Group B	40% reduction	43% reduction
Reduction in health care utilization		
Group A		96% reduction
Group B		77% reduction
Return to productivity		
Group A	42% productive	83% productive
Group B	35% productive	62% productive

medications (including narcotics). At discharge, 16 patients (76%) in group A formerly taking medications were completely withdrawn from all analgesic agents, while 17 patients (85%) in group B eliminated all analgesic intake. At 3-month follow-up, 14 of the 16 patients withdrawn from analgesic medications in Group A and 14 of the 17 patients withdrawn in group B returned for evaluation. Of those patients in groups A and B returning for follow-up evaluation, results indicated that 12 patients (86%) in group A and 11 patients (79%) in group B maintained abstinence from analgesic agents (Table 1.5).

Subjective pain intensity was rated daily by each patient on a 5-point scale of intensity, but for purposes of analysis, baseline, discharge, and follow-up ratings were compared. At discharge, 20 patients (77%) in group A and 21 (70%) in group B subjectively reported decreases in pain intensity, averaging 44% for patients suffering acute low back pain and 40% for patients suffering chronic low back pain. At 3-month follow-up, 19 of 20 patients in group A subjectively reporting decreased pain at discharge were evaluated, and 17 patients (89%) reported a continuation of pain relief averaging 72%. Eighteen of 21 group B patients originally reporting decreased low back pain as a result of treatment returned for follow-up, and 16 (83%)

reported maintenance of pain relief averaging 43% (Table 1.5).

Utilization of medical care was also sharply decreased in both treatment groups following program participation. At 3-month follow-up, one patient in group A and seven patients in group B continued under active medical care, while the remainder reported no additional visits to physicians or hospitalizations for pain with the exception of a single posttreatment evaluation appointment with the referring physician initiated by our program staff, and any appointments initiated by workers' compensation personnel. This represented a 96% reduction in group A and a 77% reduction in group B in health care utilization and expenditures (Table 1.5).

Finally, at the time of program admission, two patients in group A and four patients in group B were working daily. At the time of discharge, 10 additional group A patients (42%) and nine group B patients (35%) either returned to full-time employment or full housekeeping duties without assistance, or were attending school or vocational training. Three-month follow-up indicated that an additional 10 group A patients and seven group B patients, for a total of 20 group A patients (83%) and 16 group B patients (62%), were working or attending school daily (Table 1.5).

SUMMARY

As the facts are collected, the population with low back pain appears to be one of the most highly refractory to traditional medical care by either conservative management or surgical intervention. Despite quality medical treatment, many individuals with the onset of low back pain eventually become physically and/or emotionally disabled. It is the hope of the editors and contributing authors of this text that the interdisciplinary rehabilitative direction provided herein will have a positive impact on the comprehensive nonsurgical treatment of one of mankind's oldest and most disabling disorders.

REFERENCES

1. Turk DC, Stieg RL: Chronic pain: the necessity of interdisciplinary communication. *Clin J Pain* 3:163–167, 1987.
2. Blankenship KL: *Functional Capacity Evaluation: Work Hardening.* Macon, GA, American Therapeutics, 1985.
3. Crue BL: *Chronic Pain.* New York, Spectrum Publications, 1979.
4. Newman RI, Seres JL: The interdisciplinary pain center: an approach to the management of chronic pain. In Holzman AD, Turk DC (eds), *Pain Management: A Handbook of Psychological Therapy Approaches.* New York, Pergamon, 1986.
5. Fordyce WE: Environmental factors in the genesis of LBP. In Bonica JJ (ed), *Advances in Pain Research and Therapy.* New York, Raven Press, 1979, Vol 3, pp 659–666.
6. Crue BL: Central versus peripheral philosophies of pain. *Pain Management* 5:218–222, 1988.
7. Tollison CD: *Relief from Back Pain.* New York, Gardner Press, 1987.
8. Tollison CD, Kriegel ML, Downie GR: Chronic LBP: results of treatment at the Pain Therapy Center. South Med J 78:1291–1295, 1986.
9. Tollison CD: Diagnosing and managing chronic pain syndrome. *SC Med J* 9:449–453, 1984.
10. Tollison CD: *Managing Chronic Pain: A Patient's Guide.* New York, Sterling Press, 1982.
11. Fordyce WE, Brockway JA, Bergman JA, Spengler D: Acute back pain: a control group comparison. *J Behav Med* 9:127–140, 1986.
12. Tollison CD: Chronic benign pain: an innovative program for South Carolina. SC Med J 7:379–383, 1982.
13. Hendler N: The anatomy and psychopharmacology of chronic pain. *J Clin Psychol* 8:15–21, 1982.
14. MacDonald-Scott WA: The relief of pain with an antidepressant. *Practitioner* 202:802–807, 1969.
15. Tollison CD, Kriegel ML: Selected tricyclic antidepressants in the management of chronic benign pain. *South Med J* 5:562–564, 1988.
16. Tollison CD, Tollison JW: *Headaches: A Multimodal Program for Relief.* New York, Sterling Press, 1983.
17. Tollison CD, Kriegel ML: Comprehensive treatment of acute and chronic low back pain: a clinical outcome comparison. *Orthop Rev* 1:59–64, 1989.

Chapter 2

SURGICAL VERSUS NONSURGICAL MANAGEMENT

CLARK WATTS, MD

The title of this chapter requires an explanation in that it may lead the reader to believe there are two options, surgery and no surgery, in the management of low back pain. My thesis is that surgery is never an option for the patient with only low back pain. As someone has said in the past, "If a surgeon operates for low back pain, pain will be the result." First, I describe those syndromes of which low back pain is a component that have indications for surgery. I then define those syndromes composed largely of low back pain for which surgery has mistakenly been advocated, and attempt to explain the reasons for the error. Others in this textbook will, in more detail, outline specific nonsurgical modalities for the management of low back pain. I exempt from discussion those conditions not directly presenting with low back pain of a mechanical origin (e.g., neoplasms, trauma).

SURGICAL MANAGEMENT

LUMBAR DISK RUPTURE

The primary syndrome of which low back pain is a major component for which surgery is appropriate is that of the classic ruptured lumbar intervertebral disk. The patient with this problem is usually age 25–50 years, and has, during some exertional effort, noted the sudden onset of low back pain. Over the next several hours there is the development of pain radiating into one lower extremity. After several days of self-enforced rest at home, the patient notes some back pain but, characteristically, leg pain is out of proportion to back pain. The leg pain is in a constant distribution, usually reaching some point below the knee. Important to note is the simultaneous presence of paresthesias in the distribution

of the leg pain, which are more noticeable to the patient as the pain partially subsides with bed rest.

The physician, upon consultation, finds the patient to have some limitation of range of motion to the lower back, with spasms in the lower lumbar paravertebral musculature that are more noticeable on the side of the leg pain. Straight leg raising is most limited on the side of the leg pain and is, generally, exacerbated by dorsiflexion of the ipsilateral foot during the straight leg raising maneuver. Neurologic examination reveals appropriate hypesthesia to pinprick in the distribution of the leg pain, which the physician notes corresponds to a specific spinal dermatome. Also noted are changes in the deep tendon reflexes and weakness in muscles served by the spinal root appropriate to the previously identified dermatome.

A number of observations must coalesce during the management period for surgery to be considered (1). First, the physician must be certain the patient has a herniated lumbar disk. Back pain in such situations is invariably less than leg pain. Leg pain, although reduced, is not eliminated by inactivity that extends over several weeks (3–6), with bed rest occupying a significant portion of this time. The leg pain and the neurologic deficits must conform precisely to the distribution of an appropriate spinal root. The diagnostic studies, which include lumbar myelography, computed tomography (CT), or both, should clearly localize an extradural lesion that conforms to the location of the previously clinically identified spinal root. It must be pointed out that some are beginning to believe that magnetic resonance imaging (MRI) is offering important information in the study of back pain and lumbar intervertebral disk disease (2).

Surgical Procedures

The standard surgical procedure is that of a *lumbar laminotomy and foraminotomy.* The latter is more the partial resection of the medial aspect of the facet in order to decompress the nerve root by enlarging the recess. With the combination of laminotomy and foraminotomy the appropriate nerve root can be easily identified and retracted medially to expose the disk herniation. The segment of the disk that is herniating is removed along with a substantial portion of the disk material remaining in the ipsilateral posterior lateral quadrant of the disk. After several weeks of convalescence, during which time the patient is instructed in a gradual increase in physical activity, the patient is permitted to return to work. Recent literature reveals the surgical complication rate to be extremely low (1, 3). Morbidity or serious complications, those of nerve root injury or infection, are less than 1%. An extremely rare complication is the injury of an intraabdominal vessel anterior to the intervertebral disk, which has resulted in some deaths. The operative mortality is extremely low, with Roberts reporting no deaths directly attributable to the surgical procedure in over 15,000 patients and three deaths postoperatively secondary to arteriosclerotic disease (4).

Despite this low complication rate, the last decade has seen the introduction of procedures designed to treat the ruptured disk that are touted as being less expensive and less technical. The first of these was *microdiscectomy,* which is a modification of the standard procedure using the microscope and therefore permitting a smaller incision (5). There are no good data to suggest that outcome has been improved with microdiscectomy over that of standard discectomy, with the success rate generally reported to be 85–90% in properly selected patients (6).

After almost 20 years of development, *chemonucleolysis,* utilizing the intradiscal injection of the enzyme chymopapain for the treatment of ruptured lumbar intervertebral disk disease, was formally introduced in the early 1980s (7). In general, patients selected for this procedure resembled those selected for standard discectomy except for one very important point: Chemonucleolysis was reserved for those patients with little or no neurologic deficit. By protocol, if the patients had significant neurologic deficit they were excluded from consideration for chemonucleolysis and went directly to the standard discectomy. As one would imagine, since this decision was more judgmental than objective, a major cause of failure of chemonucleolysis was a

significant disk herniation that nevertheless was producing relatively minor neurologic deficit.

Indeed, shortly after the widespread induction of chemonucleolysis users began to become disenchanted with it because of the relatively high failure rate, which was 2–3 times that of standard discectomy (8). Contributing to this high failure rate was the fact that a number of patients were chosen who had little, if any, neurologic deficit and some with little, if any, leg pain. That is, back pain was the major reason for the decision to undergo the procedure. This decision was often bolstered by finding on discography a significant degenerative disk, even though there are no objective criteria to allow one to differentiate between a symptomatic and an asymptomatic degenerative disk by discography. The procedure rapidly lost support and is rarely done today because of the presence of serious complications in up to 2% of patients, the major complication being that of sensitivity reactions, including anaphylaxis, which led to some deaths.

However, stimulated by the simplicity of chemonucleolysis, a percutaneous procedure that permitted some patients to be discharged on the day of the procedure, the search for a mechanical percutaneous means of discectomy resulted in the introduction of *percutaneous nuclectomy* (or discectomy) (9). In this procedure a probe, hardly larger than the 18-gauge needle that was used in chemonucleolysis, is passed percutaneously into the disk and intradiscal material is removed by aspiration. Early results suggest its effectiveness to be equal to that of chemonucleolysis, with approximately 70% of patients returning to work in a few weeks pain free (10).

The procedure is based upon a well-known observation that some herniated disks, even though large enough to compress a nerve root, are confined by the superficial layers of the annulus. Both the enzyme chymopapain, which digests a significant portion of the intradiscal material, and percutaneous nuclectomy, which aspirates the material, result in an internal decompression of the nerve root. It is believed that most of the failures of these procedures are due to the inability of the physician to differentiate precisely the herniated and sequestrated disk fragment from the herniated but confined fragment. As this ability to differentiate becomes more accurate, using CT scan and MRI, it is anticipated that these procedures will become more reliable. Given the complication record of chemonucleolysis, especially regarding sensitivity reactions, it is unlikely that this procedure will be revived as accuracy improves. However, one would anticipate improvement in the results of percutaneous nuclectomy as one improves patient selection.

Patient Selection: "Referred" Versus "Radicular"

If patient selection is to be improved one must not only depend upon more accurate localization and definition of the anatomy with CT scan and MRI, but also upon improvement in clinical acumen. There is reason to believe that the patient who suffers a completely herniated and sequestrated fragment, and therefore will be best served by a standard (or micro-) discectomy, can be differentiated from the patients whose herniated fragment continues to be confined by the annulus. The findings in the former patients have been described above in the discussion of the classic lumbar intervertebral disk herniation and can be labeled the "radicular" syndrome. These patients need to be contrasted with that patient to be described, who suffers from a "referred" syndrome of intervertebral disk rupture. In order to understand the presentation of this patient, it is necessary to go back in time and analyze some clinical and anatomic data that have largely been forgotten.

Frances Murphey described a patient, a young soldier in World War II, who was suffering from back and leg pain that Murphey attributed to a ruptured lumbar intervertebral disk (11) causing an L5 radicular syndrome. While the patient was at bed rest, he contracted, and died of, meningococcal meningitis during an epidemic in the installation. At autopsy Murphey found a small herniated disk fragment confined by the annulus. In his subsequent practice Murphey made a habit of operating on the lumbar disk under local anesthesia and, during surgery, stimulating various structures in the region of the disk rupture and recording responses. He noted that stimulation of the superficial layers of the annulus or the posterior longitudinal ligament, among other structures, resulted in pain "referred" roughly in the dermatomal distribution of the nerve root at the level he was working.

Over 40 years ago Hirsh, using silver stains for nerve tissue, demonstrated nerve fibers in the superficial layers of the annulus of the intervertebral disk (12). This work has recently been confirmed (13). The source of the nerve fibers is undoubtedly the sinuvertebral nerve, which supplies the adjacent facet and dura (14). One can postulate that a small disk fragment impacted in the superficial layers of the annulus, as demonstrated by Murphey, could stimulate these pain fibers and produce a syndrome not of nerve root compression but of "referred" leg pain not unlike that demonstrated by Murphey at operation.

The question is: How would the patient present clinically? The patient should have back pain and leg pain roughly in the distribution of the appropriate spinal root, as demonstrated by Murphey. The "gate" theory of pain would suggest that although the patient would not be significantly hypesthetic in the appropriate dermatome, perception of pinprick and light touch might be altered despite the absence of significant nerve root compression (15). Reflex changes might also be altered. Recall that pain results in the diminution of ipsilateral extensor reflexes (16). However, one would not expect to find significant weakness.

Before we can accept the presence of a "referred" syndrome of lumbar intervertebral disk rupture, the patients must be clearly identified. Their disease needs to be characterized anatomically by the objective analysis of CT scans and MRI. Finally, a conscientious effort must be made to evaluate the response of these patients to treatment, whether it be conservative, with decreased physical activity, or with interventions such as percutaneous discectomy.

SPINAL STENOSIS

Spinal stenosis as a result of osteoarthritis, often associated with a congenitally small spinal canal, is another major cause of back pain associated with a syndrome that can be treated surgically. In general, the patients, who are elderly, present in one of two ways. In the first presentation the patients describe intermittent neurogenic claudication. During walking they experienced back pain and paresthesias in one or both legs that progresses, with continued activity, to pain. Upon resting, the leg pain particularly will subside in a few minutes. Upon inquiry, the physician will elicit a description of parathesias and leg pain, often in more than one dermatome. If the physician brings on the syndrome by having the patient walk up and down the hall for an appropriate period of time, the physician may find mild alterations during the examination of sensation and the reflexes, and even of strength in the distal lower extremities. Imaging studies will reveal spinal narrowing due to osteoarthritic changes in the vertebrae and in the facets, usually at multiple levels (17).

A second, less common, presentation is a progressive paraparesis in which back pain often predominates over leg pain. Imaging studies reveal stenosis at a single level secondary to the combination of osteoarthritis and a congenitally narrowed canal. The neurologic deficits present are generally not worsened by exercise.

The treatment of both these conditions is decompression of the spinal canal by a laminectomy at the appropriate levels combined with resection of the lateral recess to include the medial aspect of the facets. Given the nature of the neurologic problems and the age of the patients, the results are relatively rewarding, with complete relief of symptoms in 25% of the patients and partial relief in an additional 50%. Unfortunately, 25% are unaided by the procedure.

NONSURGICAL MANAGEMENT

One of the major problems in this country in terms of loss of work and recreational time is low back pain. The anxiety that low back pain produces in patients and physicians is extremely high, and leads to a significant amount of inappropriate treatment. This problem begins early in the doctor-patient association, because it is difficult for a physician to quantitate the degree of pain complained of by an individual patient, especially in the absence of good objective findings on the physical examination or data from diagnostic imaging studies. Because the physician is dealing with an extremely emotionally charged symptom (pain) and also dealing with a problem (low back pain) that is so intertwined in the economic and legal structure of our society (through, for example, workers' compensation plans), and because most physicians simply do not understand the management of back injury, it is easy for physicians to succumb to pressures to abandon nonsurgical management. To understand these pressures, it is helpful to examine a hypothetical case that unfortunately is all too typical.

> A 38-year-old male, semiskilled blue-collar worker (e.g., a welder), one day at work while lifting a heavy piece of metal, sustains low back pain. He is poorly insured and has only a few days of sick leave by his employment contract. He does not come to work for 3 days because of the pain, which is now radiating into the left buttock associated with an ache to the rest of the proximal lower extremity.
>
> His work supervisor, by phone, sends him to the private physician who serves as the "company" physician. The physician advises him, after examination, to take a few more days of bed rest. At 7–10 days there is some improvement in the back and hip pain at rest, so the patient returns to see the physician. The physician acknowledges that the patient is improved somewhat, but not completely. Because the patient is running

short on sick leave, he insists he be permitted to return to work and the physician reluctantly acquiesces because of the economic argument made by the patient.

After 2 days of work the patient is suffering at least as much as initially and returns to the physician demanding that something be done. The physician "believes," because the pain is not localized entirely to the lower back, that the patient may have a disk problem, so he refers the patient to a back surgeon. The surgeon determines the patient had sustained an injury that is compatible with a disk herniation. However, the physical findings are equivocal at best. The CT scan is interpreted as showing a slight "bulging" disk. The surgeon's instincts initially tell him to continue conservative therapy and not consider the economic arguments the patient makes. However, a new set of more complex pressures begin to be felt by the surgeon.

Pressure comes from the patient to "do something." The surgeon, after all, treats patients by surgery. The insurance company and the employer "believe" the patient is more likely to improve with surgery, but, even if he doesn't, a more definitive answer for disability purposes may be more rapidly obtained. The referring physician, "who has seen a lot of similar patients," encourages surgery. Therefore, the surgery is performed.

Both the initial physician and the surgeon could better withstand the nonmedically oriented pressures that are applied if they had a better grasp of the nature of the healing process undergone by the back injury that resulted in the low back pain. Pain under these circumstances is a response to injury. Injured tissue needs time to heal, whether it is abraded skin, a torn muscle, or a traumatized intervertebral disk. Studies involving the biology of wound healing suggest that those wounds that require the deposition of collagen in order to form competent scar within supporting structures require several weeks to heal (18). During this convalescent time the forming scar must be protected from mechanical stress. If it is not, the scar is poorly formed and later supplies less than adequate support. If that support needed in tendon, muscle, ligaments, or disk annulus is incompetent, one could expect stress to be transferred to those tissues not designed to supply support. This transfer of stress is signaled by pain, the body's alarm system.

The patient described above, who improves following surgery for questionable indications, does so because the surgical procedure results in a forced convalescence that is understood by all as necessary following "major surgery." During this time the patient is more willing to abide by the cautious instructions of the surgeon, and the employer and insurance company are more understanding. During the 3–6 weeks of relative inactivity, adequate wound healing occurs and the patient is healed. The same process would have occurred without surgery if the same degree of forced physical inactivity could have been undertaken.

Besides the virgin back, which is unnecessarily violated surgically because of low back pain, the most significant cause of surgery for low back pain is the failed back. The patient with the failed back is found in that group of patients who do not improve following inappropriate surgery. Here the problem of back pain is most often attributed to scar around spinal nerves in the epidural space. The patients are advised to undergo additional surgery to have the adhesions lysed and the scar resected. Despite the frequency with which this is undertaken, there is absolutely no evidence to support this procedure. There is no evidence that scar in the epidural space around the dura and around nerve roots is the source of pain. One has to recall that following all disk surgery epidural scar occurs, and yet with properly selected patients, when the procedure is properly performed, 85–90% of patients become symptom free.

The patient who continues to have pain following surgery, especially that which was performed in a patient without appropriate indications, has a very difficult and complex problem. First, the original cause of pain was not diagnosed and therefore remains unknown. Second, the psychological pressures of having gone through surgery, with loss of work time and, perhaps, loss of finances, is oppressive. Finally, the patient now has become embroiled in the social and legal machinations of workers' compensation, and possibly family rejection. It is not my purpose here to sort these problems out. Others in this textbook will attempt to do so. It is my purpose simply to advise that these patients are not candidates for surgery.

In fact, additional surgery may very well complicate the problem. First, in order to adequately explore the lower back in a patient who has undergone previous surgery, it is necessary to resect more bone, ligament, and facet. This will eventually result in low back instability, perhaps even spondylolisthesis secondary to the surgical spondylolyses. This instability can create pain because of the transfer of abnormal levels of physical stress or tension to supporting pain-sensitive ligaments. Fusion may be required. This is one of the few indications for fusion of spondylolisthesis presenting purely as back pain.

The rare progressive congenital spondylolisthesis seen in late adolescence or early adulthood is another reason for fusion. Stable congenital spondy-

lolisthesis in a mature adult or the spondylolisthesis that occasionally accompanies degenerative osteoarthritis rarely produced low back pain, and therefore is rarely a reason for fusion (19).

CONCLUSION

The title of this chapter suggests that surgery and nonsurgical management techniques are options in low back pain. I have tried to point out that, with very rare exceptions, surgery is not performed for low back pain alone. The exceptions are those patients with spondylolisthesis secondary to multiple surgical procedures or the progressive spondylolisthesis sometimes seen in late adolescence or early adulthood.

The majority of low back pain must be treated nonsurgically, and physicians must avoid the pressures to attempt to treat low back pain through interventions such as percutaneous nuclectomy, which are "less invasive, safer, and less expensive" than standard surgical procedures.

REFERENCES

1. Watts C: Disk disease. In Rosenberg RN (ed): *The Clinical Neurosciences.* Churchill Livingstone, New York, 1983, vol 2, pp 1435–1458.
2. Abram S, Blumenkopf B, Tedeschi AA, Partain CL: Differential diagnosis using MRI of severe low back pain. *Neurosurgery* 21:114, 1987.
3. Mayfield FH: Complications of laminectomy. *Clin Neurosurg* 23:435–439, 1976.
4. Roberts MP: Mortality rate of lumbar laminectomy for herniated intervertebral disc. Report of 15,378 cases. In: Proceedings of the 1984 Annual Meeting of the American Association of Neurological Surgeons, San Francisco, April 8–12, 1984, p 132.
5. Williams RW: Microlumbar discectomy: a conservative surgical approach to the origin herniated lumbar disc. *Spine* 3:175–182, 1978.
6. Wilson DH, Kenning J: Microsurgical lumbar discectomy: preliminary report of 83 consecutive cases. *Neurosurgery* 4:137–140, 1979.
7. Watts C: Mechanism of action of chymopapain in ruptured lumbar disc disease. *Clin Neurosurg* 30:642–653, 1983.
8. Watts C, Dickhaus B: Chemonucleolysis: a note of caution. *Surg Neurol* 26:236–240, 1986.
9. Friedman WA: Percutaneous discectomy: an alternative to chemonucleolysis? *Neurosurgery* 13:542–547, 1983.
10. Maroon JC, Onik G: Percutaneous automated discec-

tomy: a new method for lumbar disc removal. *J Neurosurg* 66:143–146, 1987.

11. Murphey F: Sources and patterns of pain in disc disease. *Clin Neurosurg* 15:343–351, 1968.

12. Hirsch C, Ingelmark BE, Miller M: The anatomical basis for low back pain. Studies on the presence of sensory nerve endings in ligamentous, capsular, and intervertebral disc structures in the human lumbar spine. *Acta Orthop Scand* 33:1–17, 1963.

13. Yoshizawa H, O'Brien JP, Smith WT, Trumper M: The neuropathology of intervertebral discs removed for low back pain. *J Pathol* 132:95–104, 1980.

14. Bogduk N, Long DM: The anatomy of the so-called "articular nerves" and their relationship to facet denervation in the treatment of low back pain. *J Neurosurg* 51:172–177, 1979.

15. Melzak R, Wall PD: Pain mechanisms: a new theory. *Science* 150:971–979, 1965.

16. Carew, TJ: The control of reflex action. In Kandel ER, Schwartz JH (eds): *Principles of Neural Science*, ed 2. New York, Elsevier, 1985, pp 457–468.

17. Watts C: Spinal stenosis. In Rosenberg RN (ed): *The Clinical Neurosciences*. New York, Churchill Livingstone, 1983, pp 1459–1466.

18. Madden JW, Peacock EE: Studies of biology of collagen during wound healing: III. Dynamic metabolism of scar collagen and remodeling of dermal wounds. *Ann Surg* 174:511–518, 1971.

19. Epstein JA, Epstein BS, Lavine LS, Carras R, Rosenthal AD: Degenerative lumbar spondylolisthesis with an intact neural arch (pseudospondylolisthesis). *J Neurosurg* 44:139–147, 1976.

Chapter 3

PHYSICAL EXAMINATION OF LUMBOSACRAL PAIN

STUART C. KOZINN, MD
STEPHEN J. LIPSON, MD

This chapter reviews physical examination techniques for patients who present to the orthopaedic surgeon with low back pain. It is well established that back pain is an extremely common complaint, with over 80% of studied populations affected with severe enough symptoms to seek medical attention at some time in their lives (1, 2). The actual number of patients seeking medical treatment for back pain is steadily increasing, and it has become crucial for the physician to provide an early and accurate diagnosis in order to minimize disability and overall "cost" to society.

Evaluation of lumbosacral pain presents a particular diagnostic challenge for the physician because the specific anatomic source is difficult to determine by physical examination. Paradoxically, it is the complete physical examination coupled with an exhaustive clinical history that provides the most sensitive and important information available in the evaluation of lumbosacral pain. Positive correlation of the patient's pain history with objective findings during physical examination indicates the presumptive diagnosis, and appropriate treatment can he initiated. If the diagnosis remains uncertain after complete physical evaluation, the differential may be narrowed further by a combination of available laboratory, radiologic and psychological tests.

It must be noted that acute lumbosacral injury is a common source of litigation and claims for compensation. Legal and economic issues that provide secondary gain for the ill patient make the assessment of true disability extremely difficult. It is therefore imperative for the physician evaluating lumbosacral pain to recognize inconsistent physical signs and to employ special examination techniques that expose malingering or emotional overlay.

LUMBOSACRAL PAIN

The term "discogenic disease" takes into consideration all the pathologic changes that result during the gradual process of age-related disk degeneration. It is important to recognize that disk degeneration is asymptomatic in the majority of persons. However, the deterioration of normal anatomy can predispose to pain through a variety of possible mechanisms. A number of clinical studies have attempted to demonstrate the actual sources of pain in the lower back (3–5). Smyth and Wright stimulated various anatomic structures and found that the dura, ligamentum flavum, and interspinous ligaments were insensitive, and the annulus fibrosis produced back pain and nerve roots produced sciatica when stimulated (5). Kellgren injected hypertonic saline into spinal muscles and interspinous liagaments and produced back pain with sclerotomal referral (4). Hirsch similarly injected facet joints and induced back pain (3). Injection of the disk space produced severe back pain, but injection of ligamentum flavum yielded only mild back pain. Another study demonstrated that facet irritation caused not only back pain, but also marked patterns of referred pain into the thigh and leg (6).

The usual patient presenting with low back pain does not have sciatica, and most likely the pain is related to changes in the intervertebral disks and facet joints. The nerve roots generate the pain of true sciatica, but it is important to note that a similar pain pattern can also be produced by facet joint irritation. Because of the overlap of contributing pain sources, physical examination must be done extremely carefully to differentiate and isolate the pathologically significant anatomy. If the evaluation is incorrectly performed, surgical procedures may be aimed at noncontributing anatomic structures, and they will obviously fail.

The popular terms "herniated disk," "herniated nucleus pulposus," or "slipped disk" refer to intervertebral disk material that abuts posteriorly into the cauda equina or posterolaterally into a nerve root. It has been shown that true disk herniation is actually found in only a small percentage of patients with lumbosacral pain (3). Pain from disk herniation can occur acutely after an injury, which often includes lifting, bending, or Valsalva maneuvers. It can also present more insidiously and gradually progress to a disabling level. Discogenic disease, as such, is a broader diagnosis and indicates that the etiology of pain may include segmental instability resulting from arthritic facet joints and narrowed disk spaces. If gross disk herniation is not present, pain usually remains localized to the lower back, sacroiliac region, and buttocks. However, we know that facet joint degeneration can also produce pain that radiates to the thigh.

Some common pains in the low back may be the result of lumbar muscle strain and spinal ligament sprain. Local muscle tenderness and trigger points may help distinguish these injuries from an acutely herniated disk or radiculopathy.

Spinal stenosis is a syndrome that is most commonly seen in the elderly population. In this population it involves progressive compression of the cauda equina and nerve roots by osteophytes, enlarged facet joints, hypertrophied ligamentum flavum, and bulging disks. The classic clinical symptoms include mild or moderate low back pain with more severe leg pain and sciatica that is worsened with activity. Symptoms of claudication in the elderly must be worked up to differentiate spinal stenosis from periperhal vascular disease, because their symptoms can be similar and are often confused.

Osteoporosis is often associated with spinal pain. A likely etiology of this pain is trabecular microfractures, stress fractures, and vertebral wedge compression fractures occurring in pathologically weak bone.

Osteoarthritis of the hip is occasionally mistaken for pain of lumbar spine origin. Specific examination techniques can be done to help differentiate

the true source of pain. It is also helpful to include one radiograph that shows the hip joints when evaluating lumbar pain that developed gradually.

Malignant disease, particularly myeloma and metastatic lesions, must be ruled out in elderly persons presenting with new onset of spinal pain. Primary bone and marrow tumors besides myeloma usually present in younger patients, and should always be considered in the evaluation of spinal pain in this group.

Disk space infections and vertebral osteomyelitis can cause severe back pain, which may or may not be accompanied by other systemic signs. A complete medical history will usually give insight into the diagnosis of infection.

Back pain may infrequently be referred from pathology in other internal organs. Endometriosis, pelvic inflammatory disease, pancreatitis, peptic ulcer, and dissecting aortic aneurysm can be associated with lumbosacral pain. Pregnancy is frequently associated with back pain that is relieved after birth. Herpes zoster can present as severe low back pain in an elderly patient, and the telltale skin lesions may not appear in a dermatomal distribution until after the pain is well established.

Physical examination, along with complete medical history, will help the clinician to distinguish these low back pain syndromes from one another.

MEDICAL HISTORY

The most valuable information obtained while evaluating the patient with lumbosacral pain is gleaned from a carefully detailed medical history. The history should be documented in the patient's chart so that repeated reference is available at subsequent visits. It is helpful, if there is time, for the patient to fill out a history questionnaire before seeing the physician, possibly while in the waiting area. Standard questions answered in a checklist will allow the astute clinician to spend extra time on significant positive or inconsistent responses. An evaluation of a pain diagram filled out by the patient before the visit helps the physician gain early insight into the patient's personality type. This is important because anxiety and depression have been shown to be risk factors for development of low back pain.

Of diagnostic value is the patient's age, occupation, and detailed information concerning the onset of pain. The patient's age determines susceptibility for back pain and probability of disk herniation. Typically episodic attacks of low back pain begin in the middle 20s, with major complaints occurring in the fourth decade (1, 7). Females have been shown to have an average delay of a decade over males in the onset of lumbosacral pain (2).

Occupation reflects external risk factors and helps determine disability eligibility for third parties. For example, driving motorized vehicles, heavy lifting, or work with vibratory equipment may increase the risk of back injuries. The time of onset of pain may correlate with a particular event and may document a claim made toward workers' compensation funds. Studies have shown that the typical industrial accident patient has a higher hysteria and hypochondriasis level as measured by the Minnesota Multiphasic Personality Inventory (MMPI) than does the private patient (8).

A complete review of systems should be done to acknowledge contributions to lumbosacral pain syndrome from other sources. For example, paresthesias in the distal limbs could be due to diabetes or other generalized neuropathy. Renal lesions, aortic aneurysms, peptic ulcers, and retroperitoneal tumors can produce back pain. A history elicited of deep venous thrombosis, pulmonary embolism, or any bleeding diathesis should alert a physician planning surgery.

DESCRIPTION OF PAIN

Pain in the lower back or legs is the complaint that brings the typical patient to the physician for evaluation of the lumbosacral spine. Questioning may reveal that the patient had years of intermittent low back pain before the onset of leg pain. A common history is that, with the passage of time, mild episodic pain became more frequent and intense. Some patients report that severe pain began after a physical activity or possibly after a period of prolonged sitting, standing, or lifting. Actually, only 40% of patients presenting with low back pain and disk herniation can associate a single event with the onset of pain. Even if a specific injury was associated with the onset of pain, trauma may have been a precipitating rather than a causative factor.

The evaluation of the patient's presenting complaints must be very specific in regard to the "type" and location of pain. The pain history most commonly focuses on the lower back, the sacroiliac areas, and the buttocks. The pain is often described as sharp, aching, or burning, and may radiate to and from different areas. The usual history of lumbar disk herniation is of repetitive lower back pain that is relieved by rest, which is suddenly exasperated after flexion of the spine. After this, leg pain becomes much worse than the back pain. Radiation of pain down the thigh into the legs is called sciatica. Very exacting localization of this pain should be sought by the clinician. In the presence of radiculopathy, the precise nerve root involved may be uncovered by history alone. For example, pain and paresthesia into the hallux indicates involvement of the L5 nerve root. The dermatomal distribution can be very accurate in localizing sciatic pain. Radiation of pain into the thigh alone is much more common, and sciatica should normally not be diagnosed unless the patient's pain extends below the knee. Pain from disk herniation may be relieved by rest and increased with activity or sitting, which increases intradiscal pressure. Feelings of muscle weakness and parasthesias may accompany the pain. Occasionally pain in the groin or testicle can be associated with a high midline herniation. If a disk fragment is high in the canal, rectal pain, numbness in the perineum, and paralysis of the sphincters can occur. Sudden loss of bowel and bladder control dictates emergent surgical decompression of the cauda equina by the spine surgeon.

NATURAL HISTORY OF LUMBAR PAIN

The amount of time that has passed since the pain began helps to position the patient along the time course for the natural history of low back pain. This natural history of lumbosacral pain tells us that 90% of patients can expect to have significant resolution 10–12 weeks from onset (6). Ninety-six per cent will show resolution by 6 months after onset of pain (1). Recurrence rates of 30–70% in the first year after the onset of pain have also been reported. Only a small group (about 4%) of persons with back pain progress to chronic back pain, but it is this group that incurs excessive lost time, physician's time, and rehabilitation costs.

Spinal pain in a young adult male that has progressed insidiously, is worse in the morning, and is associated with back "stiffness" suggests ankylosing spondylitis as a possible diagnosis. Pain with an insidious onset in a patient over 45 is not typical of discogenic disease and should raise the possibility of occult neoplasm. Pain of neoplastic origin is generally reported as a "deep" pain that is worse at night and is often relieved after arising and moving about. An array of supplemental questions should investigate urinary function in males and the presence of breast masses in females.

Pain that comes on and increases in intensity after prolonged activity or after walking a distance may indicate spinal stenosis. This is a much more common syndrome in elderly patients, but congenital stenosis may present in a younger patient.

Claudicating pain in the thigh and calf that is relieved slowly by sitting, and recurrent after resumption of standing and walking, is classic for spinal stenosis. In neurogenic claudication, pain lessens when the spine is flexed because the capacity of the spinal canal enlarges.

The history of pain is important when considering the value of surgical options in treatment. If spinal fusion is going to provide pain relief, the patient should have a history consistent with mechanical pain that is aggravated by movements such as bending, twisting, and prolonged sitting. Pain that is mostly in the leg will be better relieved by surgical discectomy than pain that is mostly in the low back.

PAST MEDICAL HISTORY

A history of all previous treatments and therapies for back pain should be obtained. Any previous experience that was effective in relieving pain may be worth trying again. In contrast, if the patient feels he/she "wasted" time with specific conservative modalities in the past, it may be wise to suggest other options. A history of past surgical procedures must be very specific. If pain relief was obtained for over a year after the initial surgery, new symptoms should be regarded as possibly representing independent pathology. In contrast, pain that was never completely relieved by surgery is unlikely to improve from a similar repeat procedure.

A family history of low back pain should be elicited if present. Spondylolysis, scoliosis, and osteoarthritis have been shown to have not well understood genetic components. Ankylosing spondylitis shows a very high prevalence of the human lymphocyte B27 antigen.

"PSYCHOGENIC" PAIN AND SECONDARY GAIN

Emotional factors that may contribute to disability must be taken into consideration. Secondary gain should be ruled out by careful questioning regarding employment satisfaction and compensation. It is possible for an employee on full disability to receive an income close to his/her regular salary. This may create a strong subconscious or conscious disincentive to the patient to participate in his/her own rehabilitation. Litigation that is pending from a personal injury can cloud the true presentation of symptoms. Even though most physicians would prefer not to be involved with legal battles, it is very important to know all the issues relating to the patient's pain. Psychogenic magnification of minor pain that is inconsistent with physical find-

ings should evoke caution in the surgeon who is considering surgical intervention. To help sort out emotional contributions to the patient's perception of pain, a personality "inventory" can be obtained with psychological testing. The MMPI is one such testing device. Pain "drawings" that localize the patient's pain to anatomic regions of a human silhouette also provide insight into the patient. The finding of significant psychogenic overlay in a patient with back pain indicates that a technically satisfactory intervention may be fruitless in relieving the pain.

PHYSICAL EXAMINATION

Physical examination demonstrates the applicable mechanical relationships of spinal pathology, the occurrence of postural abnormalities and truncal asymmetry, and the presence or absence of neurologic change.

OBSERVATION

The physical examination begins with inspection of the patient as he/she enters the room. Abnormalities of gait and posture should be observed. Specifically, evidence of neurologic weakness or an antalgic lurch should be noted. The patient with an acute disk herniation will hold the thigh flexed and avoid weightbearing on the leg. Patients with chronic back pain are unlikely to use a cane unless they have significant sciatica, in which case they walk with an antalgic limp, spending minimum time and placing minimum weight on the affected limb.

The general appearance of the patient can provide insight into the functional disability. Is the patient able to groom himself/herself? Is he/she concerned about dress and appearance? How much assistance does he/she need to undress for examination?

Observation continues with the patient standing in a hospital gown with the back open. The spine and stance are inspected to note lumbar lordosis, thoracic kyphosis, scoliosis, tilt or list, flexed lower limbs (to relieve nerve root tension), and muscle spasm. From a side view a gentle lumbar lordotic curve is normal, and this may be absent in the presence of paravertebral muscle spasm. Skin abnormalities such as lipomata, hairy patches, café-au-lait spots, port wine stains, or dimples over the spine may indicate the presence of spina bifida, diastematomyelia, or some other congenital malformation. Skin tags or pedunculated tumors may indicate neurofibromatosis.

In acute sciatica, the patient usually lists away from the affected side, producing a functional scoliosis. It is suggested that when a disk herniation is lateral to the nerve root, the patient will bend away from the side of the irritated root in an attempt to draw the root away from the disk fragment. When the herniation is in an axillary position, the patient will list toward the side of the lesion, also in an effort to decompress the root (9). Loss of normal lumbar lordosis is seen during the acute phase of disk herniation. Severe muscle spasm seen only on one side of the spine may indicate an extreme lateral disk protrusion.

Asymmetrical thigh and leg muscle girth or a leg length inequality may be noted. The ability to accomplish heel walking and walking on toes is a useful screening mechanism as a measure of lower extremity muscle strength and coordination.

PALPATION

After inspection, the spine is palpated to elicit those sites of tenderness that may indicate the sites of pathology. The spinous process of L4 lies above the iliac crest, and the spine of L5 can be palpated just below the crest in most people. Palpation in the midline will often elicit pain at the level of a symptomatic degenerative disk. A visible or palpable step-off from one spine to the next may indicate spondylolisthesis. It is not unusual to find tenderness laterally along the iliac crest and over the sacroiliac joint with further palpation.

If muscle spasm is present, palpation while the patient maximally extends his/her head to relax the lumbodorsal fascia will expose differences in paraspinal muscle tone. Muscle "trigger points" of maximal pain may be elicited. These points may be useful later for anesthetic or electrical blockade in an attempt to relieve pain. Pain directly over a broad area of paravertebral muscles may indicate a generalized myofascial pain syndrome. Percussion of the lumbar spine may elicit local pain, but it is not specific for disk herniation.

The sciatic nerve is fairly easy to palpate as it exits the pelvis through the greater sciatic notch beneath the piriformis muscle. It can best be felt as it passes midway between the greater trochanter and the ischial tuberosity with the patient's hip flexed. Hyperesthesia and tenderness of the sciatic nerve occurs in the presence of lumbar root irritation.

Scoliosis, structural or functional, should be determined from a rear view. A plumb line or scoliometer will help quantitate and document a spinal curve. Forward flexing of the spine accentuates an asymmetric rib hump or lumbar curve. Leg length inequality, real or apparent, should be determined

with a tape measure. While the patient is standing, it is helpful to note the effect of leveling the pelvis with calibrated wooden blocks. Gunn and coworkers have found that patients with radiculopathy had tender motor points in the myotome of the affected limb (10), and this can be misinterpreted as thrombophlebitis.

Range of spinal motion should then be determined and roughly quantitated by estimating the angles of limitation. The movements of the lumbar spine are flexion, extension, lateral bending, and rotation. Since there is a very wide range of normalcy for spine motion, numbers obtained at initial examination do not have much diagnostic value. Recorded numbers from subsequent visits should be somwhat consistent or show a pattern of improvement or worsening. The examiner must not equate flexion of the hips with flexion of the lumbar spine. It is also important to determine which of the motion postures produce pain. A patient in acute pain may be difficult to examine properly, and he/she may need to return after a week or two of bed rest for reevaluation.

In discogenic pain, forward flexion commonly causes some discomfort. It also causes reversal of spinal motion; that is, instead of smoothly raising the back from the lumbar spine when it returns from a flexed position, the patient "locks up" the lumbar spine and raises the thoracic spine. Pain from hyperextension can be nonspecific, but has classically been considered an indication of facet joint involvement. In the presence of neurogenic claudication, hyperextension for 1 min may cause radiation of pain from the back and buttocks into the extremities.

Lateral bending at rest indicates some tendency toward asymmetry of a painful lesion. Rotation is tested by steadying the iliac crests and asking the patient to rotate the shoulders. Examination of chest expansion should be done in young males. If the difference of inhalation over exhalation measurement is less than 1 inch, then ankylosing spondylitis is a possibility.

Determination of hip range of motion is important because hip pain can be referred to the low back and buttocks. A classic examination technique is Patrick's sign or the "FABERE" test, an acronym for *f*lexion, *ab*duction, *e*xternal *r*otation, and *e*xtension of the hip, which is painful in hip disease and sacroiliitis, but not in patients with sciatica.

NEUROLOGIC EXAMINATION

A thorough neurologic examination must look for objective signs of lumbar root involvement. A meticulous examination will suggest the level of root involvement, but it is not conclusive. In disk herniation, L5–S1 (involving the S1 root) and L4–5 (L5 root) are the most common. L3–4 herniation is next most common and will usually involve the L4 root. A central L4–5 disk herniation can involve both the L5 and S1 roots, and there is a 10% incidence of disk herniation at two levels (9). In extreme lateral disk herniations the nerve exiting at the same level as the disk will be involved. Superimposed facet arthritis will confuse the patterns of neurologic involvement.

Sensory Changes

Sensory findings are often confusing and must be mapped out very carefully. It is valuable to perform both pin and vibration testing to determine that all sensory columns of the cord are intact. Sensory dysfunction can have a changing picture and be quite confusing in stenosis of the cauda equina.

The sensory pattern of the thigh and buttocks is much less specific than in the distal limb. Compression of the fourth lumbar root will cause sensory abnormalities in the anteromedial leg. The sharp anterior crest of the tibia is the dividing line for the L4 and L5 dermatomes in the leg. Compression of the fifth root causes hypesthesia in the anterolateral leg as well as the medial aspect of the foot to the great toe. S1 compression causes sensory impairment in the lateral foot, posterior calf, and plantar surface of the foot. The nerves emanating from L1, L2, and L3 provide sensation over the anterior thigh in sequential band-like dermatomes.

Alterations in deep tendon reflexes are common in nerve root compression syndromes. Reflex testing can be enhanced by having the patient pull apart on his/her hands isometrically, or in the case of the gastrocnemius reflex the patient can kneel on a chair. Compression of the S1 root diminishes the gastrocnemius/ soleus or "Achilles" reflex. L5 root involvement is difficult to diagnose by reflex changes, but occasionally an asymmetric posterior tibial tendon reflex can be elicited. To obtain this reflex, the foot should be held in eversion and dorsiflexion. The posterior tibial tendon is tapped on the medial side of the foot just before it inserts into the navicular tuberosity. The patellar reflex is mediated through the L3 and L4 nerve roots. Interestingly, impairment of the quadriceps reflex, or knee jerk, has been shown to be affected more often in L4–5 herniations than in L3–4 herniations (11). It should be noted that symmetric absence of any reflex is more often a process of advanced age than a sign of radiculopathy.

Motor Changes

Nerve root compression can result in paresis or paralysis of the muscle group the nerve innervates. The patient may not be clinically aware of this weakness. The distribution of paresis in the lower extremity from a herniated disk at the L4–5 and L5–S1 levels has been studied by Weber (12), who noted that although there is a localization of paresis according to nerve root, 35% of the other muscle groups in the lower extremity can also be affected.

S1 root compression usually has no noticeable motor effect, but weakness of hallux flexion and foot eversion (peroneals) may be seen. Compression of the fifth lumbar root will result in weakness of the hallux and little toe extensors. Severe L5 compression can result in gluteus medius weakness and Trendelenberg limp. Atrophy of the anterior and lateral compartments of the leg can occur with chronic root compression. Compression of the fourth lumbar root most frequently results in diminished quadriceps muscle strength and concomitant atrophy.

Sciatic Stretch Testing

Tests that increase root tension can be grouped together as sciatic stretch tests. The most famous is that of Lasègue (3), in which the patient lies supine and one leg at a time is lifted passively by the examiner until pain or sciatica is reproduced. The angle of leg elevation relative to the table should be documented. Sciatic stretch begins at an angle of about 35° and increases rapidly until 70°, at which point practically no further stretch occurs (14). Dorsiflexing the foot at the minimum angle sharply increases the pain of sciatica because it stretches the nerve further. Internal rotation of the straight leg during elevation also increases sciatic tension via the lumbosacral plexus (15). The crossed straight leg raising test is also done by lifting the asymptomatic leg. This can cause sciatica in the symptomatic leg and has been correlated clinically with more central disk herniations. Another variant of sciatic stretch testing is called the "bowstring" sign and has been credited to Cram (16). In this test the leg is held out with the knee in extension, and compression of the sciatic /tibial nerve in the popliteal space produces radicular pain symptoms.

Irrespective of how the test is done, sciatic stretch produces a deep, aching pain that radiates down the affected limb. In severe root compression, a sharp, shooting pain may travel to the affected dermatome and be followed by local paresthesia. Absence of sciatic stretch sensitivity is very accurate in excluding a herniated disk in patients less than 30 years of age; however, older patients with a herniation may not have a positive test. Protective paraspinal muscle spasm can trigger increased back pain. Signs of tension on the sciatic nerve are found only occasionally in the spinal stenosis syndrome, and usually indicate lateral entrapment of the nerve root.

Femoral nerve stretch tests have been described that can indicate L3 or L4 radiculopathy. Placing the patient prone and flexing the knees will increase tension in the femoral nerve. This test is accentuated by placing the patient on his/her side and first extending the hip before flexing the knee of the symptomatic limb. The Ely test for rectus femoris contracture accomplishes similar stretch on the femoral nerve. The pain should radiate down the front of the thigh and stop at the knee if only L3 is involved. Stretch on the L4 root can cause pain into the lower leg.

MALINGERING AND "HYSTERIA"

Most patients have both somatic and a psychogenic component to their back problem. While deliberate feigning of illness is probably rare, emotional overlay potentiating organic symptoms is more common. Special diagnostic techniques should be used in the physical examination of back pain patients to sort out true pathology. Wiltse and Ruge have described nine rules to help the clinician spot the malingerer or hysteria-prone patient (8):

1. Dramatic description of pain, with overuse of superlatives.
2. Poor localization. "My whole left side hurts."
3. Previously prescribed treatment of no help.
4. Bizarre or undescribed action of medications.
5. Disparity of healthy appearance with protestations of pain.
6. Veiled hostility toward previous doctor.
7. Vague history with extraneous information.
8. Accompanying neurotic symptoms.
9. History of many operations on other body areas.

Specific tests can be done that rely on known anatomic relationships. A variation of Lasègue's straight leg raising test can be done in which it is noted that the patient can extend the knee while sitting, but will not allow supine leg raising. This is considered a positive "flip test," indicating non-

anatomicity of the pain. During this maneuver, plantar flexion of the foot should not increase pain because this relaxes the sciatic nerve. Dorsiflexion, conversely, should increase pain by stretching the nerve. Flexing the hip and knee toward the abdomen should not be painful until extremes of flexion, when the lumbar spine begins to move.

The flip "sign" as described by Michele (17) is a variant wherein the patient sits with his/her legs dangling off the side of the examining table. The physician places his/her open palm on the suprapatellar area of the painful thigh and depresses it forcefully into the table. With the patient's attention diverted, the examiner's other hand cups the heel of the same limb and slowly extends the knee. The malingerer will allow full knee extension but the patient with true sciatica will either not allow knee extension or will acutely reverse his/her lumbar lordosis and lean backward. Another variant is to have the patient sitting over the side of the examining table as before but with the ankle dorsiflexed. If the patient can extend the knee with the foot dorsiflexed without leaning backward, then he/she does not have sciatica. A similar test is forward bending while sitting in a chair. With the hips and knees comfortably flexed patients with chronic back pain should be able to bend forward until their chins are level with their knees.

Another flip test is rotation of the lumbar spine. Because of the sagittal position of the facet joints, the lumbar spine normally cannot rotate, and the test should therefore not be painful in an honest patient. Other physical signs that indicate nonorganic disease include superficial and nonanatomic areas of tenderness, stimulation test of axial loading, and regional disturbances in which weakness and sensory deficits are nonphysiologic ("stocking glove" distribution). Waddell et al. (18) described a group of nonorganic physical signs in low back pain. These signs are independent and separable from standard clinical signs of physical pathology. They include superficial and nonanatomic tenderness, inappropriate response to simulation tests of axial loading and rotation, distraction tests of the patient's attention, and straight leg raising. Regional disturbances such as glove anesthesia, nonanatomic weakness, and patient overreaction were also nonorganic signs. The presence of these nonorganic signs was correlated with patients who were likely to have a poor result with surgery.

A simple test of the true limits to spine motion can be obtained by watching the patient dress after the examination, particularly when bending over to pick up his/her shoes (the examiner pretends to be otherwise occupied reading the chart or on the phone). In a patient who has a true list from muscle spasm, it should remain when bending forward. The malingerer will straighten the spine as he/she bends to reach toward the floor.

Muscle weakness in the limbs can be tested under the guise of testing balance by having the patient stand alternatively on the heel and toes of each leg. If he/she can stand on the leg reported to have sciatica, it is unlikely the limb is significantly weak. Also, the patient with sciatica of long duration would be expected to have measurable muscle atrophy in the thigh or calf. The examiner must be careful not to mistake subcutaneous edema in the painful limb as normal girth.

The Burns test consists of asking the patient to kneel on a padded chair. The back of the chair is to the patient's right or left side. The patient is asked to bend at the waist and touch the floor with his/her fingertips. The examiner stands in front of the patient in case he/she falls forward. In the absence of hip disease or acute radiculopathy, the patient with chronic back pain should be able to accomplish touching the floor without difficulty. If the patient with chronic pain cannot be persuaded to try to touch the floor, there is a strong likelihood he/she is malingering.

Calliet has described the anterior tibial test for malingering as follows (8). The patient is asked to stand squarely facing the examiner, who pushes backward on the patient's sternal area. If the patient is feigning a foot drop, his/her anterior tibial tendon will fire and bowstring across the dorsum of the ankle.

SUMMARY

Physical examination should include assessment of peripheral circulation and abdominal, rectal, and pelvic examinations when deemed appropriate. Occasionally a patient's "back" pain may be originating in these areas. Having completed both the history and physical examination, the clinician should have a clear picture of the nature of the pain, its mechanical relationships, presence of neurologic symptoms, limitations of motion and function, presence of nerve root irritation, and localization of the neurologic findings. At this point a diagnostic impression is formed, and the clinician may proceed with specific therapies. If further information is necessary, laboratory, electrodiagnostic, and radiographic studies can be pursued to demonstrate abnormalities that can be corrected by surgery or otherwise. In discogenic disease, the choice of sur-

gical intervention in particular mandates acquisition of further information.

SUPPLEMENTARY DIAGNOSTIC TESTS

PSYCHOLOGICAL TESTING

Emotional factors clearly play an important role in back pain, and they should be recognized early. When personality factors are unfavorable, management will be unsuccessful, no matter how skillfully performed (19). Some emotional factors can be objectively quantitated by psychological testing. Psychological testing has been demonstrated to be a reasonable predictor or surgical and conservative treatment regardless of the etiology of spinal pain. The MMPI is the most traditional test used for this purpose. Specifically, the hysteria (Hy) and hypochondriasis (Hs) scales of the MMPI are the best prognosticators of the possibility of successful surgery for disk disease (8).

Pain diagrams are very useful because they are a simple test to administer. The pain diagram has been correlated with the MMPI and it provides a simple, rapid office assessment of those personality traits that may confuse accurate pain assessment. These tests cannot absolutely determine the presence of functional versus organic pain; instead they help the physician decide whether to pursue invasive therapy, to seek psychological or psychiatric consultation, or, in the case of chronic pain, to enter into behavioral modification by operant conditioning.

LABORATORY TESTING

When a diagnosis is not immediately obvious or warrants confirmation, screening laboratory tests are indicated to supplement the evaluation of lumboscacral pain. There is no laboratory screen for back pain, but selective testing can be of value.

An erythrocyte sedimentation rate (ESR) can be a very sensitive indicator of infection or malignancy. However, this test is not very specific and positive results could represent disease distant from the spine. A complete blood count (CBC) may suggest an anemia or a lymphocytosis of malignancy. Serum and urinary protein electrophoresis will help establish a diagnosis of myeloma, the most common primary bone malignancy in elderly patients. Elevated acid phosphatase levels in the male strongly suggest prostate malignancy as a source of spinal pain. Alkaline phosphatase levels may be elevated in Paget's disease, which can present in the spine. Baseline calcium and phosphorus levels also help screen against malignancy and metabolic bone diseases that affect the axial skeleton. The evaluation of a patient with suspected vertebral stress fractures includes a workup for osteoporosis and may necessitate a serum estrogen level in females. Rarely, human lymphocyte B27 antigen tissue typing will help clinch the diagnosis of ankylosing spondylitis in a young male. Gout can be revealed with a determination of uric acid level, and the development of rheumatoid arthritis may be picked up by immunologic screening.

Consultation with an internist, endocrinologist, rheumatologist, neurologist, or vascular surgeon should be readily sought in difficult diagnostic cases and also in the preoperative evaluation and preparation of patients with other medical problems.

RADIOGRAPHIC EXAMINATION

Very often, the complete history and physical examination are not enough to accurately localize the level of the pathology responsible for pain and disability. Supplementary diagnostic tests are indicated to confirm a clinical impression or rule out another occult pathology. Good quality plan roentgenograms can be very helpful, particularly if unusual bony pathology is present. It is presently controversial whether or not radiographs should be obtained for most patients presenting with back pain. The majority of the literature supports delaying spine radiographs until at least the second patient visit to the physician's office. This is because the diagnostic yield from plain films is quite low in the general population with lumbosacral pain. The medicolegal necessity of ruling out unusual conditions such as tumors or congenital abnormalities on the earliest possible visit to the physician is a factor in favor of early radiographs. Large studies that have evaluated spine radiographs from both symptomatic and asymptomatic individuals have shown that age-related disk degeneration occurs in everyone starting at about age 20. In a survey of films from patients over age 35, 65% of the males, and 52% of the females showed disk degeneration. However, only 13% of the patient group had symptoms of pain. Nerve root involvement occurred in only 10% of those with radiographic evidence of moderate to severe degeneration (20). In summary, plain radiographs have a high incidence of both false-positive and false-negative results for disk herniation.

Flexion and extension views can be helpful in evaluating abnormal relative motion of contiguous spinal segments. Coned-down and magnified views of a particular painful area can improve resolution.

Tomograms may be needed to help see small tumors, postsurgical pseudarthroses, or the bony defects of spondylolysis.

There has not been a demonstrated correlation between the incidence of low back pain and degenerative changes seen on plain films of the lumbar spine. Nachemson pointed out that there is no statistical significance to the following radiologic findings in the risk of developing low back pain: narrowing of a single disk space, facet arthrosis and subluxation, disk calcification, lumbarization and sacralization of the lowest segment, Schmorl's nodules, accessory ossicles, spina bifida occulta, and mild to moderate scoliosis. However, the radiographic presence of spondylolysis, retrolisthesis, severe lumbar scoliosis, and lordosis may be radiographic findings truly associated with low back pain (21).

Significant radiographic risk factors for lumbosacral pain that have been definitely established as spondylolisthesis, Scheuermann's osteochondrosis, congenital kyphosis, osteoporosis, multiple disk space narrowing, and ankylosing spondylitis.

BONE SCANNING

Bone scanning using methylene diphosphonate ^{99m}Tc uptake can define the origin of back pain when infection or tumors are suspected. Although degenerative facet disease and disk narrowing produces increased tracer uptake, no useful diagnostic information is gained when scanning for discogenic pain. Symptomatic spondylolysis can be diagnosed with a positive bone scan, particularly in a young patient.

COMPUTED TOMOGRAPHY (CT)

Computed tomography has replaced many previous methods of radiologic imaging and is still evolving in its usefulness. Excellent quality CT scans and reformatted sagittal reconstructions may obviate the need for myelography. Axial cross-section cuts are particularly informative in the evaluation of spinal canal stenosis. However, the ease of obtaining a CT scan should not make us forget its true role in diagnosis. Imaging techniques should not be used to find a lesion to provide a diagnosis, because false-positive results from asymptomatic degeneration only confuse the clinical evaluation. It has been reported that more than 35% of subjects who did not have symptoms had abnormal findings on CT. In patients older than 40 years, 50% were found to have abnormal findings on CT scans, with the most common findings being stenosis of the spinal canal and facet degeneration (22).

MAGNETIC RESONANCE IMAGING

Magnetic resonance imaging, or nuclear magnetic resonance, is rapidly evolving as a noninvasive and precise imaging modality for spine-related disease. Particularly helpful are the sagittal views of the spinal canal, which are probably now the imaging view of choice to see herniated and posteriorly bulging disks.

MYELOGRAPHY

Myelography involves the injection of iodinated contrast material into the dural sac in order to outline it on plain radiographs. Myelography was the "gold standard" for many years in the determination of spinal canal and nerve root impingement. With the advent of noninvasive imaging, the role of myelography has decreased.

Degeneration in the cervical and lumbar spine was found following myelography in 28% of patients who had no spinal symptoms and were being studied for other reasons. Myelography combined with CT allows the margins of the spinal canal to be viewed in great detail. Using this combined technique, the clinical syndrome of spinal stenosis has been correlated with an anteroposterior diameter of 10 mm or less for the dural sac.

OTHER DIAGNOSTIC TESTS

Electromyography (EMG) and nerve conduction studies can provide physiologic information about nerve root dysfunction and peripheral neuropathy. Electromyography should be used selectively, keeping in mind that it may take 6 weeks for the onset of denervation potentials. The selective use of the H reflex for the S1 reflex arc is one of the earliest changes noted and may change within days. In spinal stenosis patients, about 80% with proven stenosis will show abnormalities on an EMG. Fifteen percent of patients with disk herniation will only show paraspinal EMG changes as opposed to leg changes. Also, it is well known that EMG changes can be found without any evidence of underlying structural abnormality.

CONSERVATIVE VERSUS SURGICAL MANAGEMENT

Surgery for discogenic disease should be done in only a small proportion of patients who present with lumbosacral pain. Even when surgery is prescribed, it is most often done as an elective option of both the physician and patient. Inappropriate patient selection is the principal cause for surgical failure. However, it is important for the clinician following a conservative course of treatment to recognize the occasional patient in whom surgery is emergently indicated or who is most likely to greatly benefit from an elective procedure.

An absolute indication for lumbar decompressive spine surgery is the cauda equina syndrome, which results from massive midline disk herniation. In this syndrome, sacral roots in the midline of the dural sac are paralyzed. Functional paraparesis results, reflecting diminution of gastrocnemius, soleus, hamstring, and gluteal muscle strength. Bowel and bladder dysfunction are common. Emergent neural decompression via discectomy results in most cases in slow recovery of motor and bladder function, but perineal anesthesia and sexual function recover poorly. Another clear but relative indication for surgery is motor weakness with progressive neurologic deficit. Estimates of motor return after loss from disk herniation range from 50% to 80%; however, there is no difference in surgical or nonsurgical patients over the long term.

Relative indications for laminectomy include intolerable pain, unrelieved by conservative management over an extended period, and recurrent episodes of incapacitating pain. How long to wait before operation depends on the individual. The natural history of discogenic disease tells us that most patients will have recovered without surgery by 3 months after the acute onset of pain. Good results from surgery decrease if performed after 6 months from the onset of pain. Therefore, if surgery is the treatment of choice, the optimal time to operate is between 2 and 5 months after the onset of symptoms. Long-term studies, however, indicate that although surgery in the appropriate patient hastens recovery, the end result is not superior to one obtained by following the natural history of the disease. (12).

SUMMARY

The complete physical evaluation of the patient with lumbosacral pain is difficult and time consuming. However, it is critical to determining the correct diagnosis and the contributing anatomic sources of pain. It is important to keep in mind the full differential diagnosis of lumbosacral pain, and to understand the natural history of discogenic disease. Since the great majority of patients do improve with conservative care and the passing of time, it is important not to overtreat or prescribe surgery unless specific indications are present. The correct diagnosis is the key to successful outcome because the most appropriate treatment regimen can be initiated.

REFERENCES

1. Horal J: The clinical appearance of low back disorders in the city of Gothenburg, Sweden. *Acta Orthop Scand,* Suppl 118, 1969.
2. Kelsey JL, White A: Epidemiology and impact of low back pain, *Spine* 5:133, 1980.
3. Hirsch C, Ingelmark B, Miller BM: The anatomical basis for low back pain. *Acta Orthop Scand* 33:1, 1963.
4. Kellgren JH: Observations on referred pain arising from muscle. *Clin Sci* 3:175, 1938.
5. Smyth MJ, Wright VJ: Sciatica and the intervertebral disc: an experimental study. *J Bone Joint Surg [Am]* 40:1401, 1958.
6. Mooney V, Robertson J: The facet syndrome. *Clin Orthop* 115:149, 1976.
7. Frymoyer JW, Pope MH, Costanza MC, et al: Epidemiologic studies of low back pain. *Spine* 5:419, 1980.
8. Wiltse L, Ruge D: *Spinal Disorders: Diagnosis and Treatment.* Philadelphia, Lea & Febiger, 1977.
9. Rothman RH, Simeone FA: *Lumbar Disc Disease: The Spine.* Philadelphia, WB Saunders, 1975.
10. Gunn CC, et al: Tenderness at motor points: a diagnostic aid to low back injury. *J Bone Joint Surg [Am]* 58:815, 1976.
11. Hakelius A, Hindmarsh J: The significance of neurologic signs and myelographic findings in the diagnosis of lumbar root compression. *Acta Orthop Scand* 43:239, 1979.
12. Weber H: The effect of delayed disc surgery on muscular paresis. *Acta Orthop Scand* 46:631, 1975.
13. Lasègue EC: Consideration of sciatic pain. *Arch Gen Med* 6:558, 1864.
14. Fahrni WH: Observations on straight leg raising with special reference to nerve root adhesions. *Can J Surg* 9:44–48, 1970.
15. Briez A, Troup J: Biomechanical consideration in the straight leg raising test. *Spine* 4:242, 1979.
16. Cram RH: A sign of nerve root pressure. *J Bone Joint Surg [Br]* 35:192, 1953.
17. Michele AA: The flip sign in sciatic nerve tension. *Surgery* 44:940, 1958.
18. Waddell G, et al: Neurogenic physical signs in low-back pain. *Spine* 5:117, 1980.
19. Lipson SJ: Experimental intervertebral disc degeneration. *Arthritis Rheum* 24:12, 1981.
20. Lawrence JS: Disc degeneration: its frequency and relationship to symptoms. *Ann Rheum Dis* 28:121, 1969.
21. Nachemson A: The lumbar spine—an orthopedic challenge. *Spine* 1:59, 1976.
22. Spengler D: Degenerative stenosis of the lumbar spine. *J Bone Joint Surg [Am]* 69:305, 1987.

Chapter 4

PSYCHOLOGICAL EVALUATION OF THE LOW BACK PAIN PATIENT

LAURENCE A. BRADLEY, PhD

Chronic pain has been described as a "malefic force that often imposes severe emotional, physical, economic, and sociologic stress on the patient and his family as well as on society" (1, p. xxvii). Since the early 1970s, physicians have become increasingly aware that behavioral and psychological factors play an important role in the development and maintenance of chronic pain. As a result, physicians also have attempted to improve their abilities to recognize and respond to these factors (2). The purpose of this chapter is to review the behavioral and psychological factors that should be evaluated when patients with low back pain (LBP) present themselves to physicians and other health care professionals.

DEFINITION OF TERMS

The International Association for the Study of Pain (IASP) recently developed a standard taxonomy that defines pain as "an unpleasant sensory and emotional experience associated with actual or potential tissue damage, or described in terms of such damage" (3, p. S217). This definition recognizes that pain is both subjective and multidimensional in nature. Moreover, the definition acknowledges that one need not suffer tissue damage at a specific body site in order to perceive pain at that site (e.g., thalamic pain). Although textbooks often make clear distinctions between somatogenic and psychogenic pain, it usually is quite difficult to reliably identify patients with chronic pain due solely to organic causes with no psychological difficulties, or patients with chronic pain that is due solely to behavioral or psychological causes (4). It is necessary, then,

to acknowledge that most patients with chronic LBP will have both medical and psychological or behavioral problems that require careful evaluation.

Unlike acute pain that is "of recent onset or short duration" (5, p. 243), chronic pain is defined as "pain of at least several months duration" (5, p. 243). Regardless of chronicity, however, pain may be conceived as consisting of three levels, only one of which is observable (6). Figure 4.1 illustrates that the first level is *nociception,* which is defined as potentially tissue-damaging stimulation of the specialized endings of A-delta and C nerve fibers. The second is the *unpleasant subjective painful experience* that is associated with actual or potential tissue damage. It is clear that the first two levels of pain cannot be observed. However, the third level of pain is the *suffering* or the *observable behavior* (motor or verbal) displayed by individuals that suggests they are experiencing pain. The difficulty that physicians must confront is that the treatment of chronic pain generally must be directed toward reducing suffering and pain behavior, whereas the treatment of acute pain is directed primarily toward the other two unobservable levels. For example, if a patient seeks care from a physician for LBP due to a recent work injury, the physician usually will perform a physical examination, order various diagnostic procedures, or request consultation from other medical specialists in an attempt to identify and eventually eliminate the source of the nociceptive process. The physician often will prescribe bed rest and analgesic medication in order to reduce the patient's subjective pain experience during the diagnostic process, which may continue for several weeks. This practice is based upon the assumption that once nociception is eliminated,

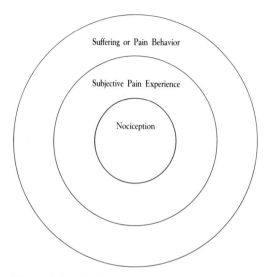

Figure 4.1. A tripartite conceptualization of pain.

the patient's pain will disappear and further treatment will be unnecessary (7).[a]

A patient with chronic LBP, however, often will seek health care even after diagnostic testing has failed to identify clearly a nociceptive source. Moreover, during the long period since the onset of pain, there will have been ample opportunity for psychological factors to begin to influence the patient's suffering. These factors may be endogenous, such as depression or anxiety, or they may be exogenous, such as the environmental consequences that follow the patient's displays of pain behavior. The environmental consequences include "positive reinforcing" events (e.g., attention from the spouse, intake of sedating or analgesic medication) as well as "negative reinforcing" events (e.g., permission to stay home in bed rather than go to work) that immediately follow the patient's behavior. In addition, the patient may not receive positive reinforcement following the display of relatively healthy behavior (e.g., family members may suggest that the patient rest rather than attempt to perform usual activities of daily living). Thus, because of the consequences that follow pain and healthy behavior, the patient may learn to display excessively dramatic levels of suffering regardless of whether or not nociception

[a]It should be noted that the prescription of prolonged bed rest recently has been challenged by data indicating that even patients with acute LBP show more positive long-term outcomes when rest is time limited and followed by resumption of activity than when cessation of rest is contingent upon elimination of pain (8, 9).

occurs (10, 11). Often the consequences delivered by physicians that are appropriate for a patient with acute pain (e.g., medication prescription, release from work duties) may contribute further to the maintenance of chronic pain and suffering. The primary focus of treatment for a chronic LBP patient, therefore, is the modification of the patient's displays of suffering rather than the elimination of the unpleasant subjective experience of pain or nociception. Indeed, Fordyce recently has noted that chronic LBP patients must be taught that (a) experiencing pain with movement does not necessarily imply that residual injury is present; and (b) their improvement depends mainly upon increasing their healthy behavior (12).

ASSESSMENT ISSUES

I previously have suggested that the psychological evaluation of chronic pain patients should include the assessment of cognitive-verbal responses, overt motor behaviors, and psychophysiologic responses (13). The following discussion is organized according to this schema.

COGNITIVE-VERBAL RESPONSES

The assessment of LBP patients' cognitive-verbal responses requires an interview as well as the administration of several self-report measures. The interview is used to evaluate the patients' suffering and the factors that may influence their suffering. The self-report measures are used to evaluate patients' affective responses, perceptions of pain, and coping strategies or cognitive distortions.

Behavioral Interview

The behavioral interview generally should involve both the patient and the spouse or some other family member. Since the interview usually is the first step in the assessment process, it is helpful to begin by explaining that the purpose of the interview is to determine how the pain has affected the patient's life and what factors may influence the pain. It also is helpful to encourage the spouse or family member to feel free to contribute his/her thoughts during the interview, even if a question is not directed specifically to the family member.

There are five important objectives to the behavioral interview. The first objective is to evaluate the patient's daily activities. It is necessary to determine (a) how the patient typically spends his/her time during the day, (b) which activities have been performed more often or less often since the onset of pain, and (c) whether any activities have been eliminated since the onset of pain.

The second objective is to identify the events that reliably precede exacerbations in the patient's pain perceptions and pain behavior as well as the events that reliably follow these exacerbations. With regard to analgesic medication usage, for example, it is important to determine whether the medication is being taken on a time-contingent basis (e.g., every 4 hours) or on a pain-contingent basis (as needed). If medication intake is contingent upon pain, it should be noted how often medication usually is required and whether medication is necessary following unpleasant or emotionally disturbing events. It also should be determined whether the patient has been gradually increasing the strength or quantity of medication over time or using the medication as a "preventive" measure (e.g., before going to bed every night or in response to small increases in pain or muscle twinges rather than severe pain). The occurrence of either of these two events would suggest that the patient may be using analgesic medication excessively. Finally, it should be noted how persons in the patient's environment respond to the patient's use of medication. Do family members bring the medication to the patient or provide reinforcement to the patient after medication usage? One example of positive reinforcement would be increased attention or nurturance (e.g., massaging the patient's back) following the intake of medication. An example of negative reinforcement might occur in a troubled marriage; in this case, reduced interaction with the spouse or children following medication intake might reward the patient for frequent usage of analgesic medication.

In addition to determining the events that influence pain behavior, it is necessary to devote attention to the events that reliably precede and follow the patient's attempts to engage in relatively healthy behavior (e.g., exercise, social activities). Some patients, particularly those with long histories of chronic pain, very rarely will try to display healthy behavior (e.g., only at times they perceive mild pain). Other patients, particularly those who have just entered the chronic phase of pain, frequently will attempt to behave in a healthy fashion even if their physical conditioning has deteriorated as a result of long periods of inactivity. Positive responses from family members following healthy behavior generally will increase the frequency with which such behavior is displayed. However, if healthy behavior is followed by increases in pain as a result of poor physical conditioning or overexertion, encouragement from others probably will not be rewarding.

The third objective of the behavioral interview is to determine the extent to which the patient may exacerbate his/her suffering. For example, a patient may report that since the onset of pain he/she has restricted or eliminated certain activities because of an expectation of increased pain. This avoidance behavior may lead to excessive disability or pain resulting from distorted gait or reduced activity levels (2). The patient may require skills training or anxiety management in order to begin the restricted activities. Conversely, a patient may describe behavior that is characterized by constant activity that is not reduced until the intensity of pain becomes severe. This patient will require instruction in appropriately modulating his/her activity level so that pain does not become a signal that automatically elicits rest, medication intake, or further avoidance of other activities (2).

The fourth objective of the behavioral interview is to evaluate the degree to which the patient is experiencing affective disturbance. Depression is commonly found among chronic pain patients (14), although there is disagreement regarding whether depression is primary (15) or secondary (16) to chronic pain. Thus, it should be determined whether the patient has experienced any change in mood or outlook on life since the onset of pain and whether the patient has experienced vegetative signs of depression such as sleep disturbance, change in food intake, or decreased desire for sexual intercourse. It commonly is found during the interview that both male and female patients report changes in sexual functioning (e.g., difficulty in achieving or maintaining erections, decreased vaginal lubrication, dyspareunia) as well as decreases in sexual desire. There also is evidence that female chronic pain patients frequently report histories of physical or sexual abuse (17). Finally, it is important to determine if changes in the marital or in other family relationships have occurred since the onset of pain.

The final objective of the interview is to determine if there are any relatives or friends in the family who suffer from chronic pain or disabilities similar to those of the patient. Careful questioning often will reveal that the patient spends a considerable amount of time with relatives or friends who also have chronic pain problems (2). Thus, the patient may have a great deal of opportunity to learn by observation maladaptive chronic pain behavior (e.g., experimenting with others' analgesic medications, inappropriate health care resource usage).

Self-Report Measures of Affective Disturbance

Although questions concerning anxiety and depression should be included in the behavioral interview, most health care professionals also administer standardized measures of affective disturbance to chronic LBP patients. The most commonly used psychological assessment instrument is the Minnesota Multiphasic Personality Inventory (MMPI). The MMPI is a 566-item questionnaire that measures 10 dimensions of psychological disturbance. Patients' raw scores on each scale are converted to standard *T* scores so that they may be compared to the scores produced by a large sample of control individuals who were administered the MMPI in the late 1930s. It should be remembered, however, that the original norms that are used for interpretation purposes are not appropriate for the assessment of chronic pain patients (4).[b] In addition, it appears that there are several items on the Hypochondriasis, Depression, Hysteria, and Schizophrenia scales that typically are answered in a pathologic fashion by patients with chronic LBP (21–24), primarily because the items describe experiences that commonly occur among patients with chronic illness (e.g., a response of "false" to "I do not tire quickly" or "I am about as able to work as I ever was").

In response to the problem of MMPI interpretation, several groups of investigators have used hierarchical clustering methods to delineate the MMPI profile patterns that are produced most frequently by chronic LBP patients and the behaviors that are associated with these patterns. Figures 4.2 through 4.4 show three MMPI profile patterns that often are generated by chronic LBP patients (25). It has been shown (25) that chronic LBP patients' profiles characterized by elevations on the Hypochondriasis, Depression, and Hysteria scales (Fig. 4.2) are associated with highly intense pain perceptions, affective disturbance, and severe disruptions in vocational, social, marital/sexual, and family endeavors. Profiles with elevations on the scales noted above as well as on the Psychopathic Deviancy and Schizophrenia scales (Fig. 4.3) tend to be associated with difficulty in giving up the positive consequences

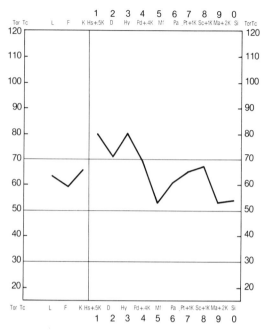

Figure 4.2. Low back pain patient's MMPI profile with elevated Hypochondriasis, Depression, and Hysteria scale scores.

received for pain behavior, relatively moderate disruptions in vocational, social, marital/sexual, and family endeavors, and high levels of psychopathology. Profiles without elevations on any of the clinical scales (Fig. 4.4) are associated with relatively few pain-related disabilities in daily functioning. These findings have received empirical support from the results of several independent investigations (26–29). It also has been shown that chronic LBP patients' responses to conservative orthopaedic management could be predicted accurately by their MMPI profile patterns (27). The proportions of accurate predictions ranged from 61 to 99% among the male patients and from 65 to 89% among the females. However, it has not been shown yet that MMPI profile patterns may be used to reliably predict outcome following interdisciplinary pain clinic treatment (30, 31).

An important factor that might account for some of the predictive error associated with clustering of MMPI profiles is excessive heterogeneity among patients with similar profile patterns (32). Henrichs (32) recently replicated the MMPI profile patterns identified in my previous research (25, 33). However, a large number of patients with similar profile patterns were classified as outliers when a stringent criterion (34) was used to evaluate profile pattern

---

[b] Recently, new norms for the MMPI have been developed with samples of contemporary adults (18, 19). One study of chronic pain patients revealed that there was a marked decrease in "psychologically disturbed" profiles when the contemporary norms were substituted for the original norms (20).

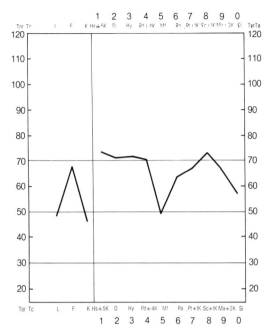

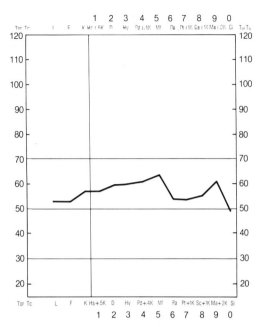

Figure 4.3. Low back pain patient's MMPI profile with elevated Hypochondriasis, Depression, Hysteria, Psychopathic Deviancy, and Schizophrenia scale scores.

Figure 4.4. Low back pain patient's MMPI profile with all clinical scale scores within normal limits.

homogeneity. Nevertheless, application of this criterion produced profile patterns that were highly associated with different behavioral correlates and responses to surgical or nonsurgical treatment. It may be possible, then, to improve the predictive power of MMPI profile patterns by further refinement of the patterns after their initial derivation by clustering methods. At present, however, the MMPI should be used to generate hypotheses regarding the psychological disturbances and behavior of chronic LBP patients that must be validated by other behavioral and interview data (2, 35).

In addition to the problems described above regarding norms, the contamination of items with physical symptoms, and the predictive validity of the profile patterns, the MMPI also has been criticized for excessive length and the use of many of the same items in multiple scales (36). Thus, some health care professionals have begun to use several newly developed psychological assessment instruments as alternatives to the MMPI. These instruments include the Illness Behavior Questionnaire (37), the Millon Behavioral Health Inventory (38), and the Symptom Checklist-90 (39). The Illness Behavior Questionnaire (IBQ) is a 62-item self-report measure that evaluates seven dimensions of illness behavior: (a) General Hypochondriasis, (b)

Conviction of Disease, (c) Psychological versus Somatic Focus of Disease, (d) Affective Inhibition, (e) Affective Disturbance, (f) Denial of Life Problems Unrelated to Pain, and (g) Irritability. It has been found that low back pain patients' scores on the Affective Inhibition, Affective Disturbance, and Irritability scales are significant predictors of their pain intensity ratings and displays of pain behavior even after controlling for the influence of demographic and medical status variables (40). However, it also has been reported that each of the IBQ scales correlates significantly with the Eysenck Personality Inventory Neuroticism scale (41). Thus, use of the IBQ may not offer any major advantage to use of the MMPI given that the IBQ might measure primarily anxiety or other neurotic disorders.

The Millon Behavioral Health Inventory (MBHI) is a 150-item self-report measure that was designed to evaluate the psychological functioning of medical patients. Its advantages relative to the MMPI are that the MBHI contains relatively few items, the items are not contaminated by symptoms of physical illness, and the norms are based on the responses of patients with a variety of medical, rather than psychiatric, disorders. Two recent investigations (42, 43) have shown that several MBHI scales are associated with chronic pain patients' responses to multidisciplinary pain clinic treatment. Both of these studies, however, revealed that patients' scores on the MBHI Pain Treatment Responsivity scale did not correlate strongly or consistently with changes in their scores on subjective and objective outcome measures across assessment periods.

The Symptom Checklist-90 (SCL-90) is a 90-item self-report measure of nine major psychological disturbances (Somatization, Obsessive-Compulsive, Interpersonal Sensitivity, Depression, Anxiety, Hostility, Phobic Anxiety, Paranoid Ideation, and Psychoticism). In addition, three global measures of psychological distress may be derived. Some investigators have begun to evaluate the utility of the SCL-90 relative to the MMPI with respect to the evaluation of chronic pain patients (e.g., 44). However, Jamison and his colleagues have adopted a more promising research strategy (45). These investigators have derived empirically three subgroups of chronic pain patients based on their SCL-90 responses. Patients with elevated scores on the majority of the scales, relative to those with scale scores within normal limits, reported the highest levels of (a) functional disability, (b) sleep disturbance, (c) sleep medication usage, (d) family conflict, and (e) emotional distress. Nevertheless, apart from the results described above, little is known regarding the clinical utility of the SCL-90 with chronic LBP patients.

Self-Report Measures of Pain Perceptions

The most commonly used methods of measuring subjective pain perceptions are numerical or verbal category scales, visual analogue scales, and the McGill Pain Questionnaire. Figure 4.5A and B illustrate a typical numerical and verbal category scale. The patient is required to choose one number or verbal descriptor that best describes the present intensity of his/her pain. Figure 4.5C shows a visual analogue scale typically used for pain measurement. The patient must indicate his/her perception of pain intensity by placing a perpendicular mark along the 10-cm horizontal line.

Category and visual analogue scales are easily administered and scored and generally are highly correlated with one another (46). However, several investigators have questioned their sensitivity to changes in the subjective pain experience (47). There also appear to be great differences among persons in their abilities to use visual analogue scales in a reliable manner (48). For example, it has been shown that older persons tend to have more difficulty than younger individuals in correctly using visual analogue scales (49). Despite the

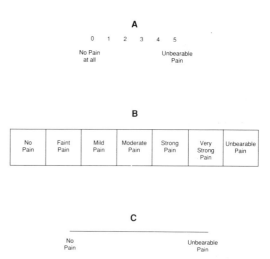

Figure 4.5. Illustrations of pain perception measures. *A,* Numerical category scale. *B,* Verbal category scale. *C,* Visual analogue scale.

difficulties described above, however, category and visual analogue scales continue to be used by many health care providers and investigators to evaluate subjective pain intensity levels.

The McGill Pain Questionnaire (MPQ) (50) is an instrument that was designed to measure multiple dimensions of the pain experience and at the same time avoid some of the problems associated with category and visual analogue scales. Figure 4.6 illustrates that the MPQ consists of 20 category scales of verbal descriptors; the descriptors within each category scale are rank ordered in terms of pain intensity. The patient must examine each category scale and choose one descriptor from each relevant scale that best describes his/her subjective pain experience at that moment. The first 11 scales assess the patient's perceptions of the sensory dimension of subjective pain. Scales 12–15 evaluate the affective dimension and scale 16 measures the evaluative or intensity dimension of the pain experience. The final four scales encompass four miscellaneous dimensions of subjective pain. The MPQ may be scored on the basis of the number of words chosen from among the 20 category scales or according to the sum of the rank values of the descriptors chosen from each of the four pain dimensions or across all dimensions (i.e., Pain Rating Index, or PRI).

A large number of investigations involving LBP patients have provided positive evidence regarding the reliability and validity of the MPQ (51). The instrument also has been shown to be sensitive to change following therapeutic interventions (e.g.,

What Does Your Pain Feel Like?

Some of the words I will read to you describe your *present* pain. Tell me which words best describe it. Leave out any word-group that is not suitable. Use only a single word in each appropriate group—the one that applies *best*.

1	2	3
1 Flickering	1 Jumping	1 Pricking
2 Quivering	2 Flashing	2 Boring
3 Pulsing	3 Shooting	3 Drilling
4 Throbbing		4 Stabbing
5 Beating		5 Lancinating
6 Pounding		

4	5	6
1 Sharp	1 Pinching	1 Tugging
2 Cutting	2 Pressing	2 Pulling
3 Lacerating	3 Gnawing	3 Wrenching
	4 Cramping	
	5 Crushing	

7	8	9
1 Hot	1 Tingling	1 Dull
2 Burning	2 Itching	2 Sore
3 Scalding	3 Smarting	3 Hurting
4 Searing	4 Stinging	4 Aching
		5 Heavy

10	11	12
1 Tender	1 Tiring	1 Sickening
2 Taut	2 Exhausting	2 Suffocating
3 Rasping		
4 Splitting		

13	14	15
1 Fearful	1 Punishing	1 Wretched
2 Frightful	2 Gruelling	2 Blinding
3 Terrifying	3 Cruel	
	4 Vicious	
	5 Killing	

16	17	18
1 Annoying	1 Spreading	1 Tight
2 Troublesome	2 Radiating	2 Numb
3 Miserable	3 Penetrating	3 Drawing
4 Intense	4 Piercing	4 Squeezing
5 Unbearable		5 Tearing

19	20
1 Cool	1 Nagging
2 Cold	2 Nauseating
3 Freezing	3 Agonizing
	4 Dreadful
	5 Torturing

Comments:

Figure 4.6. The McGill Pain Questionnaire. (From Melzack R: The McGill Pain Questionnaire: major properties and scoring methods. *Pain* 1:277–299, 1975.)

52). As a result, the MPQ has rapidly gained wide acceptance among health care providers and investigators (13) both in English-speaking countries and in countries in which translated versions of the measure have been produced (e.g., 53–56). However, several investigators have noted that patients who are unfamiliar with the English language or who come from low socioeconomic backgrounds have difficulty responding to the MPQ (4). There also has been some concern regarding whether it is more appropriate to compute a total PRI score only, given that sensory, affective, and evaluative PRI scores may be highly intercorrelated (57). Finally, the scoring of the MPQ has been criticized on the grounds that PRI scores are confounded by differences in the number of descriptors that comprise each of the 20 scales (58). Melzack and his colleagues (59) have developed an alternative, weighted-rank method for computing PRI scores that corrects for this problem. It has been shown that the use of the weighted-rank method actually increases the sensitivity of the MPQ (59).

Self-Report Measures of Cognitive Distortion and Coping Strategies

Recent research has suggested that it is very important to evaluate possible maladaptive thoughts, or cognitive distortions, and coping strategies used by LBP patients. It has been demonstrated that depressed chronic LBP patients, relative to their nondepressed counterparts, frequently attribute negative life events to internal, stable, and global causes (60). That is, these depressed individuals tend to believe that the negative events they experience are due to causes (a) for which they are personally responsible, (b) that do not vary over time, and (c) that do not vary across different situations. However, the attributions of depressed and nondepressed patients for positive life events do not differ from one another. Other investigations have examined the manner in which LBP patients interpret negative, pain-related life situations. Lefebvre (61) has shown that depressed LBP patients commonly use three cognitive distortions in interpreting these situations. The cognitive distortions are: *catastrophizing* (misinterpreting an event as a catastrophe), *overgeneralization* (assuming that the outcome of one experience applies to the same or similar future experiences), and *selective abstraction* (selectively attending to negative aspects of an experience). Lefebvre (61) has developed a questionnaire that measures cognitive distortions concerning LBP-related problems. Use of this questonnaire may aid health care providers since it recently has been reported that LBP patients' cognitive distortions, especially overgeneralization, were associated with functional disability even after controlling for depression, pain severity, and number of pain treatments (62). Thus, treatment of chronic LBP patients may be improved by altering patients' erroneous beliefs that their functional disabilities will remain stable in all future situations.

It also may be useful for health care providers to evaluate the coping strategies employed by LBP patients. A large number of investigations have indicated that the strategies used by individuals to cope with negative events may reduce or augment the impact of those stressors (63). Accordingly, Rosentiel and Keefe (64) developed a questionnaire for the assessment of chronic LBP patients' cognitive and behavioral coping strategies. Factor analysis of patients' responses to the Coping Strategies Questionnaire (CSQ) produced three related underlying dimensions: (a) Cognitive Coping and Suppression (e.g., reinterpreting pain sensations); (b) Helplessness (e.g., catastrophizing); and (c) Diverting Attention and Praying (e.g., praying and hoping). It also was reported that patients with high scores on the Cognitive Coping and Suppression or the Diverting Attention and Praying factors tended to show high levels of functional impairment. Those who produced high Helplessness scores tended to display high levels of anxiety and depression.

Turner and Clancy (65) replicated the factor structure of the CSQ among an independent sample of chronic LBP patients. Moreover, Reesor and Craig (66) have shown that, even after controlling

for differences in physical impairment and disability, chronic LBP patients with medically incongruent signs and symptoms were best discriminated from chronic LBP patients without incongruent symptoms by their tendency to use catastrophizing strategies (as measured by the CSQ) during an experimental pain induction procedure.

Brown and Nicassio (67) also have developed a measure of chronic pain coping strategies, the Vanderbilt Pain Management Inventory. However, this measure has been validated only with a sample of rheumatoid arthritis patients. Moreover, it was designed to evaluate only two classes of coping strategies, active and passive, that were defined a priori as adaptive or maladaptive, respectively. The construction of this measure, then, is not in accord with current theories of coping, which suggest that the efficacy of active and passive coping strategies may vary across individuals and situations (68).

Although the evidence reviewed above strongly suggests that LBP patients' cognitive distortions and coping strategies are associated with psychological distress and functional disability, it currently is unknown whether these cognitive processes actually produce psychological and functional impairments or result from such impairments. There also are no data concerning whether therapeutic changes in cognitive activities might reduce patients' impairments. Nevertheless, health care providers may wish to use the coping strategies and cognitive distortion measures described above as aids for planning psychological interventions with their LBP patients.

Discussion

There are a large number of techniques available for the assessment of patients' cognitive-verbal responses. The health care provider might ask, then, what techniques should be included in patients' assessment protocols. I would suggest that it is imperative to include in each patient assessment a behavioral interview, at least one self-report measure of effective disturbance, and at least one self-report measure of pain perceptions.

With regard to the evaluation of affective disturbance, I administer the MMPI, IBQ, and MBHI to my patients. I continue to rely upon the MMPI as the primary measure because of the reliable predictions concerning patient behavior that may be made with this instrument. The IBQ is a useful supplemental measure and allows one to generate some hypotheses regarding patients' pain behavior (40). Agreements between the MMPI and IBQ also lend confidence to conclusions regarding affective disturbance. Moreover, inconsistent findings, particularly with regard to patients' tendencies to overly focus on somatic complaints, should be given careful attention. I tend to give greater emphasis to the behavioral interview when the MMPI and IBQ produce conflicting results. At present, I use the MBHI primarily for heuristic and research purposes with special populations such as patients with noncardiac chest pain (69).

With respect to pain perceptions, I rely upon the MPQ for clinical assessment. Although it usually is necessary to define several verbal descriptors for patients, I find that the number of descriptors chosen by patients may provide some insights with regard to their tendencies to overdramatize or minimize their pain perceptions and suffering.

The assessment of coping strategies and cognitive distortions is a relatively recent development in the chronic pain literature. I primarily use the CSQ as a research instrument. However, the health care provider who wishes to use the CSQ for clinical purposes probably should attend primarily to responses that reflect helplessness and catastrophizing.

OVERT MOTOR BEHAVIORS

The primary benefit of evaluating overt motor or pain behaviors is that it provides the health care provider with quantifiable data regarding patients' disabilities in physical mobility and other activities that are directly related to functioning in vocational, social, and leisure endeavors (13, 51). In addition, it usually is difficult to rely solely upon the behavioral interview to determine with confidence the extent of a patient's pain behavior and the events that reliably precede and follow the patient's pain and healthy behavior (11). There often is a substantial difference between a patient's self-report of his/her behavior and more objective assessment of that behavior (70, 71). Thus, the behavioral interview described earlier in this chapter frequently serves to generate hypotheses regarding the patient's behavior and the factors that influence the behavior that must be tested using additional assessment methods. The four major methods for measuring overt motor behaviors are (a) direct behavioral observations, (b) automated measurement devices, (c) self-monitored observations, and (d) self-reports of functional disability.

Direct Behavioral Observations

Several groups of investigators recently have developed standardized protocols for measuring behaviors such as grimacing, bracing, guarded movement, and rubbing of painful body parts. Keefe and Block (72) produced the first of these protocols, which required chronic low back pain patients to perform for video recording a 10-min standardized sequence of activities (i.e., walking, sitting, reclining, and standing). Two trained observers independently viewed the video recordings and noted frequencies of guarding, bracing, rubbing, grimacing, and sighing behavior during 20-sec observation periods.

Keefe and his colleagues recently demonstrated that trained observers may generate reliable and valid frequency counts of chronic low back pain patients' motor behaviors during their physical examinations without using obtrusive video recording equipment (73). In addition, the validity and sensitivity to change of the pain behavior measurement protocol have been supported by independent investigations performed both in the United States (74) and in Sweden (75, 76). A detailed description of the use of the protocol has been provided by Keefe and coworkers (77).

Other groups of investigators have developed standardized protocols for measuring both verbal and motor behaviors indicative of pain (78–80). These protocols provide quantifiable and relatively objective measures of pain-related behaviors. However, none have been studied as extensively as the Keefe and Block (72) method.

Automated Measurement Devices

Concerns regarding the reliability of observers' recordings of patient behavior and the generalizability of patient behavior during limited observation periods have led some investigators to produce devices for the automated measurement of overt motor behavior. Sanders (81), for example, developed an inexpensive, portable automatic device for measuring patient "uptime." The instrument consisted of a miniature electronic calculator that was modified to interface with a mercury tilt switch mounted on a patient's thigh with an elastic bandage. Follick and his colleagues (82) produced an improved version of this device. The improvements included resistance to recording error associated with rapid or vigorous movements, accurate recording of time spent reclining regardless of body position, and the capacity to record time spent sitting as either "downtime" or "uptime."

Positive evidence has been produced regarding the reliability and validity of the automated devices described above. However, the clinical utility of these complex devices is restricted by the need for close supervision of patients, especially those with limited mechanical skills, high levels of emotional distress, or cognitive impairments (82). One attempt has been made to evaluate the utility of a relatively simple automated device, the actometer (83). An actometer is a modified mechanical watch that measures the amount of acceleration or G force produced by the wearer during each movement. However, the utility of this device is limited by poor reliability of measurement over time (83). It appears, then, that automated recording devices are useful primarily for research purposes at the present time. These devices should be used for clinical purposes only in conjunction with the other behavioral assessment methods described in this chapter (51).

Self-Monitored Observations

Patient self-monitoring of behavior usually is accomplished with daily pain and behavior diaries such as that shown in Figure 4.7. Self-monitoring has two major advantages over most of the direct observation and automated measurement techniques described above. First, self-monitoring requires little training of health care staff members and patients. In addition, it allows for the continuous recording of a wide variety of behaviors in addition to "uptime," "downtime," and abnormal body movements in environments other than the hospital or laboratory (84).

My colleagues and I usually ask patients to complete diary recordings for 3–7 days. When the diary is returned, it is possible to compute the time spent by the patient each day in activities that involve sitting, standing or walking, and reclining. Since the diary requires patients to record pain intensity levels and medication intake every waking hour, it also is possible to examine the relationships among the patients' activity levels, pain perceptions, and medication consumption.

Figure 4.7 shows an example of a secretary's diary recordings for one day. Examination of the early morning recordings reveals that the patient took a narcotic analgesic between 12:00 and 1:00 AM and the same medication between 4:00 and 5:00 AM. Later that morning, the patient required aspirin as her perceptions of pain intensity increased after working at her desk for approximately 1 hour. She took the narcotic analgesic during the afternoon after working at her desk for about 2 hours without rest or exercise. However, the patient's perceptions of pain intensity decreased in the evening as she divided her time fairly evenly between exercise, performing household tasks, and resting. The patient's pain, then, appears to be exacerbated by

difficulty in alternating between work, exercise, and rest activities at the job. In addition, the patient's sleep pattern appears to be disturbed; the patient actually may take narcotic medication at night primarily for sedation rather than for pain control despite her use of a small dosage of amitriptyline.

It is clear from the example above that diary recordings may be very useful in guiding treatment decisions. For example, one might consider increasing the patient's dosage of amitriptyline and perhaps changing to a schedule of multiple administrations throughout the day rather than a single administration at night. If the patient's sleep disturbance persists, one probably would consider a trial of a different antidepressant medication. One also might instruct the patient to devote 15 min during every working hour to rest or exercise (e.g., walking) in an attempt to avoid exacerbations of pain and the usage of analgesic medication. It should be noted that it usually is very helpful to discuss the diary recordings with the patient in order to provide a rationale for one's treatment recommendations. Discussion also generally improves rapport with the patient and increases the patient's motivation to remain actively involved in the treatment process. In addition, examination and discussion of a new set of diary recordings periodically during treatment provides a record of the patient's progress and indicators for modifying the patient's treatment regimen.

Despite the potential utility of patient diary recordings, there are some drawbacks to the use of this assessment technique. One drawback is that some patients find it difficult to maintain hourly recordings of their pain perceptions and behavior and will attempt to complete their diaries in a retrospective fashion. Cautioning patients about the errors that are generated by retrospective recording before they begin their first diary may help reduce the frequency of this problematic behavior. Collins and Thompson (85) also have developed unobtrusive methods of monitoring inaccurate recordings of pain perception that may be used as checks on patients' diary keeping. The second drawback associated with the use of pain and behavior diaries is that some patients will produce inaccurate recordings of their behavior even if they do maintain an hourly recording schedule as a result of impression management efforts (70, 71), as well as impaired cognitive functioning secondary to depression (14), narcotic medication dependency (86), or traumatic head/neck injury (87). Thus, patients' recordings of their behavior should be validated on periodic basis against direct observations of their

Hour Beginning	Sitting — Major Activity	Sitting — Time	Walking or Standing — Major Activity	Walking or Standing — Time	Reclining — Activity	Reclining — Time	Medications — Type	Medications — Amount	Absence 0	1	2	3	4	Unbearable 5
12:00 am	watching TV	30	in kitchen	10	in bed	20	Darvocet	2 tablets				•		
1:00					sleep	60								
2:00						60								
3:00						60								
4:00	reading	30	in bathroom	5	sleep	25	Darvocet	2 tablets			•			
5:00						60								
6:00						60								
7:00	eating/reading	40	in bathroom/kitchen	20						•				
8:00	car/desk	40	walking to work	20						•				
9:00	at desk	55	break	5			Aspirin	2 tablets			•			
10:00	at desk	60									•			
11:00	at desk/meeting	50	walking	10							•			
12:00 noon	lunch	30	walking	10	resting	20				•				
1:00	at desk	40	talking with friends	20						•				
2:00	at desk	60												
3:00	at desk	55	break	5			Darvocet	2 tablets				•		
4:00	at desk/car	30	grocery shopping	30								•		
5:00			" & in kitchen	60							•			
6:00	watching TV	30	in kitchen	30							•			
7:00	eating	40	cleaning up	20							•			
8:00	reading paper	20	walking	40						•				
9:00	on phone	30			resting/TV	30				•				
10:00							Elavil	50 mg			•			
11:00	sewing	50	ironing	10	sleep	60				•				

Figure 4.7. Example of a daily activity diary used for self-monitoring of patient behavior. (From Bradley LA: Assessing the psychological profile of the chronic pain patient. In Dubner R, Gebhart GF, Bond MR (eds): *Pain Research and Clinical Management.* (Proceedings of the Vth World Congress on Pain.) Amsterdam, Elsevier, 1988, vol 3, pp 251–262.)

behavior or medication screens (51). Comparisons of patients' recordings with family members' observations also may provide additional information regarding the events that tend to elicit or reward displays of pain behavior (2).

Self-Reports of Functional Disability

Recently, interest has developed in measuring patients' functional disability levels in activities of daily living. The Sickness Impact Profile (SIP) (88) has been used most frequently with chronic LBP patients. The SIP is a particularly promising measure since it provides a profile of patient functioning in several areas (e.g., ambulation, mobility, body care) that can provide targets for behavioral interventions (35). Follick and his colleagues (89) have provided positive evidence regarding the concurrent validity and sensitivity to change of chronic LBP patients' SIP scores. Similar findings also have been reported for a 24-item scale derived from the original 136-item SIP (90, 91).

Other investigators have attempted to develop their own measures of functional disability, such as the Chronic Illness Problem Inventory (92) and the West Haven–Yale Multidimensional Pain Inventory (93). Most of these instruments measure several variables, such as stressful life events, mood, and self-esteem, as well as functional disability. Unfortunately, none of the disability scale components of these instruments has been validated using the SIP or other accepted devices as criterion measures. Thus, health care providers who are interested in evaluating functional disability should use the SIP or other well-validated measures (e.g., Functional Status Index, Health Assessment Questionnaire). It should be noted, however, that the West Haven–Yale Multidimensional Pain Inventory may serve as a useful adjunct to these instruments because it evaluates patients' perceptions of family members' responses to displays of pain and suffering. This inventory may be particularly useful, then, if the health care provider has been unable to interview the patient or family members regarding environmental reinforcements for pain behavior (e.g., 94).

Discussion

The measurement of overt motor behaviors can provide very practical information regarding patient functioning in vocational, social, and leisure endeavors. However, the health care provider should be aware that there are several problems associated with behavioral assessment. First, the reliability of direct observations and self-monitored recordings of patient behavior must be reexamined at various intervals to ensure that the observers or patients produce accurate and consistent measurements. The need for monthly or bimonthly reliability checks may make it difficult for some health care providers to use direct observation and self-monitoring measurement methods.

The second problem associated with behavioral measurements is that it is not known to what extent direct observations, automated movement recordings, and self-monitored observations are affected by reactivity. *Reactivity* is defined as patient initiation of behavior change in response to the assessment procedure itself.

The final problem is that it is difficult to use behavioral measurements to provide information regarding the qualitative aspects of the patient's activities, such as the degree to which these activities are appropriate given the status of the patient's physical limitations or medical condition (51). It is possible to derive some of this qualitative information by examining patients' activity diaries. However, since the health care provider usually cannot observe the patient in the home or work environment, it often is necessary to rely upon interviews with the patient and spouse in order to fully understand the qualitative dimensions of the patient's behavior.

Despite the difficulties described above, I usually obtain from every patient either self-monitored observations of behavior or self-reports of functional disability. I primarily use video recordings of patient behavior as a research tool at the present time. However, I have found that showing patients video recordings of their improved behavior as they undergo treatment can be highly rewarding to them. As compact and light-weight video recording equipment becomes increasingly available at low cost, I expect that health care providers will make greater use of video recordings for clinical purposes.

PSYCHOPHYSIOLOGIC RESPONSES

The evaluation of psychophysiologic responses represents an attempt to find objective evidence of the experience of pain (95). However, no one yet has demonstrated a specific psychophysiologic response that covaries reliably with subjective reports of pain or that is free from the effects of extraneous factors such as expectations or attention.

Electromyographic Responses

The great majority of the psychophysiologic assessment studies with chronic LBP patients have been devoted to the measurement of electromyographic (EMG) activity. It generally is believed that many LBP patients tend to restrict their spinal motion and other movements and, thus, increase their paraspinal muscle tension levels for prolonged time periods. These changes, in turn, lead to a vicious cycle in which normal activities of daily living evoke increased muscle pain that leads to further restriction of motion (51). Thus, effective treatment of chronic LBP patients requires reliable and accurate measurement of paraspinal muscle EMG levels and treatments such as EMG biofeedback or relaxation training for reducing these EMG levels.

However, the assumptions described above have been challenged by several sets of inconsistent research findings. First, there have been disagreements among investigators regarding whether paraspinal muscle EMG levels can be measured reliably (e.g., 96, 97). Second, both positive (98, 99) and negative (100, 101) evidence has been reported regarding the hypothesis that chronic LBP patients show elevated EMG levels during rest or movement.

Some recent investigators have suggested the use of novel EMG assessment strategies. For example, Wolf and his colleagues (102, 103) have advocated examining the patterns rather than the absolute levels of EMG activity in paraspinal muscles during static and dynamic activities. These investigators have found that, unlike pain-free normal individuals, chronic LBP patients tend to produce abnormal EMG patterns (e.g., asymmetry of right and left paraspinal EMG levels) during both static and dynamic activities. They also have demonstrated that patients who are trained to produce more symmetric EMG patterns tend to report reduced pain perceptions and to display increased activity levels.

Findings similar to those of Wolf and his colleagues have been reported by Cram and Steger (104). Recently, however, Nouwen and his colleagues (105) failed to replicate Wolf et al.'s results, although they did find that LBP patients and pain-free controls produced different paraspinal and abdominal EMG patterns during flexion. Thus, further study of EMG patterns among LBP patients appears to be warranted.

Trigger Points and Tender Points

Myofascial trigger points are self-sustaining, hyperirritable foci located in skeletal muscle or its associated fascia that refer pain, tenderness, and autonomic changes to distant locations in patterns that are specific for each muscle (106, 107). These should be distinguished from tender points, which are hyperirritable foci that may be located in either muscular or nonmuscular tissue and that *do not*

refer pain, tenderness, or autonomic changes to distant locations (108). Trigger points often may be treated successfully by injection and stretching, but tender points rarely respond to this form of treatment (108). The distinction between trigger points and tender points is important because they are associated with different chronic back pain syndromes. Tender points are associated with fibromyalgia, a syndrome characterized by seven or more tender points, widespread pain and aching, and systemic symptoms such as morning stiffness, chronic fatigue, and sleep disturbance (108). There are several myofascial pain syndromes but all are characterized by the presence of at least one trigger point. Systemic symptoms usually are not present unless multiple trigger points have become involved and the myofascial syndrome has become chronic (107).

Until recently, identification of trigger points and tender points has been dependent upon manual palpation of the muscles. Manual palpation, however, cannot quantify the sensitivity of trigger points and tender points and thus cannot provide information relevant to assessment and treatment outcome evaluation. Fortunately, three instruments have been developed that reliably and accurately measure the sensitivity of trigger points and tender points to mechanical pressure. Fischer's pressure algometer (109) is a hand-held spring scale with a 1-cm circular, rubber-covered tip that is pressed into the skin. It is commercially available and has been the subject of several investigations. Reeves and his colleagues (110) have demonstrated the reliability of the instrument both within and between experimenters as well as the discriminative validity of the instrument. Jaeger and Reeves (106) also have shown that the pain threshold levels measured by the pressure algometer are sensitive to change following passive stretching and Fluori-Methane spraying of trigger points.

The two algometers that are not yet commercially available (111, 112) have not been studied as thoroughly as Fischer's device. Moreover, all three devices have been tested thus far only with a small number of patients suffering from head and neck pain. Thus, caution should be exercised in the use of these pressure algometers until they are tested with large patient samples, especially those with trigger points and tender points in many body areas.

Discussion

It has been very difficult for investigators to identify psychophysiologic variables that may serve as reliable markers of patients' pain experiences.

Nevertheless, the assessment of paraspinal EMG patterns as well as trigger point and tender point sensitivity represent promising attempts to provide clinically useful psychophysiologic pain markers. Indeed, my colleagues routinely evaluate paraspinal EMG patterns, although they are aware that the meaning of EMG asymmetries remains open to disagreement. My colleagues and I recently have begun to use the pressure algometer to evaluate pain thresholds. However, we currently are using this assessment method primarily for research purposes.

CONCLUSIONS

This chapter has critically reviewed the recent empirical literature concerning the psychological evaluation of the LBP patient. I have recommended that LBP patient evaluations include the assessment of cognitive-verbal responses, overt motor behaviors, and psychophysiologic responses. However, some of the methods described in this chapter are essential to any evaluation whereas others are not appropriate for routine use. Table 4.1 shows that the assessment methods that are essential to every evaluation include the behavioral interview and self-reports of affective distress, pain perceptions, and functional disability. The assessment methods that are very useful but should not be considered as mandatory include measures of cognitive distortions and coping strategies, direct observation of pain behavior, automated recordings of pain behav-

ior, self-monitored recordings of behavior, and EMG activity patterns. The only assessment methods that are not yet appropriate for routine clinical use are pressure algometer recordings of trigger point and tender point sensitivity.

It is clear that there are advantages and disadvantages associated with each of the assessment methods described in this chapter. Thus, it is desirable to use multiple measures of overt motor behavior, cognitive-verbal responses, and psychophysiologic responses in order to fully evaluate LBP patients and their treatment outcomes. For example, I recently participated in a randomized, controlled study of the efficacy of cognitive-behavioral therapy in the secondary prevention of chronic back pain among nurses (76). The investigation used a large number of outcome measures that included (a) direct observations of overt motor behavior; (b) objective recordings of work absences due to back pain; (c) visual analogue scale ratings of pain intensity; (d) self-reports of depression, anxiety, sleep distrubance, and functional disability; and (e) perceptions of control of back pain symptoms. Significant treatment effects were found on all of these outcome measures. However, the change in the experimental subjects' perceptions of symptom control was relatively small. In addition, although the experimental subjects showed a reduction in episodes of work loss as a result of back pain, the experimental and control subjects did not differ with regard to the total number of days lost as a result of back pain. These findings raise questions regarding the importance of patient cognitions in the outcomes produced by cognitive-behavioral therapy and the effectiveness of the therapy in reducing pain-related work loss. This example illustrates the need for comprehensive evaluation of LBP patients in both clinical and research settings.

Table 4.1
Assessment Methods and Their Appropriate Usage

ESSENTIAL	OPTIONAL	RESEARCH
Behavioral interview	Self-report of cognitive distortions	Trigger point pain thresholds
Self-report of affective distress	Self-report of coping strategies	Tender point pain thresholds
Self-report of pain perceptions	Direct behavioral observations	
Self-report of functional disability	Automated pain behavior recordings	
	Self-monitored behavioral observations	
	EMG activity patterns	

REFERENCES

1. Bonica JJ: Introduction to the First World Congress on Pain: goals of the IASP and the World Congress. In Bonica JJ, Albe-Fessard D (eds): *Advances in Pain Research and Therapy.* New York, Raven Press, 1976, vol 1, pp xxvii–xxxix.
2. Keefe FJ, Bradley LA: Behavioral and psychological approaches to the assessment and treatment of chronic pain. *Gen Hosp Psychiatry* 6:49–54, 1984.
3. IASP Subcommittee on Taxonomy: Classification of chronic pain: descriptions of chronic pain syndromes and definitions of pain terms. *Pain,* Suppl 3:S1–S225, 1986.

4. Bradley LA, Prokop CK, Gentry WD, Van der Heide LH, Prieto EJ: Assessment of chronic pain. In Prokop CK, Bradley LA (eds): *Medical Psychology: Contributions to Behavioral Medicine*. New York, Academic Press, 1981, pp 91–117.

5. Sternbach RA: Clinical aspects of pain. In Sternbach RA (ed): *The Psychology of Pain*. New York, Raven Press, 1978, pp 241–264.

6. Fordyce WE: Learning processes in pain. In Sternbach RA (ed): *The Psychology of Pain*. New York, Raven Press, 1978, pp 49–72.

7. Fordyce WE: An operant conditioning method for managing chronic pain. *Post-grad Med* 53:123–128, 1973.

8. Deyo R, Diehl A, Rosenthal M: How many days of bed rest for acute low back pain? *N Engl J Med* 315:1064–1070, 1986.

9. Fordyce W, Brockway J, Bergman J, Spengler D: A control group comparison of behavioral vs. traditional management methods in acute low back pain. *J Behav Med* 5:127–140, 1986.

10. Fordyce WE: Behavioral methods for chronic pain and illness. St Louis, CV Mosby, 1976, pp 26–73.

11. Linton SJ, Melin L, Götestam KG: Behavioral analysis of chronic pain and its management. In Hersen M, Eisler R, Miller PM (eds): *Progress in Behavior Modification*. New York, Academic Press, 1984, vol 18, pp 1–42.

12. Fordyce WE: Pain and suffering: a reappraisal. *Am Psychol* 43:276–283, 1988.

13. Bradley LA: Assessing the psychological profile of the chronic pain patient. In Dubner R, Gebhart GF, Bond MR (eds): *Pain Research and Clinical Management*. (Proceedings of the Vth World Congress on Pain.) Amsterdam, Elsevier, 1988, vol 3, pp 251–262.

14. Romano JM, Turner JA: Chronic pain and depression: does the evidence support a relationship? *Psychol Bull* 97:18–34, 1985.

15. Blumer D, Heilbronn M: Chronic pain as a variant of depressive disease: the pain-prone disorder. *J Nerv Ment Dis* 170:381–406, 1982.

16. Ahles TA, Yunus MB, Masi AJ: Is chronic pain a variant of depressive disease? The case of primary fibromyalgia syndrome. *Pain* 29:105–111, 1987.

17. Haber JD, Roos C: Effects of spouse abuse and/or sexual abuse in the development and maintenance of chronic pain in women. In Fields HL, Dubner R, Cervero F (eds): *Advances in Pain Research and Therapy*. New York, Raven Press, 1985, vol 9, pp 889–895.

18. Colligan RC, Osbourne D, Swenson WM, Offord KP: The ageing MMPI: development of contemporary norms. *Mayo Clin Proc* 59:377–390, 1984.

19. Hsu LM, Betman JA: Minnesota Multiphasic Personality T score conversion tables, 1957–1983. *J Consult Clin Psychol* 54:497–501, 1986.

20. Ahles TA, Yunus MB, Gaulier B, Riley SD, Masi AT: The use of contemporary MMPI norms in the study of chronic pain patients. *Pain* 24:159–163, 1986.

21. Watson D: Neurotic tendencies among chronic pain patients: an MMPI item analysis. *Pain* 14:365–385, 1982.

22. Prokop CK: Hysteria scale elevations in low back pain patients: a risk factor for misdiagnosis? *J Consult Clin Psychol* 54:558–562, 1986.

23. Moore JE, McFall ME, Kivlahan DR, Capestany F: Risk of misinterpretation of MMPI Schizophrenia scale elevations in chronic pain patients. *Pain* 32:207–213, 1988.

24. Ornduff SR, Brennan AF, Barrett CL: The Minnesota Multiphasic Personality Inventory (MMPI) Hysteria (Hy) scale: scoring bodily concern and psychological denial subscales in chronic back pain patients. *J Behav Med* 11:131–146, 1988.

25. Bradley LA, Van der Heide LH: Pain-related correlates of MMPI profile subgroups among back pain patients. *Health Psychol* 3: 157–174, 1984.

26. Armentrout DP, Moore JE, Parker JC, Hewett JE, Feltz C: Pain patient MMPI subgroups: the psychological dimensions of pain. *J Behav Med* 5:201–211, 1982.

27. McCreary C: Empirically derived MMPI profile clusters and characteristics of low back pain patients. *J Consult Clin Psychol* 53:558–560, 1985.

28. McGill J, Lawlis F, Selby D, Mooney V, McCoy CE: The relationship of Minnesota Multiphasic Personality Inventory (MMPI) profile clusters to pain behaviors. *J Behav Med* 6:77–92, 1983.

29. Rosen JC, Grubman JA, Bevins T, Frymoyer JW: Musculoskeletal status and disability of MMPI profile subgroups among patients with low back pain. *Health Psychol* 6:581–598, 1987.

30. Moore JE, Armentrout DP, Parker JC, Kivlahan DR: Empirically derived pain-patient MMPI subgroups: prediction of treatment outcome. *J Behav Med* 9:51–63, 1986.

31. Guck TP, Meilman PW, Skultety M, Poloni LD: Pain-patient Minnesota Multi-phasic Personality Inventory (MMPI) subgroups: evaluation of long-term treatment outcome. *J Behav Med* 11:159–169, 1988.

32. Henrichs TF: MMPI profiles of chronic pain patients: some methodological considerations concerning clusters and descriptors. *J Clin Psychol* 43:650–660, 1987.

33. Bradley LA, Prokop CK, Margolis R, Gentry WD: Multivariate analyses of the MMPI profiles of low back pain patients. *J Behav Med* 1:253–272, 1978.

34. Sines JO: Actuarial methods as appropriate strategy for the validation of diagnostic tests. *Psychol Rev* 71:517–523, 1964.

35. Bradley LA, Anderson, KO, Young LD, McDaniel LK, Turner RA, Agudelo CA, Salinger MC: Psychological aspects of arthritis. *Bull Rheum Dis* 35:1–12, 1985.

36. Smythe HA: Problems with the MMPI (editorial). *J Rheumatol* 11:417–418, 1984.

37. Pilowsky I, Spence ND: Patterns of illness behavior in patients with intractable pain. *J Psychosom Res* 19:279–287, 1975.

38. Millon T, Green CJ, Meagher RB: *Millon Behavioral*

Health Inventory, ed 2. Miami, Clinical Assessment Systems, 1981.

39. Derogates LR, Rickels K, Rock AF: The SCL-90 and the MMPI: a step in the validation of a new self-report scale. *Br J Psychiatry* 128:280–289, 1976.

40. Keefe FJ, Crisson JE, Maltbie A, Bradley L, Gil KM: Illness behavior as a predictor of pain and overt behavior patterns in chronic low back pain patients. *J Psychosom Res* 30:543–551, 1986.

41. Zonderman AB, Heft MW, Costa PT: Does the Illness Behavior Questionnaire measure abnormal illness behavior? *Health Psychol* 4:425–436, 1985.

42. Gatchel RJ, Mayer TG, Capra D, Barnett J, Diamond P: Millon Behavioral Health Inventory: its utility in predicting physical function in patients with low back pain. *Arch Phys Med Rehabil* 67:878–882, 1986.

43. Sweet JJ, Brewer SR, Hazlewood LA, Toye R, Paul RP: The Millon Behavioral Health Inventory: concurrent and predictive validity in a pain treatment center. *J Behav Med* 8:215–226, 985.

44. Duckro PN, Margolis RB, Tait RC: Psychological assessment in chronic pain. *J Clin Psychol* 41:499–504, 1985.

45. Jamison RN, Rock DL, Parris WCV: Empirically derived Symptom Checklist 90 subgroups of chronic pain patients: a cluster analysis. *J Behav Med* 11:147–158, 1988.

46. Reading AE: A comparison of pain rating scales. *J Psychosom Res* 24:119–124, 1979.

47. Gracely RH: Psychophysical assessment of human pain. In Bonica JJ, Liebeskind JC, Albe-Fessard D (eds): *Advances in Pain Research and Therapy.* New York, Raven Press, 1979, vol 3, pp 805–824.

48. Carlsson AM: Assessment of chronic pain. I. Aspects of the reliability and validity of the visual analogue scale. *Pain* 16:87–101, 1983.

49. Kremer E, Atkinson JH, Ignelzi RJ: Measurement of pain: patient preference does not confound pain measurement. *Pain* 10:241–248, 1981.

50. Melzack R: The McGill Pain Questionnaire: major properties and scoring methods. *Pain* 1:277–299, 1975.

51. Bradley LA, Anderson KO, Young LD, Williams T: Psychological testing. In Tollison CD (ed): *Handbook of Chronic Pain Management.* Baltimore, Williams & Wilkins, 1989, pp. 570–591.

52. Rybstein-Blinchik E: Effects of different cognitive strategies on chronic pain experience. *J Behav Med* 2:93–101, 1979.

53. DeBenedittis G, Massei R, Nobili R, Pieri A: The Italian pain questionnaire. *Pain* 33:53–62, 1988.

54. Radvila A, Adler RH, Galeazzi RL, Vorkauf H: The development of a German language (Berne) pain questionnaire and its application in a situation causing acute pain. *Pain* 28:185–195, 1987.

55. Stein C, Mendl G: The German counterpart to McGill Pain Questionnaire. *Pain* 32:251–255, 1988.

56. Vanderiet K, Adriaensen H, Carton H, Vertommer H: The McGill Pain Questionnaire constructed for the Dutch language (MPQ-DV). Preliminary data concerning reliability and validity. *Pain* 30:395–408, 1987.

57. Turk DC, Rudy TE, Salovey P: The McGill Pain Questionnaire reconsidered: confirming the factor structure and examining appropriate uses. *Pain* 21:385–397, 1985.

58. Charter RA, Nehemkis AM: The language of pain intensity and complexity: new methods of scoring the McGill Pain Questionnaire. *Percept Motor Skills* 56:519–537, 1983.

59. Melzack R, Katz J, Jeans ME: The role of compensation in chronic pain: analysis using a new method of scoring the McGill Pain Questionnaire. *Pain* 23:101–112, 1985.

60. Love AW: Attributional style of depressed chronic low back patients. *J Clin Psychol* 44:317–321, 1988.

61. Lefebvre MF: Cognitive distortion and cognitive errors in depressed psychiatric and low back pain patients. *J Consult Clin Psychol* 49:517–525, 1981.

62. Smith TW, Follick MJ, Ahern DK, Adams A: Cognitive distortion and disability in chronic low back pain. *Cogn Ther Res* 10:201–210, 1986.

63. Kessler RC, Price RH, Wortman CB: Social factors in psychopathology: stress, social support, and coping processes. In Rosenzweig MR, Porter LW (eds): *Annual Review of Psychology.* Palo Alto, CA, Annual Reviews, Inc, 1985, vol 36, pp 531–572.

64. Rosenstiel AK, Keefe FJ: The use of coping strategies in chronic low back pain patients: relationship to patient characteristics and current adjustment. *Pain* 17:33–44, 1983.

65. Turner JA, Clancy S: Strategies for coping with chronic low back pain: relationship to pain and disability. *Pain* 24:355–364, 1986.

66. Reesor KA, Craig KD: Medically incongruent chronic back pain: physical limitations, suffering, and ineffective coping. *Pain* 32:35–45, 1988.

67. Brown GK, Nicassio PM: Development of a questionnaire for the assessment of active and passive coping strategies in chronic pain patients. *Pain* 31:53–64, 1987.

68. Lazarus RS, Folkman S: *Stress, Appraisal, and Coping.* New York, Springer-Verlag, 1984.

69. Richter JE, Obrecht WF, Bradley LA, Young LD, Anderson KO: Psychological comparison of patients with nutcracker esophagus and irritable bowel syndrome. *Dig Dis Sci* 31:131–138, 1986.

70. Kremer EF, Block A, Gaylor JS: Behavioral approaches to treatment of chronic pain: the inaccuracy of patient self-report measures. *Arch Phys Med Rehabil* 62:188–191, 1981.

71. Ready LB, Sarkis E, Turner JA; Self-reported vs. actual use of medications in chronic pain patients. *Pain* 12:285–294, 1982.

72. Keefe FJ, Block AR: Development of an observation method for assessing pain behavior in chronic low back pain patients. *Behav Ther* 13:363–375, 1982.

73. Keefe FJ, Wilkins RH, Cook WA: Direct observation

of pain behavior in low back pain patients during physical examination. *Pain* 20:59–68, 1984.

74. Romano JM, Syrjala KL, Levy RL, Turner JA, Evans P, Keefe FJ: Overt pain behaviors: relationship to patient functioning and treatment outcome. *Behav Ther* 19:191–201, 1988.

75. Jensen IB, Bradley LA, Linton SJ: Validation of an observation method of pain assessment in nonchronic back pain. Manuscript submitted for publication, 1988.

76. Linton SJ, Bradley LA, Jensen I, Spangfort E, Sundell L: Secondary prevention of chronic back pain: a controlled study with follow-up. *Pain* 36:197–207, 1989.

77. Keefe FJ, Crisson JE, Trainor M: Observational methods for assessing pain: A practical guide. In Blumenthal JA, McKee DC (eds): *Applications in Behavioral Medicine and Health Psychology: A Clinician's Source Book.* Sarasota, FL, Professional Resource Exchange, 1987, pp 67–94.

78. Follick MJ, Ahern DK, Aberger EW: Development of an audiovisual taxonomy of pain behavior. *Health Psychol* 4:555–568, 1985.

79. Richards JS, Nepomuceno C, Riles M, Suer Z: Assessing pain behavior: the UAB pain behavior scale. *Pain* 14:393–398, 1982.

80. Feuerstein M, Greenwald M, Gamache MP, Papciak AS, Cook ES: The pain behavior scale: modification and validation for outpatient use. *J Psychopathol Behav Assess* 7:301–315, 1985.

81. Sanders SH: Toward a practical instrument system for the automatic measurement of "uptime" in chronic pain patients. *Pain* 9:103–109, 1980.

82. Follick MJ, Ahern DK, Laser-Wolston N, Adams AE, Molloy AJ: Chronic pain: electromechanical recording device for measuring patients' activity patterns. *Arch Phys Med Rehabil* 66:75–79, 1985.

83. Morrell EM, Keefe FJ: The actometer: an evaluation of instrument applicability for chronic pain patients. *Pain* 32:265–270, 1988.

84. White MC, Bradley LA, Prokop CK: Behavioral assessment of chronic pain. In Tryon WW (ed): *Behavioral Assessment in Behavioral Medicine.* New York, Springer-Verlag, 1985, pp. 166–200.

85. Collins FL, Thompson JK: Reliability and standardization in the assessment of self-reported headache pain. *J Behav Assess* 1:73–86, 1979.

86. McNairy SL, Maruta T, Ivnik RJ, Swanson DW, Ilstrup DM: Prescription medication dependence and neuropsychologic function. *Pain* 18:169–177, 1984.

87. Schwartz DP, Barth JT, Dane JR, Drenan SE, DeGood DE, Rowlingson JC: Cognitive deficits in chronic pain patients with and without history of head/neck injury: development of a brief screening battery. *Clin J Pain* 3:94–101, 1987.

88. Bergner M, Bobbitt FA, Carter WB, Gibson BS: The Sickness Impact Profile: development and final revision of a health status measure. *Med Care* 19:787–805, 1981.

89. Follick MJ, Smith TW, Ahern DK: The Sickness Impact Profile: a global measure of disability in chronic low back pain. *Pain* 21:67–76, 1985.

90. Roland M, Morris R: A study of the natural history of back pain: Part I: Development of a reliable and sensitive measure of disability in low-back pain. *Spine* 8:141–144, 1983.

91. Deyo RA: Comparative validity of the Sickness Impact Profile and shorter scales for functional assessment in low-back pain. *Spine* 11:951–954, 1986.

92. Kames LD, Naliboff BD, Heinrich RL, Coscarelli-Schag C: The Chronic Illness Problem Inventory: problem-oriented psychosocial assessment of patients with chronic illness. *Int J Psychiatry Med* 14:65–75, 1984.

93. Kerns RD, Turk DC, Rudy TE: The West Haven-Yale Multidimensional Pain Inventory (WHYMPI). *Pain* 23:345–356, 1985.

94. Flor H, Turk DC, Scholz OB: Impact of chronic pain on the spouse: marital, emotional and physical consequences. *J Psychosom Res* 31:63–71, 1987.

95. Chapman CR, Casey KL, Dubner R, Foley KM, Gracely RH, Reading AE: Pain measurement: an overview. *Pain* 22:1–31, 1985.

96. Ahern DK, Follick MJ, Council JR, Laser-Wolston N: Reliability of lumbar paravertebral EMG assessment in chronic low back pain. *Arch Phys Med Rehabil* 67:762–765, 1986.

97. Biedermann H-J: Comments on the reliability of muscle activity comparisons in EMG biofeedback research with back pain patients. *Biofeedback Self-Regul* 9:451–458, 1984.

98. Cobb CR, deVries HA, Urban RT, Luekens CA, Bagg RJ: Electrical activity in muscle pain. *Am J Phys Med* 54:80–87, 1975.

99. Holmes TH, Wolff HG: Life situations, emotions and backache. *Psychosom Med* 14:18–33, 1952.

100. Cohen MJ, Swanson GA, Naliboff BD, Schandler SL, McArthur DL: Comparison of electromyographic response patterns during posture and stress tasks in chronic low back pain patterns and control. *J Psychosom Med* 30:135–141, 1986.

101. Collins GA, Cohen MJ, Naliboff BD, Schandler EL: Comparative analysis of paraspinal and frontal EMG, heart rate, and skin conductance in chronic low back pain patients and normals to various postures and stress. *Scand J Rehab Med* 14:36–46, 1982.

102. Wolf SL, Basmajian JV, Russ TC, Kutner M: Normative data on low back mobility and activity levels. *Am J Phys Med* 58:217–229, 1979.

103. Wolf SL, Nacht M, Kelly JL: EMG biofeedback training during dynamic movement for low back pain patients. *Behav Ther* 13:395–406, 1982.

104. Cram JR, Steger JC: EMG scanning in the diagnosis of chronic pain. *Biofeedback Self-Regul* 8:229–241, 1983.

105. Nouwen A, Van Akkerveeken PF, Versloot JM: Patterns of muscular activity during movement in pa-

tients with chronic low-back pain. *Spine* 12:777–782, 1987.

106. Jaeger B, Reeves JL: Quantification of changes in myofascial trigger point sensitivity with the pressure algometer following passive stretch. *Pain* 27:203–210, 1986.

107. Simons DG: Myofascial pain syndromes: Where are we? Where are we going? *Arch Phys Med Rehabil* 69:207–212, 1988.

108. Wolfe F: Fibrositis, fibromyalgia, and musculoskeletal disease: the current status of the fibrositis syndrome. *Arch Phys Med Rehabil* 69:527–531, 1988.

109. Fischer AA: Pressure threshold meter: its use for

quantification of tender spots. *Arch Phys Med Rehabil* 67:836–838, 1986.

110. Reeves JL, Jaeger B, Graff-Radford SB: Reliability of the pressure algometer as a measure of myofascial trigger point sensitivity. *Pain* 24:313–321, 1986.

111. Jensen K, Andersen HO, Olesen J, Lindblom U: Pressure-pain threshold in human temporal region: evaluation of a new pressure algometer. *Pain* 25:313–323, 1986.

112. Schiffman E, Fricton J, Haley D, Tylka D: Pressure algometer for myofascial pain syndrome: reliability and validity. *Pain*, Suppl 4:S291, 1987.

Section 2
NEURAL BLOCKAGE AND NEEDLE THERAPIES

Chapter 5

DIAGNOSTIC NERVE BLOCKS

THERESA FERRER-BRECHNER, MD

Since the early 1900s, nerve blocking procedures have been used to treat patients with acute and chronic pain (1). With the advent of multidisciplinary approaches to the management of pain, including neurosurgical techniques, physical medicine, behavioral intervention, new drugs, and stimulation-induced analgesia, the appropriate role of nerve-blocking procedures for chronic pain needs to be better defined in terms of the indications and limitations of the various procedures. Anesthesiologists who limit their practice to nerve-blocking procedures for treating chronic pain immediately realize that, in certain groups of patients, local anesthetic blocking of peripheral nociceptive afferent pathways does not consistently produce pain relief and may sometimes even aggravate the pain. Recent laboratory and clinical studies have provided new information that sheds light onto the mechanisms, clinical usefulness, and application of nerve-blocking procedures (2–4).

The purpose of this chapter is to provide information on the appropriate use of diagnostic nerve block for low back pain and to define the role of such blocks in the armamentarium of comprehensive evaluative tools used to diagnose causes of acute and chronic low back pain.

BASIC MECHANISMS

To understand how diagnostic nerve blocks can block perception of low back pain, it is important to clarify the following issues:

1. What are the possible causes of peripheral nociception in the low back area?
2. What are the nonperipheral nociceptive causes of low back pain?

Causes of low back pain and radiculopathy can be complex (5). Pain could arise from trigger points in myofascial areas, from facet joints, from neural compression due to disk protrusion, from sympathetic hyperreflexia as a response to injury or bony lesions, or from a combination of these (Table 5.1). Use of diagnostic blocks can often be helpful in determining the predominant cause contributing to low back pain, especially in the chronic pain patient, in whom stress, anxiety, depression, and hysteria may modify pain experience changes with neural blocking. In 3–15% of patients with low back pain no alteration in pain report occurs even with complete sensory and motor block above the area of pain complaint (6, 7). It behooves us to utilize diagnostic blocks to rule out centrally mediated pain, since further peripheral treatments at the site of pain complaint will not be successful in relieving the patient's pain. It is also important to realize that the cause of low back pain may be multiple. For example, a patient with somatic nerve compression from a protruded disk can have a reactive myofascial pain syndrome as well as a sympathetic hyperreflexia reactionary to the somatic nerve impingement. A differential block could determine which type of pain syndrome is contributory to the total pain report.

Diagnostic nerve-blocking procedures with local anesthetic are based on the temporary interruption of specific nociceptive nerves, sympathetic nerves, and somatomotor nerves. Block of specific nociceptive or sensory fibers will relieve pain by interrupting the reflex arc of sympathetic hyperreflexia and motor fibers and establishing the dermatomal distribution of the noxious input (8). Sympathetic block will decrease the reflex vasoconstriction, and sudomotor and visceromotor hyperactivity that often contribute to the total nociceptive input. Block of

Table 5.1
Causes of Low Back Pain

    I. Myofascial pain
        A. Quadratus lumborum
        B. Iliocostalis lumborum
        C. Deep multifidi and rotatores
        D. Piriformis
        E. Gluteus maximus and medius
   II. Pain from nerve root irritation or damage
        A. Individual root involvement
        B. Multisegmented root syndromes
            1. Spondyloses
            2. Arachnoidites
            3. Taber dorsales
            4. Meningeal carcinomatoses
  III. Sympathetic mediated pain
        A. Causalgia
        B. Deafferentation pain
   IV. Centrally mediated pain

sudomotor nerves will eliminate reactive muscle spasms that can arise from musculoskeletal disorders.

To understand how diagnostic nerve block can differentiate nociceptive input from somatosensory, sympathetic, or motor nerve input, it is important to review the various sizes of these fibers and how various concentrations of anesthetic can selectively block these conducting fibers (Table 5.2).

The classic concept of differential nerve block arose from Gasser and Erlanger's work in the 1920s (9). Studying fiber representation of intact nerves by scanning the compound action potentials for blips from axons conducting impulses at different speeds, they categorized nerves into three main classes: myelinated somatic axon A fibers, myelinated autonomic axon B fibers, and myelinated C fibers. Although the classification was primarily based on electrophysiologic characteristics, other properties, such as pharmacologic response to local anesthetic, also showed a differential response. For example, conduction in nonmyelinated C fibers was more vulnerable to blockade with lower concentrations of local anesthetic than that in small-diameter A-delta fibers. This property was used to develop the differential spinal block to relieve pain of autonomic origin without affecting sensory or motor function (10–12).

Therefore, by selectively or nonselectively blocking the afferent pathway one can temporarily interrupt the reflex sympathetic and somatomotor pathways, producing prompt relief of pain in most individuals that sometimes outlasts the duration of the local anesthetics. It has been theorized that sensory block for several hours results in the cessation of self-sustaining activity of the neuron pools in the neuraxis, which could be responsible for some chronic pain states (13).

INDICATIONS

Diagnostic blocks can be one of the useful tools for the evaluation of low back pain, especially when the condition has become chronic. When pain becomes chronic, patients develop an inevitable change

Table 5.2
Sensitivity of Various Conducting Fibers to Local Anesthetic

GROUP	SUBGROUP	DIAMETER	CONDUCTION VELOCITY	FUNCTION	SENSITIVITY TO LOCAL ANESTHETIC SPINAL (PROCAINE)	EPIDURAL (LIDOCAINE)
A (myelinated)	Alpha	20 μ	100 mps	Large motor, proprioception	1%	2%
	Beta			Small motor, touch & pressure		
	Gamma			Muscle tone		
	Delta	4 μ	5 mps	Temperature, touch, pain?	0.5%	1%
B (myelinated)		3 μ	3–4 mps	Preganglionic autonomic fibers	0.25%	0.5%
C (unmyelinated)		0.5–1 μ	1.2 mps	Dull pain, temperature, touch (similar to delta but slower)	0.5%	1%

Table 5.3
Evaluation of Chronic Low Back Pain

PHYSICAL DIMENSION	AFFECTIVE DIMENSION

1. Pathophysiology of pain
   a. review x-rays; repeat if necessary
   b. thorough neurologic exam
   c. myofascial pain evaluation
2. Differential nerve blocking procedures
   a. nociceptive vs. deafferentation
   b. sympathetic mediated
   c. musculoskeletal
	1. Observe behavior with:
	   a. medications
	   b. stress
	   c. interaction with physicians and family
	2. Functionality
	   a. diaries
	   b. physical therapy evaluation
	3. Degree of depression and anxiety
	4. Psychometric testing
	   a. MMPI
	   b. Beck Depression Inventory

in their personality profile as tested by the Minnesota Multiphasic Personality Inventory (MMPI), an objective psychodiagnostic test. Elevations in the scales of hysteria, depression, and hypochondriasis in a "Conversion V" or "Neurotic Triad" has been demonstrated to be present in chronic low back pain patients in comparison to acute low back pain patients (14, 15). The presence of this triad implies that there are strong operant issues that may influence pain experience, such as medication use, spousal attention, and socioeconomic altercation with the system (i.e., workers' compensation, ongoing legal action, etc.). Therefore, the evaluation of chronic low back pain should not only include a thorough physical evaluation, but also an evaluation of the affective or emotional dimension of the pain experience (Table 5.3) (7).

Before the decision is made to utilize diagnostic blocks for low back pain, it is important to ask ourselves whether performing such procedures could lead to better understanding of the pathophysiology of the pain experience and future directions in therapy. If the result of the diagnostic block is not pivotal in diagnosis or will not influence the direction of therapy, the diagnostic block should not be performed. The therapeutic implications of diagnostic nerve blocking for low back pain are exemplified by the questions than can often be answered by performing a diagnostic nerve block:

1. Is pain centrally or peripherally generated?
2. Is the patient a placebo responder?
3. Is pain predominantly mediated by sympathetic, somatic, or somatomotor nerves?
4. Is the patient's behavior appropriate to the pain relief obtained with the diagnostic block?
5. Are the side effects of the temporary block acceptable to the patient?

Properly applied, diagnostic nerve blocks for low back pain can help ascertain the predominant and contributory pain pathways, identify the dermatomal source and distribution of pain complaint, aid in defining the mechanism of chronic pain states, and prognosticate the effect of planned neuroablative procedures.

MAXIMIZING OPTIMAL RESULTS

For diagnostic nerve blocking to be valid, careful evaluation of pain severity, pain experience, preexisting sensory, sympathetic and motor dysfunctions, and pain-provoking moments should be made before performing the procedure, and periodically afterward. Before conclusions are made regarding the effect of the block on the patient's pain experience, one must demonstrate, without question, that the intended block has been successful. For example, if an autonomic block is done, increase in temperature and/or decrease in psychogalvanic response in the region of pain complaint must be demonstrated first before performing the postprocedure measures on pain level and functionality. The same is true with somatic nerve blocks. Demonstration of decreased pinprick response in the area of pain must be demonstrated before the patient's response is evaluated. An example of a form used for evaluating the patient's response to a diagnostic block is seen in Table 5.4. These tests should be performed consistently before each injection and after the intended block is effective.

In approaching a low back pain patient for diagnostic nerve block procedure, it is important to educate the patient and his/her significant other in what is involved with the procedure, where the needle is inserted, the possible complications of the

Table 5.4
Diagnostic Nerve Block Assessment

NEUROLOGIC EXAM	PREBLOCK	POSTBLOCK (NOTE TIME)
Autonomic function		
Temperature	_____	_____
Psychogalvanic response	_____	_____
Sensory deficit	_____	_____
Motor deficits	_____	_____
Hyperesthesias	_____	_____
Trigger points	_____	_____
Pain provokers (+ or −)	_____	_____
Position	_____	_____
Palpation	_____	_____
Active movement	_____	_____
Passive movement	_____	_____
Others	_____	_____
Pain visual analog scale (in cm)	_____	_____
Pain bothersomeness (in cm)	_____	_____

procedure in the hands of the physician doing the procedure, and that the block is only temporary. Sometimes the patient unrealistically expects the diagnostic block to be the final solution to the pain problem. It is important to emphasize that the block will only lead to a possible diagnosis and/or direct the physician to a proper path of therapy. A written consent describing the procedures and potential side effects is mandatory.

For at least 2 days before the block, the patient should fill out a daily diary indicating pain scales, activity, and medications taken on a hour-to-hour basis. The same diary should be continued up to 2 days after the block to indicate the duration of pain relief, changes in medication intake, and activity.

If a patient has overwhelming anxiety related to undergoing a nerve block procedure, it might be helpful to have him/her undergo a "desensitization" process by a psychologist prior to performance of the block. This would involve two or three visits with the psychologist for relaxation therapy and repetitive education regarding the procedure. If a patient has overwhelming depression as part of the chronic pain syndrome, it is important to lift the depression by antidepressant therapy for 2 or 3 weeks prior to the nerve block, since depressed patients are known to have poor pain level discrimination (16).

ALGORITHM FOR DIFFERENTIAL BLOCKING

When a patient presents with low back pain and a differential blocking procedure is decided upon,

a frequent source of confusion is what procedure to perform first. There are two possible routes to take. One route is to perform separate blocks of various possible nociceptive pathways on different occasions, allowing evaluation of each specific nerve block for hours or days. The other route is to perform the entire differential block on one occasion, i.e., with differential epidural or spinal block.

An example of a decision tree for differential blocking procedures done on separate occasions is seen in Figure 5.1. The idea is to eliminate the various possible causes of low back pain, starting from the more obvious and proceeding to the more complicated.

TRIGGER POINT INJECTIONS

The first simple but overlooked cause of low back pain is myofascial pain syndrome. In back pain, one has to rule out a myofascial component contributory to the total pain experience. Common muscles involved in back pain are the quadratus lumborum, paraspinal, iliopsoas and piriformis muscles. Trigger points in these muscles can produce referred pain in the back and lower extremities (17). It is important to palpate these muscles carefully and, if trigger points are identified that reproduce the pain complaint, a small amount of local anesthetic (usually procaine 1%, 2–3 ml) can be injected. If pain is totally eliminated, then a myofascial program consisting of spray and stretch of the muscles involved can be planned for the patient (18). An hourly diary is then given to the patient to monitor

ALGORITHM FOR DIFFERENTIAL BLOCKING FOR BACK PAIN

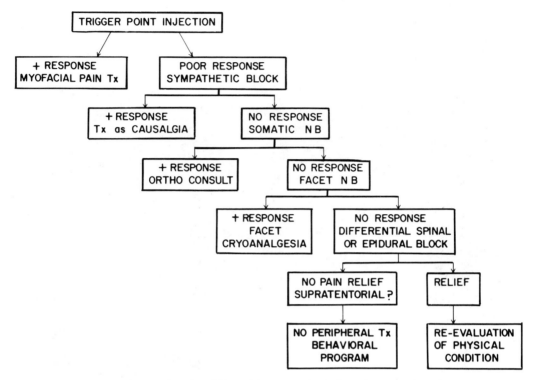

Figure 5.1. Suggested algorithm for differential nerve blocking for low back pain done on separate occasions. Cascade moves from least to most complicated, and low- to high-risk nerve blocks.

the pain level, function, and medication intake for at least 24 hours.

LUMBAR SYMPATHETIC NERVE BLOCK

If the myofascial trigger point injection does not provide pain relief, then blockade of the lumbar sympathetic nerves is indicated. In addition to pain level, measurement of temperature and/or psychogalvanic response of the area of pain complaint is a baseline measure prior to the block (19). The lumbar sympathetic chain is approached paravertebrally at the level of L2–3. The needle is inserted 6–8 cm lateral to the middle of the spinous process and pushed in slowly until it hits the vertebral body (20). It is then redirected until it lies anterolateral to the vertebral body. Ten to 20 ml of dilute local anesthetic (0.25% bupivicaine or 0.5% lidocaine) is injected after negative aspiration. Only when there is evidence of sympathetic block, such as an increase in temperature of at least 2–3°C and/or

suppression of the psychogalvanic response, should the patient's pain level be measured again. If sympathetic block relieves the patient's pain totally, then a series of sympathetic blocks can be included with the pain management.

SOMATIC NERVE BLOCK

If both myofascial and sympathetic blocks do not produce pain relief, then somatic nerve blocks can be performed under fluoroscopy. Symptomatology and review of x-rays can pinpoint which somatic nerve to block first. Blockade of the paravertebral somatic nerve has to be done under fluoroscopy since error of needle placement, in terms of level and depth, without fluoroscopic guidance is as high as 40% (21). An anteroposterior and lateral view of correct needle placement is demonstrated in Figure 5.2.

The amount of local anesthetic need not exceed 1–2 ml (usually 1% lidocaine or 0.5% bupivicaine), since larger volumes may produce a multiple par-

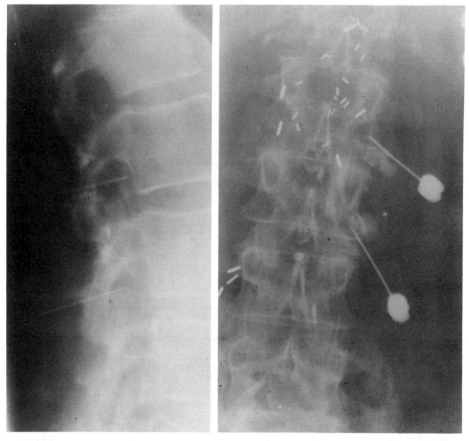

Figure 5.2 Fluoroscopic view of paravertebral somatic nerve block. Lateral view (*right*) shows needle in paravertebral foramina.

avertebral somatic nerve block and, therefore, will not isolate the nerve roots involved. After the block is completed, demonstration of decreased pinprick sensation along the distribution of the blocked somatic nerve is necessary before evaluating whether or not pain relief has occurred.

FACET NERVE BLOCK

If the above blocks do not produce pain relief, it might be worthwhile to explore the possibility of facet joint involvement by performing a block of the articular nerve of Luschka. Degenerative hypertrophy of lumbar facet joints can result in decreased size of the lateral bony nerve root canal, especially after laminectomy (22). Anatomy of the articular nerve of Luschka has been described previously (23).

Patients with characteristic facet joint involvement (pain radiating to the buttocks in a sciatic distribution but not extending distally to the knee) are ideal candidates for a diagnostic block of the facet joint (24). The patient is placed in a prone position with a pillow under the iliac crest. The tips of the spinous process are identified, and a line drawn horizontally through them (Fig. 5.3). The points mark the initial entry of the needle through the skin. The needle is inserted at an angle perpendicular to the skin. As soon as bony structure is encountered, fluoroscopy is used to confirm the needle location and the needle is repositioned to conform with the course of the facet nerve as described by Fox and Rizzoli (24). The diagnostic block is done in two stages, once with a short-acting local anesthetic such as chlorprocaine, and the other with a long-acting local anesthetic such as bupivicaine. If pain relief of at least 75% occurs

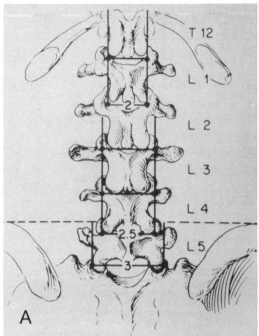
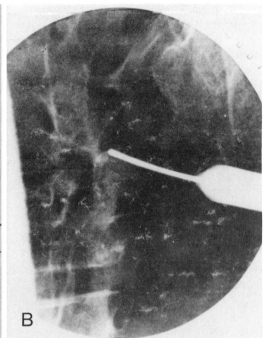

Figure 5.3. *A,* Demonstration of external landmarks for approaching articular facet nerves. *B,* Indicates location of cryoprobe tip on anteroposterior view.

with each block, then the patient can be considered for cryogenic neurolysis of the nerve of Luschka (25).

DIFFERENTIAL SPINAL OR EPIDURAL BLOCK

If the above blocks fail to produce pain relief, the occurrence of central pain needs to be ruled out. An attempt to block all sensory input generated by the source of nociception in the low back can be done by producing sensory block above the area of pain complaint. This is particularly important if there is a question of the appropriateness of further surgical procedures to relieve persistent pain. Graduated spinal block was classically done by injection of four increasing doses of procaine, administered at 10-min intervals: 0% (saline) to serve as placebo, 0.25% isobaric procaine to block the sympathetics without blocking the sensory nerves, 0.5% procaine to block sensory nerves, and 1% procaine for blocking all modalities including motor nerves (see Table 5.5). It must be emphasized that interpretation of differential spinal or epidural block may be affected by several variables, such as technical, neurophysiologic, and psychophysiologic problems (26). Technical problems include improper needle placement, resulting in uneven spread of local anesthetic, a situation that can arise in the presence of arachnoiditis or a space-occupying mass preventing the even spread of solution in the intradural or epidural space. To interpret the results of each injection, a thorough baseline neurologic exam is necessary to document any preexisting sensory deficits, hyperesthesias, trigger points in the muscles, and temperature differences and movements that provoke pain. After injection of each solution, repeat measures should be taken until pain relief occurs. At that time, the procedure can be terminated, and the patient given a pain diary to monitor duration of pain relief.

Differential epidural block is done with insertion of an epidural catheter close to the dermatomal distribution of pain. After insertion of the catheter, the following solutions are injected: saline, 0.25% lidocaine to block sympathetic nerves, 0.5% lidocaine to produce a dermatomal sensory block without motor block, 1% lidocaine for a more complete sensory block, and 1.5% lidocaine for complete sensory and motor block (Table 5.6). Sometimes it is difficult to separate sympathetic and sensory

Table 5.5
Differential Spinal Block

SOLUTION	NERVE FIBERS BLOCKED	PAIN RELIEF	THERAPEUTIC IMPLICATIONS
Saline	None	Placebo response	Maximize noninvasive techniques
0.25% procaine	Thin, myelinated B fibers Unmyelinated C fibers	Sympathetic-mediated pain	Techniques to decrease sympathetic activity, sympathetic block, TENS, biofeedback, and other relaxation techniques
0.5% procaine	Pain fibers: larger C fibers and A-delta fibers	Somatic-sensory–mediated pain (sympathetic may not be separated from somatic-sensory nerve block)	Rule out narrowing of intervertebral foramina from any cause, and arachnoiditis. If accompanied by radiculopathy, possible epidural steroids
1.0% procaine	A-alpha and A-beta fibers	Sensory and motor–mediated pain	Same as above. If no relief, rule out centrally mediated pain, organic brain syndrome by neuropsychiatric testing

block with the 0.5% concentrations of lidocaine epidurally. If separation is important, a lumbar sympathetic block can be performed separately on another day.

CASE ILLUSTRATIONS

Case A: No Pain Relief with Total Neural Interruption

A 45-year-old male construction worker sustained a head injury when a cement block fell on his head. A subdural hematoma was evacuated and the patient required neurologic rehabilitation. Three months after the injury, the patient developed lower back and extremity pains accompanied by "spasms" of the muscles in the lower extremity. Extensive workup, including myelogram, computed tomography (CT) scans, and magnetic resonance imaging (MRI) scans, did not reveal any pathology in the low back spine area. Upon entry to the clinic, a differential epidural block failed to relieve pain despite a demonstrated sensory block to the T4 level (Fig. 5.4). The MMPI demonstrated several elevated scales, indicating either severe psychopathology or organic brain syndrome. Neuropsychiatric testing confirmed the presence of organic brain syndrome, and the patient was successfully treated with amitriptyline and Tegretol, a regimen recommended for central pain.

A complete sensory and motor block above the area of perceived nociception can fail to produce pain relief in 3–15% of patients with low back pain. These patients should be carefully assessed for organic brain syndrome with neuropsychiatric cognitive testing to rule out unrecognized central lesions causing peripheral pain manifestation.

Case B: Pain Relief with Low Concentrations of Local Anesthetic

A 28-year-old white male was referred to the pain clinic because of sacral and perirectal pain. Extensive

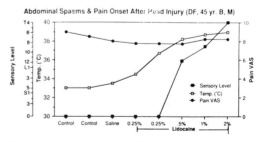

Figure 5.4. Result of differential epidural block in 45-year-old man with history of head injury, indicating no relief of pain despite sympathetic block and complete sensory block to T4 level.

Table 5.6
Differential Epidural Block

SOLUTION	NERVE FIBERS BLOCKED	PHYSICAL FINDINGS	PAIN RELIEF MEANS
Saline	None	No change	Placebo response
0.25% lidocaine	Thin, myelinated fibers Unmyelinated C fibers	Sympathetic block (increased temperature, decreased psychogalvanic response)	Sympathetic-mediated pain
0.5% lidocaine	Pain fibers: larger C fibers and A-delta	Sensory loss (increased response to pinprick)	Somatic-sensory–mediated pain
1% lidocaine	Larger C fibers and A-delta	Deceased response to pinprick	Somatic-sensory–mediated pain
1.5% lidocaine	A-alpha and A-beta fibers	Sensory and motor loss	If no relief with block above area of pain, rule out central-mediated pain

workup 6 months prior to referral, including a lower gastrointestinal tract series, CT scan, and MRI scan, failed to reveal any obvious somatic causes for the pain complaint. Differential epidural block resulted in complete pain relief with a low concentration of lidocaine that produced sympathetic block without sensory loss (Fig. 5.5). MMPI testing showed a normal profile. A repeat CT scan revealed a mass around the perirectal area that eventually was biopsied and found to be a benign tumor.

Pain relief with low concentrations of local anesthetic could indicate a visceral source of pain, since small visceral nerves are easily blocked by low concentrations of local anesthetics. Coupled with a normal MMPI, one has to rule out a missed source

of strong nociceptive input. In this case, the first CT scan failed to reveal the perirectal mass.

Case C: Pain Relief with Sensory Block

A 32-year-old white female was referred to the pain clinic because of a 3-year history of low back pain after an L5–S1 laminectomy. Repeat x-ray procedure revealed no pathology at the L5–S1 level. A differential epidural block revealed pain relief only when sensory block was extended to the L1–2 level (Fig. 5.6). The MMPI revealed scales of hysteria, depression, and hypochondriasis in an operant profile pattern, common in patients with chronic pain. A repeat MRI scan revealed a borderline disk protrusion at the L2–3 level. Pain relief was obtained after three epidural steroid injections.

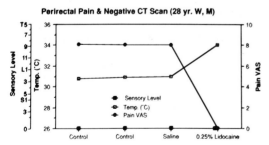

Figure 5.5. Result of differential epidural block indicating complete pain relief with low concentration of lidocaine. Pain relief with sympathetic block but without sensory loss indicated a possible visceral pathway.

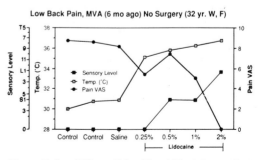

Figure 5.6. Differential epidural block in a patient with a history of L5–S1 laminectomy. Only when sensory block to the L1–2 level was reached did pain relief occur.

Pain after laminectomy can be misinterpreted as being caused by nociceptive input coming from the same level as the previous surgical intervention. Differential epidural block can be pivotal in establishing the level of involvement, which can be different from that of the original lesion.

SUMMARY

Differential nerve blocking for low back pain can be a useful diagnostic tool to establish the source of nociceptive input. Its proper interpretation is dependent upon meticulous technique and astute observation of behavioral and physiologic parameters before and after the performance of the blocks. Its concurrent use with behavioral observations and psychometric tests can maximize competent evaluation and management of acute and chronic low back pain.

REFERENCES

1. Jonica JJ: *The Management of Pain*. Philadelphia, Lea & Febiger, 1953.
2. Gissen AJ, Covino BG, Gregus J: Differential sensitivities of mammalian nerve fibers to local anesthetic agents. *Anesthesiology* 53:467–474, 1980.
3. de Jong RH: Differential nerve block by local anesthetics. *Anesthesiology* 53:443–444, 1980.
4. Ghia JN, Duncan GH, Teeple E: Differential spinal block for diagnosis of chronic pain. *Comp Ther* 8(4):55–61, 1982.
5. Frymoyer JW: Back pain and sciatica. *N Engl J Med* 318:291–300, 1988.
6. Ghia JN, Toomy TC, Mao W, et al: Towards an understanding of chronic pain mechanisms: the use of psychologic tests and a refined differential spinal block. *Anesthesiology* 50:20–25, 1979.
7. Ghia JN, Duncan G, Toomey TC, et al: The pharmacologic approach in differential diagnosis of chronic pain. *Spine* 4:447–451, 1979.
8. Levy B: Diagnostic, prognostic and therapeutic nerve blocks. Arch Surg 112:870–879, 1977.
9. Gasser HS, Erlanger J: The role of fiber size in the establishment of a nerve block by pressure or cocaine. Am J Physiol 88:581–591, 1929.
10. Sarnoff SJ, Arrowood JG: Differential spinal block. *Surgery* 20:150–159, 1946.
11. McCollum DE, Stephen CR: The use of graduated spinal anesthesia in the differential diagnosis of pain of the back and lower extremities. South Med J 57:410–416, 1964.
12. Winnie AP, Collins VJ: The pain clinic. I. Differential neural blockade in pain syndrome of questionable etiology. *Med Clin North Am* 52 (1):123–129, 1968.
13. Melzack R: Phantom limb pain: implications for treatment of pathologic pain. *Anesthesiology* 35:409–419, 1971.
14. Beals RK, Hickman NW: Industrial injuries of the back and extremities. J Bone Joint Surg [Am] 54:1593, 1972.
15. Sternback RA, Wolf SR, Murphy RW, et al: Traits of pain patients: the low back pain "loser". *Psychosomatics* 14:226, 1973.
16. Haley WE, Turner JA, Romano JM: Depression in chronic pain patients: relation to pain activity and sex differences. *Pain* 23:337–343, 1985.
17. Travell J, Rinzler SH: The myofascial genesis of pain. Postgrad Med 11:425–435, 1952.
18. Travell J, Simon DG: *Myofascial Pain and Dysfunction: The Trigger Point Manual*. Baltimore, Williams & Wilkins, 1983.
19. Graff-Radford SB: Myofascial pain: an overview. *Semin Anesthesia* 4(4):281–286, 1985
20. Lewis LW: Evaluation of sympathetic activity following chemical or surgical sympathectomy. Anesth Analg (Cleve) 34:334–337, 1955.
21. Eriksson I: *Illustrated Handbook in Local Anesthesia*. Copenhagen, Munksgaard, 1969.
22. Ferrer-Brechner T, Brechner VL: Accuracy of needle placement during diagnostic and therapeutic nerve blocks. In Bonica JJ, Albe-Fessard D (eds): *Advances in Pain Research and Therapy*. New York, Raven Press, 1976, vol 1.
23. Mooney J, Robertson JR: The facet syndrome. Clin Orthop 115:149–156, 1976.
24. Fox JR, Rizolli HV: Identification of the radiologic coordinates for the posterior articular nerve of Luschka in the lumbar spine. Surg Neurol 1:343–346, 1973.
25. Shealy CM: Percutaneous radiofrequency denervation of spinal facets. J Neurosurg 43:448–451, 1975.
26. Brechner T: Percutaneous cryogenic neurolysis of the articular nerve of Luschka. Reg Anesth 6:18–22, 1981.

Chapter 6

APPROPRIATE USE OF THERAPEUTIC NERVE BLOCKS

JOHN C. ROWLINGSON, MD

Low back pain is one of the top five presenting symptoms of hospitalized patients and second in frequency only to headaches as a chronic pain problem. Perhaps more significant, because of the socioeconomic impact, is the fact that low back pain is second only to the common cold as a cause of disability from work for workers in the United States under age 55 (1–3). Indeed, because low back pain is so common, one wonders what is wrong with those who don't have it! This prevalent and costly disease demands effective therapy to minimize not only the human suffering and disability related to it, but also the immense expense in terms of workdays lost, medical workup and treatment costs, and diagnostic tests (1).

The effective management of low back pain that does not spontaneously remit is likely only after the patient has been thoroughly evaluated and a proper diagnosis made. Patients with symptoms of short duration should expect treatment to eliminate the pain and allow a rapid return to full function. Patients with complaints that are chronic in nature still must direct their effort to regaining function, but also must accept the lack of satisfaction associated with only a partial reduction in their level of pain. The patients will likely benefit by cooperating with the therapy prescribed. However, contemporary pain management demands an active patient even though compliance is notoriously higher the more passive is the treatment. Nerve blocks offer the advantage that the patient is not responsible for their administration other than to give consent for the procedure. Patient responsibility is demanded, however, in that a therapeutic nerve block alone is unlikely to be the answer to all of the patient's intercurrent problems with pain. This

chapter clarifies the role of nerve blocks in the management of low back pain.

NERVE BLOCKS

In 1983 Spielman and Ghia (4) published data showing that in at least 90% of pain training programs, nerve blocks topped the list of modalities available to patients. That many pain facilities early on were run by anesthesiologists may have influenced this choice. Khoury and Varga (5) have recently shown that the specialty of the director does influence the treatment options used. Knowing that the injection of local anesthetics can yield prompt, temporary relief, it is not unreasonable to contemplate injection therapy for the management of low back pain. However, the temporary nature of most injections is a drawback and this must be considered. A more realistic concept, then, is to regard nerve blocks as but one component of a treatment program and not overemphasize any one option to the exclusion of the others. Each treatment modality being applied to the patient with low back pain is expected to have a therapeutic effect, with the overall result being greater than the simple sum of the parts. Contemporary management of low back pain urges us to treat the whole person, not just the spine (6).

The advantages of using nerve blocks in the management of low back pain are many (Table 6.1). In patients whose problems with low back pain are acute in nature, a nerve block may assume a greater role because the dramatic decrease in the pain quickly gets the patient on the road to recovery. The primary aim of treatment in acute pain prob-

Table 6.1

Advantages of Nerve Blocks in Low Back Pain Management

1. They involve patient interaction—an explanation of the diagnosis and the rationale for the proposed nerve block MUST precede the performance of the block. Usually a physical examination is desirable, too.
2. There are fewer risks and potential side effects than with surgery, and nerve blocks do not require a long convalescence period. Thus, the patient can return to normal function faster.
3. They can be performed on an outpatient basis.
4. They can be repeated judiciously and are not addicting.
5. The decrease in pain, even though temporary (1–4 weeks), allows:
   a. the use of fewer and/or less potent medications
   b. pain relief without central nervous system depression
   c. reduced reflex muscle spasm
   d. improved patient attitude about recovery and ability to function
   e. (perhaps) improved compliance with physical rehabilitation.

Table 6.2

Disadvantages and Possible Complications of Nerve Blocks

1. Nerve blocks ARE invasive and there ARE risks from:
   a. the needle—infection, bleeding, ligamentous/muscle trauma causing more backache, subarachnoid membrane puncture causing "spinal" headache, injury to nerve roots causing more pain, weakness or numbness
   b. the drugs injected—*local anesthetics* can cause allergic reaction, spinal anesthesia, hypotension, local anesthetic toxicity; *steroids* can cause allergic reaction, water retention, weight gain
   c. other—transient relief, increased pain, vasovagal reaction, fainting.
2. In some patients with low back pain, nerve blocks may not be appropriate. Such patients would include those with systemic infection or infection at the site of needle insertion, on major anticoagulants, following multiple back operations or trauma, and following radiation therapy.
3. A practitioner with the experience to provide the nerve block therapy may not be available to the patient and his/her doctor.
4. The physiologic trespass may not be well tolerated by the patient.

lems is to *eliminate* the pain and rapidly restore the patient to full function. In patients with chronic pain problems, the goals of treatment are necessarily different. Nerve blocks in these patients take on a more precise role and may only return the patient to his/her baseline level of chronic pain after a flare-up has occurred. Patients with chronic pain may gain more relief than this, but all involved with the patient's care must acknowledge the following objectives of treatment:

1. To decrease the frequency and intensity of the pain as much as possible, but without any further decrease in the patient's functional level.
2. To minimize the need for potent analgesic medications and perhaps to make detoxification to milder analgesic drugs feasible.
3. To prevent decisions about surgical intervention for chronic pain control being made out of desperation at the ongoing agony of the pain rather than based on sound medical judgment.
4. To create a patient who is more receptive to *all* of the contemporary management modalities (e.g., neural stimulation, physical rehabilitation, socioeconomic restoration) that will help him/her COPE with the chronic pain.
5. To provide the patient insight into the complex nature of his/her "pain" and help him/her understand the interplay between organic gen-

erators of pain and the innumerable nonphysical modifiers thereof.

Nerve blocks can maximize the conservative therapy approach to patients with low back pain. Because nerve blocks are invasive procedures and require a certain expertise, an anesthesiologist will frequently be consulted. He/she will have to evaluate the patient prior to such treatment and then perform the procedure if it is deemed to be appropriate *at* that time and *for* that patient. Table 6.2 lists the disadvantages and possible complications of the common nerve blocks that are used in patients with low back pain. Anesthesiologists are experienced with the regional anesthesia techniques and the drugs used. They are equipped to handle any untoward reactions that may occur. Their evaluation can be invaluable in helping the referring doctor and the patient decide if the nerve block is reasonable. If so, performing the therapeutic procedure in a safe, efficient environment can only increase the likelihood of its success, at the lowest risk to the patient.

THE APPROPRIATE PATIENT

The appropriate use of nerve blocks is more likely to occur when the patient has been carefully selected, as is the case when an established evaluation protocol has been followed. At the very least, the anesthesiologist must determine that none of the major contraindications to regional anesthesia (the patient is anticoagulated, has a cutaneous infection at the site of needle insertion, has blood-borne infection or chronic infection of the spine, or refuses the procedure, or there is a lack of resuscitation equipment) are present.

Less clear cut will be the use of nerve blocks in patients with relative contraindications to the application of regional anesthesia techniques. Patients with spinal deformities, the very young or very old patient, patients with any degree of impaired decision-making capacity, patients with uncorrected hypovolemia (as in "sick" patients with metastatic cancer), and even patients with active neurologic disease would fall into this category. As one comes to understand patients with chronic pain more thoroughly, to this list one would add those patients who inflexibly believe that only surgery will restore them to a pain-free state, have monetary gain through the legal system as their dominant ambition in life, or are found to have psychological problems predominant in the causation of their pain complaints. Clearly not every patient we could technically block is a candidate for such therapy! Patients on non-steroidal anti-inflammatory drugs (NSAIDs) are not necessarily to be excluded from receiving blocks. Aspirin blocks platelet cyclo-oxygenase for the duration of the platelet's existence, but other drugs in the NSAID class have a shorter effect.

It is fundamental that a diagnosis be established after the patient with low back pain has been properly evaluated. This step may be achieved prior to the referral of the patient; or the anesthesiologist, working in collaboration with pain colleagues, may contribute in the evaluation process. Because pain has recently been defined as "an unpleasant sensory and emotional experience associated with actual or potential tissue damage or described in terms of such damage" (7), one must acknowledge that we cannot divorce the perception of pain from the reaction to it. Thus, it is vital that the physical reasons for low back pain plus the patient's presentation of the complaints be carefully analyzed.

The differential diagnosis of low back pain is vast (Table 6.3). Only in some of these conditions would nerve blocks be safe, useful, and effective. Thus, part of the purpose of evaluating the patient is to determine if a nerve block is reasonable, and, if so, whether now is the appropriate time to provide it for the patient (8). The historical account by the patient of his/her pain, treatment, and medical

Table 6.3
Potential Causes of Low Back Pain

Congenital disorders
Tumors—benign and malignant
Trauma—strains, sprains, fractures
Heavy metal toxicity
Metabolic disorders
Inflammatory diseases
Degenerative diseases
Infections
Circulatory disorders
Mechanical problems
Psychological problems
Referred pain—gastrointestinal, genitourinary

history will provide some clues as to the possible etiologies of the pain and its consequences in the patient's life (i.e., work stoppage, marital discord, financial burden, etc.). Abram et al. (9) identified some features in the patient's history of low back pain that influenced the response to nerve blocks. Patients who were injured at work and out of work secondary to pain; those receiving compensation, involved with legal action, using analgesics frequently, or using tranquilizers; and those with past surgery for pain, pain of long duration, or high pain severity ratings were less likely to respond favorably to nerve block therapy. Thus, a careful history is very helpful in establishing the patient as appropriate for nerve block therapy. These items are not meant to be exclusionary but, at a minimum, to help the anesthesiologist establish realistic expectations for the response to nerve block therapy.

Data from the physical examination will help one determine the anatomic nature of pain, and neurologic assessment is mandatory prior to the use of nerve blocks and treatment. Additionally, serial physical examinations may reveal physical improvement before the patient's subjective complaints of pain are changed. The results of laboratory tests can provide the practitioner with very useful information also. The benefit of abnormal bleeding indices or various radiologic tests that reveal tumor or infection of the lumbar spine is obvious. The majority of "slipped" lumbar disks occur at the L4–5 and L5–S1 levels. Although modern medical technology has advanced, we do not have diagnostic tests for every conceivable cause of low back pain. Thus, the anesthesiologist will do well to avoid believing that negative laboratory tests mean the patient has no "real" pain. Cailliet (10) clearly pointed out that the five major sources of most low back pain are the posterior longitudinal ligament, the interspinous ligaments, the deep muscles of the low back, the facet joints, and the nerve roots and their dural coverings. Only two of these five structures are evaluated with modern-day diagnostic tests. Thus, one should recognize that laboratory data are but one source of information, and changes in laboratory tests may not explain the patient's pain.

The types of patients with low back pain that we are most frequently asked to see include those with postural low back pain, postlaminectomy syndrome, acute herniated disks, and pain from metastatic cancer. The common denominator in these pathologic conditions may be nerve root irritation with subsequent swelling, edema, and radiating pain (11–17). Under these circumstances lumbar epidural blocks with local anesthetic and depot steroid compounds may be beneficial. Classic cases of discogenic pain will be characterized by sharp, radiating pain with an impulse quality (increased pain with coughing, sneezing, and straining), dermatomal sensory change and motor weakness, appropriate reflex changes, positive straight leg raising test (radiating dermatomal pain with elevation of the straight leg), and sciatic notch tenderness. The clinician must acknowledge that every case will not be so clear cut and that judgment about the appropriateness of a patient for epidural steroid injections can only be made after distillation of data from historical, physical, and laboratory investigations.

A frequent group of patients with low back pain (80–90% compared to the 1–2% with true herniated disks) who may be referred will be those with what might be loosely termed "postural low back pain." This grouping includes patients with lumbar strain/sprain, which connotes injury to the ligaments and muscles of the low back. These patients are likely to complain of diffuse, aching low back pain rather than consistent radicular pain. There are commonly muscle spasm and subsequent stiffness and, only occasionally, neurologic changes, perhaps related to intermittent nerve root irritation.

Cailliet (10) described a logical sequence of events that explains the signs and symptoms with which these patients present and of which they complain. Ordinarily the weight of the body is supported by the column of strong, dense vertebral bones. The more delicate posterior elements of the spinal arch (lamina, pedicles, and facets) are designed for directional guidance of motion (flexion and extension) and actually limit and restrict certain movements (lateral flexion and rotation). When a patient suffers with back pain, the paraspinal muscles re-

flexly go into spasm. This reaction increases the normal lumbar lordotic curve with the following pathologic consequences:

1. A transfer of weightbearing and motion/rotation to the posterior spine structures.
2. Stress on the posterior longitudinal ligament, which normally is thinnest between L2 and L5.
3. Increased sheer stress on the disks and bony articulations.
4. Increased intradiscal pressure with the likelihood of posterior bulging because the annulus of the disk is thinnest posteriorly.
5. Increased pressure at the facet joints.
6. Potentially a relative narrowing of the intravertebral foramen, one-third to one-half of which is normally occupied by the nerve root.
7. Nerve root irritation due to the narrowed foramen, intermittent pressure anteriorly from a bulging disk, or particular motions or body positions that pinch a swollen nerve root in the intervertebral foramen.
8. Chronically, there can be osteophyte formation, ligament distortion, and incoordination of muscle groups (paraspinals, hamstrings, abdominals) that are necessary to make the lumbar spine function as the machine it is.

Patients with low back pain that is truly chronic and/or the postlaminectomy or "failed back" syndrome frequently have features of chronic postural low back pain plus scar tissue from one or more surgical procedures on the lumbar spine. There is diffuse, ill-defined, dull, achy pain that is located in the low back and hips more than the legs. These patients have interference with spinal mobility because of pain and muscle shortening. There can also be changes in the neurologic exam representing residua of past surgery.

It is hard to propose strict guidelines for declaring a patient to be appropriate for nerve block intervention. Sometimes instinct and intuition enter into what has to be a calculated clinical decision. For instance, even though a young patient may not have more than a recent history of radicular pain, if he/she is going to work and doing all necessary life activities as best he/she can in spite of persistent low back pain, and not lying back and wallowing in inactivity or showing excessive pain behavior, he/she may be a reasonable candidate for epidural steroid injections. The motivation of the patient is a crucial variable in the decision. Table 6.4 summarizes the types of patients who are likely to be appropriate for nerve block therapy.

Table 6.4
Appropriate Patients to be Considered for Nerve Block Therapy

1. Patients with a history of radicular pain and an associated neurologic deficit. The shorter the duration of symptoms, the better the result. However, 2–6 weeks should be allowed for conservative therapy without nerve blocks in most cases. Some patients will have pathologic conditions (e.g., extruded disks) in which the anti-inflammatory effect of the steroids cannot provide enough clinical effect to reduce the symptoms.
2. Active patients with chronic low back pain who suffer an acute flare-up of pain that exceeds their "usual" pain and have at least radiculoid features.
3. Some selected patients with postural low back pain who are maintaining activities, are motivated to avoid dysfunction, and manifest irritation of the posterior primary division of the spinal nerve rather than the classical anterior division.
4. Some selected cases of chronic low back pain in which the nerve block is a part of a comprehensive treatment program that also addresses the gamut of the patient's problems with pain and identifies potentially significant detractors of success.

TREATMENT

Because pain is so complex and the possible etiologies for low back pain are so numerous, it is easily understood how no one treatment can be expected to "cure" low back pain. Patients with acute pain are logically more likely to respond quicker and more thoroughly to treatment than those with more chronic conditions, but even chronic patients will benefit more extensively when a continuum of treatments is provided. Surely in the patient with chronic low back pain, a treatment program, with each component contributing a percentage reduction in the total pain, is necessary. One cannot treat all pain (i.e., acute versus chronic) in the same way, but some modalities are versatile enough to benefit patients with either condition.

Conservative therapy is the generic name given to all treatment for low back pain that is nonsurgical in nature. There are many therapies available, but documentation of definitive effect is needed for most (18). With the components of bed rest and traction, the lumbosacral spine is immobilized to allow a reduction in inflammation of neural and musculoskeletal low back structures. Narcotic and nonnarcotic analgesics may be provided, as may be sedatives or muscle relaxants. These agents decrease pain and also contribute to the physical and emotional rest the patient may need. Sensory modulation therapies, such as heat, cold, massage, transcutaneous electrical nerve stimulation (TENS), diathermy, and ultrasound, can decrease pain and can be used in conjunction with a physical therapy program that demands the patient be actively involved in graduated exercise. Ultimately, life-style recommendations may need to be provided for the patient, such as avoiding the debility of bed rest, changing from jobs that demand constant sitting or repetitious heavy lifting, and maintaining weight loss. There is a window in which returning the patient to work is likely, so successful treatment early on is crucial. Low back pain may be more a problem of prevention of the primary injury and recurrent injury than treatment, since most cases get better (19).

EPIDURAL STEROID INJECTION

The now-familiar evolution of concepts about radicular low back pain date to the 1930s. Mixter and Barr (20) proposed then that compression of nerve roots caused the pain, so it seemed entirely reasonable to peform laminectomies to relieve the compression. In 1956 Kelley (11) modified this theory by saying that inflammation of the nerve roots from the compression caused the pain and neurologic changes. Thus, the concept of using steroids to decrease the inflammatory reaction to the compression became popular. Recent evidence affirms an inflammatory reaction in neural tissue caused by contact with nucleus pulposus material (21, 22).

In the late 1920s Hench used cortisone to treat patients suffering from arthritis (23). This was one of the first uses of systemic corticosteroid compounds for indications other than adrenocortical insufficiency. Since then many naturally occurring and synthetic corticosteroid drugs have been used for various medical purposes, including that of decreasing inflammation. These potent drugs can suppress both the early (edema, fibrin deposition, capillary dilatation, white blood cell migration, and phagocytic activity) and late (capillary and fibroblast proliferation, deposition of collagen, cicatrization) manifestations of the inflammatory response (23). In the specific use of perispinal (subarachnoid and epidural) steroids, one must determine if the patient's symptoms are due to inflammatory changes in nerve roots or secondary to scarring, because steroids are less likely to positively influence the symptoms due to the latter.

Several authors (11, 17, 24, 25) have proposed that low back pain with typical sciatica is caused by inflammatory irritation of nerve roots secondary to mechanical compression by herniated disk material or bony contact. This concept originally led Goebert et al. (26) in the late 1950s to add 125 mg of hydrocortisone, a potent anti-inflammatory drug, to 30 ml of procaine administered into the caudal epidural space for the treatment of sciatica. Patients with sciatica given this combination of drugs improved more than those who received only the local anesthetic. This phenomenon was more recently reported by Breivik et al. (27) and Bourne (28).

Subsequent reports of the use of perispinal steroid drugs with minor modifications of this basic technique followed and dictated practice in the United States (29). In general these studies with large volume injectates (as above) administered primarily in the caudal epidural space resulted in *at least* good improvement for *at least* 4 months in approximately 60–70% of patients. The conclusion gained from this research was that the combination of local anesthetic and steroids was a useful adjunct in the treatment of sciatica. This degree of improvement was duplicated by Carron (1976, unpublished data) and, more recently, by Berman et al. (16). Berman's group gave 367 patients with radicular pain 100 mg of methylprednisolone and 10ml of 0.5% marcaine in the lumbar epidural space after 2 weeks of conservative therapy had not helped their pain. The study showed that 66% of the patients were improved with the epidural steroid injection (ESI) if the symptoms were less than 6 months in duration, but only 33% were improved with symptoms of more than 1 year's duration.

The decrease in volume of solution injected from the early 1960s to Berman's study was based upon a growing appreciation for the mechanism of action of the ingredients of the injectate. Originally Goebert et al. (26) were using 100 ml of saline in the caudal epidural space. This was modified to only 30 ml of procaine and eventually to that volume plus the additional small volume of hydrocortisone. Winnie et al. (13) wanted to clarify the need for such large injectates and the mechanism of action of ESIs. They studied 20 patients with active sciatica who each received basically only 80 mg of methylprednisolone in a lumbar epidural injection. The questions to be answered by the study were whether the large volumes were necessary to lyze adhesions in the epidural space, the local anesthetics were interrupting an RSD-like syndrome, or the steroids were really exerting an anti-inflammatory effect. The work basically demonstrated that only the steroid was necessary as long as it was placed at the level of suspected nerve root inflammation. Since then the application of 40–80 mg of methylprednisolone acetate (Dep-o-Medrol, UpJohn) or 25–50

mg of triamcinolone diacetate (Aristocort Intralesional, Lederle) has been a popular form of treatment provided by a growing number of anesthesiologists in the conservative management of patients with low back pain. Benzon's (17) analytic review of this topic accurately noted that many past studies of the effectiveness of ESIs have failed to have an appropriate control group. However, he quoted five scientifically valid, well-controlled studies that support the usefulness of ESIs in selected patients with sciatica. As Abram and Anderson (30) have well shown, the longer the pain complaints are present the more likely it is that factors other than the original tissue damage (e.g., trigger points, psychosocial issues) will influence the complaints and response to therapy.

This author's current protocol (15, 31) (Table 6.5) proposes performing ESIs at the level of suspected nerve root involvement using 4–6 ml of local anesthetic (in our outpatient pain management center the drug is usually 1% xylocaine or 2% chloroprocaine) mixed with 50 mg (2 ml of 2.5% solution) of triamcinolone diacetate at 2-week intervals to a maximum of three blocks. Whenever improvement occurs, the patient is continued solely with other components of his/her therapeutic program (e.g., anti-inflammatory medications and graded exercise).

The local anesthetic is not absolutely necessary. However, it does provide temporary analgesia that may interrupt the pain–muscle spasm–pain cycle and bias the patient's impression that something really can be done for the pain. It also helps the steroids spread to the affected nerve root and, in a teaching setting, provides positive feedback that the steroid was properly placed (we must *technically* accomplish *epidural* placement of the drug before

Table 6.5
Protocol for Epidural Steroid Injection for Low Back Pain

Decubitus position with the involved side down
LOR technique to identify the epidural space—then a
  negative aspiration test
Injection of local anesthetic or saline or deposteroid, mixed
  or separately
Possible transient radicular pain
Clear the needle of steroid to avoid a fistulous track
Maintain the decubitus position for 10 min
Test for improvement in straight leg raising if local anesthetic was used
Caution the patient about the interval during which the
  local anesthetic effect will wear off and the steroid effect will not have become manifest

we can reasonably ask the patient if it worked) It is noteworthy, too, that the doses of steroids being injected are not inert in the body, as suggested in Table 6.2 and in the studies by Sehgal et al. (32) and Gorski et al. (33). The drugs can produce a suppression of endogenous steroids for 2–3 weeks. Caution is necessary in that, although not associated with epidural steroid use so far, patients have developed Cushing's syndrome from exogenous steroid administration by other routes for therapeutic purposes (34).

We usually place the patient in a decubitus position with the side of his/her pain complaints the down side. After routine prepping and draping of the back and the placement of a skin wheal, the epidural space is located by a loss of resistance (LOR) technique. After a negative response to a 2-ml test dose of local anesthetic drug and a negative aspiration test for cerebrospinal fluid, the local anesthetic and steroid drugs are injected separately or as a mixed injectate. It is not uncommon that the patient's symptoms of radicular pain will be temporarily reproduced with this positive pressure injection. Preservative-free saline can be substituted for the local anesthetic drug or only the steroid injected if one so desires. Whether the needle must be cleared of steroid to avoid possible fistula formation is unclear, but is strongly advocated, most recently by Longmire and Joyce (35).

The decubitus position is maintained for approximately 10 min after the epidural procedure is completed to let the "heavy" steroid (it is heavier than the local anesthetic and begins to separate from the mixture in a matter of minutes) bathe the affected nerve roots. When the patient is placed supine, if local anesthetic has been used, the most sensitive indicator of proper placement of the drug mixture is improvement in the straight leg raising test. The patient must be informed that he/she may experience a temporary increase in pain after the local anesthetic effect has worn off and before the steroid action begins (usually in 24–48 hours). The epidural block can be repeated when the patient's decrease in pain reaches a plateau or when pain recurs, but usually is not done at closer than 2-week intervals.

When nerve blocks are used as part of a comprehensive pain management program according to this protocol, one finds that the success can't help but vary somewhat with the accuracy of the diagnosis and the duration of symptoms. Intuitively, the shorter the period of follow-up, the better the results for any treatment. Arnhoff et al. (36) determined 2 years after treatment that nerve blocks were helpful, but gender-associated differences in life function contributed to the complexity of factors involved in outcome assessment. Toomey et al. (37) reassessed Arnoff's patients 3 years later and concluded that there had not been any significant change in the number of patients with further improvement, but neither had there been a major backslide in terms of the subjective ratings of pain, the percentage of patients having further surgery, or an increase in work ability. Thus, nerve blocks can be an important component of pain management, but appraisal of outcome of any treatment is difficult (38).

With the burgeoning understanding of the site of the action of opiates and the increasing experience with their clinical effects when applied to the epidural and intrathecal spaces, several authors have studied the use of epidural morphine and steroids in the treatment of low back pain. Because there is an interval of return of low back pain after an ESI (during which the analgesia from the local anesthetic has worn off and before the deposteroid exerts an obvious clinical effect), it is worthy to seek a drug that will remain active until the steroid takes effect. Cohn et al. (39) enthusiastically reproted 50–100% pain relief lasting 6–24 months in 20 patients with intractable postoperative, recurrent low back pain when 8 mg of morphine and 80 mg of methylprednisolone were sequentially injected.

Using a more scientific, double-blind, crossover design, Dallas et al. (40) could not duplicate Cohn's results. The patients did get more relief of postlaminectomy low back pain with morphine and steroid when compared to steroid alone, but only 65% of their 20-patient sample had any relief at all and the pain relief lasted only 1 day to 6 weeks. Brechner (41) found he could not "come within a country mile of the results reported by Dr. Cohn . . ." when he applied the same treatment protocol to 30 patients. Thus, the combination of epidural morphine and deposteroids for even chronic low back pain is still controversial and demands further scientific study before it can be recommended.

Because epidural steroids have been used subsequently in the generic treatment of low back pain for many causes, the success rate has varied greatly. Cuckler et al. (42) have published the most recent study that fails to show a positive effect of epidural steroid use. In a prospective, randomized, double-blind study of 73 patients in whom at least 2 weeks of conservative therapy had failed to improve the symptoms of lumbar radicular pain, no therapeutic efficacy of epidural methylprednisolone in the treatment of acute or chronic neural compression syndrome was found. One can question the clinical relevance of this study, however, because a number of people did in subsequent letters to the editor in the same journal. For instance, all drugs (procaine, methylprednisolone, or saline) were injected at the same L3–4 level without regard to the level of pathology. The authors waited only 24 hours for a "steroid effect," whereas it can take up to 72 hours for this to become manifest. Also, they included patients with spinal stenosis in their study. This is a mechanical anatomic problem, but not necessarily one with inflammatory neural pathology. Nonetheless, scientific challenge is healthy and prevents complacency.

The most recent critique of ESIs for patients with complaints of low back pain is the Quebec Task Force report (2). These authors generally agreed that a lot of work has been reported on low back pain, but much of it is not too good. As for ESI, the extensive literature review placed the therapy in the "common practice but no scientific evidence" category. No invasive therapeutic procedures were recommended until 4 weeks after the onset of acute low back pain, and chronic low back pain is now deemed to exist after only 3 months of symptoms.

ALTERNATE TECHNIQUES

Some patients will have had surgery or severe trauma that will preclude safe entry into the epidural space at the lumbar level where nerve root irritation is suspected. It is also possible that a patient with pain secondary to metastatic cancer will have radicular symptoms but should not be injected at the offending level because of the presence of tumor. In these situations it is not uncommon to return to the techniques of old and inject steroids into the caudal epidural space. Understandably, scar tissue and anatomic derangement in the lumbar epidural space can limit the cephalad spread of the bolus injected, so one may only get the drug to the L5–S1 or L4–5 level.

When the caudal approach is used, 8–15 ml of solution may be needed just to fill the caudal space before any lumbar ascension occurs. The same dose of deposteroid is used as for lumbar placement. Occasionally, selective transsacral blocks, especially at the S2 or S3 level, will be beneficial to those who have had lumbar fusions to the sacrum from which scarring and fibrosis may compromise nerve root motion and function. These are performed with standard technique using 25–50 mg of triamcinolone diacetate and 2–3 ml of local anesthetic solution (43).

Another approach to consider when access to a specific spinal level centrally is not anatomically or functionally possible is that of paravertebral block (10). This will deposit a bolus of drug (e.g., 5–7 ml of local anesthetic and 1–2 ml of depsteroid) distal to the intervertebral foramen and depends upon retrograde flow of the bolus back through this opening to yield a clinical effect.

The application of steroids in the intrathecal space was popularized years ago (32, 44) in the treatment of lumbar radiculopathy and has also been used historically for arachnoiditis and multiple sclerosis. Gardner et al. (44) reported that the injection of 40–80 mg of methylprednisolone was safe, only a transient increase in pain symptoms were reported, and cerebrospinal fluid analysis showed only a transient pleocytosis. Perhaps more significant was that the drug stayed in the cerebrospinal fluid for at least 1 week. Abram (45) published a report indicating that such use may benefit those patients who have shown a partial response to epidural steroid administration but that the primary use of subarachnoid steroids for low back pain met with very limited success. In his study of 19 patients, five of six with a partial response to ESIs had further, slight improvement with intrathecal triamcinolone, but only one of 13 without previous benefit from ESI s had any further noticeable improvement.

It is noteworthy that no corticosteroid preparation has Food and Drug Administration approval for intrathecal or epidural use and that the Depo-Medrol package insert specifically states that the product is "not recommended" for subarachnoid use. In Bernat's (46) review of this whole topic, it is accurately noted that the hazards of intrathecal steroid use are not due to the steriod itself, but rather to the accompanying bacteriostatic agents or the solubility-altering vehicles in the depot forms commonly used to produce a prolonged clinical effect. The intrathecal use of corticosteroid drugs seems to be diminishing as concern over the side effects increases and evidence for an exceptional, additional benefit is lacking (45, 47, 48). Kepes and Duncalf (48) espouse the opinion that in this age of accountability, subarachnoid steroid use should be condemned.

INTERESTING MECHANISMS OF LOW BACK PAIN

Winnie et al.'s (13) research seems to plausibly identify the anti-inflammatory action of steroids as the active effect of ESI therapy. Although the extensive clinical experience of 25 years seems to have indicated this, only recently have Delaney et al. (49) shown in a cat model that the epidural injection of triamcinolonoe diacetate is safe because it lacks histologic evidence of damage to neural tissue. This study involved only one epidural injection and demonstrated a mild inflammatory reaction that was resolved in 120 days after placement of drug. Caution is certainly warranted in the extrapolation of these results to man. Wood et al. (50) showed that after five injections of methylprednisolone around the sciatic nerve in rats, there was evidence of structural nerve damage when compared to controls given only needle insertions, local anesthetics, or no injections. The groups receiving steroids had microscopic evidence of axonal degeneration, loss of myelin, and endoneural fibrosis. The clinical significance of these changes was undetermined since none of the affected rats had neurologic changes prior to being sacrificed.

Edwards et al. (51) reported that 41% of 43 patients with radicular pain responded effectively to the intravenous infusion of lidocaine with pain relief of greater than 1 week's duration. That this might be so would seem to detract from the anti-inflammatory theory. However, because this same therapy was also shown to treat various peripheral neuropathies, one can't help but wonder if the local anesthetic isn't having an additional, and as yet unexplained, neurophysiologic effect in the central nervous system. Patients with mechanical low back pain and myofascial syndrome did not improve with the same therapy.

More recent scientific investigation shows a return to the concept of an inflammatory etiology for radicular low back pain (21, 22). Even small amounts of nucleus pulposus material produce an inflammatory response upon contact with neural tissue. If this is consistently so, the positive results of ESIs in cases that are less than classic for radicular pain may be explained. That is, the patient would not have to have a persistent defect on diagnostic testing, but rather only intermittent contact of a bulging disk with a nerve root or the release of small quantities of nucleus pulposus to set up a possible inflammatory reaction. Pountain et al. (52) studied 34 patients with chronic low back pain. They found that fibrinolysis was significant in these patients when they were compared to matched controls and suggested that the abnormal fibrinolytic activity led to fibrin deposition and chronic inflammation.

Interesting, too, is the idea proposed by Loeser (53) in 1985. His opinion was that chronic microtrauma to neural and musculoskeletal structures of the low back after lumbar surgery could result in

the formation of neuromas. These small masses of twisted terminal nerve branches are characteristically very sensitive to mechanical stimuli and circulating catecholamines. Devor et al. (54) showed in a rat sciatic nerve model that the spontaneous discharge from neuromas and the exaggerated reaction to physical and chemical stimuli could be rapidly suppressed by the topical application of steroids. Again, then, ESIs may be of benefit in patients with less than classic signs and symptoms of herniated disk not only because of their potent anti-inflammatory effect, but also because of the direct action on the membranes of ectopic nocioceptive foci of an injured nervous system.

CONCLUSION

Low back pain is a ubiquitous problem. As with any pain problem, the patient requires a careful workup that will lead to a comprehensive diagnosis—one that takes into account the physical generators of *and* the nonphysical contributions to the total pain problem. Once the patient understands the diagnosis and the rationale for the proposed therapy, educated decisions about therapy can be made and a treatment course embarked upon. In most cases, limited use will be made of potent analgesics, surgery, and activity restriction. Rather, a program that includes anti-inflammatory medications, neural stimulation, progressive exercise, and rehabilitation to full function will be encouraged. In patients with chronic low back pain, psychosocial rehabilitation may also be necessary since just taking the pain away does not immediately eliminate all of the adverse consequences the pain perpetrates on the patient's attitudes, behavior, and life-style.

Therapeutic nerve blocks, used alone, *occasionally* have remarkable results in patients with low back pain. More commonly, they are but one component of a treatment program. The use of local anesthetic and steroid drugs in the epidural space is a successful modality of treatment in the management of cases in which there is reasonable evidence that inflammation of nerve roots is causing the patient's symptoms. The epidural route of drug administration is usually chosen because fewer complications from the steroid drug have been reported, post–lumbar puncture headaches are avoided, and many pathologic conditions produce inflammatory changes of the nerve roots in this space. There seems to be an ever-decreasing indication for the use of steroid drugs with or without local anesthetic in the subarachnoid space. Some alternate forms of injection are occasionally necessary. Until more accurate diagnostic techniques, discriminating surgical procedures, and successful, conservative therapy measures are developed, the use of nerve blocks will remain an important therapeutic intervention when judiciously applied in selected patients with back pain.

REFERENCES

1. Bonica JJ: The nature of the problem. In Carron H, McLaughlin RE (eds): *Management of Low Back Pain.* Boston, John Wright and Sons, PGS Inc, 1982, pp 1–15.
2. Quebec Task Force: Magnitude of the problem. *Spine* 12(7S):S12–S15, 1987.
3. Loeser JD: Low back pain: Introduction to plenary session. In Bonica JJ, Liebeskind JC, Albe-Fessard DG (eds): *Advances in Pain Research and Therapy.* New York, Raven Press, 1979, vol 3, pp 631–633.
4. Spielman FJ, Ghia JN: Pain control teaching in anesthesia residencies. *Reg Anesth* 8:154–157, 1983.
5. Khoury G, Varga CA: Does the frequency of utilization of nerve blocks in pain clinics vary with the specialty of the director? *Pain* 33:265, 1988.
6. Waddell G: A new clinical model for the treatment of low-back pain. *Spine* 12:632–644, 1987.
7. International Association for the Study of Pain: Classification of chronic pain. *Pain* 24(Suppl 3):S217, 1986.
8. Swerdlow M: Medicolegal aspects of complications following pain relieving blocks. *Pain* 13:321–331, 1982.
9. Abram SE, Anderson RA, Maita-D'Cruze AM: Factors predicting short-term outcome of nerve blocks in the management of chronic pain. *Pain* 10:323–330, 1981.
10. Cailliet R: Low back pain. In Cailliet R (ed): *Soft Tissue Pain and Disability.* Philadelphia, FA Davis Co, 1977, pp 41–106.
11. Kelley M: Pain due to pressure on nerves? Spinal tumors and the intervertebral disc. *Neurology* 6:32–36, 1956.
12. Swerdlow M, Sayle-Creer W: A study of extradural medication in the relief of the lumbosciatic syndrome. *Anaesthesia* 25:341–345, 1970.
13. Winnie AP, Hartman JT, Meyers HL, et al: Pain clinic II: intradural and extradural corticosteroids for sciatrica. *Anesth Analg (Cleve)* 51:990–999, 1972.
14. Murphy RW: Nerve roots and spinal nerves in degenerative disc disease. *Clin Orthop* 129:46–60, 1977.
15. Carron H, Toomey TC: Epidural steroid therapy for low back pain. In Stanton-Hicks M, Boas R (eds): *Chronic Low Back Pain.* New York, Raven Press, 1982, pp 193–198.
16. Berman AT, Garbarino JL, Fisher SM, Bosacco SJ: The effects of epidrual injection of local anesthetics and corticosteroids on patients with lumbosciatic pain. *Clin Orthop Rel Res* 188:144–151, 1984.
17. Benzon HT: Epidural steroid injections for low back pain and lumbosacral radiculopathy. *Pain* 24:277–295, 1986.
18. Deyo RA: Conservative therapy for low back pain. *JAMA* 250:1057–1062, 1983.
19. Deyo RA, Tsui-Wu Y: Descriptive epidemiology of low-back pain and its related medical care in the United States. *Spine* 12:264, 1987.
20. Mixter WJ, Barr JS: Rupture of the intervertebral disc with involvement of the spinal canal. *N Engl J Med* 211:210, 1934.
21. Jaffray D, O'Brien JP: Isolated intervertebral disc resorption. *Spine* 11:397, 1986.
22. McCarron RF, Wimpee MW, Hudkins PG, Laros, GS: The imflammatory effect of nucleus pulposus. *Spine* 12:760–764, 1987.
23. Hayes RC Jr, Murad F: Adrenocorticotrophic hormone: adrenocortical steroids and their synthetic analogs; inhibitors of adrenocortical steroid biosynthesis. In Gilman AG, Goodman LS, Rall TW, Murad F (eds): *The Pharmacologic Basis of Therapeutics.* New York, Macmillan Publishing Co, Inc, 1985, pp 1459–1489.
24. Lindahl O, Rexed B: Histological changes in the spinal nerve roots of operated cases of sciatica. *Acta Orthop Scand* 20:215–225, 1951.
25. Hakelius A: Prognosis in sciatica. A clinical follow-up of surgical and non-surgical treatment. *Acta Orthop Scand* 129(Suppl):1–73, 1970.
26. Goebert HW, Jallo SJ, Gardner WJ, et al: Sciatica: treatment with epidural injections of procaine and hydrocortisone. *Cleve Clinic Q* 27:191–197, 1960.
27. Breivik H, Hesla PE, Molnar I, Lind B: Treatment of chronic low back pain and sciatica. Comparison of caudal epidural injection of bupivacaine and methylprednisolone with bupivacaine followed by saline. In Bonica JJ, Albe-Fessard DG (eds): *Advances in Pain Research and Therapy.* New York, Raven Press, 1976, vol 1, pp 927–932.
28. Bourne IHJ: Treatment of chronic back pain comparing corticosteroid-lignocaine injections with lignocaine alone. *Practitioner* 228:333–338, 1984.
29. Goebert HW, Jallo SJ, Gardner WJ, et al: Painful radiculopathy treated with epidural injections of procaine and hydrocortisone acetate. Results in 113 patients. *Anesth Analg* 40:130–134, 1961.
30. Abram SE, Anderson RA: Using a pain questionnaire to predict response to epidural steroids. *Reg Anesth* 5(3):11–14, 1980.
31. Rowlingson JC: The evaluation and management of acute low back pain. *Curr Con Pain* 1(7):3–6, 1983.
32. Sehgal AD, Gardner WJ, Dohn DF: Pantopaque "arachnoiditis" treatment with subarachnoid injection of corticosteroids. *Cleve Clinic Q* 29:177–188, 1962.
33. Gorski DW, Rao TK, Glisson SN, McDowell D: Epidural triamcinolone and adrenal response to stress. *Anesthesilogy* 55(3):A147, 1981.

34. Hughes JM, Hichens M, Booze GW, Thorner MO: Cushing's syndrome from the therapeutic use of intramuscular dexamethasone acetate. *Arch Intern Med* 146:1848–1849, 1986.
35. Longmire S, Joyce TH: Treatment of a duro-cutaneous fistula secondary to attempted epidural anesthesia with an epidural autologous blood patch. *Anesthesiology* 60:63–64, 1984.
36. Arnhoff FN, Triplett HB, Pokorney B: Follow-up status of patients treated with nerve blocks for low back pain. *Anesthesiology* 46:170–178, 1977.
37. Toomey TC, Taylor AG, Skelton JA, et al: Stability of self-report measures of improvement in chronic pain: a five year follow-up. *Pain* 12:273–283, 1982.
38. McArthur DL, Cohen MJ, Gottlieb HJ, Naliboff BD, Schandler SL: Treating chronic low back pain. II. Long-term follow-up. *Pain* 29:23–38, 1987.
39. Cohn ML, Huntington CT, Byrd SE, et al: Epidural morphine and methylprednisolone. *Spine* 11:960–963, 1986.
40. Dallas TL, Lin RL, Wu W, Wolskee P: Epidural morphine and methylprednisolone for low-back pain. *Anesthesiology* 67:408–411, 1987.
41. Brechner VL: Letters. *Spine* 12:827, 1987.
42. Cuckler JM, Bernini PA, Wiesel SW, et al: The use of epidural steroids in the treatment of lumbar radicular pain. *J Bone Joint Surg [Am]* 67:63–66, 1985.
43. Carron H, Korbon GA, Rowlingson JC: *Regional Anesthesia: Techniques and Clinical Applications.* Orlando, FL, Grune & Stratton, Inc, 1984, pp 64–66.
44. Gardner WJ, Goebert HW, Sehgal AD: Intraspinal corticosteroids in the treatment of sciatica. *Trans Am Neurol Assoc* 86:214–215, 1961.
45. Abram SE: Subarachnoid corticosteroid injection following inadequate response to epidural steroids for sciatica. *Anesth Analg* 57:313–315, 1978.
46. Bernat JL: Intraspinal steroid therapy. *Neurology* 31:168–171, 1981.
47. Sheely CN: Dangers of spinal injection without proper diagnosis. *JAMA* 197:1104–1106, 1966.
48. Kepes ER, Duncalf D: Treatment of backache with spinal injection of local anesthetics, spinal and systemic steroids. A review. *Pain* 22:33–47, 1985.
49. Delaney TJ, Rowlingson JC, Carron H, Butler A: The effects of steroids on nerves and meninges. *Anesth Analg* 59:610–614, 1980.
50. Wood KM, Arguelles J, Norenberg MD: Degenerative lesions on rat sciatic nerves after local injection of methylprednisolone in sterile aqueous solution. *Reg Anesth* 5(1):13–15, 1980.
51. Edwards WT, Habib F, Burney RG, Begin G: Intravenous lidocaine in the management of various chronic pain states. A review of 211 cases. *Reg Anesth* 10:1–6, 1985.
52. Pountain GD, Keegan AL, Jayson MIV: Impaired fibrinolytic activity in defined chronic back pain syndromes. *Spine* 12:83–86, 1987.
53. Loeser JD: Pain due to nerve injury. *Spine* 10:232–235, 1985.
54. Devor M, Govrin-Lippmann R, Raber P: Corticosteroids suppress ectopic neural discharges originating in experimental neuromas. *Pain* 22:127–137, 1985.

Chapter 7

TRIGGER POINT AND RELATED INJECTION THERAPIES

LAWRENCE W. FRIEDMANN, MD, FACA, FICA

There are a number of injection and needle methods of treating back pain, some of which are used commonly and some of which are used rarely. Under proper circumstances each can be extremely useful for both diagnosis and treatment. They may be classified in a number of ways. I find that separating them into techniques to be used when the patient has radiculopathy, as opposed to when the patient does not have radiculopathy, makes it easier to understand when to use which technique.

RADICULOPATHY TECHNIQUES

The techniques to be used when the patient appears to have irritation of a specific nerve root or roots may be divided into blocks of the nerves themselves, blocks of the nerve roots at their exit from the spinal canal, or blocks within the spinal canal, either epidural or intradural.

NERVE BLOCKS

Nerve blocks are described in detail in Chapters 5 and 6, and are not described here, except to state that the author has had favorable experiences.

NERVE ROOT BLOCKS

Nerve root blocks are done to diagnose whether pain is originating from the posterior primary division of the spinal nerve. The posterior primary division originates from muscles, ligments, or facets in the spinal segment distribution. This usually occurs in patients with no neurologic deficit. In these patients, the straight leg raising test is usually within normal limits. If a local anesthetic blocks the patient's pain when the injection is done, then the pain is originating from a structure innervated by the posterior primary division at that nerve root. The injection is usually done at the levels of L3, L4, or L5 at the level of the intertransversus ligament. For therapy of inflammation, steroids may be included. An occasional repeated block may prove useful. If the patient has temporary relief, but the pain is resistant even to repeated blocks, electrocautery of the posterior primary ramus may be useful.

Specific injection of the facets or other inflamed structures is also useful and may be done simultaneously or independently.

EPIDURAL INJECTIONS

Epidural injections are done both for pain that is radicular and also for pain not truly radicular in origin. The latter pain, which is transmitted through the recurrent sinuvertebral nerve distal to the foramen, has been termed "pseudoradicular." The stimuli that are transmitted by the recurrent sinuvertebral nerve generally come from irritation of the posterior longitudinal ligament, the anterior dura, or the apophyseal joints. These pains are not relieved by anesthesia of the posterior primary ramus. Generally, in these patients the neurologic examination is negative. The patient's pain ordinarily does not radiate to below the knee. The straight leg raising test is usually equivocal. These patients frequently benefit from an epidural injection of corticosteroids with a local anesthetic. The method is to inject between 10 and 30 ml of a 0.25% solution of procaine with a soluble corticosteroid. If desired, a 0.5% solution of Pontocaine (tetracaine) may be used.

INTRADURAL INJECTIONS

Intradural injections are performed specifically for diagnosis and, less commonly, for therapeutic reasons. The author finds diagnostic blocks extremely useful when there is a serious question of what proportion of the patient's complaints are somatosensory, autonomic, and emotional if they are performed in alert, cooperative patients with relatively normal intellect. The diagnostic intradural injection must be done extremely carefully to get the information desired. The patient must be tested by all sensory modalities in the distribution of the area to be blocked. The sensory modalities must include, as a minimum, pinprick, light touch, and skin temperature. The muscles in the nerve distribution to be blocked must be graded. These tests of sensation and motor pwoer must be repeated after each phase of the injection.

The method is to insert a spinal needle, usually between L4 and L5, with the usual spinal tap technique. The spinal needle is left in place after each phase. The patient is not told what solutions are being used at each phase. The procedure must be indentical after each injection. For that reason the diagnostician must know whether he/she will use a hyperbaric solution for phases 2 and 3 or a hypobaric solution. If he/she uses a hypobaric solution then the patient will be placed in Trendelenburg after each injection. If he/she uses a hyperbaric solution then the patient will be seated after each injection.

Phase 1

After the patient has been tapped, he/she is given an injection of 5 ml of sterile normal saline. After the injection a 5-min wait occurs and the patient is asked whether his/her pain has changed, and is tested for sensory and motor changes. If the patient reports significant pain relief after the saline injection, it is clear that there is a large psychological component to the patient's pain, since normal saline will not relieve pain except as a placebo. In addition, the results of the sensory and motor examinations should be identical to those made prior to the injection of the saline. If there are differences these are also due to psychological causes.

Phase 2

While the needle is still in the patient's intradural space, 5 ml of 0.2% procaine or 0.05–0.1% tetracaine in sterile isotonic saline are injected. If one wishes to use a hyperbaric solution, 10% glucose solution is used instead of the isotonic saline. This concentration of local anesthetic blocks the sympathetic nerves selectively. If the patient has pain relief then treatment of the sympathetic nervous system may be of value. Further testing is not needed. One may consider the use of anticholinergic medications, paravertebral sympathetic blocks, and/or surgical sympathectomy for treatment of the pain. If the patient has no relief of his/her symptoms then it may be that the pain is mediated through the sensory spinal roots, or it may have an emotional component, or both. One then proceeds to Phase 3.

Phase 3

While the needle is still in the intradural space one injects 5 ml of either 0.5% procaine or 1% tetracaine in 10% glucose if one wishes a hyperbaric solution. This gives complete anesthesia and thus blocks the sensory roots. If the patient's pain is relieved this verifies somatosensory nerve root pain. However, if the patient says that pain is not relieved it indicates a very strong psychological component to the patient's pain.

Therapeutic Intradural Injections

Therapeutic intradural injections may also be used. In this case, soluble corticosteroids, usually mixed with an anesthetic, are injected. If there is inflammation of the nerve root and its dural sheath, such as might occur with a herniated nucleus pulposus or arachnoiditis, the patient will have some relief.

NONRADICULOPATHY TECHNIQUES

FACET INJECTIONS

Facet joint abnormalities may cause back pain, sciatica, or both (1). Injection of the facet may be done with only an anesthetic for diagnostic purposes, but if done therapeutically is usually done with steroids. The injection is done under fluoroscopic control. Obviously injection of the facet interrupts pain that originates in the facet and nowhere else. Irritation of a facet does not cause a true radiculopathy but because of stimulation of the posterior primary ramus, frequently the pain mimics a true radiculopathy. The capsule of the facet only holds about 3–5 ml of fluid. Often much more fluid is injected, which then ruptures the capsule. There is some evidence that capsular rupture may enhance the success rate of the injection.

TRIGGER POINT INJECTIONS

There is considerable discussion in the medical literature about the nature of trigger points. Physicians with experience have palpated local areas of tenderness in muscles and fascia for many years. They are sometimes accompanied by muscle spasm, and their treatment often includes measures designed to reduce muscle spasm, since the total pain experience is then diminished. If one defines the trigger points as very localized areas of exquisite tenderness, with the surrounding ropy and tender muscles being in protective muscle spasm, then the treatment becomes more specific. Some biopsy studies over the years have sometimes found a physical lesion, whereas others have found only normal tissue. While the controversy remains as to what trigger points (and muscle spasm, for that matter) are, we know that certain treatments are effective in the relief of pain.

This author speculates that trigger points are local areas of muscle edema, possibly inflammatory, which give rise to spontaneous pain, muscular tenderness, and often reactive muscle twitching on palpation. In addition, they frequently cause surrounding muscle spasm, all of which may be quite disabling. While trigger points may occasioally be found in the areas where the acupuncture points have been described, others are not over such points. They often give rise to radicular or pseudoradicular pain as described by Kraus when he termed the radiating pain the "psuedodisk syndrome" (2). Some differentiate between tender points, which do not radiate, and trigger points, which have radiating pain (3). I do not think they are significantly different.

A fairly complete, although still controversial, description of trigger points and their treatment is found in the book by Travell and Simons (3).

Types of Trigger Point Treatment

There are many treatments for trigger points. The appropriate management of myofascial pain syndrome consists of educating patients on how to prevent and deal with recurrences as well as specific myofascial therapy, which may include trigger point injection. Injection is most useful when a limited number of trigger points remain that are unresponsive or inaccessible to other modes of therapy. Precise trigger point injection with a suitable local anesthetic can be depended on to inactivate trigger points that are encountered by the needle, but may not eliminate the ones that are missed, even though they may be missed only narrowly. There are numerous technqiues used in trigger point injection. While injection therapy has been utilized for many years, no standardized method is used by various physicians. This is undoubtedly because no study showing the superiority of one method over the others has been reported until recently (4).

The fastest way to the resolution of trigger points is by injection. However, many patients resist injection because of the pain involved. For that reason the author prefers to start treatment with the vapocoolant spray–and-stretch technique. If that doesn't work, ultrasound with subsequent stretch is often useful but takes considerably more time in many instances. There are many variations to using the spray-and-stretch technique. Travell and Simons (3) sometimes use a stretch technique without a vapocoolant spray. One can use passive stretch, or rhythmic stabilization with alternate contraction of the agonist and antagonist muscle groups, which utilizes reciprocal inhibition, or a combination of the two.

Travell prefers Fluori-Methane vapo-coolant spray because it is not flammable and is not a general anesthetic. She sprays basically in the direction of the muscle fibers. She recommends parallel sweeps moving in one direction only. She stresses that one does not wish to cool the underlying muscle. After the skin is cooled, the muscle is stretched. Apparently it is the stretching that provides most of the relief. The vapo-coolant spray provides a short period of hypalgesia.

Kraus (2) and this author (5) prefer ethyl chloride spray, which in our experience is much more effective than the Fluori-Methane spray, despite the disadvantages of being a general anesthetic and flammable in contrast to Fluori-Methane spary. We find some cooling of the underlying muscle very helpful. I do not find unidirectional spraying better than bidirectional. Freezing of the skin is contraindicated. The stretch is the therapeutic maneuver, while the spraying makes the stretch less painful and thus the person resists the stretch less.

Another treatment is sustained pressure over the trigger point with a knuckle or other hard object. This is similar to Shiatzu (6) or acupressure (7). Acupuncture is also effective (see Chapter 8). Acupuncture has many theories as to its action (8). The reason it is mentioned here is that many claims have been made for acupuncture and many of them have been disputed. While I do not do acupuncture, I have seen many cases in which I am absolutely convinced that the beneficial effect is real, and not merely placebo.

Other treatments that have been proposed are heat (dry and wet), cold without stretch, massage, medications (for analgesia, anti-inflammation, or muscle relaxation), biofeedback, and transcutaneous electrical nerve stimulation. In my opinion these treatments are helpful for the muscle spasm that often accompanies trigger points, but are not useful for the trigger points themselves.

Injection Techniques

Various trigger point injection techniques are used. The main objective of injection is to accurately localize and disrupt each individual trigger point with the needle. Dry needling of a trigger point is very effective treatment. Exactly why this is so is speculative, but many authors have confirmed the finding (2, 9, 10). The afterpain, however, appears to be worse. Different authors have recommended various solutions for insertion. This author uses sterile saline in allergic patients, and anesthetic alone in diabetics, with a good result but with some increase in afterpain in both.

Despite the wide range of variability of results with different agents or no agent at all, it is important to inactivate the affected sites with precision. Although procaine (0.5%) does shorten the duration of pain when the needle contacts a trigger point, it does not block the referral of pain from the trigger point at the moment of needle contact; this is important for locating all trigger points in a group. Procaine also has the least myotoxicity of the local anesthetics in common use, which property can reactivate or worsen trigger point areas; moreover, it does not obscure the local pain reaction of a trigger point during localization.

Varying techniques are used by different authors. Travell and Simons (3) palpate the trigger point, fixate it between the fingers while compressing the vessels, and inject after spraying.

Travell uses a 1.5-inch needle, usually 22-gauge but sometimes thinner, but always uses a needle long enough to reach the trigger point, which, on ocasion, may require a 3.5-inch spinal needle.

Travell says that one identifies a trigger point by palpation as the most tender spot in the palpable band. She then places the muscle on stretch and tries to localize it by feeling the band roll back and forth between two fingers. She does not mark the skin. She then tries to immobilize the trigger point by pinning it down between the fingers and separating the fingers forcefully. She uses Fluori-Methane spray prior to the insertion of the needle. Travell does not add corticosteroids to the procaine solution when injecting trigger points unless the patient has bicipital tendonitis or adhesive capsulitis. Travell peppers the area in a fanlike manner in the method of Berges (11). Berges described the method in which the needle is inserted at only one point of entry, then directed at different angles

until the most sensitive region is contacted. The "tactile vision approach" is another method used by Travell and Simons wherein the needle is inserted at only one point of entry. The trigger point is carefully located with the finger and then, after inserting the needle subcutaneously, the trigger point is pressed against the finger to accurately localize it until finally the needle tip is inserted into the trigger point and the anesthetic injected by this "tactile vision" method.

For trigger points located in superficial layers of muscle, the tactile vision approach may have the advantage of accurate needling because these trigger points can be localized precisely with the finger. It is also probably useful in muscles that can be grasped (e.g., latissimus dorsi) between fingers to define trigger points on the side of the muscle opposite the puncture site. Taut bands in the superficial iliocostalis lumborum, but not the deep rotarores and multifidi, are probably helped by this particular method.

In another method akin to the fanlike approach, when a trigger area is found, the needle is moved rapidly back and forth in this region until the whole area has been "peppered" with the solution (12).

Travell always stretches after the trigger point injection. She says that this is an integral part of the procedure. Travell follows the injection with the application of a hot pack.

Russek (1959, personal communication) used a 1½-inch, 22-gauge needle after finding the trigger point. He did this after spraying vapo-coolant on the skin, without skin marking. Russek injected local anesthetic with steroids on the way in as he attempted to hit the trigger point. This method is the direct approach, in which the needle is inserted at only one point of entry in an oblique angle (about 60°) and injection of the anesthetic is begun subcutaneously, and thereafter continued as the needle is advanced to maximal depth, where the trigger point is located. This technique was used since the patient did not feel the injection. My experience with this method is that the trigger point was missed more often than with the techniques that did not inject until the trigger point was hit. Accurate localization with the needle much improves the success rate. When the trigger point is hit, the patient usually screams with pain and/or jumps. The pain is not only local, but along the referral path as well. That is when the fluid should be injected. With Russek's direct approach the patient feels nothing when the trigger point is hit, and the clinician has no idea when to inject.

Kraus (1962, personal communication) palpates

the trigger point and when he has located it places a scratch "X" over it. He then sterilizes the area with Tincture of Merthiolate in light-skinned individuals, which is then wiped off with alcohol. In light-skinned individuals the "X" stands out in red and the trigger point can then be injected with a no-touch technique. Ethyl chloride spray is used to cool the "X" and the needle is inserted. In the deeper muscles in the low back, Kraus uses a 22-gauge, 3.5-inch spinal needle. He then peppers the various trigger points, but in a circle. After the trigger point injections, Kraus stretches the muscle and then gives the patient 3 days of aftercare with electrical stimulation using both continuous tetanizing and surging sinusoidal electrical stimulation.

The technique the author prefers is a mixture of the above techniques. I locate the trigger point manually. Where there is doubt as to whether there is a trigger point, I prefer not to inject but to use preliminary treatment such as electrical stimulation using both continuous tetanizing and surging sinusoidal stimulation with or without superficial heat to reduce the surrounding muscle spasm. I then locate the trigger point as accurately as possible with a finger. It is important to realize that if one moves one fingerbreadth away from a trigger point, the area should be completely nontender.

While the bands that Travell describes occasionally exist, in many instances these bands can be relaxed by heat or electrical stimulation and the trigger point then can be more accurately localized. When it is localized I place a scratch in the shape of an "X" over the point of maximal tenderness. I use Tincture of Merthiolate to sterilize and to darken the "X" and then use alcohol sponges to sterilize and to clean off the Tincture of Merthiolate every place but in the scratch. This is useful for all lightskinned individuals and shows up the area of injection as a bright red "X." The purpose of the scratch is twofold: not only is the physician able to inject with the no-touch technique, but also the "X" is visible for 2–3 weeks after the injection. If the patient is cured then the "X" has served its first purpose. However, if the patient continues to complain of pain the examiner then can reexamine the person's back a few days later and see whether the injected trigger point was missed and is therefore still tender or whether the patient is complaining of tenderness from surrounding trigger points. No one can remember exactly where he/she injected a few days later unless there is some physical sign to indicate where the injection was. The "X" serves that purpose. Very often the patient says that he/she feels exactly the same as previously, but one can see that the trigger point that is now tender is anywhere between 0.5 and 2 inches away from the previous site of injection. The new sites of injection are then marked and injected as previously.

For the gluteal muscles I routinely use a 3.5-inch, 22-gauge spinal needle, which is disposable. It is important to know that when one injects in the thorax one should use a 25- or 27-gauge needle no longer than 1 inch. This is so that if by chance the pleura is punctured, the hole is small and it can seal readily. I have had two cases of pneumothorax in my career. They are frightening both to the patient and the physician. In one, the patient had a spinal deformity with scoliosis. The danger of getting a penumothorax impels me to try to use conservative measures prior to the trigger point injections.

Comparison of Injection Techniques

The precise technique of needling has recently been studied by Bocobo et al. (4). Twenty-two patients with myofascial pain syndrome underwent one of three different injection techniques. These were the direct, the fanlike, and the tactile vision methods. Responses in muscle spasm tenderness and eight pain-related categories were determined before treatment and 2 days and 5 days after treatment. The fanlike method was found to be most effective in relieving muscle spasm and was superior in alleviating tenderness. It was also preferred over the other two techniques in several pain-related categories. This indicated that the pain relief was not only due to the type of agent used, but could be enhanced by the injection method.

When one injects a solution rather than using the dry needling technique, the volume of the solution is more important than the solution used in my opinion. We have found that in patients who are allergic or diabetic, steroids or procaine or other local anesthetics, while shortening the afterpain, do not influence the efficacy of the injection. The volume of the solution is important, and I routinely inject anywhere between 5 and 12 ml in any trigger point or group of trigger points using the peppering circle method of injection.

Latent trigger points are those what do not cause pain during normal activities, but cause pain when palpated. Satellite trigger points are those that are located in muscles that are in the zone of pain referral from an active trigger point. No study has shown the actual incidence of those two types of trigger points among individuals affected by active trigger points; however, a method that introduces the local anesthetic at different points while inside the muscle affected would be more beneficial than one that introduces the anesthetic at only one point in the presence of these two types of trigger points. When multiple trigger points are present in one region of a muscle, all tender spots in that region should be eliminated before leaving it.

The fanlike method appears to be the superior method in relieving the tautness of the muscle in which there are trigger points (4). The fanlike method may have more effect in mechancially disrupting the trigger points or free nerve endings, which are the sensory and motor components of the feedback loop responsible for self-perpetuation of trigger point activity. Because of the greater extent of needle reach with the fanlike technique, another mechanism could possibly be greater release of intracellular potassium as a result of damage of muscle fibers, which could cause a depolarization block of the nerve fibers in areas where extracellular potassium reached sufficient concentration. Since injection by the direct method involves release of the anesthetic starting at the subcutaneous level, this would theoretically cause less volume of the anesthetic to reach the muscle layers (especially in obese individuals). It is noteworthy to remember that another possible mechanism is the "washout" of any nerve-sensitizing substances, which would reduce the irritability of the trigger point and inactivate neural feedback mechanisms.

For trigger points located in superficial layers of muscle, the tactile vision approach may have the advantage of accurate needling because these trigger points can be localized precisely with the finger. It is also probably useful in muscles that can be grasped (e.g., latissimus dorsi) between fingers to define trigger points on the side of the muscle opposite the puncture site. Taut bands in the superficial iliocostalis lumborium, but not the deep rotarores and multifidi, are probably helped by this particular method.

Reasons for failure of injection in patients may include: overlooking other active trigger points in the myotatic unit; injecting a latent trigger point and not the responsible active trigger point (3); injecting the area of referred pain and referred tenderness (13); and needling the vicinity of the trigger point, including needling of the tense band, but actually missing the trigger point itself (14). The last reason may actually irritate or worsen the patient's condition.

Despite findings indicating no significant differences in most of the parameters between the injection methods, almost all patients followed showed a prolonged response. Possible mechanisms include interruption of reflex trophic circuits; endogenous opioids; release and depletion of substance P, kinins, or histamine from primary nerve fibers; altered electrical impedance of myofascial tissue; changes in sympathetic tone; lysis of peripheral nerve fibers; and vascular uptake of injectate with systemic effects in patients with prolonged response (15).

OTHER INJECTION TECHNIQUES

Many different injection techniques have been used to relieve pain, with the proponents all claiming success. This author believes that there is a good reason for this variability.

Injection therapies are part of a broad spectrum of pain-relieving methods that this author believes act through similar mechanisms. Pain perception and tolerance are affected by the central excitatory state (16) of the brain and spinal cord and possibly other synapses. Modification of the central excitatory state by any means changes both the threshold of pain and the intensity and quality of the sensation. Modification can be obtained by sensory input from the skin via sensors for touch, vibration, and temperature, and by muscle sensors, tendon organs, proprioceptors, and the like. Since we now know that the autonomic nervous system is not autonomic, but can be controlled by the will, it is clear that the systems are integrated. Sensations from internal organs are appreciated by the central nervous systems, and they modify the central excitatory state. Many stimuli cause the release of endorphins, cortisol, and other endogenous analgesics and anti-inflammatories. They also interfere with pain transmission, modulation, and appreciation. They may also afect mood and expectation, all known modifiers of pain tolerance (15). This theory seems to unify and explain why widely divergent treatment methods appear to be effective. Further research in all of these methods is needed urgently.

There have developed pain treatment methods based on stimulation of the dermatomes, the myotomes, and the sclerotomes. They include injection and noninjection techniques.

Acupuncture (17) stimulates the dermatomes. This changes the central excitatory state in the central nervous system. Shiatzu (6) and acupressure (7) are almost identical in effect when they are effective. Zone therapy, reflexology, and Rood sensory stimulation are all effective. They probably work on a similar basis of stimulating the dermatomes and changing the central excitatory state and endogenous substance release. It is hard to find another reason that they work when the techniques are otherwise so different. I have seen the methods

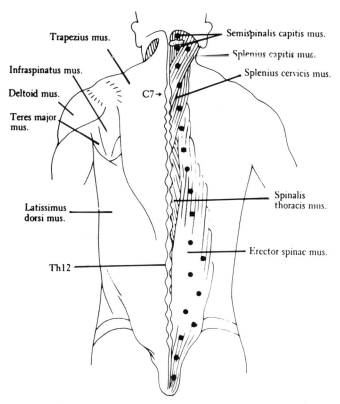

Figure 7.1. Common back tender points benefited by Edagawa therapy.

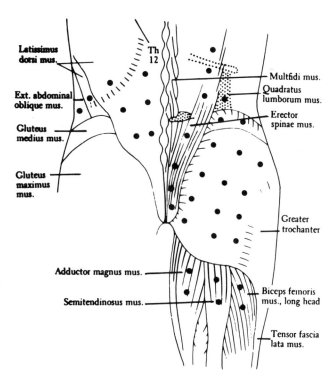

Figure 7.2. More detailed lower back and upper thigh tender points helped by Edagawa treatment. Many are also trigger point locations and/or acupuncture points.

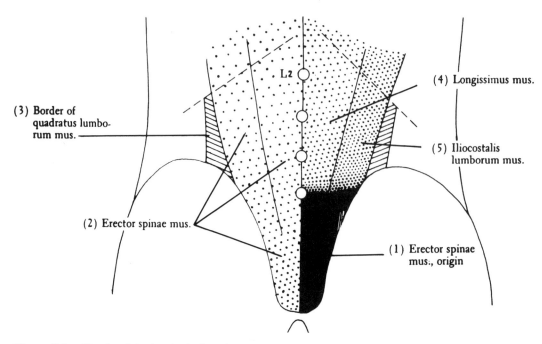

(3) Border of
quadratus lumbo-
rum mus. ——

(4) Longissimus mus.

(5) Iliocostalis
lumborum mus.

(2) Erector spinae mus.

(1) Erector spinae
mus:, origin

L2

Figure 7.3. Muscls of the low back that should be injected. The deep and superficial layers should all be injected.

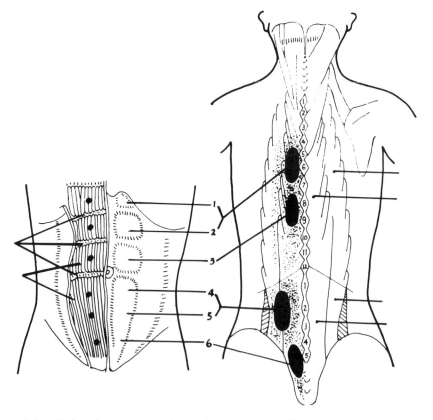

Figure 7.4. Back with common tender areas and corresponding abdominal injection sites.

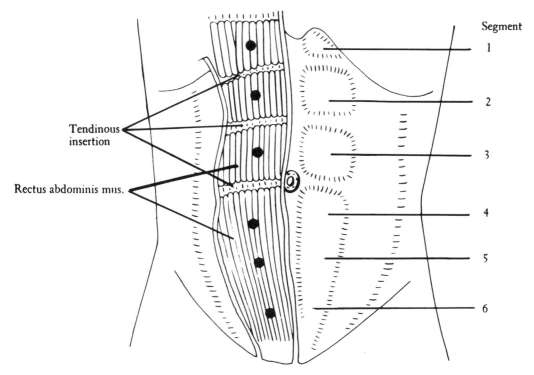

Figure 7.5. Abdominal injection sites to stimulate sensory fibers of anterior primary ramus.

give pain relief. The practitioners are not fakers, and the patients are getting more than placebo therapy.

Osteopuncture (18–20) uses electrical stimulation of the periosteum to relieve pain in the back and elsewhere. This appears to me to stimulate the sclerotomes and thus modify the central excitatory state in the spinal cord. The pain relief is not only local, but also fairly widespread. The distribution of the relief is different from that of acupuncture. It relieves the deep, boring, poorly localized pain that some patients have. Osteomassage is to osteopuncture what acupressure is to acupuncture (21).

The new myotomal stimulating Edagawa techniques (22) involves the injection of a dilute solution of soluble steroids and local anesthetic into the muscles that are tender (Fig. 7.1). The injection is done on the contralateral side as well (Fig. 7.2) so as to increase the stimuli at the appropriate spinal cord level(s) and in both the back muscles (Fig.7.3) that are innervated by that posterior primary ramus and the limb and abdominal muscles (Fig. 7.4) innervated by the same anterior primary ramus. The injections are thus in the limbs, back, abdomen (Fig. 7.5), and/or head and neck. This has been extremely effective in my experience in reliev-

ing back pain and the vague complaints that many patients have. The muscles stimulated are those in specific spinal segments.

While the details of all of these methods cannot be described in this short chapter, the references will lead the reader to explore them to benefit his/her patients.

REFERENCES

1. Mooney V, Robertson J: The facet syndrome. *Clin Orthop* 115:149–156, 1976.
2. Kraus H: *Clinical Treatment of Back and Neck Pain.* New York, McGraw-Hill, 1970.
3. Travell JG, Simons DG: *Myofascial Pain and Dysfunction: The Trigger Point Manual.* Baltimore, Williams & Wilkins, 1983.
4. Bocobo CR, Friedmann LW, Shapiro D: Myofascial pain syndrome: a comparison of different techniques. Poster Presentation, International Federation of Physical Medicine and Rehabilitation, Xth Congress, Toronto, Canada, April 11–15, 1988.
5. Friedmann LW, Galton L: *Fredom From Backaches.* New York, Simon & Schuster, 1973.
6. Irwin Y, Wagenvoord J: *Shiatzu.* Philadelphia, JB Lippincott, 1976.

7. Chan P: *Finger Acupressure*. New York, Ballantine Books, 1975.

8. Melzack R, Stillwell DM, Fox EJ: Trigger points and acupuncture points for pain: correlations and implications. *Pain* 3:3–23, 1977.

9. Lewit K: The needle effect in the relief of myofascial pain. *Pain* 6:83–90, 1979.

10. Travell J: *Office Hours: Day and Night*. New York, World Publishing Co, 1968.

11. Berges PU: Myofascial pain syndromes. *Postgrad Med* 53(6):161–168, 1973.

12. Gold H, Travell J: Cornell Conference on Therapy: management of pain due to muscle spasm. *NY State J Med* 45:2085–2097, 1945.

13. Zohn DA, Mennell JMcM: *Musculoskeletal Pain: Diagnosis and Physical Treatment*. Boston, Little, Brown and Co, 1976.

14. Bardeen CR: The musculature. In Jackson CM (ed): *Morris's Human Anatomy,* ed 6. Philadelphia, Blakiston's Son & Co, 1921, sec 5.

15. Hameroff SR, Crago BR, Blitt CD, et al: Comparison of bupivacaine, etidocaine, and saline for trigger-point therapy. *Anesth Analg* 60:752–755, 1981.

16. Sherrington CS: *The Integrative Action of the Nervous System*. New Haven, CT, Yale University Press, 1906.

17. Gunn CC: Type IV acupuncture points. *Acupuncture* 5:51–52, 1977.

18. Lawrence RM: A new method of pain control by stimulation of the periosteum of the bone. *Am J Acupuncture* 4:37–40, 1976.

19. Lawrence RM: New approach to the treatment of chronic pain: combination therapy. *Am J Acupuncture* 5:59–62, 1978.

20. Lawrence RM: The periosteum: neurophysiology and its role in treatment. *Ann Sport Med* 3:2:85–87, 1987.

21. Lawrence RM, Rosenberg S: *Pain Relief with Osteomassage*. Santa Barbara, CA, Woodbridge Press, 1982.

22. Edagawa N, Friedmann LW: *The Treatment of Disordered Function—from Pain to Sexual Complaints*. Smithtown, NY, Exposition Press, 1981.

Chapter 8

ACUPUNCTURE

GEORGE A. ULETT, MD, PhD

Acupuncture is a neurophysiologic phenomenon. Major work from China in support of this statement has been beautifully summarized by Han in a collection of papers detailing work done at the Beijing Medical College between 1973 and 1987 (1). Numerous studies from the laboratory of Pomeranz are summarized, along with other important studies, in a chapter entitled, "Scientific Basis of Acupuncture" that appeared in 1987 (2). My own small book in support of this thesis appeared in 1982 and is entitled *"Principles and Practice of Physiologic Acupuncture"* (3). Prior to this the vast majority of published texts were mainly repetitions of metaphysical explanations given in the over 3000-year-old *Nei Ching* (4). This ancient text was the written work compiling the observations and explanations given by many generations of Chinese healers. Although their keen observations were of diseases and treatment reactions that have been unchanged over centuries, the explanations were formulated at a time when there was no knowledge of anatomy, physiology, or biochemistry. Hence, their theories, based upon Taoistic religious beliefs, superstition, and numerology, have little relevance today. There is much scientific knowledge that now explains acupuncture in terms of what actually happens in the body when an electrical stimulus is given through a needle inserted in such a manner as to access the nervous system. Such stimulation of the nervous system is what acupuncture is all about.

It is unfortunate that the scientific mechanisms that modify pain pathways were not well known when acupuncture was first introduced into the Western world. There is still in the United States great confusion over what acupuncture actually is and by whom it should be practiced.

HISTORICAL NOTES

This ancient method for the control of back pain and other maladies had its origin in China some 4000 years ago. In approximately 300 AD acupuncture was brought to the attention of Europeans at a time when Western medicine was still concerned with the harsher procedures of blistering and phlebotomy. By the year 1880, there was considerable interest in acupuncture in Europe. In 1825, Chevalier Sarlandiere demonstrated the application of an electric current from Leyden jars to inserted needles. It has been reported that Gennai Hiraga in Japan had similarly used electroacpuncture in 1764. By 1840, Leed's Infirmary in England became a center for the treatment of rheumatism by acupuncture. From England it spread to the United States. Mention of its use here was made in a surgical treatise by Billroth in 1863. In 1916 Sir William Osler, in the eighth edition of *"Principles and Practice of Medicine,"* stated that "For lumbago acupuncture is, in acute cases, the most efficient treatment" (5). There was then a hiatus of some 60 years before this advice was again taken seriously by physicians in the United States. This was not so in other parts of the world.

Treatment by acupuncture continued in Europe, particularly in France and Germany, where it is widely used. In the United States it received little or no attention throughout most of the 20th century until the visit of President Nixon to China in 1972. At that time a member of the Press Corps, James Reston, had an emergency appendectomy performed in China. He reported upon his relief from postappendectomy pain by means of acupuncture. At that time, with the parting of the bamboo curtain, there was considerable interest in things Chinese and the idea that tiny needles could relieve pain widely fascinated the American public. Its use as an anesthetic in surgical procedures created great interest. Reports in the popular press presented acupuncture as a "cure-all." This created an instant demand for such treatments by patients with chronic pain of varied etiology.

Explanation of the acupuncture phenomenon in terms of Yin/Yang and other Oriental metaphysical and superstitious ideas was unacceptable to American physicians. They were quick to explain its action as hypnosis or placebo or simply an Oriental stoicism. The American Medical Association, in 1972, cautioned against acupuncture quackery and since then has labeled acupuncture an "experimental procedure."

The public, however, was not to be put off. Patients with chronic pain sought this treatment with great hope, and rising to meet their need were hundreds of persons with no formal medical training. Such practitioners immersed themselves in the theories of ancient Chinese metaphysical methods of diagnosis and treatment. This resulted in a pressure that produced premature decisions by poorly informed legislators. Upward of a dozen states passed legislation licensing the practice of acupuncture as a treatment specialty but, at the same time, without limitation on its usage by persons with no medical qualifications. In California, applicants for such certification are not even required to know the English language because examinations can be taken in Chinese. As a result of this confusion, and because available books and courses are simply repetitions of ancient philosophical concepts, American physicians have been most reluctant to add this treatment to their clinical practice, thus depriving their patients of a valuable and effective treatment.

ACUPUNCTURE IS NOT HYPNOSIS

Two leading hypnotists with vast experience in hypnosis, but little with acupuncture, stated early on that acupuncture was a kind of Oriental induction ceremony (6, 7). As one becomes more familiar with acupuncture, such opinions can certainly change. Patrick Wall stated in 1972, "My own belief is that . . . acupuncture is an effective use of hypnosis" (8). In 1974, after a study tour of China, he retracted that statement (9). Ronald Katz stated, "I have assisted at four operations under acupuncture anesthesia and many more than that under hypnosis. The patients behave differently. Those

under hypnosis are . . . seemingly unaware of what is going on about them. Patients under acupuncture were part of the team, joking, laughing, and commenting freely" (10).

My own experience has been similar. When I first read of acupuncture, I, too, believed that it must be a form of hypnosis. My coworkers and I were awarded the first NIH grant[a] to study the relationship between acupuncture and hypnosis. We studied healthy female volunteers using cold pressor (water bath) pain and also the pain of electrical stimulation used for eliciting somatosensory-evoked potentials. We used the protective effects of hypnotic suggestion and of acupuncture needles inserted at both specific (acupuncture) points and nonspecific (false) points. We used acupuncture both with and without electrical stimulation. We compared the analgesia that was produced by 10 mg of morphine sulfate given intramuscularly and the administration of analgesia by hypnosis. We found that hypnosis, electroacupuncture, and morphine sulfate were all able to reduce experimental pain at a level of statistical significance (11, 12) (Fig. 8.1). While needle insertion alone was somewhat effective, needles inserted at true acupuncture points with electrical stimulation produced a more significant amount of analgesia (13).

Thus, it was our conclusion that electroacupuncture, given at specific acupuncture points with electrical stimulation, was an effective agent for reducing experimental pain. We concluded also that hypnotic susceptibility does not account for the effectiveness of acupuncture (14).

In our clinical experience with some patients in whom acupuncture failed, we have turned to hypnosis with good results. In that regard, it has become increasingly clear that hypnosis and acupuncture act in different ways upon the complex pain mechanisms within the central nervous system.

In our work we were able to identify some points on the skin that had a standing electrical potential different from that of surrounding tissue (15, 16). Some of these points had locations identical to those of classical acupuncture points, and others did not. In view of this, and upon learning of the work of Liu (17), the conclusion seemed obvious that what the early Chinese had discovered were the motor points. This fitted in with observations of Gunn (18) regarding the importance of points on Golgi tendon organs and of Travell's (19) use of

---

[a] Grant NIGMS-CPS-1-RO1-GM-20621 (1972).

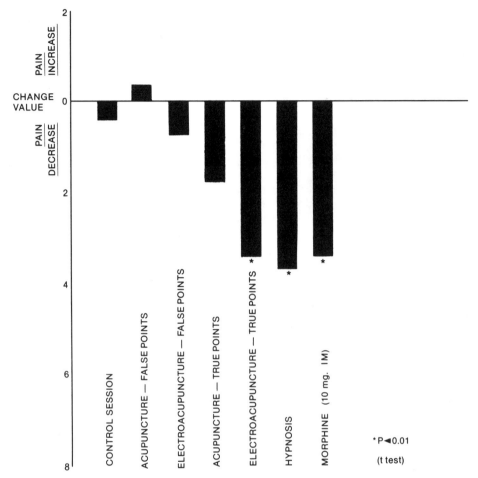

Figure 8.1. Comparison of changes in subjective experience of experimental pain with difficult pain challengers in 20 subjects.

trigger points, which coincide with the "ah shih" points of acupuncture as clearly expounded by Chung (20).

We concluded, therefore, that the most useful acupuncture points had nothing to do with a mysterious energy "chi" traveling over nonexistent meridians, but rather that we were dealing with trigger points, motor points, points over Golgi tendon organs and adjacent to major nerve trunks. In reality, then, it appeared to us, from our own experience and the findings of others, that the essence of what acupuncture is all about has nothing to do with hypnosis but rather has an acceptable scientific explanation. Acupuncture is thus concerned with the best way to get a stimulus into the central nervous system. I have expressed this view repeatedly (21–27) and use it in my teaching of medical students. It is only recently, however, that

there has been sufficient exploration of the neurochemistry of the nociceptive system to piece together a scientific explanation that is acceptable to Western-trained physicians.

SCIENTIFIC STUDIES AND THEORIES OF ACUPUNCTURE ACTION

NEUROCHEMICAL MECHANISMS OF ACUPUNCTURE

Systematic studies on the neurochemical mechanisms of acupuncture have been conducted by Dr. Ji-Sheng Han and his associates at Beijing University (1). This outstanding work has not only removed the veil of metaphysics from the over 3000-year-old Chinese medical treatment, but has vastly advanced knowledge of the brain's circuitry concerned with pain perception and its modulation. Initially, observations made of the rate of recovery of surgical patients after receiving acupuncture analgesia prompted the use of crossinfusion of cerebrospinal fluid in two cats, one of which received electroacpunucture and the other only the spinal fluid perfusate. Both cats experienced a change in pain threshold (28). Encouraged by the new techniques of neurobioassay (29), Han then embarked upon a series of experiments aimed at discovering which neurohumors were responsible for this transfer of analgesic properties.

Early studies (28) showed that, of the classical neurotransmitters, serotonin was the most important for mediating acupuncture analgesia. It was found that the effect of acupuncture analgesia was markedly decreased when the brain was depleted of 5-hydroxytryptophan (5-HTP), the serotonin precursor (30). Similarly, chlorimipramine, a tricyclic compound that selectively facilitated serotonergic transmission, potentiated the effect of acupuncture analgesia (31). The central catecholamine, norepinephrine, was found to have an antagonistic effect upon acupuncture in the brain (32), but was essential for the mediation of acupuncture analgesia in the spinal cord.

Enhancement of the action of the endorphin system and, thus, enhancement of acupuncture analgesia, may be induced by D-amino acids (33), such as D-phenylalanine (34).

The role of midbrain monoamines is of importance. Parachlorphenylalanine (PCTA), which blocks the biosynthesis of serotonin, blocks acupuncture analgesia in the rabbit (35). Methysergide, which blocks serotonin receptors, has been shown to have a similar effect in mice (36). Han et al. (31), showed that forebrain serotonin is more important than spinal cord serotonin for acupuncture analgesia. Yohimbine, a norepinephrine α-antagonist, given systemically, blocks acupuncture analgesia (37). Hammond (38) combined intrathecal antagonists (methysergide for serotonin and phentolamine for norepinephrine) and produced marked antagonism of descending analgesia from brainstem stimulation. Thus, there is good collective evidence that the monoamines serotonin and norepinephrine play a role in acupuncture analgesia.

In the 1950s, Chang (39) discovered that the site of analgesic action of morphine was in the brain. Knowledge of nature's own morphine-like substance, the endorphins, opened up a whole new chapter in pain research.

There is much evidence to support the role of endorphins in acupuncture analgesia. Mayer et al. (40) studied laboratory-induced tooth pain in humans, producing acupuncture analgesia by manual twirling of needles in LI-4, the first dorsal interosseus motor point of the hand. In a double-blind study, they found that naloxone blocked this analgesia while saline did not.

Microinjection studies of naloxone into the periacqueductal gray or intrathecally over the spinal cord decreased acupuncture analgesia in rats and rabbits (41). Other sites that do not contain endorphins show no such naloxone effects. It was found that the opioid peptides could be grouped into the enkephalins, endorphins, and dynorphins. Working with Terenius, Han (42), using the antibody injection technique, showed that enkephalins were mediators for acupuncture analgesia in both the brain and spinal cord, whereas β-endorphin was effective in the brain but not in the spinal cord. In a carefully conducted experiment Han and Xie (43) also showed that dynorphin antiserum blocked acupuncture analesia in rabbits.

It was found that dynorphins (44) were effective in the spinal cord but not in the brain. Thus, in summary, it could be seen that acupuncture could release β-endorphins and enkephalins in the brain and dynorphins and enkephalins in the spinal cord.

Peetz and Pomeranz (45) bred a strain of mice with a congenital deficiency in endorphin receptors. These mice produced less than half the electroacupuncture analgesia seen in normal strains of mice. These workers hypothesized that the 30% of humans who do not respond to acupuncture analgesia may well have a genetic deficiency in opiate receptors in the central nervous system.

Important correlates of the endorphin acupuncture analgesia hypothesis are found in the reports by Sjolund et al. (46) that endorphins are increased in cerebrospinal fluid with acupuncture stimulation. A doubling of the endorphin level in cerebrospinal fluid occurred within 30 min of stimulation. Similarly, an increase of 50% in blood cortisol occurred with stimulation at acupuncture points but there was no such increase with stimulation at nonacupuncture points (47).

Traditional acpuncturists have observed that different types of needle manipulation at the same point could bring about different results. Needling at St-36 (anterior tibialis motor point) could, for example, treat diarrhea in one case and constipation in another. Following this lead, a possible explanation was found when it was shown that low-frequency (2–4 Hz) stimulation could cause profound release of met-enkephalin whereas high frequency (80–100 Hz) stimulation would release dynorphins.

Pomeranz and Cheng (48) showed that naloxone would block low-frequency (4 Hz) electroacupuncture. Acupuncture analgesia produced by low-frequency stimulation is endorphinergic (49, 50). Acupuncture analgesia produced by high-frequency stimulation is not affected by naloxone but is monoaminergic and can be enhanced by the serotonin precursor 5-HTP (31).

It was shown by Pomeranz (51) and Watkins and Mayer (52) that antagonists such as maloxone work best when given before the acupuncture treatment and may fail to reverse the acupuncture analgesia once it is established. This may well be due to the fact that naloxone binds poorly to kappa receptors and, hence, may have difficulty overcoming the effect of dynorphin.

Since the analgesic effect of met-enkephalin is mediated mainly by mu and delta receptors and that of dynorphins by kappa receptors, it becomes apparent that by using specific parameters of electrical stimulation of acupuncture needles, one may switch on and off the activity of various peptidergic systems of the central nervous system for different therapeutic purposes.

The work of Han has clearly shown that it is the frequency rather than the intensity of the stimulation that is of the utmost importance in producing acupuncture analgesia (53), and thus it may be that lack of response to electroacupuncture could well be overcome by finding the proper parameters of stimulation for each individual. Because the acupuncture effect depends upon manipulation of biochemical systems that have widespread effects throughout the central nervous system, it has become apparent that the effectiveness of acupuncture stimulation is not dependent upon the specific placement of needles. It is only important perhaps that some locations have a greater overall effect than others. Thus a needle placed in Hoku (doral interosseus motor point of the thumb), or any other motor point distal on the upper extremity, may produce widespread analgesic effects through actuating the β-endorphinergic and enkephalinergic systems. Simultaneous stimulation of another point, for example, Tsu San Li on the leg (tibialis anterior motor point), might produce an additive effect. On the other hand, if one wishes to stimulate the release of dynorphins for local effect mediated by spinal cord nerves, stimulation of motor points in the neurotome supplying the area of pain could

conceivably add yet another dimension of analgesia.

The work of Han also demonstrated the importance of the phenomenon of acupuncture tolerance (54). With continuous stimulation acupuncture analgesia may be completely abolished within 6 hours. It appears that γ-aminobutyric acid and cholecystokinin-8 may be important in antagonizing acupuncture analgesia. The implication here is that electroacupuncture stimulation should be given intermittently. Therefore, clinically, electroacupuncture stimulation is often given for periods of 20–30 min daily with a stimulus that delivers alternating low (2–4 Hz) and high (80–100 Hz) frequencies.

The work of Han has clearly delineated anatomic areas that are important way stations in the central nervous system network responsible for mediation and control of noxious input. Four nuclei—accumbens, amygdala, habenula, and the periacqueductal gray—were found to be sensitive areas where naloxone was most effective in blocking acupuncture analgesia. It became clear that there was a mesolimbic loop (55) with connections between accumbens, habenula, and periacqueductal gray, and if this loop was broken at any of the nuclei the impulses necessary for the modulation of pain at the dorsal horn neurone of the spinal cord would be interrupted.

It was also found that the hindbrain neural circuits are essential for control of the spinal gating mechanisms. If the upward flow from acupuncture stimulation is blocked supratentorially there is considerable interference with the analgesic effect (55).

The role of the hypothalamus is clearly indicated. All of the β-endorphin cells of the brain are found in the arcuate nucleus of the hypothalamus and in the pituitary gland (56). From the arcuate nucleus β-endorphins are released that stimulate long-reaching axons to affect midbrain pain control mechanisms (57). Lesions in the arcuate nucleus can abolish acupuncture analgesia in a rat (58).

Brain and blood levels of β-endorphin are elevated by stress (59). Although we are concerned mainly with the effect of acupuncture on pain in this discussion, it is important to note that other effects of acupuncture, such as upon infections and the immune system, may be attributed to the fact that the precursor molecule for β-endorphin is the same precursor molecule from which adrenocorticotropic hormone (ACTH) is formed. Thus, for every molecule of β-endorphin produced by electroacupuncture stimulation, simultaneously a molecule of ACTH is released.

In summary, acupuncture stimulates the endogenous pain-modulating system to release serotonin, opioid substances, and other transmitters at three levels of the central nervous system—the spinal cord, the thalamus, and the cerebral cortex—thus serving to dampen the perception and transmission of nociceptive signals. How these impulses enter the central nervous system to produce the neurochemical effects demonstrated above is, of course, of the utmost importance to an understanding of the acupuncture phenomenon.

PERCEPTION AND TRANSMISSION OF PAIN SIGNALS

Melzack and Melinkoff (60) raised the pain threshold by stimulating the cat's midbrain reticular formation. Andersson concluded that stimulation of the muscle afferents at intensities activating high-threshold nerves can produce acupuncture effects (61). A sensation of "Teh Chi" (swelling, drawing, soreness, and numbness), said to be essential for obtaining therapeutic effectiveness of acupuncture, arises from A-delta fibers and, thus, is mainly derived from muscle nerves. As noted injection of novocaine into the skin does not block the acupuncture effect whereas deep injection into the muscle tissue often does.

Once pain signals have entered the dorsal horn of the spinal cord they spread widely throughout the central nervous system. Andersson and coworkers in Göteborg (62–65), working with pain from tooth pulp stimulation in the cat, ascertained that information interpreted as pain reached the cortex by multiple paths, some spreading diffusely and some proceeding directly over the thalamocortical pathways and ultimately terminating in laminae IV of the cortex. Studies from China (66) showed that these stimulated potentials in the sensory cortex could be abolished by stimulation of the acupuncture point LI-4 (motor point of the dorsal interosseus muscle).

The widespread nature of pain responses has also been confirmed by observations of an increased cerebral blood flow over large regions of the cerebral cortex after a noxious stimulus (67). This has also been beautifully demonstrated by the work of Hand (68), who indexed pain pathways throughout the central nervous system by means of labeled deoxyglucose. He then studied the powerful acupuncture point Tsu San Li (anterior tibialis motor point) and detected a statistically significant decrease in neuronal activity at representative points throughout the central nervous system pain network when acupuncture was delivered simultaneously with the pain stimulus. Taken together,

such explanations clearly demonstrated the effect of acupuncture as an electrophysiologic event modifying pain impulses.

While such explanations may serve to describe the modulation of acute, ongoing, pain phenomena, they still leave questions regarding the perception and control of chronic pain.

When acupuncture is used as an analgesic for surgery, stimulation is started 20–40 min prior to the operation to permit a build-up (recruiting, deepening) of sufficient analgesia to allow surgery with sensation but without pain. When the analgesia-producing electroacupuncture stimulation is stopped, it has been observed that, while diminishing, the effect lasts over a period of 30 min or more. What, then, might be the mechanism for relief from chronic pain over even longer periods of time or permanently?

It seems probable on the basis of known physiology that, in establishing conditions of chronic pain, the ancient, slowly conducting system of C fibers takes dominion over the more phylogenetically recent, rapidly conducting large myelinated fibers. With continuing stimulation from tissue damage or irritation, the pain becomes continuous or chronically intermittent. Such continuous bombardment of the neuraxis by noxious stimuli could well produce a kindling effect (69) within eurone pools of the central nervous system such that reverberating circuits are created with self-perpetuation or continuation of the pain sensations. This type of self-sustaining activity was described by Lorente de No (70) and Dusser de Barenne and McCulloch (71). Such circuits at the spinal cord level have been described by Loeser et al. in the deafferented spinal cord in a patient with continuing paraplegic pain (72). This self-generated abnormal bursting activity in the spinal cord has also been described by the above workers in the cat with chronic deafferentation.

Such spinal reverberating circuits could serve to constantly activate midbrain and cortical pain mechanisms via ascending pathways. This might explain the continuing memory of pain in the central nervous system long after the original tissue injury has been repaired. In the case of phantom limb pain, it would appear that the activity continues to reverberate in the central circuits previously utilized by the now nonexistent limb.

An alternative mechanism could be a malfunction of the system for production and control of brain hormones that relate to the pain experience. Thus, the noxious impulses could well produce a dysregulation of those homeostatic mechanisms that are normally responsible for a return to the resting stage after the sensation of acute pain has given a warning for the location and extent of tissue damage. A continuing or very intense pain stimulus could presumably result in either an excessive production of the peptides responsible for the transmission of pain impulses or a breakdown in the function of those structures responsible for the production of enkephalins necessary for suppression of neuronal activity in the pain pathways.

Another possible scenario occurs when the pain impulse spreads to involve the anteromediolateral column of the spinal cord and sympathetic nervous system neurones located there are activated. Dysregulation here results in causalgia (73) with burning pain, trophic changes (glossy skin), and often a local rise in temperature. If left untreated hyperalgesia occurs, muscles become fibrosed, osteoporosis develops, and there may occur accompanying emotional symptoms.

Other posttraumatic pain syndromes as described by Livingston (73) include a peculiar distribution of pain. He speaks of "mirror image" pain in which pain develops in the noninvolved side at the precise mirrored location of the contralateral lesion. Such phenomena are explained by the spread of uncontrolled pain by neurons crossing the midlines or by spread of excitation by neurohumors to involve other neuron galaxies in the spinal cord within the same segment but on the opposite side. Livingston has also emphasized the importance of recognizing neurotome distribution, which I believe is an important principle in acupuncture treatment. An example is his "multifidus triangle syndrome." Here the innervation of the multifidus muscle by S1–3 may refer pain to both the lateral thigh and the sciatic distribution in the lower leg.

Livingston pointed out that, "In many of the causalgic states which have long been established, the higher centers become affected and all manner of physiologic and even organic changes may take place in parts of the body far removed from the original focus of irritation." In some clinical syndromes there may be a combination of somatic, visceral, and psychic irritation each contributing to the central process. Once a vicious cycle is established the process tends to become self-sustaining.

The term "pain memory" has been utilized by Melzack and others to describe such long-term chronic pain. The intensity of chronic pain may gradually abate under the application of repeated acupuncture treatments given over a period of days or weeks. This physiologic effect could thus represent a kind of kindling of activity that inhibits the reverberating pain circuits, or it may be that repeated acupuncture treatments stimulate those neuropharmacologic pain control mechanisms that somehow had been lulled into relative inactivity. Acupuncture stimuli then brings new life, as it were, into nature's own mechanism for the release of pain-inhibiting neurohumors.

NEEDLES AND NEEDLING

Acupuncture means, literally, "needle penetration," or needles through the skin. The earliest recorded acupuncture needles were of stone and were described as "stone borers." In the *Book of Mountains and Seas,* written over 2000 years ago, there is a passage that reads, "in the Kaoshigh mountains are rich deposits of jade underlaid with stones suitable for making needles." Other early needles of various types were introduced. Some were arrow- or wedge-shaped and used for blood letting. Acupuncture needles of gold and silver have been found in tombs from the Han Dynasty (206 BC to 221 AD). Such needles are still used, especially in France, where special mystical curative properties are attached to each metal, stimulation for silver and sedation for gold.

Today, acupuncturists use needles made from stainless steel. Most common are the "Hao" needles, filiform in shape and available in a variety of gauges from 26 (0.45 mm) to 32 (0.26 mm). Gauges 28 and 30 are most popular. Needles vary in length from 1 to 10 cm. Needles from 1 to 2 inches in length are most commonly used. Typically, the handles of these needles are double-wound with silver. This allows for a better grip for the twirling and twisting between forefinger and thumb that propels the needle through the skin with a drilling type of motion. The above types of needles are commonly reused and should, therefore, be carefully autoclaved.

Most recently, and with the common fear of spreading infections such as AIDS, disposable needles have become widely used. Some of these have plastic handles and come presterilized, each in a small plastic tube. For insertion, the tube is placed tightly against the skin. A sharp tap of the finger causes the needle to painlessly penetrate the skin. The tube is then removed and the needle twisted and pushed deeper into the muscle tissue.

There is little or no pain associated with proper needle technique. The more rapid the insertion the better. The fingers and skin area to be penetrated should be cleaned with alcohol prior to needle insertion. The depth of insertion must be governed by the size of the muscle mass to be penetrated in order to reach the area of stimulation. It is not possible to give a figure for the safe depth of insertion at each point because there is so much variation from one person to another. A sound knowledge of anatomy is therefore necessary for the proper practice of acupuncture. In this regard, an atlas of cross-sectional anatomy can be of particular assistance. Whenever possible, the tip of the needle should approximate a motor point. When the point is reached, the patient may experience a feeling of pressure, heavy soreness, or distention. Such sensations are termed "De Qi" or "Teh Chi." This awareness of the needles is usually not described as painful. It results from stimulation of the receptors in the muscle, including those nerves involved in proprioception and mechanoreception. This sensation occurs within a few seconds of insertion and may remain localized or can spread along the distribution of the nerve trunk. It is then experienced as a brief "electrical shock."

Most needles may be inserted vertically at 90° perpendicular to the skin. In order to bypass certain bones and organs, a 45° angle of insertion may sometimes be necessary. For points about the face and head, needles are inserted under and even more parallel to the skin surface.

COMPLICATIONS

Acupuncture is a very safe method for the treatment of back pain. Complications and side effects are far less than those seen with the administration of pain-killing drugs. If general precautions are taken no complications occur. However, because acupuncture is often done by persons with no medical training the literature describes a number of instances of untoward happenings.

Dizziness and circulatory shock (fainting) can occur, especially in persons receiving acupuncture for the first time. This may be due to emotional stress, tension, fatigue, hunger, or a liable autonomic nervous system. Be wary of patients who are highly neurotic or who experience profuse sweating and tachycardia and have a weak, thready pulse. Such patients should lie flat on the table.

Rarely needle grasp may occur, making it difficult to withdraw the needle. This is due to muscle tension or the gamma reflex and can be overcome by relaxing the patient or by the application of a second needle at an angle and adjacent to the impounded needle.

Should a needle bend, simply change the pa-tient's position and withdraw the needle in the direction of the curve. I have never experienced a broken needle. This complication can be avoided by careful selection and discarding of eroded or defective needles. With the newer disposable needles this complication should never occur.

Upon removal of the needles, each point should be carefully inspected for bleeding, which may appear even after the delay of a minute or two. Surface bleeding can be seen and controlled by pressure. Small ecchymoses may occur some hours later at the point where the needle was inserted. These are of no importance, but the patient should be informed of such possible occurrence. We have treated hemophiliac patients without this complication.

With autoclaved needles and clean technique or with the use of disposable needles, infection should never occur. I have not had a single occasion in several thousand patients. Transmission of viral hepatitis has been reported when needles have been inadequately sterilized.

In the hands of unskilled practitioners with poor knowledge of anatomy, penetration of organs, especially the intestines, bladder, lungs, and peritoneum, has been reported. Atelectasis has been reported following treatment of shoulder areas where the acupuncturist has failed to realize that the apex of the left lung in thin females may be within reach of a 2-inch needle. Selection of needles should be appropriate to the depth of muscle and the area to be treated. Too shallow penetration is less effective and too deep penetration dangerous.

Some pain or discomfort may occur with clumsy, inept technique or when blunt or hooked needles are inserted. If the patient moves during or after needle insertion, small muscle tears and pain may result. It is important, therefore, that the patient be in a position of comfort for the duration of the treatment. Needling around the face and ear or the tips of the extremities is more painful than elsewhere.

Contraindications to acupuncture include patients who are inebriated and tense or who are perspiring freely. In pregnant women, electroacupuncture should not be used in the lumbosacral outflow or on the abdomen below the umbilicus. One should always avoid swollen or infected areas and large blood vessels.

PATIENT SELECTION AND PREPARATION

I have treated patients of all ages with acupuncture. Although acupuncture is usually given in the physician's office, hospitals are increasingly tolerant of acupuncture procedures. Some insurance companies will reimburse, at last in part, for acupuncture, particularly if it is explained to them in terms such as "similar to transcutaneous electrical nerve stimulation."

There is no way to predict which patients will respond to electroacupuncture stimulation. While it has been reported that hypnotizable subjects do better than nonhypnotizable subjects, this would seem to be part of the generalization that positive suggestion added to any treatment will increase the yield. In our research and that of others, poorly hypnotizable subjects have had good results from acupuncture (14). A positive attitude is said to be predictive, but we have not found this to be universally true. We have successfully treated patients who were openly skeptical and who came to the office reluctantly at the urging of a spouse. Less positive results are found in patients who have had previous surgery. Success on the first treatment has some positive predictive value.

Patients should be psychologically prepared by some discussion of the nature of acupuncture, including the near absence of side effects, no great pain, and so forth. Patients should be placed in a comfortable position and cautioned against any gross movements of the body. The bladder should be emptied prior to treatment. The patient should have no alcohol or drugs active on the nervous system prior to treatment.

Often for the initial treatment we use very few needles and no electrical stimulation.

PLACEMENT OF NEEDLES FOR THE TREATMENT OF LOW BACK PAIN

First the patient should be examined for trigger point areas where finger pressure can reproduce the patient's typical pattern of pain either locally or referred to a distant area. Such points are described by the Chinese as "ah shi" points. This is the first choice for needle placement. If such points are not discovered needles may then be placed in paravertebral points along the muscle mass in neurotome areas that pertain to the outflow of the roots making up the distribution of the sciatic nerve. Such points are termed "bladder points" in the classical acupuncture literature and lie approximately 2 inches lateral to the vertebral column. Needles should be inserted deeply into the muscle mass in order to stimulate the motor points of the erector spinae and lower trapezius muscles.

A point on the buttocks that is frequently used lies one-third of the distance up a line drawn from the prominence of the greater trochanter to the lower tip of the sacrum. Depending upon the depth of insertion and strength of electrical stimulation here, one may activate motor points of the glutei, obturator internus, gemelli, or piriformis muscles.

Other points along the sciatic distribution can activate motor points of the long head of the biceps femoris, gastrocnemius, and flexor hallicus longus. A widely used and effective point on the lower extremity known as Tsu-San-Li (St-36) is actually the motor point of the tibialis anticus muscle.

A guide to the location of these points used in the treatment of low back pain is shown in Figure 8.2.

STIMULATION OF THE NEEDLE

Early on, and even at the present time, especially in Asia and Europe, stimulation of the acupuncture points was accomplished by manual manipulation of the needles. Rotation of the needles clockwise and counterclockwise while lifting and thrusting was a commonly described technique.

In an attempt to intensify the stimulation hundreds of years before electricity was known, the practice of moxibustion was introduced. This consists of the application of heat to acupuncture points. Moxa is a punk-like substance made from the herb *Artemesia vulgaris* (mugwort). This is mixed with tinder and then formed into small cones that are burned either directly on the skin or upon a layer of soybean paste or a small slice of ginger root. Pellets of moxa may be squeezed on the handle of acupuncture needles and ignited. Moxa is also sold and formed into sticks (cigars) that are ignited and held over the spots to be healed. This type of counterirritation formed of itself a specialty of treatment that proposed to give a greater stimulus to acupuncture treatments at a time when electricity was not yet available. Many persons with burn scars at acupuncture points testify to the ongoing popularity of this method of treatment in the Orient. Moxibustion, however, is simply another way of applying heat to the body.

Most acupuncture today is accomplished by the use of electrical stimulation. It is certainly easier to apply than manual manipulation, especially for the long periods of stimulation required for surgical analgesic techniques. Our own studies (11) have shown electrical stimulation to be 100% more effective than simple needling techniques. Because electroacupuncture produces a stronger stimulation it is often reserved for the second and subse-

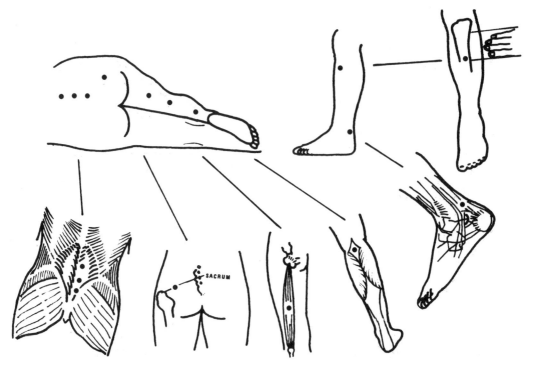

Figure 8.2. Suggested points for needle placement for electroacupuncture stimulation for the treatment of low back pain.

quent sessions, especially in patients who are initially apprehensive. With electrical stimulation some benefit can be achieved even if the needle is not precisely located because of the spread of current through the tissues.

The stimulation is brought to the needles by small wire leads from the stimulator, which in turn are attached to the needles by small clips. The paired wires are usually affixed to needles that are nearby each other, although no definite rules have been developed for such selection. The number of needles stimulated depends upon the number of lead jacks in the stimulator. These are usually three or four in number, and hence six or eight needles can be connected at one time.

A great deal of investigation remains to be done to ascertain the ideal parameters of stimulation for different types of illness. Currently, it is thought that useful stimulation can occur with currents varying from 0.5 to 50 mA. Voltages are from 0.3 to 9 V, usually produced by a 9-V dry-cell source. The waveforms vary but customarily are square waves of exponentially rising or falling form and from 0.1 to 0.3 msec in duration and occurring in

trains. Thus, these are pulsating direct-current (DC) potentials.

Pulses from 1 to 1000 Hz have been used. Some workers believe that slow pulsations (1–20 Hz) are best for acute pain and fast (80–120 Hz) pulsations are best for chronic pain. This belief is not universally held (74).

Most of the electroacupuncture equipment on the market produces a square wave output. In this case the "needle sensation" elicited from the negative electrode is much stronger than that induced from the positive lead. Polarization may be induced by long-term stimulation. To overcome such problems asymmetric, biphasic, modified square wave currents have been used, but these have afforded only a partial solution. A more successful apparatus utilizes identical wave forms with alternating polarity, thus ensuring equally intense stimulation at both electrodes.

Stimulating equipment usually gives a choice of impulse patterns, with waves being continuous or coming initially in bursts with the impulse frequency being adjustable. In dense-disperse (D-D) stimulation, a slow dispersion (e.g., 2/sec) alternates with a burst of dense (80–100 Hz) waves. I prefer this setting for all treatments.

Sessions of stimulation are typically from 15 to 30 min in duration. Although there are few data in the scientific literature to support any specific amount of stimulation, most reports indicate that improvement will occur within six to eight treatments. Some patients will improve after only one or two treatments whereas others require many more. Occasionally patients get no therapeutic response until after 10–12 treatments. Initially, some patients are treated two to three times a week; later one treatment a week is sufficient. In patients with severe pain, treatment may be given two times a day, 5 days a week. In other patients (e.g., those with chronic arthritis), it has been useful, after an initial course, to continue with maintenance treatments on a once-a-month schedule. We have found that such a schedule may prevent relapse. Other patients obtain complete relief after six or eight treatments and do not require more. Pain relief is usually cumulative with successive treatments, although here, too, the course of recovery may be irregular. If there is no relief after eight to 10 treatments, acupuncture is probably an inappropriate modality for that patient.

The duration of relief from a single treatment varies greatly. Vierck et al. (75) found in monkeys that the suppression of pain from a single treatment could last up to 70 hours, but that the pain threshold showed a major fluctuation during that time. With chronic pain, at times the greatest relief may appear 1 or 2 days after the treatment. On occasion the pain seems to increase for a few hours following the treatment before a long period of abatement.

The level of stimulation required varies from patient to patient and for the same patient from day to day. The patient should be able to feel the stimulation but it should not be at an uncomfortable level. Often there is muscle fibrillation. The current is adequate when either of the above occurs. As treatment progresses the patient may state that the stimulus is no longer felt. This is simply the result of body accommodation, with the level of stimulation remaining the same. Such accommodation is less likely to occur with a dense-disperse type of stimulating current. In susceptible individuals reddening of the skin can occur even with simple placement of the needle, but is more often seen with electroacupuncture stimulation. With careful adjustment of the current, skin burns are never seen. On theoretical grounds and because of the possible danger of inducing cardiac fibrillation, one should avoid using electrostimulation around the precordium or in any patient with an implanted pacemaker.

RESULTS OF CLINICAL STUDIES

Controlled studies of acupuncture are difficult because the insertion of needles even into non-acupuncture points can reduce pain (11). The placebo effect alone can account for 30–35% of the relief.

Good studies have shown that acupuncture is effective in 55–85% of patients with chronic pain. Review of clinical reports worldwide (76) show figures hovering around the 70% success rate. Two studies have reported results specific for back pain. One was by Matsumoto, Professor of Surgery at Hahnemann Medical School (77); the study included 78 patients with lumbosacral osteoarthritis, with total or satisfactory improvement in 83%. Stux, from Dusseldorf, Germany, treated 60 patients with a variety of etiologies of low back pain with 88% success (78).

My own experience has included over 1000 patients running the gamut from low back sprain with myalgia, radiculitis with sciatica, osteoarthritis, and fibrositis to ruptured disks. I have brought pain relief to many patients in all these categories with an overall estimate of some benefit to 70%. I would agree with Matsumoto and others that patients with continuing pain despite previous surgery are less responsive, possibly as the result of scar tissue.

Some 30% of patients fail to respond to acupuncture treatments. This is approximately the same number who fail to respond to the administration of morphine (79). Like Pomeranz' rats, these persons possibly have some inherited defect in their opiate receptor system. The administration of DL-phenylalanine can convert some patients from nonresponders to responders, but more work remains to be done to determine how best to help this group of patients.

SUMMARY

In summary, acupuncture is effective in controlling chronic back pain. This has been well documented both by clinical experience and by controlled studies. Treatment models for the mechanisms of action have now been developed. When eight to 10 treatments are given once or twice a week one can expect to see some relief of chronic back pain in 70% of patients.

REFERENCES

1. Han JS: *The Neurochemical Basis of Pain Relief by Acupuncture. A Collection of Papers 1973–1987*. Beijing, China, Beijing Medical University, 1987.
2. Pomeranz B: Scientific basis of acupuncture. In Stux G, Pomeranz B (eds): *Acupuncture Textbook and Atlas*. New York, Springer-Verlag, 1987.
3. Ulett GA: *Principles and Practice of Physiologic Acupuncture*. St. Louis, Warren Green Publisher, 1982.
4. Veith I: *Huang Ti Nei Ching Su Wen. The Yellow Emperor's Classic of Internal Medicine*. Berkeley, University of California Press, 1949.
5. Osler W: *The Principles and Practice of Medicine*, ed 8. New York, D. Appleton and Co, 1916.
6. Spiegel H, Spiegel D: *Trance and Treatment*. New York, Basic Books, 1978.
7. Kroger WS: Hypnotism and acupuncture. *JAMA* 220:1012, 1972.
8. Wall P: An eye on the needle. *New Scientist* 55:129–131, 1972.
9. Wall P: Acupuncture revisited. *New Scientist* 64:31–34, 1974.
10. Katz RL, Kao CY, Spiegel H, Katz GT: Acupuncture and hypnosis. *Adv Neurol* 44:819–825, 1974.
11. Parwatikar S, Brown M, Stern J, Ulett GA, Sletten IW: Acupuncture, hypnosis and experimental pain. I. Study with volunteers. *Acupunct Electrother Res* 3:161–190, 1978.
12. Ulett G, Parwatikar S, Stern JA, Brown M: Acupuncture, hypnosis and experimental pain. II. Study with patients. *Acupunct Electrother Res* 3:191–201, 1987.
13. Saletu B, Saletu M, Stern JA, Sletten IW, Ulett GA: Hypno-analgesia and acupuncture analgesia: a neurophysiological reality? *Neuropsychobiology* 1:218–242, 1975.
14. Ulett GA: Acupuncture is not hypnosis: recent physiological studies. *Am J Acupunct* 11(1):5–13, 1983.
15. Brown ML, Ulett GA, Stern JA: Acupuncture loci: techniques for location. *Am J Chin Med* 2:67–74, 1974.
15. Brown ML, Ulett GA, Stern JA: The effects of Acupuncture on white blood cell counts. *Am J Clin Med* 2:383–398, 1974.
17. Liu YK, Varela M, Oswald R: The correspondence between some motor points and acupuncture loci. *Am J Clin Med* 3:347–358, 1975.
18. Gunn CC: Reprints on pain, acupuncture and related subjects. From the Worker's Compensation Board of British Columbia. (Privately published.)
19. Travell J: Referred pain from skeletal muscle. *NY State J Med* 55:331–340, 1955.
20. Chung C: *Ah-shih Point*. Taipei, Taiwan, Republic of China, Chen Kwan Book Co, Ltd, 1983.

21. Ulett GA: Acupuncture and medical practice. *Mo Med* 77:12–14, 1975.
22. Ulett GA: Acupuncture—a technique for the regularly licensed physician. *Fed Bull* 62:334–343, 1975.
23. Ulett GA: Control of chronic pain by acupuncture. *Psychiatr J Univ Ottawa* 2(3):143–146, 1977.
24. Ulett GA: Acupuncture: pricking the bubble of skepticism (editorial). *Biol Psychiatry* 13:159–161, 1978.
25. Ulett GA: Acupuncture treatments for pain relief. *JAMA* 245:768–769, 1981.
26. Ulett GA: Acupuncture—time for a second look. *South Med J* 76(4):421–423, 1983.
27. Ulett GA: Acupuncture update—1984 (editorial). *South Med J* 78:237–238, 1985.
28. Research Group of Acupuncture Anesthesia, Peking Medical College: The role of some neurotransmitters of the brain in finger-acupuncture analgesia. *Sci Sin* 17:112–130, 1974.
29. Myers RD: Transfusion of cerebrospinal fluid and tissue bound chemical factors between the brains of conscious monkeys: a new neurobiological assay. *Physiol Behav* 2:373–377, 1967.
30. Research Group of Acupuncture Anesthesia, Peking Medical College: The effect of PCP and 5-HTP on acupuncture analgesia in the rat. *J New Med Pharmacol* 3:133–138, 1976.
31. Han C-S, Chou P-H, Lu C-C, Lu L-H, Yang T-S, Jen M-F (Research Group of Acupuncture Anesthesia, Peking Medical College): The role of central 5-hydroxytryptamine in acupuncture analgesia. *Sci Sin* 22:91–104, 1979.
32. Xie GX, Han JS, Hollt V: Electroacupuncture analgesia blocked by microinjection of anti-beta-endorphin antiserum into periaqueductal grey of the rabbit. *Int J Neurosci* 18:287–291, 1983.
33. Cheng R, Pomeranz B: A combined treatment with D-amino acids and electro-acupuncture produces a greater anesthesia than either treatment alone: naloxone reverses these effects. *Pain* 8:231–236, 1980.
34. Ehrenpreis S: Analgesic properties of enkephalinase inhibitors: animal and human studies. *Prog Clin Res* 192:363–370, 1985.
35. Kaada B, Jorum E, Sagvolden T: Analgesia induced by trigeminal nerve stimulation (electro-acupuncture) abolished by nuclei raphe lesions in rats. *Acupunct Electrother Res* 4:221–234, 1979.
36. Shimizu T, Koja T, et al: Effects of methysergide and naloxone on analgesia produced by peripheral electrical stimulation in mice. *Brain Res* 208:463–467, 1981.
37. Cheng R, Pomeranz B: Monoaminergic mechanisms of electroacupuncture analgesia. *Brain Res* 215:77–92, 1981.
38. Hammond DL: Pharmacology of central pain modulating networks (biogenic amines and non-opioid analgesics). In Fields H, Dubner R, Cervero F (eds): *Advances in Pain Research and Therapy*. New York, Raven Press, 1985, vol 9, pp 499–511.
39. Chang HT: Integrative action of thalamus in the

process of acupuncture for analgesia. *Sci Sin* 16:25–60, 1973.

40. Mayer DJ, Price DD, Raffii A: Antagonism of acupuncture analgesia in man by the narcotic antagonist naloxone. *Brain Res* 121:368–372, 1977.

41. Zhou ZF, Du MY, Han JS, et al: Effect of intracerebral microinjection of naloxone on acupuncture and morphine-analgesia in the rabbit. *Sci Sin* 24:1166–1178, 1981.

42. Han JS, Xie GX, Zhou ZF, Fokesoon R, Terenius L: Enkepahlin and B-endorphin as mediators of electro-acupuncture analgesia in rabbits. An antiserum microinjection study. *Adv Biochem Psychopharmacol* 33:369–377, 1982.

43. Han JS, Xie GX: Dynorphin: important mediator for electro-acupuncture analgesia in the spinal cord of the rabbit. *Pain* 18:367–377, 1984.

44. Han JS, Xie GX, Goldstein A: Analgesia induced by intrathecal injection of dynorphin B in the rat. *Life Sci* 34:1573–1579, 1984.

45. Peets J, Pomeranz B: CXBX mice deficient in opiate receptors show poor electro-acupuncture analgesia. *Nature* 273:675–676, 1978.

46. Sjolund B, Terenius L, Eriksson M: Increased cerebrospinal fluid levels of endorphins after electro-acupuncture. *Acta Physiol Scand* 100:382–384, 1977.

47. Masala A, Satta G, Alagna S, et al: Suppression of electro-acupuncture (EA)-induced beta-endorphin and ACTH release by hydrocortisone in man. Absence of effects on EA-induced anesthesia. *Acta Endocrinol (Copenh)* 103:469–472, 1983.

48. Pomeranz B, Cheng R: Suppression of noxious responses in single neurones of cat spinal cord by electro-acupuncture and its reversal by the opiate antagonist naloxone. *Exp. Neurol* 64:327–341, 1979.

49. Cheng R, Pomeranz B: Electro-acupuncture analgesia could be mediated by at least two pain relieving mechanisms: endorphin and non-endorphin systems. *Life Sci* 25:1957–1962, 1980.

50. Sjolund BH, Erikson BE: The influence of naloxone on analgesia produced by peripheral conditioning stimulation. *Brain Res* 173:295–301, 1979.

51. Pomeranz B: Acupuncture neurophysiology. In Adelman G (ed): *Encyclopedia of Neuroscience*. Birkhauser, Boston, 1986.

52. Watkins LR, Mayer DJ: Organization of endogenous opiate and non-opiate pain control systems. *Science* 216:1192–2285, 1982.

53. Hans JS: Progress in the pharamcological studies of acupuncture analgesia. In Paton SW, Mitchell J, Turner P (eds): *Proceedings IUPHAR Ninth International Congress of Pharmacology*. London, Macmillan, 1984. vol 1, pp 387–394.

54. Han JS, Ding XZ, Fan SG: Cholecystokinin octapeptide (CCK-8): antagonism to electro-acupuncture analgesia and a possible role in electro-acupuncture tolerance. *Pain* 27:101–115, 1986.

55. Han JS, Yu LC, Shi YS: A mesolimbic loop of analgesia. III. A neuronal pathway from nucleus accumbens to periaqueductal grey. *Asian Pacific J Pharmacol* 1:17–22, 1986.

56. Bloom F, Guillemin R, et al: Neurons containing B-endorphin in rat brain exist separately from those containing enkephalin: immuno-cytochemical studies. *Proc Natl Acad Sci (USA)* 75:1591–1595, 1978.

57. Watson SJ, Barchas JD: Anatomy of the endogenous opioid peptides and related substances. In Beers RF (ed): *Mechanisms of Pain and Analgesic Compounds*. New York, Raven Press, 1979, pp 227–237.

58. Sato T, Usami S, Takeshige C: Role of the arcuate nucleus of the hypothalamus as the descending pain inhibitory system in acupuncture point and non-point produced analgesia (in Japanese, English summary). In Takeshige C (ed): *Studies on the Mechanism of Acupuncture Analgesia Based on Animal Experiments*. Tokyo, Showa University Press, 1986, p. 627.

59. Rossier J, Guillemin R, Bloom FE: Foot shock-induced stress increases B-endorphin levels in blood but not brain. *Nature* 270:618–620, 1977.

60. Melzack R, Melinkoff RF: Analgesia produced by brain stimulation. Evidence of a prolonged onset period. *Exp Neruol* 43:369–374, 1974.

61. Shyu BC, Andersson SA, Thoren P: Endorphin mediated increase in pain threshold induced by long-lasting exercise in rats. *Life Sci* 8:833–840, 1982.

62. Roos A, Rydenhag C, Andersson SA: Activity in cortical cells after stimulation of tooth pulp afferents in the cat. Extracellular analysis. *Pain* 16:49–60, 1983.

63. Roos A, Rydenhag B, Andersson SA: Cortical responses evoked by tooth pulp stimulation in the cat. *Pain* 3:247–265, 1982.

64. Rydenhag B, Olausson B, Andersson SA: Projection of tooth pulp afferents to the thalamus of the cat. I. Focal potentials and thalamocortical connections. *Exp Brain Res* 64:37–48, 1986.

65. Rydenhag B, Olausson B, Shyu BC, Andersson S: Localized responses in the midsuprasylvian gyrus of the cat following stimulation of the central lateral nucleus in thalamus. *Exp Brain Res* 62:11–24, 1986.

66. Peking Acupuncture Anesthesia Coordinating Group: Preliminary study of the mechanism of acupuncture anesthesia. *Sci Sin* 16:447–456, 1973.

67. Lassen NA, Ingvar DH, Skinh JE: Brain function and blood flow. *Sci Am* 239:62–71, 1978.

68. Hand PJ, Huang Y-H, Liu C-N: Use of the (^{14}C)-deoxyglucose method in acupuncture analgesia studies (abstract). *Acupunct Electrother Res* 10(4):364, 1985.

69. Gaito J: The kindling effect. *Physiol Psychol* 2:45–50, 1965.

70. Lorente de No R: Analysis of the activity of chains of internuncial neurone. *J Neurophysiol* 1:207–244, 1938.

71. Dusser de Barenne JG, McCulloch WS: Factors for facilitation and extinction in the central nervous system. *J Neurophysiol* 2:319–355, 1939.

72. Loeser JD, Ward AA, White LE: Chronic deafferentation of human spinal cord neurons. *J Neurosurg* 29:48–50, 1968.

73. Livingston WK: *Pain Mechanisms.* New York, Macmillan, 1943, p. 253.
74. Bowsher D: Role of the reticular formation in responses to noxious stimulation. *Pain* 2:361–378, 1976.
75. Vierck CJ Jr, Lineberry CG, Lee PK et al: Prolonged hyperalgesia following acupuncture in monkeys. *Life Sci* 15:1277–1289, 1974.
76. Lu G-D, Needham J: *Celestial Lancets.* Cambridge,
England, Cambridge University Press, 1980, p. 427.
77. Matsumoto T: *Acupuncture for Physicians.* Springfield, IL, Charles Thomas, 1974, p. 204.
78. Stux G: Acupuncture in the treatment of chronic locomotor disorders. *Pain* Suppl 4, S363, 1987.
79. Beecher HK: Placebo analgesia in human volunteers. *JAMA* 159:1602–1606, 1955.

Section 3
PHYSICAL MEDICINE TREATMENTS

Chapter 9

ROLE OF PHYSICAL MEDICINE MODALITIES

RAJKA SORIC, MD, MSc, FRCPC

Low back pain is the most frequent cause of functional disability and work absenteeism in the population of industrialized societies. It is second only to headaches among the leading causes of pain. With an annual incidence of 5%, its lifetime prevalence ranges from 60 to 90% (1). The most recent epidemiologic data suggest that more than 90 million work days are lost in the United States each year because of back pain, with the combined cost for diagnostic procedures and treatment exceeding 5 billion dollars (2).

In most instances the causes of chronic low back pain are of a benign nature. Consequently, various tests usually performed in an attempt to identify the underlying pathology yield negative results and are useful only to exclude possibly reversible conditions.

ETIOLOGY AND DIAGNOSIS

Pain in the low back must always be regarded as a symptom rather than a diagnosis. A thorough history and physical examination will frequently enable the physician to focus investigations in a particular direction. Unremitting pain, particularly when present at rest, should make one suspicious of either a primary or secondary malignancy. Metabolic bone disease must also be considered in such cases. Associated systemic signs with an elevated temperature make a localized septic process very likely, whereas severe "shooting" pain in the radicular distribution implies in most cases a herniated nucleus pulposus as the cause for the patient's symptoms.

As with any other medical specialty, identifying the exact etiology of the low back pain allows the physician to administer treatment for the underlying pathology, thereby eradicating the cause of the pain. This may mean complete resolution of the patient's symptoms. Often, however, this is not possible. If a history and physical examination in conjunction with various laboratory and radiologic investigations fail to provide the exact diagnosis, symptomatic therapy remains the only option.

The development of ergonomics, or human engineering, helped a great deal in revealing the complex relationship between the mechanics of the human body and vocational and avocational activities (3). Simultaneous development of sophisticated diagnostic tools and better understanding of spinal biomechanics enabled the medical professionals to more accurately identify the underlying causes for "mechanical back pain." This syndrome is often diagnosed in patients who present with a history of minor trauma, overuse, or poor posture. By and large it is aggravated by movement and relieved by recumbency (3). Current thinking is that an abnormal posture, weakness of the supporting soft tissues, and apophyseal joint abnormalities directly or indirectly cause faulty spinal biomechanics, resulting in low back pain.

An exaggerated lumbar lordosis is one of the most common examples of mechanically induced pain in the low back. Women in the late stages of pregnancy hyperextend their back in order to maintain the center of gravity within the base of support. Obese people, particularly those with protuberant abdomens, do the same. This puts additional stress on the facet joints, stretches the anterior longitudinal ligament, and may compromise the patency of the intervertebral foramina. A similar problem can be seen in individuals with hip flexion contractures or in women wearing high-heeled shoes. Although the cause of the exaggerated lumbar lordosis in the given examples is quite different, the end result is the same.

A leg length discrepancy is another frequent condition that leads to mechanical back pain. Compensatory scoliosis that results if the difference in the leg length is significant causes asymmetric loading of the facet joints that in itself is a painful condition. If the leg length discrepancy is not corrected, a secondary complication of ligamentous and muscle fiber shortening may occur, eventually leading to a structural spinal deformity and further aggravation of the pain.

There are numerous other examples of mechanical factors resulting in low back pain that are beyond the scope of this chapter.

TREATMENT

Before attempting to vigorously treat a patient suffering from low back pain, physicians should bear in mind that in only 10–20% of all patients with back pain will the exact pathoanatomic diagnosis be established. The chosen treatment, therefore, will be an attempt to provide symptomatic relief, to improve the patient's overall function, and to whenever possible prevent the development of secondary complications that may further enhance the patient's disability.

The physical modalities are probably the most frequently utilized treatment options for various types of low back pain. The frequency of physiotherapy prescriptions is most likely surpassed only by the use of analgesics. In spite of such frequent use of the different physical modalities, convincing evidence for their effectiveness is still sadly lacking (1). This may be explained at least in part by a scarce number of reported prospective randomized trials. Furthermore, the natural history of the disease makes it difficult to differentiate what improvement resulted from the treatment as opposed to spontaneous resolution.

In most instances the indications for the use of physical modalities are symptomatic pain relief, relief of muscle spasm, strengthening and endurance training, and restoration of spinal mobility, as well as postural reeducation. This in itself clearly identifies the additional importance of physical medicine as a preventive measure in low back ailments. Unfortunately, the prescription of physical modalities is often abused. Patients are sent from one clinic to another and are treated for extended periods of time with various agents and exercise programs without any benefit. Such management only reinforces the patient's sense of disability. Regular follow-up and a careful evaluation of the therapy program is mandatory if such occurrences are to be minimized.

REST

Bed rest is the most frequently prescribed type of treatment for sufferers of acute low back pain. It provides relief by virtue of unloading the painful spinal segment and by decreasing the intradiscal pressure. Nachemson demonstrated an 86% drop in intradiscal pressure achieved by recumbency (4, 5). In a case of a compressed spinal nerve, edema of the perineural sheath is thought to be the reason for pain (6). Recumbency allows the edema to subside, thus contributing to the pain relief.

Duration of bed rest has been disputed for a long time. It should be long enough to allow the inflammatory reaction to subside, yet short enough to maintain the patient's compliance and prevent the adverse effects of bed rest. The latter is particularly important for elderly patients, whose overall well-being may be severely compromised by prolonged bed rest. Over the past decade, there has been an obvious tendency to shorten the period of recumbency. Deyo and coworkers have shown that 2 days of bed rest are just as effective as 7 days (7). Most authors still advocate 2 weeks of bed rest as an initial treatment that is followed by gradual mobilization. This applies to patients who suffer from severe pain due to either soft tissue derangement (e.g., acute ligamentous overstretch, herniated nucleus pulposus) or a compression fracture.

In chronic back sufferers, however, bed rest as a method of treatment will most likely not produce a significant improvement or long-term benefit. In addition to the psychological dependency, it may cause muscle atrophy and generalized deconditioning (2). Currently, there is very little convincing evidence to suggest that recumbency is beneficial for this group of patients at all, because the complications of such treatment outweigh the possible benefit of muscle relaxation (1, 8).

THERMAL THERAPY AND CRYOTHERAPY

These modalities are of benefit mostly as an adjunct to other types of treatment. Superficial heat is relaxing, soothing, and pleasant. Ice, conversely, provides a longer lasting analgesic effect and is more effective in reducing muscle spasm.

Therapeutic Heat

The physiologic effects of heat are well known. In conditions characterized by muscle spasm, it achieves the therapeutic effect by producing vasodilatation that allows rapid removal of cell metabolites from the tonically contracted muscles (9). Its nonspecific counterirritant effect also contributes to analgesia, because it acts as an afferent stimulus operating via the gate mechanism in the substantia gelatinosa. Lehmann and coworkers claimed that heat produces analgesia by increasing the pain threshold (10).

In most instances of chronic low back pain, heat is used as an adjunct to other physical modalities. Hydrotherapy, for example, combines the effects of heat, buoyancy of the water, and counterirritant phenomena. When the body is immersed in the deep end of the pool, the effect of buoyancy is sufficient to almost overcome the effect of gravity. This greatly diminishes the weightbearing stress on the lumbar spine. alleviating the pain and permitting the patient to follow the therapist's instructions with more ease. The temperature of the water relaxes and sedates the patient, further contributing to compliance with the prescribed exercise program.

Therapeutic Cold

Cryotherapy is gaining popularity in the treatment of painful conditions. Chilling from ice applied to the low back region penetrates through the skin, subcutaneous tissue, and fat, cooling the superficial layer of the muscle. This decreases the muscle spasm and alleviates the pain (11). Because of the superior insulating properties of the fat tissue the resulting analgesia and diminished muscle spasm will be longer lasting (12). The counterirritant effect of the ice further contributes to its analgesic effect.

EXERCISE

Exercise as a therapeutic modality is prescribed for a patient with low back pain in order to improve flexibility, strength, endurance, and overall level of function. Exercise reduces the pain by stretching the muscles in spasm, and may also minimize the chance of recurrence (1). Extensive review of the various exercise programs postulates their beneficial effects on disk nutrition, pain modulation, and spinal column biomechanics (2). The three most frequently used types of exercises are hyperextension exercises, mobilization exercises, and flexion exercises.

In 1937 Williams advocated flexion exercises, the purpose of which was to open the intervertebral foramina, thus relieving compression of the nerve and reducing the pain and inflammation of the neural sheath. Although studies evaluating this proposed mechanism are lacking, it seems unlikely that the intermittent relief of pressure that may occur with lumbar flexion would suffice to decompress the spinal root sufficiently to allow its healing and reversal of symptoms (13). David advocated the flexion exercise program as a method to increase the intraabdominal pressure and to diminish mechanical stress of the lumbar spine (14).

McKenzie's extension routine is based on the hypothesis that lumbar lordosis may lead to a shift of the nucleus pulposus away from the spinal nerve (15). Other proponents of the extension routine feel that maintenance of the physiologic lumbar lordosis and strengthening of the paravertebral musculature enhances the ability of the lumbar spine to withstand the axial compression produced by the superincumbent body weight (13).

Aerobic fitness programs that are not directed to a particular part of the body are gaining in popularity as a method of treating low back pain. Activities such as bicycling, swimming, brisk walking, and jogging help keep the patient in good physical shape and enhance a sense of well-being. An improved level of fitness has been associated with a lower rate of recurrence and diminished intensity of the symptoms in patients already suffering from back pain (16). Furthermore, Bell and Rothman have shown that such activities performed four times a week for 20–30 min each time lead to the increased production of β-endorphins found in the peripheral circulation (6). nevertheless, care must be taken in interpreting these findings. Production of the β-endorphins in the plasma and the cerebrospinal fluid is under separate control. One should not, therefore, readily conclude that aerobic exercise can be considered as a central pain–reducing mechanism (13).

An important factor in prevention of mechanical low back pain is postural reeducation. When sitting, the low back should be supported, but care should be taken not to exaggerate the lumbar curve, because this may enhance the stress on the facet joints and possibly overstretch the anterior longitudinal ligament. When standing, frequent weight shifting may alleviate the discomfort in the low back.

Three types of exercises have been developed in an attempt to improve the patient's posture: pelvic tilt, strengthening of the abdominal muscles, and stretching of the lumbosacral musculature. Even though patients by and large report improvement in their condition after regularly performing these exercises, there is no evidence to support the claims that this occurs as a result of corrected posture. Furthermore, the available data suggest that exercise alone cannot alter the posture (10).

Several authors have provided strong evidence that flexibility of the lumbar spine provides a mechanical advantage and efficiency while performing various activities (e.g., bending, lifting). The intravertebral disk, which is the only a vascular segment of the spinal functional unit, depends upon this movement for its nutrition (17). The same is true for the synovium-lined facet joints (18). The critical level of lumbar spine mobility necessary to maintain tissue nutrition and provide mechanical efficiency is not known (13).

When prescribing an exercise program, it is important that the patient is informed not to expect remarkable results immediately. The benefit of exercise can be appreciated only if it is carried out over a longer period of time on a regular basis.

MOBILIZATION, TRACTION, AND MANIPULATION

Mobilization

Mobilization is a group of therapeutic modalities where a passive force is used to restore joint mobility and tissue extensibility and achieve tissue perfusion. It consists of gentle pressure and controlled passive oscillations of the joint within the existing range of motion. For low back pain, oscillations are achieved by rhythmically applied pressure over the spinous or transverse processes that enhances movement of the joints in the anteroposterior direction (19).

Traction

The purpose of spinal traction is to stretch the spinal musculature and to distract the vertebral bodies. Sutides have suggested that the applied weight must be at least 25% of the total body weight in order to overcome inertia and the resistance of the recumbent body (8). If one is to achieve changes in the intradiscal pressure, the weight applied must be at least 60% of the total body weight.

Lumbar traction may be applied as a manual technique or may be achieved by mechanical or gravitational forces. It can be applied in a continuous manner or intermittently. Best results are reported with the use of mechanical devices that apply the traction force intermittently. Claims that

disk herniations can be reduced by traction are generally not accepted (20).

Spinal Manipulation

This is a technique of applying sudden, low-amplitude thrust that takes the joint beyond the existing range of motion (19). The direction of this movement is still somewhat controversial, but most often it is done initially in the direction opposite to the one that causes the most pain (21). If a patient has pain with rotation to the left at the outset of the treatment, thrust should be applied to the right.

Two types of manipulations apply to the treatment of low back pain. With the "direct" technique, manipulative thrust is directed to a particular joint (e.g., facet joint), whereas with "indirect" manipulation, force is applied to the remote part of the body, causing movement in the lumbar spine (22).

At least four different trials were done comparing the effects of manipulation to other types of treatment for low back pain (6, 23–26). None of these has demonstrated long-term effectiveness of this treatment. This is rather remarkable considering that out of 75–120 million annual visits to chiropractors in the United States, at least 50% are made because of low back pain (24).

In patients who have low back pain with objective clinical evidence of a radicular involvement, manipulation may in fact cause further progression of a neurologic deficit (27). However, this remains a controversial issue.

BIOFEEDBACK

Even though electromyographic biofeedback can theoretically be of help in the treatment of low back pain by helping patients achieve the ability to relax and contract various muscles at specific times, it is not a frequently used physical modality in the treatment of low back pain.

SPINAL ORTHOTICS

Two characteristics of spinal orthotics are to be considered when prescribing these devices for the treatment of low back pain. An appliance that fits snugly around the body will primarily unload the spine by increasing the intraabdominal pressure and allowing part of the superincumbent body weight to be transmitted through the abdominal wall. Rigid orthoses, conversely, contribute to the control of low back pain by reducing the amount of spinal movement. In both cases, the lumbar lordosis is decreased. Whether this further contributes to pain relief is still debatable. It may do so in patients with degenerative changes of the facet joints by virtue of transferring part of the stress to the anterior functional segment. A corset or a rigid brace serves as a reminder to the patient to consciously reduce the amount of spinal movement. This sensory "feedback" is yet another mechanism that explains the pain-relieving effect of spinal orthotics.

Choice of lumbar support differs depending upon the condition that is thought to cause the pain. A patient with acute back pain resulting from a compression fracture or a compromised spinal root will experience fairly rapid and significant pain relief with a tight-fitting corset, whereas a patient following spinal instrumentation requires a rigid orthosis to decrease the amount of spinal movement.

While spinal orthoses may be of help in the management of spinal disorders, their use, particularly if long term, may create problems. In addition to the well-recognized weakness and eventual atrophy of the abdominal and paraspinal muscles (8), Chapman and Ralston have documented alteration of the gait pattern and increased energy expenditure in patients wearing spinal orthotics (28). Another side effect of the spinal appliance is its tendency to cause increased motion of the segment adjacent to the ends of the orthosis (29). One should also remember the possibility of developing psychological dependency and the possibility of skin breakdown, particularly when dealing with a patient who has a neurologic and/or vascular compromise or inadequate soft tissue coverage over the bony prominences.

REFERENCES

1. Deyo RA: Conservative therapy of low back pain. *JAMA* 250:1057–1062, 1983.
2. Keim HA, Kirkaldy-Willis WH: Low back pain. *Clin Symp* No. 2, 1988.
3. Sheon RP, Moskowitz RW, Goldberg VM: *Soft Tissue Rheumatic Pain,* ed 2. Philadelphia, Lea & Febiger, 1987.
4. Nachemson AL: The load on lumbar disc in different positions of the body. *Clin Orthop* 45:107–122, 1966.
5. Nachemson AL: The lumbar spine. An orthopedic challenge. *Spine* 1:59–71, 1976.
6. Bell GR, Rothman RH: The conservative treatment of sciatica. *Spine* 9:54–56, 1984.
7. Deyo RA, Diehl AK, Rosenthal M: How many days of bed rest for acute low back pain? N Engl Med 316:1064–1070, 1986.
8. Quintet RJ, Hadler NM: Diagnosis and treatment of backache. *Semin Arthritis Rheum* 8:261–287, 1979.
9. Lehmann JF, DeLateur BJ: Therapeutic heat. In Lehmann JF (ed): *Therapeutic Heat and Cold,* ed 3. Baltimore, Williams & Wilkins, 1982, pp 404–562.
10. Lehmann JF, Brunner GD, Stow RW: Pain threshold measurements after therapeutic appliation of ultrasound, microwaves and infrared. *Arch Phys Med Rehabil* 39:560–565, 1958.
11. Lippold OCJ, Nicholls JG, Redfearn JWT: A study of the afferent discharge produced by cooling a mammalian muscle spindle. *J Physiol* 153:218–231, 1960.
12. Hartvikson K: Ice therapy for spasticity. *Acta Neurol Scand* 38(suppl 3):79–84, 1962.
13. Jackson CP, Brown MD: Is there a role for exercise in the treatment of patients with low back pain. *Clin Orthop Rel Res* 179:31–45, 1983.
14. Davis PR: The use of intra-abdominal pressure in evaluating stresses on the lumbar spine. *Spine* 6:90, 1981.
15. McKenzie R: *Treat Your Own Back,* ed 3. Melbourne, Wright & Carman Ltd, 1986.
16. Cady LD, Bischoff DP, O'Connell ER, Thomas PC, Allan JK: Strength and fitness and subsequent back injuries in firefighters. *J Occup Med* 21:269, 1979.
17. Kramer J: Pressure dependent fluid shifts in the intervertebral disc. *Orthop Clin North Am* 8:211, 1977.
18. Enneking WF, Horowitz M: The intra-articular effects of immobilization on the human kene. *J Bone Joint Surg [Am]* 54:973, 1972.
19. Mannheimer JS, Lampe GN: *Clinical Transcutaneous Electrical Stimulation.* Philadelphia, FA Davis Company, 1985, pp. 463–495.
20. Frymoyer JW: Back pain and sciatica. *N Engl J Med* 318:291–300, 1988.
21. Maigne R: The concept of painlessness and opposite motion in spinal manipulation. *Am J Phys Med* 44:55, 1965.
22. Basmajian JV (ed): *Manipulation, Traction and Massage,* ed 3. Baltimore, Williams & Wilkins, 1985.
23. Godfrey CM, Morgan PP, Schatzker J: A randomized trial of manipulation for low back pain in a medical setting. *Spine* 9:301–304, 1984.
24. Brunarski DJ: Clinical trials of spinal manipulation: a critical appraisal and review of literature. *J Manipulative Physiol Ther* 7:243–249, 1984.
25. Ottenbacher K, DiFabio RP: Efficacy of spinal manipulation mobilization. *Med J Aust* 2:672–673, 1983.
26. Nachemson A: Work for all: for those with low back pain as well. *Clin Orthop* 179:77–85, 1985.
27. Dan NG, Saccasan PA: Serious complications of lumbar spinal manipulation. *Med J Aust* 2:672–673, 1983.
28. Chapman MW, Ralston MJ: *Effects of Immobilization of Back and Arms on Energy Expenditure during Level Walking.* Technical Report 51. University of California Biomechanics Laboratory, June 1964.
29. Norton PL, Brown T: The immobilizing efficiency of back braces; their effect on the posture and motion of the lumbosacral spine. *J Bone Joint Surg.* 39:111, 1957.

Chapter 10

TRANSCUTANEOUS ELECTRICAL NERVE STIMULATION AND ELECTROTHERAPY

RAJKA SORIC, MD, MSc, FRCPC

The use of electrical energy for therapeutic purposes dates back several centuries. Scribonius Largus (46 AD) is credited with one of the earliest recorded descriptions, the use of decapitated torpedo fish in the treatment of headaches and gout (1). In the 18th and 19th centuries, man-made devices began replacing the natural sources of electrical energy. Galvanic current soon became a panacea for many human ailments (1, 2). During these times very little effort was spent looking into the mechanism of achieved benefits induced by electrical stimulation. They were largely attributed to the special properties of electricity itself rather than its effect on the nervous system.

In the early 20th century, however, use of electrical current for treatment purposes lost its popularity. It was not until intensive neurophysiologic research began in the 1950s that electrotherapy was revived (3). Two principle effects of electrical energy—stimulation of excitable tissue and generation of heat—soon became the mainstay of physical medicine. The introduction of the "gate theory" in the mid-1960s fostered the development of electrical stimulation as a mechanism of achieving symptomatic analgesia (2). In 1967, Mortimer and Shealy developed a dorsal column stimulator for the treatment of chronic pain. The high failure rate that was observed prompted a further search for a transcutaneous electrical device that would help predict the efficacy of the implanted stimulators (1). As clinicians soon found out, this device provided adequate pain relief, and it soon became a popular and preferred mode of treatment.

MECHANISM OF ACTION

Transcutaneous electrical nerve stimulation (TENS) is a procedure of applying electricity of defined intensity and frequency to the skin with the purpose of achieving an analgesic effect. It is by now well accepted that the single most important physical effect of electrical stimulation is its ability to alter neuronal activity (4). The exact mechanism of this action, however, remains to be determined.

A few theories currently exist to explain the analgesic action of TENS. Francini, Melzack, and Zoppi entertained the possibility of electrical stimulation altering the sensitivity of the peripheral receptors (5–7). However, this hypothesis remains unproven. Campbell and Taub proposed that TENS antidromically alters the transmission of the noxious stimuli from the periphery (8).

The most popular theory explains the effect of TENS on the basis of the "gate theory." In the substantia gelatinosa, terminal branches of thick, myelinated A fibers transmitting the sensation of pressure and light touch interact with small nonmyelinated C fibers that transmit pain. If the afferent input via C fibers predominates, cells in the substantia gelatinosa are inhibited, leading to reduced presynaptic inhibition that opens the gate for the noxious stimuli to ascend along the neuraxis. Eventually, a painful sensation is perceived. TENS selectively stimulates the thick, myelinated A fibers that activate the interneurons of the substantia gelatinosa, thus presynaptically inhibiting further transmission of pain (2). This may further be mediated to a certain degree by the release of γ-aminobutyric acid (GABA) (9). In 1971, Melzack postulated that TENS produces analgesia via the central biasing mechanism located in the midbrain (10). This theory explains the success of TENS in controlling the pain that results from the loss of afferent input.

The neuropharmacologic theory deserves special attention. The "conventional" TENS units were noted to raise the concentration of enkephalins in the cerebrospinal fluid. These are the short-chain peptides that are endogenously produced and possess morphine-like properties. Enkephalins are widespread throughout the peripheral and central nervous systems (11, 12). Analgesia produced in this manner is not reversible by naloxone (13). Conversely, the "acupuncture-like" TENS enhances the release of β-endorphins, the long-chain peptides that have a longer half-life and are concentrated in the central nervous system. Their analegesic effect can be reversed by the intravenous administration of naloxone (13). Elevated levels of plasma cortisol have also been reported with the use of "acupuncture-like" TENS. It is concluded, therefore, that TENS used in this manner produces analgesia by a combination of neuromodulation secondary to the enhanced release of endogenous opiates, as well as a systemic anti-inflammatory effect (5, 9). It should be noted that healthy people and patients with pain of a documented physiologic cause have normal or low levels of enkephalins and endorphins, whereas the level of these peptides in patients with psychogenic pain is high (14). This is a very important finding since TENS has very little effect in pain of psychogenic origin.

TECHNIQUE

The most frequently used type of TENS (conventional mode) uses a high rate, narrow pulse width, and moderate intensity of stimulus. It selectively stimulates large-diameter, myelinated afferent fibers. An analgesic effect is produced quickly, but its duration unfortunately is short. When applied correctly, patients report feeling a tingling sensation over the area of pain.

In "acupuncture-like" TENS, the stimulation is characterized by a low rate, wide pulse width, and high intensity. It must produce visible muscle contraction of the myotomes over which the electrodes are placed. Stimulation of at least 20–30 min is necessary if suprasegmental endorphin release is to occur. Once the analgesic effect is achieved, it lasts

appreciably longer than does pain relief induced by conventional modes of stimulation.

The placement of the electrodes is still done largely on an empirical basis. Initially, it was suggested to apply the electrodes over the trigger points, along the course of the peripheral nerve supplying the painful area or acupuncture meridians (15, 16). The most common location for the treatment in case of nonradiating low back pain is over the lumbosacral junction. If the pain is radicular in nature, the electrodes may be placed over the dermatome involved. The major advantage of the "conventional" TENS unit is that it provides the rapid onset of analgesia, and the "conventional" TENS is by and large better accepted by patients. It produces rapid pain relief and the stimulation causes only paresthesiae that are generally well tolerated (17). Unfortunately, tolerance develops relatively quickly. With the use of the "acupuncture-like" TENS, strong muscle contractions may not be well tolerated by patients and, considering the rather slow onset of pain relief, the incidence of rejection is higher. This problem may be avoided if the "conventional" TENS mode is used at the onset of the trial treatment (18).

Although the onset of the analgesia following the application of TENS should occur after 30 min of stimulation, in some patients several days may pass before any improvement can be appreciated. The treatment should therefore not be discontinued after the first unsuccessful trial (18, 19). Procacci reported that the success of TENS in the treatment of low back pain was primarily dependent on the presence of trigger points and intact afferent fibers (1).

PATIENT SELECTION

Throughout the 1970s and early 1980s, numerous studies have demonstrated that electrical stimulation produced more than the placebo response in patients with chronic pain (19–22). The "acupuncture-like" TENS is generally considered to be of more benefit in the treatment of chronic painful conditions than the high-frequency stimulation, which is more appropriate in acute conditions.

Although TENS as a treatment modality produces symptomatic analgesia only, before its administration one should make an effort to fully understand the patient's complaint of pain and to identify the various factors that may influence the success of the treatment. Patients with psychogenic pain often have an elevated concentration of endorphins in the cerebrospinal fluid. The chances are, therefore, that the "acupuncture-like" TENS will be of no benefit to these patients at all. It is by now well recognized that depression and anxiety are the major contributors to chronic low back pain. The use of TENS in such patients either will be ineffective or may in fact aggravate the pain. Psychotherapy in conjunction with behavioral modification is more likely to succeed in controlling the symptoms in such a patient. Kosterlitz and Hughes (23), as well as Wei and Loh (24), have reported a diminished production of enkephalins and endorphins in patients dependent on narcotics. This was further confirmed by Solomon and his coworkers (25). The effectiveness of TENS treatment in these patients is therefore diminished. This is an important factor to keep in mind since many patients suffering from low back pain do have a tendency for long-term use of narcotic-containing analgesics.

There are a very few contraindications for the use of TENS. Patients with cardiac dysrhythmia should be closely monitored at the onset of the treatment, as should patients with demand-type pacemakers. Electrode placement over the carotid sinus may trigger the vasovagal reflex (2, 17). Although one should keep these precautions in mind, it is not very likely that the cited contraindications would preclude the use of TENS for the control of low back pain.

SIDE EFFECTS

As with any treatment modality, the physician should carefully consider the possible adverse reactions when prescribing TENS. The most common problem experienced by the patient is contact dermatitis, due either to tape allergy or to intolerance of the coupling agent. Hypoallergenic substances have been introduced in recent years, but unfortunately this inevitably leads to an increased cost for the unit. Micropunctate burns occasionally have been reported, particularly with chronic use of the device. The same holds true for occasional hyperpigmentation of the skin at the site of the electrode placement. Clearly most of the adverse side effects are not related to the current itself.

MONITORING USE OF THE DEVICE

To achieve the full therapeutic effect of TENS, proper use of the machine is mandatory. This does not present a problem while the patient is undergoing "trial" treatments under medical supervision, since the electrodes are placed by a therapist who also adjusts the settings on the machine. If TENS proves to be effective in the control of the pain, the patient must be thoroughly educated regarding its use. Periodic follow-up visits may be necessary to ensure that the proper technique is maintained.

With the long-term use of TENS, the degree of pain control may decrease. If this occurs, a repeated visit to the therapist may reveal an inappropriate technique of its application or, less frequently, a malfunctioning unit. Should this not be the case, nerve adaptation (accommodation) must be considered. With ongoing electrical stimulation, the membrane of the afferent fibers may become less excitable. This occurs more frequently with the "conventional" TENS. The problem can be resolved by changing the stimulation parameters (pulse width and frequency). Newer models of TENS units have this modulation feature already built in. One or more parameters can be modulated either in isolation or simultaneously. If modulation of the pulse width and frequency does not restore the effectiveness of the unit, placement of the electrodes may have to be changed.

CONCLUSIONS

Even though studies have documented the overall efficiency of TENS to be lower in patients suffering from chronic conditions, this still remains an effective treatment modality for patients with low back pain, particularly if care is taken to select the appropriate candidates and to closely monitor the use of the device. This would ensure that the possible technical errors are brought to a minimum. The best results are achieved if TENS is introduced as a treatment modality early on in the course of the disease. Mannheimer and Lampe suggest that in patients with low back pain, if "acupuncture-like TENS" is to be used, electrodes be placed over the gastrocnemius/soleus muscles (1). Bilateral stimulation has been proven more effective. If the patient does not obtain any pain relief, simultaneous bimodal stimulation is indicated. "Conventional" TENS can be applied to the lumbosacral region while strong, low-rate stimulation is applied to the lower extremities (18). This can be achieved either by the simultaneous use of two different units or by using a TENS unit that allows complete channel separation with one channel providing the "conventional" and the other "acupuncture-like" stimulation (17, 18).

Low back pain remains the most frequent indication for the use of TENS. It is a safe and easy-to-use modality that allows the patient to be in charge of his/her own treatment. Even when not completely successful in controlling the pain, TENS may significantly contribute to pain reduction when used in conjunction with other types of treatments, thereby minimizing the patient's disability.

REFERENCES

1. Mannheimer JS, Lampe GN: *Clinical Transcutaneous Electrical Nerve Stimulation*. Philadelphia, FA Davis Company, 1985, pp. 1–4.
2. Soric R, Devlin M: Transcutaneous electrical nerve stimulation. *Postgrad Med* 78(4):101–105, 1985.
3. Lichts S: Therapeutic electricity. In Stillwell GK (ed): *Therapeutic Electricity and Ultraviolet Radiation*. Baltimore, Williams & Wilkins, 1983.
4. Warfield CA, Bargston R: Physical therapy for pain relief. *Hosp Pract* Aug, 84E–84S, 1984.
5. Francini F, Maresca M, Procacci P, Zoppi M: The effects of nonpainful transcutaneous electrical nerve stimulation on cutaneous pain threshold and muscular reflexes in normal men and in subjects with chronic pain. *Pain* 11:49–63, 1981.
6. Procacci P, Zoppi M, Maresca M, Francini F: Hypoalgesia induced by transcutaneous electrical stimulation. A physiological and clinical investigation. *J Neurosurg Sci* 4:221–228, 1977.
7. Zoppi M., Francini F, Maresca M, Procacci P: Changes of cutaneous sensory thresholds induced by nonpainful transcutaneous electrical stimulation in normal subjects with chronic pain. *J Neurol Neurosurg Psychiatry* 44:708–717, 1981.
8. Campbell JN, Taub A: Local analgesia from percutaneous electrical stimulation: A peripheral mechanism. *Arch Neurol* 28:347–350, 1973.
9. Warfield CA, Stein JM: Pain relief by electrical stimulation. *Hosp Pract* March, 207–218, 1983.
10. Melzack R: Prolonged relief of pain by brief, intense transcutaneous somatic stimulation. *Pain* 1:357, 1971.
11. Johansson F, Almay BG, von Knorring L, et al: Predictors for the outcome of treatment with high frequency transcutaneous electrical nerve stimulation (TENS) in patients with chronic pain. *Pain* 9:55–61, 1980.
12. Schuster GD, Infante MC: Pain relief after low back surgery: the efficacy of transcutaneous electrical nerve stimulation. *Pain* 8:299–302, 1980.
13. Cheng RS, Pomeranz B: Electroacupuncture analgesic could be mediated by at least two pain-relieving mechanisms; endorphin and non-endorphin systems. *Life Sci* 25:1957–1962, 1978.
14. Gersh MR: Postoperative pain and transcutaneous electrical nerve stimulation: a model to critique literature and develop documentation schema. *Phys Ther* 58:1463–1466, 1978.
15. Rao VR, Wolf SL, Gersh MR: Examination of electrode placements and stimulating parameters in treating chronic pain with conventional transcutaneous electrical nerve stimulation (TENS). *Pain* 11:37–47, 1981.
16. Mannheimer JS: Electrode placements for transcutaneous electrical nerve stimulation. *Phys Ther* 58:1455–1462, 1978.
17. Mannheimer JS: Electrode placements for transcutaneous electrical nerve stimulation. *Phys Ther* 58 (12):345–352, 1978.
18. Mannheimer JS: Electrode placements for transcutaneous electrical nerve stimulation. *Phys Ther* 58 (12):338–345, 1978.
19. Rutkowski B, Niedzialkowska T, Otto J: Electrical stimulation in chronic low back pain. *Br J Anaesth* 49:629–632, 1977.
20. Andersson SA: Pain control by sensory stimulation. In Bonica JJ, Liebeskind JC, Albe-Fessard DG (eds): *Advances in Pain Research and Therapy*. New York, Raven Press, 1979, vol 3, pp. 569–585.
21. Jeans ME: Relief of chronic pain by brief, intense transcutaneous electrical stimulation. A double-blind study. In Bonica JJ, Liebeskind JC, Albe-Fessard DG (eds): *Advances in Pain Research and Therapy*. New York, Raven Press, 1979, vol 3, pp. 601–606.
22. Moritz, U: Physical therapy and rehabilitation. *Scand J Rheumatol (Suppl)* 43:49–55, 1982.
23. Kosterlitz HW, Hughes J: Some thoughts on the significance of enkephalins, the endogenous ligand. *Life Sci* 17:91, 1975.
24. Wei I, Loh H: Physical dependance on opiate-like peptides. *Science* 193:1262, 1976.
25. Solomon RA, Viernstein MC, Long DM: Reduction of postoperative pain and narcotic use by transcutaneous electrical nerve stimulation. *Surgery* 87:142, 1980.

Chapter 11

MANIPULATION AND MOBILIZATION OF THE LUMBAR SPINE

JERRY C. LANGLEY, DC

With increased research and understanding, spinal manipulation is growing in acceptance. Over the years, manipulation has often proven controversial and, at times, the practitioners of the methods have been cast outside the primary area of health care. This alienation of manipulators primarily has been due to the absence of clinical research and the presence of incomprehensible theories, as well as socioeconomic and political reasons. As the acceptance of spinal manipulation by the medical and physical therapy professions grows, the gap between clinical observations of manipulators and that of documented research continues to narrow.

Manipulation of the spine has been practiced in some fashion since Hippocrates first described manipulative techniques (1). Primitive forms of manipulation appear to have been available and widely used by almost every society in recorded history, from the ancient Romans and Greeks through the Middle Ages to modern times (2). In today's society manipulation is primarily provided by chiropractors, since most medical physicians have neither the time nor the inclination to master the art and skill of manipulative therapy. However, there are still some osteopaths, a few medical physicians, and a growing number of physical therapists who employ the procedure. It appears that conflict will continue between practitioners of different training. There are differences in the skill, standards of practice, and theoretical emphasis among clinicians who practice manipulative therapy (3).

CLINICAL RESEARCH

Interestingly, chiropractors have claimed that poor manipulative skills have produced substandard performance results in many of the earlier medical studies and that superior manipulative skills employed by chiropractors would have a more positive effect on test results. It has been noted that the number of hours of specific training in manipulation is far greater for chiropractors than for any other group of practitioners (4). Additionally, manipulation is the full-time vocation of the chiropractor, and his/her frequent, repetitive use of manipulative techniques increases progressive skills (5).

In general, the consensus from past studies has been that spinal manipulation performs well in acute back pain when compared to traditional alternatives. Practitioners in their private offices tended to report improvement following manipulation in more than 90% of their ambulatory patients with lower back pain (6). Evans et al. performed a crossover trial comparing manipulation with analgesia and found that patients tended to show greater improvement during periods when they were receiving spinal manipulation than during periods when they were only receiving analgesics (7).

Rassmussen compared manipulation with short-wave therapy in a small number of patients by a single-blinded method (8). He found that at both 7 and 14 days the manipulated group showed markedly improved spinal mobility and symptoms as compared to the control group. It should be noted that some studies suggest that manipulation combined with other treatment methods may be more effective than manipulation alone. For example, Coxhead et al. demonstrated that manipulation was only slightly better than traction, exercise, and corsets individually, but that symptoms were significantly improved as these treatment approaches were combined (9).

While the data demonstrating the success of manipulation in the treatment of the acute back pain patient have been somewhat impressive, earlier studies have failed to demonstrate the effectiveness of manipulation in the more difficult chronic patient. However, two recent studies have found chiropractic manipulation to perform well with low back pain in comparison to controls (10) and to the use of medical alternatives (11) in the treatment of the patient with chronic back pain. Additionally, recent trials indicate the superiority of manipulative skills that employ low-amplitude, short-lever, high-velocity, specific manipulation over that of the nonspecific long-lever techniques. Thabe utilized electromyography (EMG) studies to demonstrate that specific short-lever manipulation physiologically out performed mobilization (12). His studies indicated that abnormal muscle activity accompanying joint dysfunction was resolved immediately and completely by specific manipulation, whereas mobilization failed to completely resolve the abnormal activity.

MANIPULATION VERSUS MOBILIZATION

Broad concepts in the definition of manipulation have been conceived over the years. One early form of manipulation required that the patient be tied to a ladder with ropes so that two people could shake it, thereby facilitating what is perceived to be a crude form of manipulation. It was also thought that American Indians would wrap their "patient" in a blanket and roll him/her down a hill to facilitate manipulation. Today, varying concepts of the definition of manipulation still remain.

Many times the definition of manipulation is offered to include all procedures in which the hands are used to massage, mobilize, adjust, or manipulate the osseous structures of the body and their surrounding tissue. This broad concept of manipulation is partly due to the fact that extensive myofascial and soft tissue techniques are required along with manipulation to produce effective pain

control and to reduce musculoskeletal dysfunction.

However, this liberal concept of manipulation has generated some misconceptions regarding the distinction between manipulation and mobilization. Cassidy et al. provided a very good understanding of the distinct difference between the two procedures (13). Mobilization involves taking the joint to its limit of passive range of motion while manipulation goes beyond the passive range of motion into the paraphysiologic zone. Extension beyond the paraphysiologic zone can induce damage to the articular ligaments. Therefore it is evident that in order to deal safely and effectively with mechanical joint dysfunctions by utilizing spinal manipulation, a complete and thorough knowledge of joint kinematics and joint examination is required.

NATURE OF THE PRIMARY MANIPULABLE LESION

One of the most interesting aspects surrounding manipulation today is the contrast in thinking regarding what actually constitutes a primary manipulable lesion. In earlier years the theory supported by many manipulators was that of a static spinal lesion such as a vertebra out of alignment. However, current research is bringing about a change toward a concept of a dynamic lesion wherein static anatomic relationships might very well be normal but the movement of a particular segment is altered.

Burnarski used a group of functional biomechanical tests, including dynamic lateral bending x-rays, to identify patients with mechanical low back pain. (14). He noted, however, that the test in fact had poor specificity in that it gave a high number of false positives in many patients who did not have low back pain. Yet, Grice argued that the normal dynamic lateral bending is the initial dysfunction that precedes the development of mechanical low back pain (15). Scientific studies evaluating the improvement in dynamic lateral bending x-rays following manipulation in both asymptomatic and symptomatic individuals support the concept of decreased aberrant mobility being a significant component in the primary manipulable lesion (14, 16).

The contrast regarding the primary manipulable lesion is somewhat divided by simple somatics and the terminology used to describe the lesion itself. Schafer described the spinal subluxation complex as the alteration of the normal dynamic, anatomic, and physiologic relationships of continuous articular structures (17). This lesion is accompanied by some degree of articular dysfunction, neurologic insult, and stressed muscles, tendons, and ligaments. Once the lesion is produced it becomes a focus of sustained pathologic irritation, and a flood of impulses flow into the spinal cord, where internuncial neurons receive and relay the impulses to the motor pathways. The lesion, along with the joint dysfunction, is reinforced, perpetuating the condition.

Johnston referred to the manipulable lesion as a biomechanical fault (18). He indicated that the condition includes palpable muscle tension, structural or positional irregularities, and altered mobility. Neuman referred to the disturbance as a somatic dysfunction (19). This dysfunction has a group of components that include a disturbance to the joint, intervertebral disk, muscles, and/or nervous system.

The common underlying feature of the manipulable lesion is the loss of clinical stability. White and Panjabi defined clinical stability as being the ability of the spine to prevent initial or additional neurologic damage, intractable pain, or gross deformity (20). Therefore, the concept of the manipulable lesion would include not only positional or postural changes but also any aberrant or restricted motions along the spinal segments.

MANIPULATION IN THE REDUCTION OF PAIN

Manipulation has been proven effective in producing relief in lower back pain, neck pain, and headaches. However, the exact pathway of manipulative pain relief is still somewhat controversial. Denslow and Hassett (21) and Korr (22) projected the role of muscle spindle afferents in both sustaining and abolishing segmental central fasciculation. These authors believe that spinal manipulation produces short-term bursts of proprioceptive sensory bombardment that produces an inhibition of the pain pathways. This bombardment could occur as a result of instantaneous stretch of the articular and myofascial receptors as their elastic barriers are exceeded in manipulation. Glover found zones of hyperesthesia lateral to the facet joints at painful segments that he believed were due to fasciculation of cutaneous pain reflexes by nociceptive impulses from the joint receptors (23). He found the zones to disappear following rotational manipulation along the involved segment.

Neurophysiologically, the proposed alteration that is precipitated by local joint hypermobility is a lack of stimulation of joint mechanoreceptors that normally inhibit nociceptive or pain afferentation. Lack of joint movement prevents the normal input into the neuron pool that blocks pain afferents from conducting impulses in higher levels. Although nociceptive impulses cannot be measured directly, it has been demonstrated that local joint restriction induces abnormal EMG changes and that spinal manipulation normalizes the response concurrently with the correction of joint dysfunction (12). A positive gain in muscle strength as recorded by EMG has also been documented through spinal manipulation in asymptomatic patients (25).

Terrett and Vernon measured cutaneous pain threshold and tolerance to electrical current (26). Areas of spinal joint hypermobility were manipulated and pain threshold and tolerance remeasured. Those manipulated had a 140% increase in pain tolerance versus nonmanipulated control patients.

With the rapid growth of knowledge concerning pain modulation by endogenous opioids and endorphins in the central nervous system, the possibility of more central and indirect effects of spinal manipulation exists. Vernon et al. have demonstrated a statistically significant increase in serum β-endorphin for a short period of time following spinal manipulation (27).

A RATIONAL APPROACH TO MECHANICAL DYSFUNCTION

Basically there are six areas that must be considered when approaching and evaluating a neuromuscular problem prior to manipulation. These six areas must be evaluated thoroughly, with the results of the evaluation being the determining factor as to what procedure is to be used in facilitating the optimum results and returning the patient to a more normal function. These six areas are: (a) osseous structure and related capsules, (b) ligamentous structures that give support and strength to the joints, (c) tendons, (d) muscles, (e) neurologic structures, and (f) the disk component with its effect on the neurologic aspect as well as the ligaments, tendons, and muscles. While each area mentioned can be a primary source of pain, it is more common to find a concomitance of the underlying aspects. If the diagnosis is thorough and complete there is reasonable assurance that treatment will be directed toward the primary source rather than toward secondary components, which treatment can lead to less desirable results and a dissatisfied patient.

The first and foremost goal of any diagnostic process is to determine if there are any contraindications to manipulative therapy. Any underlying organic lesions, fractures, or unacceptable degenerative changes must be ruled out.

The clinician who believes he/she can understand the patient's perception of pain is most likely mistaken. He/she can only seek to understand the patient's reaction to it. This is true whether the pain is isolated or generalized, local or referred. Pain that can be purely isolated as a structural, functional, or emotional effect is rare. Most likely, all three are superimposed upon and interlaced with each other in various degrees of status. Therefore an important phase of the data-finding portion of the evaluation of musculoskeletal pain begins with pain pattern drawing. Ensure that the patient is as specific as possible in determining the exact location of pain and its related referral patterns. A description of the type of pain will guide the examiner to a more accurate diagnosis. With musculoskeletal components it is extremely important to pay particular attention to perpetuating factors and aggravating circumstances that may have initiated the patient's pain. Often these will play an important part in the diagnostic phase.

Examination begins with a general visual observation of the painful area. Review the patient's general posture, examining it for postural weaknesses such as a forward head carriage, round shoulders, and pronation disorders. Proceed with both bony and soft tissue palpation. Place the joints through static and motion palpation, carefully noting the movement and glide of articulations. Pain over a joint upon static palpation can indicate ligamentous involvement in the absence of fracture and other pathologies. Carefully note any tender areas and trigger points associated along the involved levels. Both active and passive muscle testing is an essential part of the evaluation.

Unfortunately, our present taxonomy of illness is oriented toward disease rather than mechanical functional analysis. While differential diagnosis to rule out disease processes is mandatory prior to manipulation, a comprehensive approach in searching for mechanical faults is also essential. A thorough examination and investigation into the structures of the lumbar spine that are subjected to mechanical stress is very important. The lumbar vertebra motion unit consists of two lumbar vertebrae, each with a body, pedicles, transverse processes, articular processes, facet joints, and spinous

process together with innervating intervertebral disks. Additionally, there are other structures that can mechanically influence the nerve root, such as the posterior longitudinal ligament, intervertebral disk, ligamentum flavum, and facet joint. Since the classic report of Mixter and Barr (28) the herniated disk has received much attention. Currently, we recognize three types of intervertebral disk disorders:

1. A *prolapsed* intervertebral disk describes the condition in which some of the nucleus pulposus passes through the fissures in the annulus fibrosis of the vertebral endplate, resulting in narrowing of the interverebral disk space and bulging of its lateral aspects.
2. The *extruded* intervertebral disk occurs when nuclear material extrudes through and creates bulging of the disk periphery.
3. The *sequestrated* intervertebral disk is the condition wherein nuclear material is found within the spinal canal.

While the intervertebral disk receives a great deal of attention, a diagnosis of prolapse or displacement is made only in 15% of back pain patients presenting to general practitioners (29).

Murphy indicated that the pathophysiology of the nerve root includes compression and inflammation (30). Additionally, Marshall et al. cited the potential for a change in the immune response (31). Knowing and understanding muscle innervations and dermatome patterns is an essential part of musculoskeletal diagnosis. With nerve root compression there may be changes in the deep tendon reflexes, strength of muscle groups, bowel and bladder function, nerve stretch signs, and pain distribution.

To say that the clinician must be fully competent to recognize even subtle differences in pain distribution patterns, muscle strengths, and basic clinical findings is an understatement. Oftentimes these subtle changes will determine manipulative procedures and/or may exclude manipulation as a mode of treatment. The following scenario is a perfect example of these subtle differences. Frequently, pain radiates to the posterior hip and thigh with biomechanical faults at the posterior facets of the lumbar spine or with a sacroiliac syndrome. These are conditions that respond very favorably to manipulation, and a clinician should expect a high success level with these patients. However, if the distribution of pain extends below the knee, there is greater suspicion of a more significant nerve root compression, which would necessitate a more refined skill in manipulation.

Since varying conditions affecting the musculo-skeletal system result in similar symptoms, it is important for the physician to have and maintain an orderly examination process. A comprehensive examination allows the physician to clarify not only the nature, but also the extent of the involved lesion. Additionally, examination establishes a basis whereby the physician is able to ascertain the progress of the patient as well as the success or failure of the treatment.

Examination of the lumbar spine should include standard orthopaedic and neurologic tests. Special attention is given to the deep tendon reflexes. Absence of the patellar reflex is frequently associated with the L4 nerve root. Likewise, a change in the Achilles reflex suggests a disturbance to the function of the S1 nerve root.

Muscle strength and weakness should be assessed. Heel walking evaluates the strength of the tibialis anterior and extensor muscle groups (L4–5 disk, whereas toe walking assesses the gastrocnemius and soleus function (L5–S1 disk). The overall condition of the hamstrings and quadriceps should be noted. Hypertonus or spasm along these muscles could indicate a loss of joint play in the hip or sacroiliac joint.

The pelvic girdle and lumbar region should be visually examined for relative symmetry. The iliac crest and greater trochanters should be noted for postural balance.

Restricted pelvic mobility is assessed by noting the movement of the posterior superior iliac spines. While palpating the posterior superior iliac spines in a standing position, have the patient lean forward. Any abnormal cephalic or anterior movement indicates a restricted pelvic movement. A comparison test can be done with the patient in the seated position. Once again, palpate the posterior superior iliac spines and have the patient lean forward, keeping the feet flat on the floor with the arms between the knees. If the movement of the posterior superior iliac spines is different from that in the standing version of the test, close examination into the possibility of a lower extremity dysfunction is necessary.

The Trendelenburg test is performed with the patient once again in the standing position while the clinician palpates the posterior superior iliac spine. Have the patient flex one knee and hip. The iliac crest should rise on the side of flexion. However, if the hip lowers on the side of flexion there is indication of a lesion to the opposite side.

The test for Kemp's sign can be performed with the patient either standing or in the seated position.

Sitting increases intradiscal pressure and therefore maximizes stress to the disk, whereas standing increases weightbearing and maximizes stress to the facets. The test for Kemp's sign should be performed in both positions. Kemp's sign can be positive for facet irritation or compression of a bulging nucleus against a nerve root. Normally speaking, a medial disk will produce greater pain when the patient is flexed away from the side of radicular involvement and lateral disk protrusions produce greater pain when the patient is flexed toward the side of radicular involvement.

Variations of the straight leg raising test may produce significant information for the examining physician. Normally, the degree of elevation of the leg at which pain is produced is noted by the physician, pain production being the positive sign. However, Breig and Troup made specific notations of certain aspects of pain production by the leg raising test (32). These authors suggested that after noting the level of pain on straight leg raising, the examiner should lower the extremity a few degrees to relieve the pain and dorsiflex the ankle while medially rotating the hip. Medial hip rotation places greater stretch on the lumbar and sacral nerve roots and accentuates the straight leg raising sign. If the pain that limits straight leg raising is elicited by dorsiflexion and medial hip rotation, increased nerve root tension is indicated, and the site of pain may assist in locating the level of a potential disk lesion.

Edgar and Park studied 50 patients over a 2-year period and concluded that the pattern of pain on straight leg raising was closely related to the central or lateral position of disk protrusion (33). Clinically, myelographic and operative observations were carried out on 50 patients to investigate the relationship between the pattern of pain in straight leg raising and the site of disk protrusion. In general it was noted that lateral disk protrusions produced pain along the lower extremity upon straight leg raising. Medial disk protrusions produced pain along the lower back, and medial (subrhizal) protrusions produce both back and leg pain.

Additional orthopaedic and neurologic tests will allow the physician to determine the process of a primary manipulative lesion. Clinical correlations are also important in determining contraindications for manipulation. Spinal manipulation is not a totally innocuous procedure. By far the major portion of severe complications arise from injuries to the cerebral circulation or spinal cord following cervical manipulation (34). Injuries to the lumbar spine are much less common. The most common complication to the lumbar region with manipulation appears to be the accentuation of disk injury. These complications are most likely due to the use of long-lever, high-force, nonspecific rotational manipulations. Additionally, costovertebral and costochondral joint strains maybe associated with nonspecific manipulation.

SPINAL BIOMECHANICS

Many practitioners of manipulation make fine measurements of vertebral positional relationships prior to manipulation. The prime reason for determining these relationships, and vertebral positions, is to determine the direction in which the manipulative thrust should be given. Vertebra position takes into consideration the slope of the facets and the position of the vertebra, which can allow a less dramatic force in producing the desired correction. Hildebrandt and Howe made in in-depth listing of biomechanical changes and positions in accordance with the static and kinetic aspects of the involved vertebral motor units (35).

Perhaps the most widely held view of joint dysfunction is that of a restriction, fixation, or blockage along a specific joint (36). The location and characteristics of the fixation must be determined prior to manipulation. Consideration should be given to any decrease and/or increase in the normal range of motions of the joints. Also, it is important to note and take into consideration any aberrant motion of the spine. Aberant motion can be described as movement of a vertebra out of the normal phase with a segment above and below the involved unit. Specific methods for palpating vertebral motion have been developed and taught (36). Interestingly, Johnson found that there was a high degree of correlation between the palpatory findings of different clinicians using similar palpatory techniques (37).

Palpation of paraspinal soft tissue changes is an important aspect. Tenderness, muscle spasm, and trigger points have been noted by clinicians who treat spinal dysfunctions. The detection of soft tissue changes should be considered an important indicator in the presence of a manipulative lesion (38). The presence of muscle contractions and muscle imbalance cannot be ignored because many manipulative techniques are directed toward muscles rather than joints and ligaments (39). The goal of these techniques is to relax the spasm or contraction and balance synergistic or opposing muscle groups.

TYPES OF MANIPULATION

Joint manipulation, as any other clinical art, represents a practical skill. To the casual observer it may appear quite simple. However, a wealth of practiced manual dexterity combined with an ability to concentrate on the changing status of the soft tissues of the patient is required. Skilled manipulators are able to develop effective techniques that require small amounts of force and reduce amenable reactions to the procedures.

A thorough review of manipulation reveals two integral types of techniques. Manipulation can be categorized as either general or specific. A general spinal manipulation is considered to be a regional type of manipulation and is actually a stretch performed to more than one joint and over more than one spinal segment. General manipulation has an increased chance of failure because it is applied to nonspecific points and may mobilize joints that have normal motion and hyperextend joints that have hypermobility. Specific manipulation is directed toward only one joint. This type of manipulation minimizes force to surrounding and uninvolved spinal segments. In general this type of manipulation is considered to be a safer and more effective technique, but also requires a greater skill by the manipulator.

The categorization of manipulation may be further divided into direct versus indirect manipulation. Direct manipulation involves manipulation into the direction of motion restriction whereas indirect manipulation produces movement in the opposite direction of motion restriction. Indirect manipulation is considered to be a safer technique and, perhaps, is less painful for the patient (40). Normally manipulators will not attempt direct manipulation until all possibilities of correction by indirect manipulation have been exhausted. While direct manipulation may be painful for the patient, there are some specific indications for the utilization of direct manipulation, and in the presence of these indications the utilization of the technique by the manipulator is both a logical and effective choice.

Other types of manipulative techniques are those of the contact or noncontact technique. Contact manipulation requires the hand or the finger to make contact with the involved segment. Contacts are frequently made along the spinous process or mamillary process of the lumbar spine. In noncontact techniques there is no direct contact with the hand or finger over the site of involvement. Normally these techniques are used when greater force is necessary to release a joint.

SPECIFIC TYPES OF MANIPULATION

For the sake of simplifying our discussion of manipulative techniques the following definitions will be used:

1. *Contact hand:* the hand used by the manipulator to deliver the thrust.
2. *Segmental contact point:* the point of the patient that is to be contacted by the contact hand.
3. *Contact point:* the part of the contact hand that is directly over the segmental contact point.
4. *Stabilizing hand:* the hand away from the contact hand; it is used in stabilization.
5. *Segmental stabilizing joint:* the part of the patient that comes in contact with the stabilizing hand and is used for stabilization.

A widely used technique for the correction of lumbar lesions and sacroiliac joint dysfunctions is the specific short-lever, high-velocity spinal manipulation. An example of this technique would be the double thenar manipulation. To perform this manipulation the patient should be lying in the prone position. The technique is performed best when utilizing a specific table that allows the pelvic area to be stabilized while permitting the thoracic and abdominal region to drop away. Once the direction or line of drive of the correction is determined the manipulator stands on the side in which the correction is to be made. The contact point is the thenar process of the contact hand. Stabilization would be achieved by placing the thenar portion of the stabilizing hand over the segmental stabilizing point (the mamillary process opposite the side of involvement). In this particular move, the line of drive of the correction is the most important aspect, along with any torque that may be induced to facilitate the correction. The manipulation is delivered in a high-velocity, low-amplitude thrust (Fig. 11.1).

A short-lever, high-velocity manipulation can also be carried out with the patient in the sidelying position. Several variations exist and are effective. The levers used in the sidelying position are normally the spinous process or the mamillary process of the lumbar vertebrae. If utilizing the spinous process, the patient should be in the sidelying position with the side of the vertebra rotation placed downward and the superior leg flexed. The contact

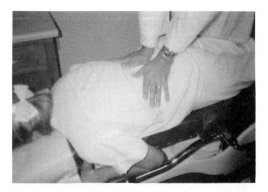

Figure 11.1. Double thenar manipulation.

hand is the inferior hand. The contact point is the tip of the fingers along the contact hand. The segmental contact point is the inferior side of the spinous process to be manipulated. Using the superior hand, the clinician contacts the superior shoulder of the patient (segmental stabilizing point) and slightly rotates posteriorly to bring the spine to tension. The hip is simultaneously flexed downward with the thigh portion of the manipulator's leg. The high-velocity thrust is with a pulling motion along the desired line of correction (Fig. 11.2).

A similar type of manipulation that can be effective for rotational malpositionings and/or fixations can be achieved with a pushing action. Once again the patient is placed in the sidelying position with the side of spinous rotation placed downward. The contact hand is the inferior hand. The contact point is normally the pisiform process of the contact hand. The segmental contact point is the mamillary process of the vertebra to be corrected. Once again using the shoulder as the segmental stabilizing point, the spine is brought to tension. The high-

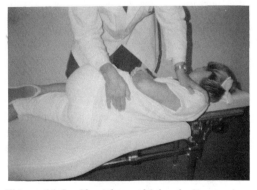

Figure 11.2 Short-lever, high-velocity manipulation with patient in the sidelying position.

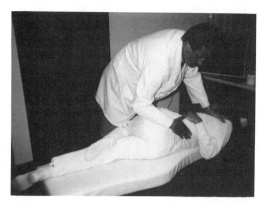

Figure 11.3. Manipulation for correction of rotational malpositionings and/or fixations.

velocity thrust is made along the desired line of correction and torque can be utilized to correct inferiority or superiority (Fig. 11.3).

The sacroiliac joint dysfunctions may be corrected with short-lever manipulations. The patient is placed in the sidelying position with the involved joint up. If the ilium is rotated posteriorly, the segmental contact point will be the posterior superior spine of the ilium. The contact hand is the inferior hand. The contact point is the pisiform of the contact hand. The shoulder (segmental stabilizing point) is rotated posteriorly to bring the spine into tension. The thrust is made from the posterior to the anterior toward the shoulder. If the ilium is rotated anteriorly, a push along the ischium in a posterior and inferior manner may bring the ilium back into position (Fig. 11.4).

Once the primary manipulative lesion is detected, the direction in which motion is lost has been determined, and the facet placings and structural relationships between the vertebrae are known, it is possible to formulate a technique that will theoretically correct the lesion. It should be noted, however, that crude, nonspecific manipulations are potentially dangerous. Skilled and refined art with knowledge of the changing state of the soft tissues around the spine is essential to prevent injury to the patient.

NONSPECIFIC LONG-LEVER MANIPULATIONS

Long-lever manipulations are described as manipulations that utilize and exert force on a part of the body some distance from the area that is expected to receive the beneficial effect. Long levers used in this type of manipulation include the leg, the shoulder, the pelvis, and the thoracic spine. The most commonly used long-lever technique for

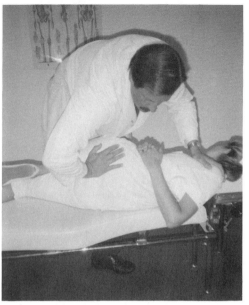

Figure 11.4. Short-lever manipulation for correction of sacroiliac joint dysfunctions.

the lumbar spine is the rotational manipulation as described by Cyriax (40). The patient is placed in the sidelying position with the involved side up. The hip and the superior leg are flexed while the inferior leg is held in extension. The clinician stands in front of the patient and stabilizes the shoulder of the superior hand. The contact hand is placed on the buttock of the patient and is used to roll the patient's pelvis forward. With this particular technique a general rotation is placed along the lumbar spine in a nonspecific fashion.

The long levers make it very difficult, although not impossible, to make a specific manipulation. Generally speaking, the force is exerted into the entire region of the lumbar spine. The vertebral level that receives most of the mobilization is often the one that is hypermobile rather than the one at which motion is restricted.

DISTRACTION MANIPULATION

Distraction techniques can be utilized in the treatment of lumbar disk protrusion, spondylolisthesis, facet syndrome, subluxation, and scoliotic curves of a nonsurgical nature, and can be utilized to restore the normal range of motion along the lumbar spine. Cox described the Cox Flexion Distraction manipulation as a form of chiropractic spinal manipulative therapy that increases the intervertebral disk height to remove annular distortion, allows the nucleus pulposus to assume its central position, restores vertebral joints to their physiologic relationships of motion, and improves posture and locomotion while relieving pain (41).

Distraction techniques utilize specific tables that allow the physician to place the patient through the specific ranges of motion of flexion, extension, lateral bending, rotation, and circumduction and further allows for distraction of the lumbar spine.

This technique can be extremely beneficial in the case of a lumbar disk herniation. The technique uses low force and can be employed to the patient's tolerance, which allows for an effective and general way of dealing with the patient with severe lower back pain and/or radiation of pain to the lower extremities.

SOFT TISSUE MANIPULATION

Soft tissue manipulation and/or pressure point manipulation can also be effective in reducing lower back pain. Light pressure with the thumbs and/or elbow over the trigger point and muscle tenderness as well as deep goading of the muscle groups can be effective in reducing contractures and balancing lower extremity muscles. Special attention should be given to the piriformis muscles because their contractions can produce significant pain to the lower back and lower flank region.

CONTRAINDICATIONS TO MANIPULATION

It is generally considered that the most severe complications from manipulation arise from injury to the cerebral circulation following cervical manipulation. Injuries to the lumbar spine are much less common and usually can be prevented by employing proper diagnostic procedures and proper techniques (42). The most frequently experienced complication of lumbar manipulation is the prolapse of a herniated intervertebral disk, resulting in cauda equina syndrome (43). The most common forebear of failed manipulation of the lumbar spine is inadequate examination to rule out contraindications or the use of crude manipulative techniques that are nonspecific in the hands of unskilled and untrained manipulators.

REFERENCES

1. Withington ET (ed): *Hippocrates with an English Translation,* Cambridge, MA, Harvard University Press, 1959, vol 3, pp 278–307.
2. Schafer RC: *Chiropractic Health Care,* ed 2, Des Moines, IA, Foundation for Chiropractic Education and Research, 1976.
3. Kirkaldy-Willis WH, Cassidy JD: Spinal manipulation in the treatment of low back pain. *Can Fam Physician* 31:535–540, 1985.
4. Dvorak J: Manual medicine in the United States and Europe in the Year 1982. *Manual Med* 1:3–9, 1983.
5. Wood J, Adams AA: Comparison of forces used in selective adjustments of the low back by experienced chiropractors and chiropractic students with no clinical experience: preliminary study. *Res Forum* 1:18, 1984.
6. Fisk JW: Manipulation in general practice. *N Z Med J* 74:172, 1971.
7. Evans DP, Burke MS, Lloyds KN, Roberts EE, Roberts GM: Lumbar spinal manipulation on trial. Part I. Clinical assessment. *Rheumatol Rehab* 17:46, 1978.
8. Rassmussen GG: Manipulation in low back pain: a randomized clinical trial. *Manual Med* 1:8, 1977.
9. Coxhead CE, Inskip H, Meade TW, North WRS, Troup JDG: Multicentre trial of physiotherapy in the management of sciatic symptoms. *Lancet* 1:1065, 1981.
10. Waagen GN, Haldeman S, Cook G, Lopez D, Deboer J: Short term trial of chiropractic adjustments for the relief of chronic low back pain. *Manual Med* 2:63–67, 1986.
11. Bronfort G: Chiropractic treatment of low back pain: a prospective survey. *J Manipulative Physiol Ther* 9:99–112, 1986.
12. Thabe H: Electromyography as a tool to document diagnostic findings and therapeutic results associated with somatic dysfunctions in the upper cervical spinal joints and sacroiliac joints. *Manual Med* 2:53–58, 1986.
13. Cassidy JD, Kirkaldy-Willis WH, McGregor M: Spinal manipulation for the treatment of chronic low back and leg pain: an observational study. In Buerger AA, Greenman PE (eds): *Empirical Approaches to the Validation of Spinal Manipulation.* Springfield, IL, Charles C Thomas, 1985, pp 199–150.
14. Burnarski DJ: Chiropractic biomechanical evaluations: validity in myofascial low back pain. *J Manipulative Physiol Ther* 5: 155–161, 1982.
15. Grice AS: Radiographic, biomechanical and clinical factors in lumbar lateral flexion. Part I. *J Manipulative Physiol Ther* 2:26–34, 1979.
16. Carrick FR: Treatment of pathomechanics of the lumbar spine by manipulation. *J Manipulative Physiol Ther* 4:173–178, 1981.
17. Schafer RC; *Chiropractic Management of Sports and Recreational Injuries.* Baltimore, Williams & Wilkins, 1982, pp 273–274.
18. Johnston WL: Inter-rater reliability on the selection of manipulable patients. In Buerger AA, Greenman PE (eds): *Empirical Approaches to the Validation of Spinal Manipulation.* Springfield, IL, Charles C. Thomas, 1985, p 107.
19. Neuman H: A concept of manual medicine. In Buerger

AA, Greenman PE (eds): *Empirical Approaches to the Validation of Spinal Manipulation.* Springfield, IL, Charles C. Thomas, 1985, p 267.

20. White AA, Panjabi M: The role of stabilitation in the treatment of cervical spine injuries. *Spine* 9:229–238, 1984.

21. Denslow JS, Hassett CC: The central excitatory state associated with postural abnormalities. *J Neurophysiol* 5:393–402, 1942.

22. Korr IM: Proprioceptors and the discussion of mechanisms of manipulative therapy. In Korr IM (ed): *Neurobiologic Mechanisms in Manipulative Therapy.* New York, Plenum, 1978.

23. Glover JR: Back pain and hyperesthesia. *Lancet* 1:1165–1169, 1980.

24. Buerger AA: Experimental neuromuscular models of spinal manual techniques. *Manual Med* 1:10–17, 1983.

25. Rebechini-Zasadny H, Tasharski CC, Heinze WJ: Electromyographic analysis following chiropractic manipulation of the cervical spine: a model to study manipulation-induced peripheral muscle changes. *J Manipulative Physiol Ther* 4:61–63, 1984.

26. Terrett ACJ, Vernon H: Manipulation and pain tolerance: a controlled study of the effects of spinal manipulation on paraspinal cutaneous pain tolerance level. *Am J Phys Med* 63:217–225.

27. Vernon HT, Dhami MI, Hawley TP, Annett R: Spinal manipulation and beta-endorphin: a controlled study of the effect of a spinal manipulation on plasma beta-endorphin levels in normal males. *J Manipulative Physiol Ther* 9:115–122, 1986.

28. Mixter WJ, Barr IS: Rupture of the intervertebral disc with involvement of the spinal canal. *N Engl J Med* 211:210–215, 1934.

29. Wood PHN, Badley EM: Epidemiology of back pain. In Jayson M (ed): *The Lumbar Spine and Back Pain,* ed 2. Tunbridge Wells, Kent, England, Pittman Medical Publishing Co, 1980, pp 29–55.

30. Murphy RW: Nerve roots and spinal nerves in degenerative disc disease. *Clin Orthop Rel Res* 129:46–60, 1977.

31. Marshall LL, Trethewil ER, Curtain CC: Chemical radiculitis. *Clin Orthop* 129:61–67, 1977.

32. Breig A, Troup JDG: Biomechanical considerations in the straight leg raising test. *Spine* 4:242–250, 1979.

33. Edgar MA, Park WM: Induced pain patterns on passive straight leg raising in lower lumbar disc protrusions. *J Bone Joint Surg [Br]* 56:4, 1974.

34. Loach AA: *The Chiropractic Theories,* ed 2. Baltimore, Williams & Wilkins, 1986.

35. Hildebrandt RW, Howe JW: *Spinal Biomechanics and Subluxation Classification.* Lowbrand, IL, National College of Chiropractic, 1974.

36. Gillet H, Liekens M: *Belgian Chiropractic Research Notes,* ed 10. Brussels, Self-published, 1973.

37. Johnson WL: Interexaminer reliability in palpation. *J Am Osteopath Assoc* 76:286, 1976.

38. Tavell J: Myofascial trigger points. Clinical review. In Bonica JJ, Albe-Fessard DG (eds): *Advances in Pain Research and Therapy.* New York, Raven Press, 1976, vol 1, p 919.

39. Haldeman S: Spinal manipulation therapy: a status report. *Clin Orthop Rel Res* 179:62–70, 1983.

40. Cyriax J: *Textbook of Orthopaedic Medicine,* Vol 2, ed 8. London, Bailliere-Tindall, 1971.

41. Cox JM: *Low Back Pain: Mechanism, Diagnosis and Treatment,* ed 4. Baltimore, Williams & Wilkins, 1985.

42. Terrett AG: Vascular accidents from cervical spine manipulation: the mechanics of chiropractic. *J Chiropractic* 25(5):59–74, 1988.

43. Jennet WB: A study of 25 cases of compression of the cauda equina by prolapse IVD. J Neurol Neurosurg 79:109–116, 1956.

Chapter 12

BIOFEEDBACK AND RELAXATION THERAPIES

JEFFREY R. CRAM, PHD
THOMAS H. BUDZYNSKI, PHD

Biofeedback is slowly coming to be viewed within the context of applied psychophysiology. Biofeedback is a multifaceted set of procedures, describing the process in which biologic information is "monitored" and "fed back" to the patient in an attempt to reestablish or "relearn" homeostasis. It is commonly used adjunctively with relaxation procedures (or relaxation may be utilized by itself). Luthe (1) and Jacobson (2) introduced relaxation techniques during the early 1900s as the means to achieve homeostasis.

When biofeedback is used, it usually involves a two-stage process. The first stage, physiologic monitoring, should lead to a description of the pathophysiology (3). How and where the physiologic system is monitored will set boundaries for the clinical or diagnostic findings. The second stage, biologic feedback, is typically directed at the pathophysiology observed during stage one. The external feedback is intended to functionally replace the faulty "negative feedback" loop found within the patient's physiologic system (4).

When biofeedback and relaxation are applied to pain-related disorders, the musculoskeletal or neuromuscular system is of primary interest. To adequately work within this system, one would want to diagnostically consider, and potentially treat, the three following areas: the neuromuscular system's capacity for emotional displays, the primary role it plays in postural support, and the contributions to pain arising from the muscle organ itself.

The clinical application of biofeedback through general relaxation techniques is limited to the treatment of the emotional displays embedded as part of the pain cycle. The emotional displays may extend well beyond the central nervous system (CNS) (muscles) to include the arousal of various aspects of the autonomic nervous system (ANS) as well. In addition, the cognitive, sensory, and affective domains of pain may be explored through relaxation therapies, to better teach the patient how to cope with the pain, and fear of it.

The postural and muscular aspects of pain may also be considered. To work with the neuromuscular system, one should appreciate and understand some of its complexities. For example, the sensory system for the muscles (muscle spindles, Golgi tendon organs, Ruffini terminals, and free nerve endings) informs the CNS of the instantaneous status of each muscle, while strongly modulating the output of the final common pathway of the motor unit, by pushing nd pulling on the two motor systems (alpha and gamma). The primary function of the skeletal muscles is postural support. Once posture is assumed, the secondary function of movement may take place. Posture and movement patterns may be altered by a shortened resting length of the muscle, by muscle splinting, or by a learned protective guarding pattern to prevent pain. All of these aspects may be quantified and potentially treated with the aid of electromyography (EMG) biofeedback instruments.

This chapter focuses primarily upon the use of surface EMG in the diagnosis and treatment of back pain. In the discussion of general relaxation techniques this focus is necessarily broadened to include autonomic indicators. A brief review of each of the three areas of potential investigation and treatment

Table 12.1
Diagnostic Frameworks[a]

DIAGNOSTIC LEVEL	DIAGNOSTIC PROCEDURE	TREATMENT OPTIONS
No diagnosis	None	Treat everybody the same
Emotional		
General	Stress profile (typically frontal site)	General relaxation, recliner chair therapy
Specific	EMG scan, stress profile (site-specific recording)	Site-specific relaxation, transactional psychophysiology
Organicity		
Metabolic	EMG scan, dynamic movement, symmetries assessed	Myotherapy, site-specific relaxation
Resting length	EMG scan, dynamic movement, symmetries assessed	Stretch to relax, site-specific feedback
Postural	EMG scan, dynamic movement, gravitational	Postural change, biomechanics

[a] From Cram JR: Surface EMG recordings and pain related disorders: a diagnostic framework. *Biofeedback Self Regul* 13:125, 1988.

is given. The diagnostic procedures are described, the different levels of findings reviewed, and the implications for differential treatment explored. Treatment strategies and protocols are briefly described. Particular emphasis is placed on the interaction between diagnostic findings, diagnostic procedures, and the array of possible treatment procedures. Table 12.1 provides the reader with four different levels of diagnosis and associated treatment protocols. The basic philosophy that guides the use of surface electromyography and relaxation in the treatment of pain-related disorders is: Differential diagnosis should lead to differential treatment.

THE "NO DIAGNOSIS" MODEL

The "No Diagnosis" model would be invoked when a practitioner or researcher utilizes the same muscle site (e.g., frontalis), the same relaxation procedure (e.g., guided imagery), and/or the same posture (e.g., recliner chair) with *all* patients who present for evaluation, treatment, or study. In other words, treatment of the patient is the same because variations in the presenting problem have not been considered.

This type of diagnostic thinking and treatment planning suffers from the overutilization of both the "patient uniformity" and "treatment uniformity" myths (5). It is this type of thinking that led earlier reviewers (6) to conclude that the clinical efficacy for EMG or relaxation therapies in the

treatment of pain was poor. More recent reviews (7), however, have cast away this simplistic thinking, and have clearly acknowledged and elaborated upon the multiple etiologies of myogenic (back) pain, considering multifaceted diagnostic and treatment procedures.

THE GENERAL EMOTIONAL MODEL AND RELAXATION TRAINING

The general emotional model is the oldest and best known model for the biofeedback researcher and clinician. The physiologic aspects of this model have grown out of the early work on general activation theory (8–10). Jacobson (2) and Sargent (11) initially extended this clinically, by laying down the foundations that increased muscle tension, and therefore painful muscles, may spring from ineffective coping with environmental and emotional stress. This has been supported by later studies (12, 13). The increased anxiety and concomitant static increase in muscular tension lead to a state of muscular fatigue characterized by initial muscle ischemia, followed by hyperemia (14), both potentially stimulating nociception. With increased nociception, the ANS may come into play. In the acute pain phase, there is a shift in autonomic balance to sympathetic dominance (stress pattern). With a chronic condition, the recovery phase may not occur.

A second aspect of the general emotional model is a psychological one. Any clinician who has evaluated chronic pain patients has observed that the level of pain and the degree of stress experienced by the patient are positively correlated. Chronic pain is itself a stressor, and adds to additional stressors experienced by the patient. These include the round after round of sometimes painful and time-consuming medical tests, physical therapy, vocational rehabilitation, psychiatric and psychological testing, and possibly psychotherapy. The loss of income often contributes to family or marital discord. Moreover, there is the very real possibility that the former job will not be waiting for the chronic pain patient in the event that he/she does recover enough to go back to work after some time. Friendships are strained or destroyed because the pain patient no longer enjoys many of the formerly shared activities. In most cases there is a deterioration of sexual functioning. Finally, there is the agony of not knowing if part or all of the pain is "all in the mind," as many patients are brought to believe. Self-esteem is eroded as a result and further contributes to the stress of the patient.

In assessing the back pain patient, a careful clinical interview is needed to clarify the level of stress the patient is experiencing. From a biofeedback point of view, the monitoring of both CNS (muscle) and ANS (hand temperature, electrodermal activity, heart rate, blood volume pulse, respiration) indicators during "stress profiling" or a "pain interview" is indicated. From this two-pronged approach, the relative emphasis on relaxation and/or stress management during treatment may be determined. Relaxation alone is seldom indicated. If relaxation is indicated by hyperactive or chronic activation patterns in the emotional display patterns of the muscles or ANS, the next major choice entails selecting the appropriate relaxation technique.

Davidson and Schwartz (15) argued that one should match the technique to the patient's individual style. If the patient is a squirming, fidgeting pain patient then the stress profile more likely than not indicates the muscular system should be treated using a Jacobsonian Progressive Relaxation (2). If the interview indicates a very strong ruminative cognitive style, a more mental form of relaxation such as autogenics (1), meditation (16), or open focus (17) would be suggested. In such patients, psychotherapy will also tend to play a larger role. Finally, if the patient is more autonomically bound, one might consider respiration training (18) to help quiet the overall system. Lang et al. (19) pointed out that the physiologic systems are loosely coupled. Treating one system may not alter other systems. It has been noted by some (20), however,

that during muscle relaxation training, there will be a shift in autonomic balance from apparent sympathetic dominance (stress pattern) to a pattern characterized by an increase in parasympathetic activity (rest pattern).

Audiocassette home relaxation programs often combine several of the above-mentioned techniques so that patients can later choose the one they prefer. Moreover, one of us (T.H.B.) has found that use of subliminal processing in the form of audiocassettes is very helpful in the reduction of pain (see later in this chapter).

PROGRESSIVE MUSCLE RELAXATION

Developed by Edmund Jacobson (2) the 1930s, progressive muscle relaxation (PMR) has been applied to a great variety of pain and stress-related disorders and remains to this day one of the most widely used relaxation training systems. It involves a tensing and relaxing of the muscles. The practice develops a fine "muscle sense" that enables patients to be very aware of the inappropriate tensing of the skeletal muscles. Electromyographic biofeedback is commonly used in an adjunctive fashion with this technique. Here, the feedback provides an objective measure of muscle activity that the patient may use to refine his/her internal sensory awareness.

Progressive muscle relaxation is a very good starting point for patients who are "squirmers," or have a poor muscle sense or little awareness of the tension in their muscles. For an excellent description of the procedures associated with PMR see Catalano (21). One word of caution concerning chronic pain patients using this technique: The patient must be cautioned not to overdo the tensing of a painful muscle group!

AUTOGENIC TRAINING

Based on the work of Johannes Schultz and Wolfgang Luthe (1), autogenic training involves a series of phrases that, when repeated over and over mentally and with the correct attitude, produce a relaxation of the skeletal muscles and a shift in autonomic balance from sympathetic toward parasympathetic dominance.

Unlike PMR, autogenic training involves passive mental exercises so there is little chance of the pain patient hurting him/herself. These phrases are designed to produce specific changes in the physiology when repeated silently. However, it is crucial that the trainee adopt the correct focus of attention. If the trainee tries too hard to produce the suggested change the opposite reaction will often take place. This type of incorrect attitude must be changed to one that is more passive in nature. It is a very subtle change and one that is sometimes difficult to convey to the patient/trainee. While mentally repeating the phrases and thinking of the body part involved, the patient learns to "just allow" the suggested change to happen. The monitoring of the patient's physiology with biofeedback instruments objectifies the shift in physiologic functioning.

Most biofeedback therapists have icnorporated just a few of the total number of autogenic training phrases into their relaxation-oriented work. The phrases most often employed involve heaviness in the limbs and warmth in the hands and feet. For a detailed account of the phrases and procedures associated with autogenic training, see Catalano (21). As with PMR, the autogenic training phrases should be practiced for roughly 20 min twice a day.

MEDITATION

Some patients will be more successful with a form of meditation than with PMR or autogenic training. A previous history of successful use of one or the other sometimes provides a clue. If necessary, the patient may need to try each of these three procedures while monitoring the physiologic effect of each. On this trial-and-error basis, the one that produces the deepest relaxation may be selected for further development of skills. In any event, biofeedback plays the role of verifying the pattern of change, rather than actively leading the person to the relaxed state.

As with PMR and autogenic training, the patient will need to be given a rationale for doing meditation each day. It is helpful to explain that the mental process of repeating a mantra or phrase tends to produce a state of wakeful relaxation with a shift away from the stress pattern into one of rest. The choosing of a mantra should be done with the patient's involvement. For further information on the procedures associated with meditation, see Benson (16).

RESPIRATION TRAINING

Everyone would probably agree that breathing patterns are affected by stress and pain, but few realize how influential respiration can be in the development of relaxation skills. In his excellent text *The Hyperventilation Syndrome,* Robert Fried (18) details the theory, research, and application of breathing patterns. His major thesis is that stressed and distressed human beings hyperventilate.

Hyperventilation is a fast, shallow, upper chest or thoracic breathing pattern. Fried has noted that hyperventilation is the most frequently observed breathing disorder in persons who suffer from emotional or psychophysiologic disorders. Moreover, respiration patterns are altered by the presence of pain. As part of an activation pattern acute, severe pain produces fast, shallow thoracic breathing. Even moderate pain seems to result in a thoracic, as contrasted to a diaphragmatic, pattern.

If pain is located in the low back or abdominal area, respiration pattern may be chronically altered in a thoracic fashion as a pain-avoidance behavior. The diaphragm is a dome-shaped muscle that separates the thorax from the abdominal/visceral region. When relaxed, the diaphragm is in its dome shape, vaulted upward into the lower space filled by the lungs. In normal respiratory patterns, the diaphragm is contracted during the inspiration phase, and the dome is collapsed downward, causing a negative pressure so that the lungs may fill. During this phase, the abdominal region below the diaphragm is pushed downward and outward. During normal expiration phase, the diaphragm relaxes, moving back to its dome shape, and the pressure on the abdomen is released and it flattens out. It is not uncommon to see a thoracic respiration pattern in low back pain patients as a means to avoid movement of a painful area. Unfortunately, this adds to their painful condition by "turning on" a sympathetic dominance.

If a dysfunctional respiratory pattern is noted during the diagnostic evaluation or if a high level of sympathetic activation is noted, training of the respiratory system is indicated. Interestingly enough, monitoring heart rate along with respiratory patterns allows assessment for the presence of a respiratory sinus arrhythmia (RSA). In a healthy person, there is an increase in heart rate with inspiration and a decrease with expiration. This normal periodic acceleration and deceleration is known as RSA, and is indicative of a low level of sympathetic arousal and normalized vagal tone. Fried has observed the absence of RSA in a number of anxiety- and psychosomatic-related disorders. In virtually every case where breathing retraining was accompanied by a reduction of symptoms, the RSA was restored.

Biofeedback training may be used to teach abdominal breathing and RSA in the pain patient. Computerized biofeedback screens can display beat-by-beat heart rate along with thoracic and abdominal respiration patterns. The patient watches the varying heart rate and respiration signal on the computer screen and, and with the gentle coaching of the biofeedback therapist, learns to shift the breathing from the thoracic to the abdominal region. The heart ate trace then begins to oscillate in a rough sinusoidal fashion showing the RSA pattern. Often, at the start, the production of the RSA seems foreign to the patient and a lightheadness may result from inhaling too deeply. When done properly, the lightheadedness goes away.

Once the RSA pattern is learned, generalization must bepursued. There is a need for the patient to be able to maintain the RSA as the therapist talks to him/her. When the patient can do this, the next phase is to develop the capacity to maintain the RSA while imagining a variety of personally stressful scenes. Finally, there is the problem of transfering the skill to real-life situations. The patient must be reminded to be aware of the breathing during the busy day. Small, brightly colored stick-on dots that can be obtained in any office supply store may be placed on the telephone, steering wheel, and so forth as reminders.

Breathing from the diaphragm is a very important skill to be learned by the pain patient. It tends to break the habit of maintaining a high level of chronic tension in the abdominal and low back musculature as well as other skeletal msucles. Once learned, patients often report a decrease in pain. Moreover, the RSA pattern helps shift the autonomic balance from sympathetic toward parasympathetic dominance. Nuernberger (22) noted that during thoracic breathing the motion of the lungs keeps the arousal mechanism activated, continuously creating an unnecessary level of stress.

To summarize, upper chest, thoracic breathing appears to be associated with a number of pathologic conditions and chronic pain as well. This type of breathing also seems to help maintain a state of sympathetic dominance or stress in the individual. The development of a diaphragmatic breathing style is associated with a more relaxed physiology and lessened degree of pain. The appearance of the RSA during abdominal breathing signals the proper breathing pattern. The training of the pain patient in this respiratory style is an important first step in the overall pain relief program

CASSETTE TAPE PROGRAMS FOR HOME PRACTICE

The difficult problem of transferring the relaxation and stress management skills into daily life is at least partialy solved by the use of audiocassettes. The home practice sessions help bridge the time between biofeedback sessions. Our experience has been that patients are more willing to use cassette tapes than to simply attempt to remember the verbal instructions given in the office training ses-sion. The tapes provide precise instruction on the details of relaxation practice.

The tape program by one of us (T.H.B.) has been used by a large number of clinicians over the years. It consists of six phases of training. The first phase is an abbreviated form of PMR. Its purpose is to develop a good "muscle sense" in the user. The second phase involves a more refined variation of the first phase. The third phase of training begins with a brief form of autogenic training. Phases four and five continue with autogenic training, with the fifth phase specialized for the relaxation of facial and jaw muscles. The sixth phase, titled "Stress Management," focuses on a form of systematic desensitization. The goal of this phase is the successful transfer of the relaxation to daily life. Follow-up results confirm the fact that patients will tend to fall back on daily listening to the tapes months or years after the training if symptoms should return.

Over the last 8 years one of the authors (T.H.B.) has made use of subliminal processing cassette tapes with the goal of increasing self-esteem, decreasing pain, and priming positive thinking (23). The rationale for the use of such a process involves a model of brain function that incorporates both a conscious and an unconscious. A dynamic model of the mind that can support the concept of subliminal processing is based partly on unconscious functioning. Emmanuel Dochin (24), a leading researcher in the study of cognitive psychobiology, emphasized that information processing is largely preconscious or not available to awareness. With the hypothesis that pain patients, as well as others, suffer from low self-esteem and negative thought processes, the use of a simple positive phrasing operation on the unconscious level may just prime a positive change in attitude in the patient. This, in fact, is what seems to happen when the tapes are used over a period of at least several weeks. Patients report an increase in positive mood and often a decrease in pain. They begin to have the feeling that they can improve their condition. The subliminal tapes thus constitute a way of establishing a more positive unconscious base in individuals who are often damaged on this level as well as consciously.

THE SPECIFIC EMOTIONAL MODEL AND TREATMENT OPTIONS

The development of a more *specific emotional model* flows from the writings of Lacey and Lacey

(25) on response stereotypy. They presented data on individual patients who responded in only one physiologic system, to a variety of stressors, over many years of study. In the biofeedback arena, several researchers (26–28) have noted the weakness of applying the "key muscle" hypothesis of activation to all cases. The specificity model essentially states that the EMG activation pattern may be found in specific muscle groups, as well as the more general frontalis recordings. Dysfunctional activation patterns, then, may be specific to one muscle group rather than indicative of a general arousal problem.

The specificity paradigm utilizes the psychophysiologic stress profiling procedure directed at specific muscle groups or sites. Consider the EMG recordings from the right and left aspects of the trapezius of a single patient (Fig. 12.1). Here, an individual patient was asked to rest, engage in a serial mental arithmetic task out loud (mild stress), and then relax to the best of her abilities. The recordings clearly show a "specific" EMG activation pattern. The left aspect responds to the mild stressor while the right aspect does not. In this particular case, the patient had injured her left shoulder in a fall some 6 months prior. She reported a very strong relationship between stress and the intensity of the pain in her left shoulder. This type of response pattern might fall under the "weakened organ" or the "diathesis stress" models (29), where a structurally weak organ becomes the primary pathway for physiologic responses to stress.

It is also possible to conduct psychophysiologic

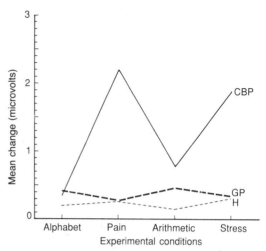

Figure 12.2 Psychophysiologic stress profile from the low back. *CBP,* chronic back pain patients; *GP,* general pain patients; *H,* healthy controls. (From Flor H, Turk D, Birbaumer N: Assessment of stress-related psychophysiological reactions in chronic back pain patients. *J Consult Clin Psychol* 53(3):359), 1985.)

stress profiling of the low back muscles. Figure 12.2 presents data taken from a very well-controlled group study by Flor et al. (29). In this study the frontalis, along with the right and left aspects of the L3 paraspinals, were monitored by EMG in a set of well-matched patients subjects. Chronic back pain patients, general pain patients, and healthy controls were asked to engage in four events while sitting unsupported in a chair. The results of the study indicated that the general activation associated with frontalis EMG recordings did not differentiate between the groups. The L3 paraspinal recordings, however, indicated significant activation patterns during the two personally relevant stressors (discuss your pain; discuss a recent stressful event). Again, this type of response pattern falls under the diathesis stress model (29) for idiopathic back pain.

The treatment offered individuals who display this type of specific activation should logically follow from the diagnostic findings. Given the lack of generalization of EMG-assisted relaxation training from the frontalis site to muscles of the torso or limbs (26, 31), the frontalis site would be a poor selection. More specificc feedback to the trapezius or erector spinae muscles would be indicated. The patient would be offered specific relaxation training for the specific site of activation: left trapezius for the first patient example and L3 paraspinals for the

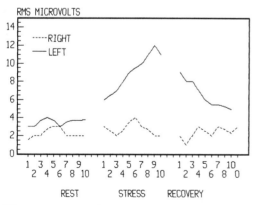

Figure 12.1 Psychophysiologic stress profile of right and left trapezius in an individual patient. (From Cram JR: Surface EMG recordings and pain related disorders: a diagnostic framework. *Biofeedback Self Regul* 13:127, 1988.)

second patient example. This relaxation training is then generalized from the "quiet state" through visualization of stressful events or by giving EMG feedback during stress/pain management sessions in which the impact of coping with the pain is being discussed. When activation patterns are "provoked" during the discussion, this is acknowledged and a brief quieting response is conducted.

Specific activation patterns may also lateralize to one side at a specific site. In the Flor et al. (30) study, there was a "more robust" left-sided activation pattern. Cram and Engstrom (32) have noted that the *left* low back clearly separates chronic back pain patients from normal subjects, but only in the standing posture. Why the left aspect? Two theoretical frameworks may be used to explain these left-sided findings. The first is an emotional one. It is possible to argue that negative emotions (or pain) are represented primarily in the right hemisphere of the brain (33). In addition, it has been observed that patients with "hysterical" symptoms tend to display these symptoms primarily on the left side of the body (34). The second, more parsimonious framework is a biomechanical one. It essentially assumes that the majority of the population is right-handed, and thus "overutilize" the left low back muscles as they move off their center of gravity to operate in their world. This overuse pattern sets the stage for neuromuscular or mechanical disturbances on the left aspect. The diathesis stress model proposed by Flor et al. (3) takes this one step further, suggesting that environmental or psychological stress would tend to find its expression in these weakened muscular structures.

THE ORGANICITY MODEL

The organicity model has grown out of interest in the muscle as an organ in and of itself. When one attempts to understand the phenomenon of muscle tension pain, several organ-specific parameters should be considered: the nature of the pain receptor, the circulation and metabolism of the muscle, nodules or other structural changes in the muscle, the resting length of the muscle, and splinting guarding patterns.

For muscle-related pain to exist, there needs to be an anatomic prerequisite. Within the muscle, there exist free nerve endings that primarily surround the arteries and arterioles supplying the muscle. These are sensitive to acidotic conditions or mechanical stimulation caused by swelling. Lack of adequate clearance of the metabolite lactic acid

is associated with ischemia. The nocioception associated with this type of disturbance comes on fairly quickly. If the event or activity causing this environment ceases, the pain typically subsides in a short period of time (a few hours maximum). Severe or prolonged reductions in oxygen will lead to an increase in the release of bradykinin, prostaglandin, and serotonin (35, 36). These lower the threshold for nocioception associated with swelling, edema, and the buildup of muscle metabolites (37). As a result of these metabolic changes, even moderate muscle contractions may now lead to pain.

Interestingly enough, the pain associated with a disturbance in circulation and metabolism that leads to swelling and edema is associated with a "temporal dislocation" of pain. This is commonly termed "delayed-onset muscle soreness" or DOMS. Here, the muscular effort responsible for the circulation-metabolism imbalance may have occurred hours or the day before the actual experience of the pain. This phenomenon has created some probelms in the study of headache and other related pain (38, 39).

To complicate things further, prolonged diminished oxygen supply can cause necrosis of muscle tissue, creating a nodule, "taut band," or "trigger point" (40). Travell has clearly documented that these trigger points may refer pain to locations away from the source of stimulation. Travell and Rinzler (41), for example, have demonstrated how pain in the head or face may be associated with trigger points in the neck or shoulders. More recently, Travell and Simons (42) have published a comprehensive map of referred zones for the torso, neck, and head. It is important to note that this "spatial dislocation" of pain will tend to create problems in pain-related research and diagnostic procedures. If one attmepts to identify pathophysiology at the site of reported pain, one may or may not find it. Phillips (38), for example, observed only a 40% concordance between the strongest pain and the highest level of muscle activity.

In addition, one needs to consider the phenomenon of splinting and protective guarding (43). In the acute phase when a joint or area is initially injured, the muscles of the surrounding area tighten down to provide a "muscular splint." This "reflexive spasm" has a strong biologic advantage, preventing further injury to the area or joint. If the splinting persists for a prolonged period of time, however, it may merge into a self-sustaining "pain-spasm-pain" cycle (44). This is one of the proposed mechanisms for the development of trigger point nodules (45). This longer term process may merge into a protective guarding pattern (43), in which the patient learns to favor the injured area, motorically moving away from the source of pain. In the acute splinting phase one would expect to see specific EMG activation patterns at the reported site of pain. In the more chronic phase of protective guarding, one would expect to see the specific EMG activation pattern in a homologous muscle group away from the pain.

Given these phenomena, it would seem naive to assume that the EMG activation pattern will be found at the site of reported pain. Perhaps it is this nature of the neuromuscular system that led Goldstein (46) to suggest that one should sample from multiple sites of the muscular system. Hudzynski and Lawrence (47), for example, reported that site of "electrode placement" was a major factor in separating headache patients from non–headache patients, and headache periods from non–headache periods. In addition, Cram and Steger (48) have introduced, and Cram and Cahn (49) have reviewed, the development of an EMG muscle scanning technique. This technique allows the practitioner to rapidly sample the "static" activation patterns of the neuromuscular system for: sites of activation; asymmetrical pattern of splinting or guarding; and postural disturbances.

The muscle scanning technique (50) is considered the first stage of evaluation in identifying possible "organicity" factors. Palpation (of trigger points) and/or dynamic movement–oriented EMG procedures provide a second tier of diagnostic information. The total constellation of diagnostic information may suggest that myotherapy (51), or spray and stretch (42) may be indicated. If muscle activiation patterns are noted during the evaluation phase, or following one of the more structurally oriented therapies, specific or general relaxation training is clearly indicated. It is not uncommon to hear a patient report that the clinical effects of the stuctural therapies lasted for only a few hours or days. It is speculated by the authors that concurrent EMG biofeedback relaxation training would extend the therapeutic effects of these therapies by teaching the patient to minimize the activation patterns that are in part responsible for the alteration of the muscle tissue or environment.

Finally, it is possible for a muscle to feel hard to the touch (palpation), yet be electrically silent during a surface EMG muscle scanning procedure. In this case, the hardness of the muscle to touch would be due to a *shortened resting length* rather than reflex muscle spasm. The static surface EMG assessment provides the basis for a very nice differ-

ential diagnostic finding. If the muscle is hard to the touch and is electrically active, relaxation-oriented biofeedback, perhaps initially in conjunction with muscle relaxants or other tranquilizing medications, is clearly indicated to treat the muscle spasm. If the muscle is hard to the touch and is electrically silent, relaxation alone is *not* indicated. In this latter case, one might consider using EMG biofeedback during a stretching program (50). Visual or auditory EMG feedback may be used to guide a long, slow stretch of 30 sec or more. If one allows gravity to guide the intensity of the stretch, and encourages the patient first to "breathe into the stretch," and then to relax into the stretch, one would expect to see reductions of EMG activity during the stretch over time. Interestingly enough, this form of EMG feedback might be considered as the only way in which the gamma motor system might be trained using EMG biofeedback. In the head and neck region, the stretches suggested and displayed in Robin McKenzie's *Treat Your Own Neck* (52) have been found to be very helpful. They are modified only to the extent that a slow, gravity-guided stretch is encouraged.

THE POSTURAL MODEL

The postural aspects of the neuromuscular system may involve both emotional and biomechanical aspects. Neither should be ignored. The emotional aspects of posture were elegantly described by Patton (53), when he stated, "Mammals react to stressful events with three mechanisms: Glandular secretions; Movements; and Postural Adjustments" (p. 69). In the animal kingdom, the fixed action pattern of the arched back of the cat is an obvious example of fight or flight. The frozen posture of the rabbit in response to a sudden noise might best represent the conservation withdrawal pattern. With humans one only needs to ponder the elevated shoulders of the anxious patient, or the slumped shoulders of the depressed patient. Whatmore (3, 54) has investigated and proposed a theory of "dysponesis" to help conceptualize the role of the neuromuscular system in pathophysiology of affective and physical states. The diagnostic and treatment considerations of emotional displays have been considered in a previous section of this chapter.

The biomechanical aspects of posture come into focus once man moves from a supine posture to an erect one. At this point, his body is subjected to gravitational influences according to the laws of Newtonian physics. Once erect, the intrinsic, postural muscles of the back are considered to have the primary function of stabilizing the spine against gravity (55). In general, the muscles of the back should come into play only when the spine moves off its center of gravity (37). Otherwise, the spine should be adequately supported by the ligaments (56), while the soleus muscles provides balance at the ankles.

In the classic paper by Floyd and Silver (57), the electrical activity of normal back muscles is described as being quiet during "static," quiet standing. Basmajian (55) has also described low levels of electrical activity in the erector spinae muscles when the weight of the torso is distributed over the spinal column. These types of findings, however, are probably found only in "well-postured" individuals. Floyd and Silver observed, for example, that even minor postural adjustments of the head, arms, or torso were enough to recruit paraspinal activity. A significant increase in tonic paraspinal activity was observed by Cram and Engstrom (32) to occur between quiet, unsupported sitting and quiet, unsupported standing postures in a large sample of "normal" subjects. Perhaps it is not as easy to "go out onto ligament support" or to find our biomechanical center of gravity as we are led to believe. For example, an altered sense of our center of gravity may stem from muscle shortness, lack of adequate tone, and the poor postural habits that naturally developed out of the sedate nature of the modern life-style. Indeed, Wolf et al. (58) have observed limited mobility in range of motion for men ages 30–39 working in sedate vocations.

Given the above, one would assume that paraspinal activity associated with static postures provides clinically relevant diagnostic information for the back pain patient. Wolf et al. (59) noted that chronic back pain patients often assume abnormal static postures. These patients typically stand with the trunk bent forward, the shoulders rounded and protracted, and the pelvis derotated. Several studies (60–62) noted higher levels of EMG activity in chronic pain patients compared to normal subjects during prolonged quiet standing. Such activation patterns may also be asymmetrical in nature. Cram and Engstrom (32), for example, observed that L3 paraspinal EMG activity separates normal subjects from chronic pain patients, but only on the left side, and only in the standing posture.

It would appear that having the muscular system bear weight increases the likelihood of observing abnormal patterns of "static" EMG activity in the back. Table 12.2 presents the findings of a "static" evaluation on an individual patient using the muscle scanning technique developed by Cram (50). Notice how "specific" the activation patterns are, and how they are "augmented" when the patient bears weight in the standing posture. The asymmetries clearly suggest either splinting or protective guarding patterns in response to pain.

The static evaluation procedures have been described in detail by Cram (50). There are two main approaches: muscle scanning, which samples from the right and left aspects of multiple muscle sites; and attached electrodes studying the left and right aspects of one muscle group. The major clinical

Table 12.2
Muscle Scan Protocol on an Individual Low Back Pain Patient[a]

MUSCLE SITE	SITTING		STANDING	
	LEFT	RIGHT	LEFT	RIGHT
Frontalis	3.5	3.8	1.2	1.3
Temporalis	3.5	3.5	4.6	3.6
Masseter	1.3	1.5	1.5	1.6
Sternocleidomastoid	1.2	1.5	0.8	0.9
Cervical paraspinals	1.6	1.7	1.9	1.9
Trapezius	2.2	2.3	3.0	2.5
T1 paraspinals	1.5	1.5	1.3	1.1
T6 paraspinals	3.7	3.5	4.7	4.4
T10 paraspinals	9.6[b]	19.2[b]	44.8[b]	59.2[b]
L3 paraspinals	2.2	11.2[b]	19.2[b]	30.4[b]
Abdominals	1.3	1.5	1.6	1.8

[a]From Cram JR: *Clinical EMG: Muscle Scanning and Diagnostic Manual for Surface Recordings.* Seattle, Clinical Resources, 1986, p. 91.
[b]Surface EMG findings that are outside the normal and expected ranges.

"manipulation" in both procedures is to ask the patient to sit, and then to stand in a "comfortable, unsupported" fashion. One avoids directive language, such as "stand up straight," or physical prompting to place the patient over the center of gravity. Instead, a more naturalistic observation is made of the EMG activity in both postures. The data obtained during the case study should be compared to normative data to facilitate clinical decisions. An example of the normative data available for the muscle scanning procedure conducted on the J&J EMG (models M-53, M-57, and M-58) instruments using the narrow (100–200-Hz) filter setting may be seen in Table 12.3. With this table, the nature of abnormalities at any give site may be determined. Quantitative rules regarding the "ratio" of EMG activity during the seated and standing postures need to be more firmly developed. Clinically, however, once a given muscle reaches the criterion of one standard deviation above the mean (mild elevation), a 200% increase or 50% decrease from sitting to standing is currently used to describe a postural disturbance as seen in EMG activity.

Once discovered, these static abnormalities may be treated using a biofeedback postural change method (50, 59, 63). Initially, the patient is taught to find his/her center of gravity by observing what happens to the erector spinae muscle when the patient moves off this center. The patient is asked: "What happens when one raises the arms, leans forward, etc.?" Next, the patient is encouraged to "deiscover" appropriate postures that are associated with normalized levels and symmetries of surface EMG activity. While standing, this may entail the utilization of pelvic tilt, a wider base stance, slight flexion of the knees, and the like.

In addition to the "static" evaluation, a "dynamic" evaluation of the back musculature during movement yields an additional set of diagnostic information concerning biomechanics. This procedure was first described by Price et al. (43), when they reported their observation of abnormal "patterns" of EMG activity in back pain patients during movement. These were described as abnormally high or low EMG levels, as well as left-right asymmetries. Wolf and Basmajian (64) also reported abnormal patterns of muscle activity in low back

Table 12.3
Normative Data for Muscle Scanning Procedure Using the J&J M-53/57 Electromyograph Set at a 100–200-Hz Filter[a,b]

MUSCLE SITE	POSTURE	MEAN	MILD	MODERATE	RADICAL
Frontalis	Sit	1.9	3.9	5.9	7.9
	Stand	2.1	4.1	6.1	8.1
Temporalis	Sit	2.4	4.5	6.6	8.7
	Stand	2.3	4.4	6.5	8.6
Masseter	Sit	1.7	3.0	4.3	5.6
	Stand	1.6	3.1	4.6	6.1
Sternocleidomastoid	Sit	1.3	2.8	4.3	5.8
	Stand	1.4	3.0	4.6	6.2
Cervical P.S.	Sit	1.9	3.1	4.3	5.5
	Stand	1.8	3.7	5.6	7.5
Trapezius	Sit	2.2	4.8	7.4	10.0
	Stand	3.1	5.9	8.7	11.5
T1 paraspinals	Sit	2.2	4.1	6.0	7.9
	Stand	2.9	5.7	8.5	11.3
T6 paraspinals	Sit	2.5	5.2	7.9	10.6
	Stand	2.3	5.2	7.5	9.8
T10 paraspinals	Sit	2.2	5.0	7.8	10.6
	Stand	3.0	6.1	9.2	12.3
L3 paraspinals	Sit	1.9	4.5	7.1	9.7
	Stand	3.3	6.7	10.1	13.5
Abdominals	Sit	1.0	2.5	4.0	5.5
	Stand	1.1	2.1	3.1	4.1

[a] From Cram JR: *Clinical EMG: Muscle Scanning and Diagnostic Manual for Surface Recordings.* Seattle, Clinical Resources, 1986, p. 81.
[b] Mean, mild, moderate, and radical refer to relative levels of EMG activation; mean = average level of EMG activation, mild = elevation of EMG activation of 1 SD above the mean, and moderate and radical = elevations of EMG activation of 2 and 3 SD above the mean, respectively.

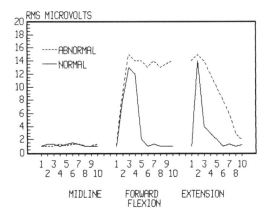

Figure 12.3. Dynamic evaluation during forward flexion of the low back. (From Cram JR: Surface EMG recordings and pain related disorders: a diagnostic framework. *Biofeedback Self Regul* 13:135, 1988).

pain patients compared to normal controls during the structured movement patterns of forward flexion and rotation of the trunk. Figure 12.3 shows the EMG activity recorded on a single patient. During the forward flexion assessment, the patient is instructed to lean forward as if to touch his/her toes. In the normal back, there is a decrease in the EMG activity as the torso goes out onto ligament support at approximately 45° of forward flexion. The inability to show this reduction in EMG activity is considered abnormal. During the rotational patterns, the hips are stabilized by the therapist, and the patient is instructed to turn to the left, return to midline, turn to the right, and return to midline. Synergistic muscle patterns are assessed. Co-contractions of the right and left aspects during rotation are considered abnormal.

If abnormalities are observed during this evaluation, an extension of the postural training techniques described above is used. In this treatment protocol, the patient is taught to display "normalized" patterns of EMG activity during both static and dynamic movements commonly used during everyday life. Strengthening and stretching along with postural changes are usually needed to assist the patient in using the back in a biomechanically efficient and safe way.

SUMMARY AND CONCLUSION

This paper has attempted to present a diagnostic framework for EMG-oriented biofeedback and general relaxation-oriented therapy. It has placed an emphasis upon the role of differential diagnostic considerations for emotional, organ-related, and postural aspects. These are not meant to be viewed in an orthogonal fashion, and may indeed overlap. The diagnostic techniques reviewed included diagnostic interview, static muscle scanning, dynamic movement evaluations, and psychophysiologic profiling. Each of these techniques samples from, and develops diagnostic information about, a different level of the neuromuscular system. Negative findings from any one technique do not necessarily rule out the possibility of positive findings from a second assessment technique.

The diagnosis of pain-related problems is complex, and necessitates a comprehensive assessment approach. As Dolce and Raczynski (7) pointed out in the conclusion of their review of the area, "a complete and in-depth electromyogrpahic assessment may be useful when dealing with myogenic back disorders to differentiate accurately the extent and type of muscular pathology" (p. 518). In addition, one should consider other maintaining or causative aspects of pain. Discogenic factors may play the primary role in the report of pain, with muscle activation patterns occurring as a secondary response. Only after an adequate passage of time to allow for healing (estimate 6 months) do pain-related disorders move from the acute to the chronic phase. It is after this point that one wants to consider how environmental/operant factors may have come to maintain pain behaviors in the absence of nociception (65). At any point along this time course, however, one will want to consider the stress of continuing pain on psychological, social, and monetary structures.

In addition, we have attempted to link each level of diagnostic findings with a companion therapeutic technique. This is based on the belief that a differential diagnosis should lead to differential treatment of the problem. It is hoped tht future applied clinical research will consider the differential efficacy of these and other techniques for each diagnostic set of information known. The techniques reviewed have included traditional general relaxation training, specific relaxation training, transactional psychophysiology, myotherapy, stretch to relax, and postural change. The effects of EMG biofeedback treatments have been observed to be very specific (31). This specificity includes not only the site of EMG feedback, but also the posture in which it was trained. There is very little "nonspecific" generalization of EMG activation reduction from one muscular region to the next, and very little spontaneous transfer of EMG activation reductions from one posture to the next (e.g., reclining to standing). Because of this, one needs to carefully match the site(s) and posture(s) of treatment to the nature of the dysfunctions. Much work is needed to develop and extend these diagnostic and therapeutic procedures to their fullest potential. A very crucial aspect of this development will be the linkage of the correct treatment procedure to the diagnostic findings.

REFERENCES

1. Luthe W: *Autogenics Therapy*, vols I–V. New York: Grune & Stratton, 1969.
2. Jacobson E: *Progressive Relaxation*. Chicago, University of Chicago Press, 1938.
3. Whatmore G, Kohli D: *The Physiopathology and Treatment of Functional Disorders*. New York, Grune & Stratton, 1974.
4. Schwartz G: Towards a comprehensive theory of clinical biofeedback: a systems perspective. In Vandyke C, Temashk L, Zegang L (eds): *Emotions in Health and Illness: Applications to Clinical Practice*. Orlando, FL, Grune & Stratton, 1984.
5. Kiesler D: Some myths of psychotherapy research and the search for a paradigm. *Psychol Bull* 66:110–136, 1966.
6. Turner J, Chapman D: Psychological interventions for chronic pain: a critical review (I, II). *Pain* 12:1–46, 1982.
7. Dolce JJ, Raczynski JM: Neuromuscular activity and electromyography in painful backs: psychological and biomechanical models in assessment and treatment. *Psychol Bull* 97(3):502–520, 1985.
8. Cannon J: *The Wisdom of the Body*. New York, WW Norton, 1932.
9. Malmo RB: Activation: a neuropsychological dimension. *Psychol Rev* 66:367–386, 1959.
10. Duffy E: The psychological significance of the concept of "arousal" or "activation." *Psychol Rev* 64:265–275, 1975.
11. Sargent MM: Psychosomatic backache. *N Engl J Med* 234:427–430, 1946.
12. Fowler R, Kraft G: Tension perception in patients having pain associated with chronic muscle tension. *Arch Phys Med Rehab* 55:28–30, 1974.
13. Jacobs A, Felton G: Visual feedback of myoelectric output to facilitate muscle relaxation in normal persons and patients with neck injuries. *Arch Phys Med Rehab* 50:34–39, 1969.
14. Bancroft H, Millen J: The blood flow through muscle during sustained contraction. *J Physiol (Lond)* 97:17, 1939.
15. Davidson R, Schwartz G: The psychobiology of relaxation and related states: a multi-purpose theory. In Mostalsky D (ed): *Behavior control and the modification of physiological Activity*. Englewood Cliffs, NJ, Prentice-Hall, 1976.
16. Benson H: *Your Maximum Mind*. New York, Times Books, 1988.
17. Fehmi L: EEG biofeedback, mutlichannel synchrony training and attention. In Surgerman A (ed): *Expanding Dimensions of Consciousness*. New York, Springer-Verlag, 1975.
18. Fried R: *The Hyperventilation Syndrome: Research on Clinical Treatment*. Baltimore, The Johns Hopkins University Press, 1987.
19. Lang P, Levin D, Miller G, Kozak R: Fear behavior, fear imagery, and the psychophysiology of emotion: the problem of affective response integration. *J Abnorm Psychol* 92:276–306, 1983.
20. Budzynski T, Stoyva J, Peffer K: Biofeedback techniques in psychosomatic disorders. In Goldstein A, Foe E (eds): *Handbook for Behavioral Interventions: A Clinical Guide*. New York, John Wiley & Sons, 1980.
21. Catalano E: *The Chronic Pain Control Workbook*. Oakland, CA, New Harbinger Publication, 1987.
22. Nuernberger P: *Freedom from Stress: A Holistic Approach*. Honsesdale, PA, The Himalayan International Institute of Yoga Science and Philosophy of the USA, 1981.
23. Budzynski T: Clinical applications of non-drug induced states of consciousness. In Wolman B, Ulmann M (eds): *Handbook of States of Consciousness*. New York, Van Nostrand Reinholt, 1986.
24. Dochin E: Personal communication. In Goleman D: *Vital Lies, Simple Truths: The Psychology of Self-Deception*. New York, Simon and Schuster, 1985.
25. Lacey J, Lacey B: Verification and extension of the principle of autonomic response-stereotypy. *Am J Psychol* 71:50–73, 1958.
26. Alexander AB, Smith DD: Clinical applications of EMG biofeedback. In Gatchel RJ, Price KR (eds): *Clinical Applications of Biofeedback: Appraisal and Status*. New York, Pergamon Press, 1979.
27. Carlson J, Basilio C, Heaukulani J: Transfer of EMG training: another look at the general relaxation issue. *Psychophysiology* 20:530–536, 1983.
28. Suarez A, Kohlenberg R, Pagano R: Is EMG activity from the frontalis site a good measure of general bodily tension in clinical populations? *Biofeedback Self Regul* 4:293, 1979.
29. Turk DC, Flor H: Etiological theories and treatments for chronic back pain. II. Psychological factors and interventions. *Pain* 19:209–233, 1984.
30. Flor H, Turk DC, Birbaumer N: Assessment of stress related psychophysiological reactions in chronic back pain patients. *J Consult Clin Psychol* 53(3):354–364, 1985.
31. Cram JR, Freeman CW: Specificity in EMG biofeedback treatment of chronic pain patients. *Clin Biofeedback Health* 8:39–48, 1985.
32. Cram JR, Engstrom D: Patterns of neuromuscular activity in pain and non-pain patients. *Clin Biofeedback Health* 9:55–61, 1986.
33. Davidson RJ,Fox NA: Asymmetrical brain activity dis-

criminates between positive and negative affective stimuli in human infants. *Science* 218:1235–1237, 1982.

34. Ferenczi S: An attempted explanation of some hysterical stigmata. In *Further Contributions to the Theory and Technique of Psychoanalysis.* 1929.

35. Ulmer HV: Arbeitsphysiologie-Umweltphysiologie. In Schnidt RF, Thews G (eds): *Physiologie des Menschen.* Berlin, Springer-Verlag, 1977.

36. Rodbard S: Pain in contracting muscles. In Crue BL (ed): *Pain: Research and Treatment.* New York, Academic Press, 1975.

37. Calliet R: *Soft Tissue Injury and Disability.* Philadelphia, FA Davis, 1977.

38. Phillips C: The modification of tension headache pain using EMG biofeedback. *Behav Res Ther* 15:119–125, 1977.

39. Bischoff C, Traue H: Myogenic headache. In Holroyd K, Schlote B, Zenz H (eds): *Perspectives in Research on Headache.* New York, CJ Hogrefe, 1983.

40. Travell J: Myofacial trigger points: clinical review. In Bonica JJ, Albe-Fessard D (eds): *Advances in Pain Research and Therapy.* New York, Raven Press, 1976, vol 1, p 919.

41. Travell J, Rinzler S: The myofascial genesis of pain. *Postgrad Med* 11:425–434, 1952.

42. Travell J, Simons D: *Myofacial Pain and Dysfunction: The Trigger Point Manual.* Baltimore, Williams & Wilkins, 1983.

43. Price JP, Clare MH, Ewerhardt RH: Studies in low backache with persistent muscle spasm. *Arch Phys Med Rehab* 29:703–709, 1948.

44. Bonica JJ; Introduction to Symposium On Pain. *Arch Surg* 112:357, 1957.

45. Fisher A: Documentation of myofascial trigger points. *Arch Phys Med Rehab* 69:286–291, 1988.

46. Goldstein B: Electromyography: a measure of skeletal muscle response. In Greenfield N, Sternbach R (eds): *Handbook of Psychophysiology.* New York, Holt, Reinhart & Winston, 1972.

47. Hudzynski L, Lawrence G: Significance of EMG surface electrode placement models and headache findings. *Headache* 28;30–35, 1988.

48. Cram JR, Steger JS: EMG scanning in the diagnosis of chronic pain. *Biofeedback Self Regul* 8:229–242, 1983.

49. Cram JR, Cahn TS: EMG muscle scanning: a diagnostic protocol for back pain. *Pain Management* 2:28–39, 1988.

50. Cram JR: *Clinical EMG: Muscle Scanning and Diagnostic Manual For Surface EMG.* Seattle, Clinical Resources, 1986.

51. Prudden B: *Pain Erasure: The Bonnie Prudden Way.* New York, Ballantine Books, 1980.

52. McKenzie R: *Treat Your Own Neck.* Lower Hut, New Zealand, Spinal Publications, 1983.

53. Patton H: Muscles and neuromuscular transmission. In Patton H, Sundsten J, Crill W, Swanson P (eds): *Introduction To Basic Neurology.* Philadelphia, WB Saunders, 1976.

54. Whatmore G, Ellis R: Some neurophysiologic aspects of depressed state. *Arch Gen Psychiatry* 1:70–80, 1959.

55. Basmajian JV: A fresh look at the intrinsic muscles of the back. *Am Surg* 42:685–690, 1976.

56. Carmichael SW, Burkart SL: Clinical anatomy of the lumbar complex. *Phys Ther* 59:966–968, 1979.

57. Floyd WF, Silver P: The function of the erector spinae muscles in certain movements and postures in man. *J Physiol (Lond)* 129:184–203, 1955.

58. Wolf S, Basmajian J, Russe T, Kutner M: Normative data on low back mobility and activity levels. *Am J Phys Ther* 58(5):217–229, 1979.

59. Wolf S, Nacht M, Kelly J: EMG feedback training during dynamic movement for low back pain patients. *Behav Ther* 13:395–406, 1982.

60. Hoyt WH, Hunt HH, De Pouw MA, Bard D, Shaffer F, Passias JN, Robbins DH, Runyon DD, Sermrad SE, Symonds JS, Watt KC: Electromyographic assessment of chronic low back pain syndrome. *J Osteopath Assoc* 80:57–59, 1981.

61. deVries H: Electromyographic fatigue curves in postural muscles, a possible etiology for idiopathic low back pain. *Am J Phys Med* 47:175–181, 1968.

62. Jayasinghe W, Harding R, Anderson J, Sweetman B: An electromyographic investigation of postural fatigue in low back pain. *Electromyogr Clin Neurophysiol* 18:191–198, 1978.

63. Jones A, Wolf S: Treating chronic low back pain. *Phys Ther* 60(1):58–63, 1980.

64. Wolf S, Basmajian JV: Assessment of paraspinal electromyographic activity in normal subjects and chronic back pain patients using a muscle biofeedback device. In Asmussen E, Jorgensen K (eds): *International Series On Biomechanics.* Baltimore, University Park Press, 1978, vol 6B.

65. Fordyce W: *Behavioral Methods for Chronic Pain and Illness.* St. Louis, CV Mosby, 1976.

Section 4
PHARMACOLOGIC TREATMENT

Chapter 13

OPIOID THERAPY

RUSSELL K. PORTENOY, MD

Intense controversy surrounds the use of chronic opioid therapy in the management of low back pain and other nonmaligant pain syndromes. Emphatic rejection of this approach is the norm, a situation justified in the opinion of many practitioners by the potential for opioid toxicity and physical dependence, loss of efficacy due to development of tolerance, and psychological dependence (addiction). These perceptions are buttressed by governmental regulation and monitoring of the medical use of these drugs, reports of sanctions placed on physicians who have "overprescribed" opioids, and the dramatic depiction in the media of the social costs of drug addiction and efforts to police it. In sum, conventional thinking has viewed opioid maintenance therapy as a potentially unsafe and ineffective option in the treatment of chronic nonmalignant pain.

Without denying a priori the potential validity of any of these perceptions, it is nonetheless true that the enormous advances of the past two decades in the scientific understanding and clinical management of chronic malignant and nonmalignant pain have provided a new impetus to a dispassionate and critical reappraisal of these beliefs. The controversy will certainly not disappear, but there is a compelling need for professionals involved in pain-related research and treatment to engage in open discourse about the issues involved. Specifically, it is within medical purview to critique relevant data about opioid maintenance therapy, clarify those areas in need of further investigation, and draw distinctions between medically appropriate use of drugs with abuse potential and their misuse. This input is needed to avoid the implementation of laws and policies regulating the availability and use of these drugs without due consideration of the needs of patients with pain. Without it, decisions are made

blindly by individuals in government whose concern for the social impact of drug abuse has historically taken precedence over the medical requirements of patients.

This chapter evaluates the proposition that there are a group of patients with chronic nonmalignant pain syndromes, a subgroup of whom have low back pain, who can obtain substantial and sustained relief of pain from the long-term administration of opioid drugs, without significant risk of opioid toxicity or addiction. A review of this controversial notion first requires definition of the salient issues. Following this, a detailed description of patients managed by this approach is presented. This is essential in establishing the phenomenon of opioid maintenance therapy and highlighting the most clinically relevant issues from the many raised by this approach. The final section of this chapter addresses the most important of these issues in depth.

DEFINING THE ISSUES

An evaluation of the utility of chronic opioid therapy in nonmalignant pain raises many disparate points of discussion. The most immediately relevant relate to the pharmacologic and medical considerations inherent in this treatment approach. Others refer to the more general role played by opioid drugs in medical practice and in society at large.

OPIOID THERAPY IN NONMALIGNANT PAIN: CRITICAL ISSUES

Three issues must be addressed to assess the potential of opioid maintenance therapy. First is the potential for therapeutic efficacy. This is a deceptively complex issue that must be divided into its component parts to be understood. It must be determined that chronic nonmalignant pain syndromes, including each of the many types of low back pain, are responsive to opioid drugs. More specifically, the range of response, if any, among different types of pain, and the nature of the benefits that accrue to individual patients, must be considered. It must also be established that benefits, if any, can be sustained, or more particularly that pharmacologic tolerance to opioid effects will not inevitably compromise the long-term efficacy of therapy. Finally, and more controversial yet, the definition of efficacy within the context of chronic pain treatment must be addressed: Should opioid efficacy be judged solely in terms of analgesia, or should it be evaluated from the perspective of its impact on other, equally important goals of pain therapy, such as return to work, increased activity, enhanced social interaction, or reduced use of medical resources?

The second issue relevant to the therapy itself relates to the potential for adverse pharmacologic outcomes from chronic opioid therapy. As with the issue of efficacy, important distinctions must be drawn here. Pharmacologic outcomes can be divided into expected physiologic effects, which may or may not be therapeutic but do not undermine the health or function of the patient; side effects, which are expected negative outcomes without substantial risk of damage to the patient; and adverse effects, which can be unexpectedly severe side effects or toxic effects that place the patient at significant risk. In the use of the opioids, an evaluation of adverse pharmacologic outcomes must assess the risks of major organ dysfunction and intolerable and persistent side effects. Of the latter, one of the most important considerations is the potential for subtle neuropsychological disturbances that may compromise the function of the patient.

The third issue, the risk of psychological dependence or addiction, is the most difficult to evaluate. Most discussions of this issue are characterized by doctrinaire pronouncements unsupported by empirical literature. A fair and balanced assessment depends first on clarifiction of the relevant terminology. Since confusion or imprecision in the use of terms, such as addiction or dependence, impedes efforts to evaluate this risk, and indeed may make a prominent contribution to the controversy, the definitions must be clearly stated at the outset. Once accomplished, the potential for the development of this phenomenon among patients with chronic pain treated with opioid drugs can be addressed.

RELATED ISSUES

Opioid drugs have long been accepted in the managment of acute pain, such as that following surgery. Recent decades have also brought widespread acceptance of chronic opioid therapy for patients with pain due to cancer (1–14), for more than three-quarters of whom it may provide substantial comfort (1, 2, 5). The World Health Organization and various bodies representing organized medicine in the United States fully support the availability and expanded use of these agents for cancer pain patients (9–14). It is thus clear that there are bona fide medical uses for opioid drugs. The discussion of the fundamental issues enumerated above will derive in part from experience in the populations with acute pain and chronic cancer pain. It is useful to note at the outset, however, that the medical experience with opioid drugs also presents a number of other issues that are indirectly related to the evaluation of opioid therapy for nonmaligant pain. These provide a context for the discussion that follows and appropriately suggest the need for ongoing review of the larger medical and societal considerations raised by this treatment approach.

Nonanalgesic Uses

Several surveys have demonstrated the potential value of chronic opioid therapy in the management of specific movement disorders and intractable dyspnea. Like the experience in chronic nonmalignant pain described below, these surveys raise questions about the inherent risks involved in long-term administration to patients with medical disease.

Hening et al. (15) reported on five patients with refractory restless legs syndrome who were successfully treated with opioid drugs, including propoxyphene (130–260 mg/day), codeine (30–120 mg/day), and methadone (5–20 mg/day), for up to 6 years. No evidence of tolerance or psychological dependence developed. A companion study reported similar results in a group of patients with neuroleptic-induced dyskinesias (16). A more recent survey (17) described six patients with restless legs syndrome unresponsive to multiple pharmacologic agents who improved dramatically with opioid administration; during 12 months of treatment, only one patient developed evidence of tolerance.

Chronic opioid therapy has also been used in the treatment of intractable dyspnea (18, 19). Although a controlled long-term trial has not been performed, and anecdotal evidence in support of the therapy is equivocal (19), no evidence of psychological dependence to the drug was observed in patients followed for prolonged periods.

This experience, albeit small, reflects on two of the most salient characteristics of opioid drugs, the potential for tolerance (with resultant loss of long-term efficacy) and abuse liability. It is thus notable that neither outcome has been a significant problem among these patients with nonpainful medical disorders.

Undertreatment of Pain

There is ample evidence that both acute pain and chronic cancer pain are substantially undertreated with opioid drugs. Insofar as these data reflect negative attitudes toward this class of drugs, inadequate knowledge of their pharmacology, or pressures from regulatory agencies, they provide insight into the potential use of these agents in the long-term treatment of chronic nonmalignant pain.

Surveys of postoperative patients have noted pain of moderate intensity or greater in up to 75% of patients after surgery (20, 21), despite data suggesting that adequate relief is possible in nearly all (22). Among cancer patients, extensive epidemiologic data indicate a pain prevalence of approximately 50% of those at all stages of disease and over 70% of those with advanced disease (23, 24). Compared to data that suggest the potential for adequate relief in more than 70% using simple drug regimens alone (25) and anecdotal reports of much higher rates of success (26), this extraordinary prevalence clearly demonstrates the inadequacy of current treatment.

Although the failures of clinical pain management can occasionally be ascribed to the refractory nature of the pain syndrome, there is compelling evidence that undertreatment by medical practitioners is the primary cause (20, 21, 23, 24, 27, 28). In general, overestimation of the risk of toxicity and concern about dependence, both physical and psychological, interact with the failure to assess and monitor pain to yield an approach to the patient characterized by the administration of inappropriately low doses of opioids at intervals longer than their duration of action (20, 21, 23, 27–30).

These data, therefore, indicate that the appropriate use of opioids is compromised even in populations widely believed to be proper recipients for this class of drugs. While the specific issues of toxicity and abuse liability in the population with chronic nonmalignant pain is addressed below, it is likely that the perceived utility of these drugs will be influenced by the same deficiencies that

impede their effective use in those patients with acute and chronic malignant pain.

Global Availability of Opioid Drugs

Some of the attitudes underlying the medical undertreatment of pain in settings in which opioid use is sanctioned are a reflection of broad social concerns about the abuse potential of these drugs. Practitioners are subject to the same social and cultural pressures about the abuse potential of opioids as the lay public, which includes policymakers responsible for the regulation of these and other psychoactive agents. The ambivalence resulting from these pressures, which in one way is manifest by undertreatment, may also be evidenced by the failure of medical practitioners to actively engage in efforts to influence these policymakers on issues related to the treatment of pain with opioid drugs. This is most exemplified by the global status of opioid availability for cancer pain management.

Although it is now widely accepted among practitioners that the precepts of effective and humane medical care mandate the unimpeded availability of opioid drugs to patients with cancer pain, the unfortunate reality is that opioid analgesics are not readily available in most countries (31, 32). Many developing countries provide no potent oral opioids to the populace whatsoever, and many others sanction only the use of agents in the agonist-antagonist subclass, drugs generally eschewed by experts in cancer pain management (5, 6). In the United States, a number of opioids are commercially available, but the clinician is often hampered by the failure of pharmacies to maintain a supply (33), strict limits in the quantities dispensed, and the burden of recordkeeping, in many states through a triplicate system. The implementation of a triplicate system, for example, may be associated with a dramatic reduction in the prescription of opioids by practitioners, over 60% in one survey (34). Although the degree to which the use of such systems limits appropriate prescribing has not been assessed, it is difficult to attribute a reduction in drug use of this magnitude only to diminution in inappropriate prescribing, particularly in light of the undertreatment of pain already extant.

The Risks of Sanctions

A little-discussed influence on professional behavior as it relates to the chronic administration of opioid drugs is the perceived threat of sanctions. Reports of legal action against physicians who undertake this therapy, either by individuals in government or oversight medical groups, have appeared (35, 36). The impact of these reports are exacerbated by an untold number of cases, in most instances unverified, that are discussed word-of-mouth among physicians, pharmacists, and other professionals engaged in the care of patients with nonmalignant pain. This word-of-mouth transfer of information from physician to physician is a cardinal element of medical education and has been held responsible for the perpetuation of a number of unsubstantiated concerns about opioids and misconceptions about their appropriate use (37). Fears about intrusive monitoring by zealous law enforcement agencies are further fueled by the implementation of triplicate recordkeeping and other requirements specific for the use of these drugs, and by occassional stories in the media about the prosecution of alleged drug-related wrongdoing by a physician or other professional. While the majority of physicians may agree with the need for careful monitoring of opioid prescription (38), and probably none would find fault with the vigorous identification and punishment of professionals engaged in criminal behavior, the net effect of all these perceptions is to suggest that a degree of personal risk, particularly to the physician and pharmacist, attends the administration of opioid drugs to patients.

Research is needed to determine the true disparity between actual and perceived risk to those who administer opioids for chronic back pain and other nonmalignant pain syndromes. The specific impact of perceived risk on prescribing behavior is also conjectural at the present time and should be clarified through careful surveys of professional behavior. A reasonable hypothesis supported by clinical experience is that the level of perceived risk correlates directly with the perception of the abuse liability of opioid drugs, and that each of these factors, as well as their combination, relates directly to both the rejection of chronic opioid therapy for nonmalignant pain and the likelihood of opioid undertreatment in the medically condoned settings of acute and chronic cancer pain. Inasmuch as the rejection or acceptance of chronic opioid therapy for nonmalignant pain should be made on medical grounds, rather than on the basis of the fear of sanctions, and it is agreed that efforts should be made to reverse the factors responsible for opioid undertreatment in accepted settings, the influence of perceived risk on prescribing practices should be clarified and approached as an independent problem in medical care.

OPIOIDS IN NONMALIGNANT PAIN: PUBLISHED EXPERIENCE

In recent years, several surveys have been published detailing the experience of patients chronically maintained on opioid drugs for the treatment of nonmalignant pain syndromes. As survey data, this material is most useful in a descriptive sense, identifying a phenomenon and helping to clarify the specific issues that must be addressed to confirm or deny the long-term efficacy of the approach. From a pharmacologic standpoint, survey data are also useful in determining the toxicity of the treatment, at least within the parameters defined in the patient sample. Candid reports detailing the incidence and course of management problems also provide a sense of the potential for psychological dependence and addictive behaviors among patients treated in this manner. Although definitive conclusions about abuse liability in the general population cannot be drawn given the selection biases inherent in survey data of this type, careful review of cases chosen for presentation may nonetheless indicate the generalizability of the results. Finally, this experience may be useful in positing a set of guidelines, which may be helpful to others who decide upon a trial of opioid therapy.

PREVIOUS LITERATURE

The largest survey yet published describes 313 personally treated patients with chronic intractable pain of nonmalignant origin who were maintained on opioid drugs for up to 6 years (39). The specific diagnoses of these patients were not enumerated. A variety of medications were used, including methadone, oxycodone, codeine, and meperidine. The average maintenance dose was equivalent to 10–20 mg of oral methadone per day and the maximum maintenance dose was equivalent to 40 mg of oral methadone per day. No major organ toxicity was observed, and although efficacy data are sparse, the comment is made that no patient suffered uncontrolled spontaneous pain while on opioids. Baseline doses did not increase more than 25% during the follow-up period, although an unreported number of patients did approach or exceed this level for a short time. In all these cases, doses were reduced to baseline during hospitalization and maintenance was resumed at the lower dose.

Thirteen of the 313 patients in this survey presented management problems. Three of these patients had been established in the drug abuse subculture in the past or at the time of treatment, five were said to be marginally related to this subculture, and five were unrelated. The types of problems encountered among the first two groups included prescription forgery, heroin abuse, excessive "loss" or theft of medication, and consumption of medication during the first 2 or 3 days of the prescription period. The problems observed among the third group included alteration of a prescription, repeated excessive consumption of drug early in the prescription period, and the intravenous administration of doses prescribed for intramuscular use. The author of this survey notes that the exclusion from chronic opioid therapy of those with a prior history of substance abuse would have resulted in a prevalence of management problems of only 1.5%. Close observation identified all these cases and strict rules were established for managing them (39).

More detail is provided in another report, in which opioid maintenance therapy was used as a component of multidisciplinary pain treatment in 16 patients with nonmalignant pain, all but one with low back pain (40). The mean duration of pain was 6.5 years, with a range of 2–14 years. All but four patients had a diagnosable psychiatric disease, in six cases a major affective disorder. Twelve patients were using opioid drugs at the time of admission to the program. Concurrent with the institution of other pain-control measures, these patients were provided opioid drugs (codeine, oxycodone, or methadone) at a mean dose equivalent to 8 mg oral methadone per day (range 3–20 mg). Reported pain relief was 50–74% in three patients and 75–99% in 13 patients at the time of discharge from the program. During a mean follow-up period of 13 months (range 6–22 months), opioid efficacy was fully maintained in six patients, slightly decreased in six, and markedly decreased in four. Opioid doses were increased in only five patients. Twelve of the 16 patients increased their activity level at home or returned to work. Neither opioid toxicity nor drug-seeking behavior was observed in any patient.

Two other surveys report similarly favorable results, but provide less exhaustive detail. In one report, brief mention is made of 22 patients with chronic intractable nonmalignant pain who had failed a variety of pain clinic approaches and were then offered chronic opioid therapy (35). Fifteen were able to return to work and all reduced medical visits. Another survey describes the use of methadone (10–20 mg/day) in the treatment of five patients with chronic phantom limb pain (41). At the time of discharge from the pain program, four patients reported more than 50% relief of pain. At the end of a follow-up period of 12–26 months (mean 22 months), all patients reported more than 50% relief. Only one patient noted a reduction in the degree of pain relief from that experienced initially; each attempt to temporarily withdraw the opioid was followed by an increase in pain. There was no clinically significant toxicity, no alteration of mood, and no evidence of abuse.

OTHER EXPERIENCE

Two additional surveys of opioid maintenance therapy for nonmalignant pain have been published (42, 43). Both were undertaken as retrospective reviews of patients with chronic nonmalignant pain who were managed with opioid drugs by pain specialists within multidisciplinary pain treatment centers. In both cases, all patients at each pain clinic who were currently under treatment with this approach werre included in the survey. Patient selection, choice of drug, and dosing regimen were determined on an individual basis by the treating physician. As retrospective surveys of clinical experience that spanned many years, these descriptive data are most useful to demonstrate the spectrum of this therapeutic approach as practiced by these specific clinicians. Additionally, these data can provide important information about drug toxicity, the circumstances of medication abuse and its management in a highly selected population, and a broad description of the degree and persistence of analgesia. The data cannot be used to assess the comparative value of the therapeutic approach against others, its utility in different types of patients, or the relative benefit of different drugs or dosing regimens.

The initial survey (42) included patients who were treated with opioids on a continuing basis for a minimum of 6 months by physicians on the Pain Service of Memorial Sloan-Kettering Cancer Center. Clinical data were extensive in 19 of these cases and provided information adequate to evaluate efficacy, toxicity, and evidence of abuse. Five of these patients and 19 additional patients managed in a similar fashion underwent testing with two psychometric measures, the Minnesota Multiphasic Personality Inventory (MMPI) and the 16 Personality Factor Questionnaire (16PFQ). Additional data about these latter 19 patients were limited to demographics and drug-related history. In sum, this first survey yielded demographic and drug-related history in 38 patients, data from two psychometric measures in 24 patients, and salient clinical details related to the potential efficacy and adverse consequences of therapy in 19 patients.

The second survey (43) comprised 20 patients with chronic nonmalignant pain who were managed with opioid maintenance therapy by physicians on the Pain Service of the Albert Einstein College of Medicine. Exhaustive clinical detail was available for each of these cases.

With the exception of age and sex ratio, the patients in each of these surveys had remarkably similar demographic profiles. The 38 patients in the first survey had a median age of 52 years (range 25–82 years), and those in the second had a median age of 44 years (range 21–69 years). The male-female ratios in the first and second surveys were 13:25 and 13:7, respectively.

Chronic low back pain was the most common diagnosis in both, comprising 20 of the 58 total patients. A large number of other diagnoses were represented among the rest (Table 13.1), including such neuropathic pain disorders as phantom limb pain, postherpetic neuralgia, and thalamic pain syndrome. The duration of chronic pain ranged from 2 years to over 2 decades.

As described previously, clinical detail was adequate in 39 cases from the two surveys combined to evaluate the pain history, prior drug use, and psychosocial profiles of the patients before the institution of formal opioid maintenance therapy. Thirty-four patients had no history of drug abuse. Of the remaining five patients, one had abused several nonopioid drugs (including sedative/hypnotics, marijuana, and LSD), one reported aberrant use of an opioid and sedative/hypnotic drugs, and

Table 13.1
Diagnoses in 58 Patients Maintained on Opioid Drugs for Chronic Pain

Chronic back pain		20
Discogenic + surgery	14	
Traumatic	4	
Other	2	
Chronic pain of unknown etiology		13
Neuropathic pain		12
Postherpetic neuralgia	3	
Stump pain	2	
Thalamic pain	3	
Phantom pain	2	
Causalgia	2	
Benign tumor		5
Arthritis		3
Other		5
Total		58

Table 13.2
Opioid Drugs Used in the Long-Term Treatment of 58 Patients with Chronic Pain

Oxycodone	24
Methadone	11
Levorphanol	5
Meperidine	5
Oxycodone/methadone	3
Propoxyphene	2
Propoxyphene/oxycodone	2
Codeine	2
Pentazocine	1
Pentazocine/propoxyphene	1
Levorphanol/codeine	1
Hydromorphone	1

two described specific problems with single opioids in the past (one oxycodone and one pentazocine). There had been no recent history of these behaviors at the time opioids were begun for the treatment of pain.

Thirty of the 39 patients had no chronic pain history preceding the present pain complaint. Five had chronic headache, and one patient each reported painful joints due to hemophilic hemarthroses, persistent abdominal pain due to colitis, and chronic pelvic pain of unknown etiology. Six patients had a history of significant psychiatric disease, including major depression in four and manic-depressive disorder in two.

Twenty-five patients were married at the time therapy was begun; most of the 14 unmarried patients had been divorced. Prior to opioid maintenance therapy, 23 of the 39 evaluable patients were employed. Of the 16 unemployed patients, 11 were considered potentially employable by virtue of age and lack of overwhelming physical disability. Twelve patients were receiving disability payments.

Information about opioid dosing was available from all 58 patients included in the two surveys. The most commonly used drugs were methadone and oxycodone, although a large number of other opioids and combinations were selected in specific patients (Table 13.2). Forty patients received a daily opioid dose less than that equivalent to 20 mg intramuscular morphine (Table 13.3). The duration of formal opioid administration ranged from 9 months to more than 10 years. Thirty-nine patients had been treated for more than 2 years at the time of the surveys; 16 had been treated for more than 5 years (Table 13.3).

An assessment of outcome was adequate in the 39 patients for whom extensive clinical details were

Table 13.3
Duration of Opioid Maintenance Therapy and Drug Dosage in 58 Patients with Chronic Pain

DURATION OF USE (YEARS)	NO.	DOSE[a]	NO.
<2	19	<10	17
2–3	15	10–20	23
4–5	8	21–30	0
6–7	7	31–40	5
8–10	4	41–50	4
>10	3	51–60	1
Unknown[b]	2	>61	3
		Unknown[b]	5

[a] Dose is expressed as number of milligrams equianalgesic to intramuscular morphine consumed per day. Although fluctuation in the dose was common, a stable baseline was maintained in nearly every patient (see text).
[b] Precise duration or dose was not evident in review of the patient's record.

available. There was no evidence of opioid toxicity in 35 cases. Two patients each reported a personality change and myoclonus, respectively, that were attributed to the use of the opioid.

As noted, 24 patients in the initial survey underwent formal evaluation with the MMPI and 16PFQ while receiving opioid maintenance therapy. Since scores on these tests were not available from the time before implementation of opioid therapy, these results cannot be interpreted as an outcome of the therapy. Nonetheless, they describe a spectrum of psychological problems and traits that characterized the patients under treatment. Scores on two validity scales (F and K) and three clinical scales (Hysteria, Depression, and Hypochondriasis) of the MMPI and all subscales of the 16PFQ were compared with those from 13 other patients with nonmalignant pain who were treated without opioids and 26 patients with malignant pain, most of whom were also managed with opioid drugs. On the MMPI, this comparison revealed a trend in all groups toward elevated scores on all three clinical scales, with those from the patient group with nonmalignant pain treated with opioid drugs significantly higher than those from the nonmalignant pain patients treated without these drugs on the F and Depression scales, and significantly higher than the malignant pain patients on the three clinical scales. There were no significant differences on the 16PFQ.

Four patients developed abuse behaviors, including unsanctioned dose escalation in three and drug diversion in one. All of the patients who increased their opioid intake without medical imprimatur did

so during periods of great psychological distress, including a psychotic episode in one. In two of these cases, the treating clinician decided that the relationship between the patient and the pain clinic was strong enough to allow reinstitution of therapy at the lower baseline dose after restating the prohibition against such behavior and warning that further episodes would lead to the cessation of treatment. In both cases, baseline doses were resumed without further management problems during more than 2 years of follow-up in each case.

All patients treated with opioid maintenance therapy had failed the usual approaches employed in a pain clinic setting. Unfortunately, records were inadequate to detail these prior treatment efforts. As noted in Table 13.1, 14 of the 20 patients with chronic back pain had undergone surgery at least once without relief of pain.

Although survey data of this type do not permit definitive statements about therapeutic efficacy, an effort was made to discern the degree of pain relief experienced by patients at repeated points during the period of opioid maintenance therapy, specifically as it compared to prior efforts to provide analgesia. Although the records typically attributed the analgesia experienced by the patient to the opioid, it should also be noted that many of these patients received other interventions concurrently during their lengthy courses and all experienced the psychological benefits that the commitment of a single concerned practitioner and stable support staff can provide.

Pain relief was broadly divided into three categories. Adequate relief was defined as sustained improvement in pain with no more than occasional brief periods of severe pain. Implicit in this definition is the observation that complete analgesia was extremely rare in this population and that chronic nonmalignant pain of all types commonly fluctuates over time, often without clear exacerbating or palliative factors. Of the 39 patients with adequate clinical detail to judge, this outcome was achieved by 16. Partial relief was defined as improved baseline pain with more frequent periods of severe pain. This outcome occurred in 16 patients as well. Finally, inadequate relief was defined as continued periods of severe pain, whether or not the intervals between them were improved over the baseline prior to the institution of therapy. This was noted in seven of the 39 cases. Thus, partial to adequate analgesia occurred in 80% of patients treated with opioid drugs in this setting.

Transitory fluctuation in dosage, accomplished with the guidance of the treating physician, was common among these patients. Almost always, however, baseline levels were regained. Hospitalization was sometimes used to provide a respite for patients during periods of pain exacerbation, particularly when the physician agreed that increased doses of opioids would be helpful but difficult to monitor in an outpatient setting. No patient developed the gradual loss of efficacy anticipated with the development of tolerance.

Unfortunately, the data from these surveys are inadequate to fully judge other criteria of successful treatment, such as increased activity levels, enhanced involvement with significant others, improvement in mood and vegetative signs, and reduction in medical visits. The records did reveal that there was no significant improvement in employment or need for disability payments among these patient. Twenty-three of the 39 valuable patients were working prior to the sustained use of opioid drugs, but only 19 were working at the last evaluation. Although the meaning of this statistic is unclear given the lengthy follow-up periods involved, it did not appear that the improved comfort described by many patients enhanced employability. The records also demonstrated that no patient underwent pain-related surgery during the follow-up periods.

PUBLISHED EXPERIENCE: CONCLUSIONS, IMPLICATIONS, AND QUESTIONS

The published surveys of patients with nonmalignant pain treated with chronic opioid therapy suggest that there is a subpopulation of these patients who can obtain sustained partial relief of pain from the administration of opioid drugs. In these patients, opioid toxicity and clinically significant tolerance did not compromise the analgesic benefits of therapy. Although marked improvement in functional status was not a reliable concomitant of this analgesia, behaviors consistent with drug abuse were very uncommon among this selected group, and within the controlled therapeutic context described in these surveys, the development of these behaviors was rapidly identified and managed.

These data raise many questions. How is this responsible subgroup who may benefit from therapy identified, and how large is it relative to the full population of patients with chronic nonmalignant pain? Clinical experience suggests that relatively few patients who are offered chronic administration of opioids fail quickly, either from complete lack of efficacy, intolerable toxicity, or the development of drug abuse. Moreover, few patients posed management problems subsequently. These observations suggest both that the nature of the therapy may be more benign that generally considered, as discussed below, and that the clinical judgment that guides the empirical selection of patients is generally sound, at least as it has been demonstrated by the pain specialists who managed the therapy of the patients included in these surveys. Research is needed to clarify these issues.

Furthermore, these survey data cannot address the causality of the observed phenomena. Is it the drug, the physician-patient relationship, the therapeutic context, the additional therapies provided within that context, or some combination that leads to the low prevalence of adverse consequences and the benefits observed in these groups of patients? Is the specific drug, methods of dosing, or absolute dose important?

Finally, these data emphasize the important issue of functional gain versus analgesia alone. Although some investigators report clear improvement in function (35, 40), others fail to note it. If it can be confirmed that enhanced comfort does little to improve function among these impaired patients, it is reasonable to consider whether the potential benefits of therapy are ever greater than the possible risks. Of course, the answer to this question depends on a valid estimation of the risks, as discussed below. In addition, it is extremely important to note one other possibility, that the failure to improve functionally, and indeed the deterioration of some patients during therapy, may in fact be due to the opioids. That is, is it possible that the provision of opioids may compromise function, perhaps through subtle neuropsychological effects, even as they provide comfort in these impaired patients with chronic nonmalignant pain?

CRITICAL ISSUES REVISITED

These survey data thus depict a phenomenon the very existence of which is held in question by many practitioners: the long-term administration of analgesic doses of opioid drugs to selected nonmalignant pain patients without the development of addictive behaviors, toxicity, or signs of tolerance. As noted, this observation cannot systematically address the many questions it raises, the most salient of which relate to the issues of efficacy, adverse consequences, and drug dependence. Although most of these issues will remain open until well-controlled clinical trials of chronic opioid administration to pain patients are done, a review of the relevant literature provides additional insight.

EFFICACY

The issue of efficacy is complex and controversial. Narrowly defined, the concept can be understood to refer only to the ability of the treatment to provide analgesia and the likelihood that analgesia will persist over time in patients with chronic pain. The latter question relates specifically to the development of pharmacologic tolerance. More broadly, efficacy can also be evaluated from the perspective of the overall goals of pain treatment.

Response to Opioids

Although there have been no controlled studies to assess the degree of responsiveness of different types of pain syndromes to opioid maintenance therapy, the issue of analgesic efficacy must first attempt to address the overall responsiveness of chronic nonmalignant pain, and then of specific pain syndromes. This is particularly important in light of anecdotal reports that suggest that some groups of patients, such as those with deafferentation pain (44), do not obtain analgesia from opioid drugs. Clinical experience in the cancer pain population also suggests that some patients do respond poorly to these drugs, even with appropriately aggressive upward dose titration. This has also been attributed to the existence of a deafferentation component to the pain, as well as to other factors (45).

These observations notwithstanding, the published experience with opioid maintenance therapy fails to identify a group of patients likely to fail. This experience has also demonstrated that a subgroup of patients with chronic low back pain, many of whom have pain with neuropathic contribution as a result of nerve root compression, respond to opioid analgesics (40, 42, 43). Controlled studies will be needed to assess the possibility that some pains are inherently unresponsive to opioid drugs. At the present time, there are data to suggest that chronic pain of any type can potentially be ameliorated with these analgesics.

Development of Tolerance

Equally important to the concept of chronic opioid therapy, however, is the persistence of the salutary effects of the drug, that is, the likelihood that tolerance will compromise the long-term efficacy of treatment. Tolerance is a pharmacologic property defined by the need for increasing doses to maintain drug effects (46)). It is apparent that opioid maintenance therapy for chronic nonmalignant pain would not be a viable option if it were demonstrated that pharmacologic tolerance to the analgesic effects of the drug regularly developed at such a rate

that effective pain relief waned with time or could be maintained only by rapid escalation of doses to unacceptable levels.

True pharmacologic tolerance is due to poorly understood alterations at a receptor level and is an extremely complex phenomenon with protean clinical manifestations. Extensive experience in the cancer population indicates that clinically significant tolerance to the analgesic effects of opioid drugs does not uniformly occur and that tolerance to different opioid effects occurs at varying rates (3, 5, 47, 48). A substantial proportion of patients with cancer pain can be maintained on stable oral doses of an opioid for very prolonged periods (47, 48). In surveys of cancer patients in which a gradual increase in average daily consumption of oral opioid is demonstrated, the overall size of the increment is relatively small and does not compromise treatment (49). A study of continuous opioid infusion in the management of cancer pain identified distinct patterns of response, which included a group of patients who required rapid escalation of doses to maintain effects and another who remained comfortable for many days on stable doses (45). Opioid tolerance, therefore, is not a uniform phenomenon among cancer patients, and indeed, escalating doses in these patients is most often correlated with progression of the underlying disease or increases in psychological distress.

The lack of clinically significant tolerance to the analgesic effects of the opioids in those with stable pain problems is also suggested by the surveys of opioid maintenance therapy in patients without cancer. Reports in which chronic opioid therapy was used in the treatment of dyskinesias (15) and those in which analgesia was the goal (39–43) have noted the persistence of effects, in some cases for many years. While no study has attempted to evaluate the development of tolerance directly, this experience suggests that concern about waning efficacy due to pharmacologic tolerance is overstated.

Goals of Therapy

The issue of efficacy is rendered more controversial by efforts to define it more broadly. It is possible to evaluate opioid efficacy using criteria that define the success of the overall treatment program for the chronic pain patient. In this view, efficacy of opioid maintenance therapy is judged within the context of a range of treatment goals for the patient, including increased activity, return to work, enhanced social interaction, and reduced use of medical resources. The decision to apply analgesia alone or a set of criteria in the determination of opioid efficacy in patients with nonmalignant pain represents a value judgment, which is most stark when obversely stated: Is chronic opioid therapy efficacious if all it does is provide some analgesia to the patient, who does not then develop an associated improvement in function. While admittedly a bias, implicit in this review is the perspective that the efficacy of treatment with an opioid drug should be primarily determined by the provision of analgesia. While the other goals of pain treatment may be equally, if not more, important than comfort alone, and enhanced comfort must always be used as a lever to pry additional function from the globally impaired patient, it is not reasonable to evaluate the results of a specific therapy according to outcomes it alone is not designed to attain. Clearly, however, if opioids compromised the other goals of therapy, as suggested by some authors (50–53), treatment with these drugs should not be considered even if enhanced comfort was achieved.

Only surveys and case reports are available to assess this important issue. Some of the reports of opioid maintenance therapy for nonmalignant pain make mention of improvements in function (35, 40), whereas others cannot confirm this (42, 43) or fail to assess it (39, 41). Surveys originating from pain clinics present data that support a relationship between substantial opioid use and a greater number of prior hospitalizations and operations, more physical impairment, greater psychological disturbance, potential misuse of analgesic drugs, and poorer outcome of therapy (52–55).

This information suffers from the usual problems inherent in survey data. The populations described, whether successfully managed by opioids or seemingly damaged by their use, are highly selected. Just as clinicians begin opioid therapy only in those patients likely to benefit and manage the drugs responsibly, many patients are referred to pain clinics because they have already demonstrated a problem with prescription drugs. It is also true that the relationships derived from these data are correlative and causality cannot be imputed from them. Thus, both opioid use and its adverse concomitants may result from a third factor, such as a more severe pain syndrome or a more aggressive, help-seeking personality, and may not be causally linked. Similarly, patients who appear to benefit from opioid drugs may in fact improve as a result of the particular ambiance or associated treatments offered by the physician. Indeed, it has been postulated (42) that the long-term commitment of one or more practitioners that has characterized opioid maintenance therapy in all the aforementioned surveys

may contribute more to the improvement of the patient than the use of the drug itself.

Surveys of pain clinic patients, from which the strongest criticism of chronic opioid therapy derives, are further compromised by the methodologic flaws apparent in many of the published outcome studies, most notably the lack of long-term follow-up (56, 57). Moreover, the use of definitions for drug-related behavior that do not conform to current standards compromises the validity of some of these reports. For example, one survey (53) that purports to demonstrate a high rate of drug abuse and poorer outcome among those who abuse drugs defines drug abuse as "no medical explanation . . . that ordinarily warrants the sustained use of the drug and one of the following: (1) use of narcotic medication . . . on a daily basis for more than a month, (2) use of nonnarcotic pain-related medication . . . at the maximum recommended dose or above on a daily basis for more than a month, (3) simultaneous use of four or more pain medications on a daily basis for more than a month." The arbitrary nature of this definition undermines the stated conclusions and prevents group comparisons across studies.

In sum, conflicting survey data do not permit definitive conclusions regarding the relationship between chronic opioid administration and functional gains from therapy. Furthermore, much of the survey data available may evaluate an unrepresentative sample of patients. There is a fundamental distinction between the controlled administration of an opioid drug by a primary care physician and the typical situation encountered by the pain specialist in a multidisciplinary pain clinic, that is, uncontrolled polypharmacy in patients receiving no other interventions designed to ameliorate physical and psychological function. The most reasonable hypothesis suggested by the surveys extant is that opioids by themselves neither substantially improve nor damage function; they may become part of the problem in some patients with chronic intractable pain and globally impaired function who consume them without clearly defined medical direction, but may enhance the comfort without further compromising the function of other patients monitored carefully in a controlled setting. Further studies are needed to evaluate this hypothesis.

ADVERSE PHARMACOLOGIC OUTCOMES

As described previously, the adverse consequences of particular importance to chronic opioid therapy pertain to the risk of persistent side effects, major organ dysfunction, and more subtle neuropsychological disturbances that may compromise concurrent rehabilitative efforts. Such consequences could not be justified in a population of patients with normal life expectancy for whom the dual goals of therapy are enhanced comfort and improved function. In addition, the possibility that physical dependence on opioid drugs is itself an adverse consequence of therapy must be addressed.

Persistent Side Effects

Opioid drugs have protean pharmacologic effects on a large number of physiologic systems. In addition to the well-appreciated effects on central nervous system function, changes in the hypothalamic-pituitary axis, peripheral vasculature, gastrointestinal tract, urinary tract, skin, and possibly immune system can be observed after acute administration of these drugs in man (58). Many of these effects are not experienced overtly by the patient, while some produce aversive phenomena, such as nausea, constipation, or confusion. With chronic administration of these drugs, tolerance develops at different rates to each effect. The evaluation of long-term safety, therefore, depends on the prevalence of sustained opioid effects and the risks associated with each, whether experienced by the patient or not.

The most detailed assessment of this issue has been done in the methadone maintenance population (59–61). Studies of these patients have demonstrated persistent constipation, insomnia, and decreased sexual function in 10–20% of patients and the complaint of excessive sweating in a somewhat higher proportion. Elevated plasma proteins often persist, and occasionally sustained abnormalities of hypothalamic-pituitary regulation, particularly abnormalities in the level and fluctuation of prolactin, are observed. While some of the clinical effects can be troubling to the patient, none of the biochemical abnormalities has ever been associated with symptomatic disease (61). Clinical experience in the cancer population indicates that constipation is the most common opioid effect for which tolerance develops so slowly that persistent problems ensue (5, 6).

Long-Term Toxicity

In addition to these sustained effects, the possibility of major organ toxicity must also be evaluated. Major organ toxicity due to prolonged exposure to opioid drugs has not been observed among cancer patients or those on methadone maintenance. In one study of patients receiving methadone, hepatic dysfunction did not occur in the absence of viral hepatitis or ethanol abuse (62).

Neuropsychological Impairment

In the absence of significant organ toxicity or adverse metabolic effects from chronic opioid administration, the issue of subtle neuropsychological impairment consequent to the long-term use of these drugs becomes paramount. Although sedation or other cognitive impairment is observed commonly after acute administration of opioid drugs, clinical experience in the cancer population suggests that tolerance to these effects develops rapidly and that full cognitive and psychological functioning is compatible with the long-term administration of these drugs (5). This experience, however, may not translate to the population without cancer. Surveys of patients admitted to pain programs who are dependent on opioids and other prescription drugs (63, 64), as well as surveys of heroin addicts (65) and methadone maintenance patients (66–68), have demonstrated clinically evident sedation or abnormalities on neuropsychological testing. Another survey of methadone maintenance patients has not confirmed these findings (69), however.

The generalizability of the conclusions implicit in the studies that have demonstrated neuropsychological deficits in patients on opioids is suspect because of the failure to control for the concurrent use of other drugs, particularly sedative/hypnotics, and the occurrence of premorbid cognitive deficits or head trauma (65, 70, 71). Indeed, a study in which patients dependent solely on opioids were compared to a group dependent only on benzodiazepines revealed substantial cognitive deficits only in those receiving the sedative/hypnotic drug (71). Although the number of patients in the latter study was relatively small and far more extensive and sophisticated testing could have been performed, the results suggest nonetheless that cognitive impairment may not result from the opioid per se in those who consume these drugs chronically. This finding and the clinical experience recounted above suggest that the prevalence of cognitive impairment after chronic administration of opioids alone in otherwise intact individuals, and the impact it has on the ability to function, is probably less than commonly believed. Additional investigations are needed to clarify this issue. At the present time, data are inadequate to attribute this adverse effect reliably to the opioid drug during long-term administration.

DRUG DEPENDENCE

The fear of dependence on opioid drugs pervades the social fabric and has profound influence on patterns of medical behavior and expectations of patients. Most people perceive a direct link between the street addict who abuses opioid drugs and the patient offered these agents for their analgesic effects. Although heroin addiction is a relatively uncommon phenomenon, with a stable prevalence of 400,000–600,000 individuals nationwide (72), it is often viewed as the potential outcome of all but the most limited efforts to treat pain with opioid drugs. If this relationship were borne out, it would represent an extremely strong contraindication to the use of opioid maintenance therapy for nonmalignant pain. If negated, a shift in attitude must be encouraged among patients, policymakers, and physicians so that a more rational approach to the management of these drugs can ensue.

Terminology of Drug Dependence

The terminology related to dependence and abuse of opioid drugs must be clearly defined to avoid significant confusion about the risks involved in chronic administration. More than three decades ago, the World Health Organization recognized the difficulties inherent in the classification and terminology used to describe these phenomena (73). In 1964, the World Health Organization suggested that the word "dependence" be substtituted for "addiction," in an effort to reduce the confusion about the latter term (74). Disagreements about nomenclature have continued to impede discourse about these issues, however (75), and in 1983 the American Medical Association's (AMA) Council on Scientific Affairs' Panels on Alcoholism and Drug Abuse established a Task Force whose goal was the development of a consensus on terminology associated with substance abuse disorders. The conclusions of this Task Force have been recently published (76)); unfortunately, some of the more important definitions, such as that determined by the term "addict," diverge excessively from respected standards (75) and are destined to perpetuate the misunderstandings that have heretofore plagued professional discourse about the medical use of opioid drugs.

From the viewpoint of chronic opioid therapy for nonmalignant pain syndromes, including chronic back pain, the largest problem has been the confusion between the physiologic outcome of opioid use known as physical dependence and the aberrant use of opioid drugs, which has been variably described as addiction, drug abuse, drug dependence, compulsive use, and psychological dependence. Misidentification or mislabeling of the former phenomenon as the latter can compromise the care of the individual patient and inhibit the fair evaluation of the therapy as a whole.

Physical dependence is a pharmacologic property characterized by the occurrence of an abstinence syndrome after abrupt discontinuation of the drug or administration of an opioid antagonist (46, 75, 77, 78). While the definition propounded by the AMA Task Force notes as well that this phenomenon is usually also characterized by the development of tolerance (76), it has been generally agreed that the emergence of a withdrawal syndrome is the sine qua non for the use of this term (75). Physical dependence, therefore, does not imply drug craving or abuse of the drug. While it is certainly appropriate to debate the impact physical dependence should have on the decision to institute chronic therapy, it is incorrect to assume that this phenomenon in any way defines the aberrant psychological state and behavior of the "addicted" or "drug-abusing" patient. Specifically, neither the use of relatively high doses for long periods (if appropriately prescribed), the development of tolerance to opioid effects, nor the occurrence of withdrawal indicates that the patient is "addicted," although such signs are common in those who do fit the criteria for this term.

A number of terms can be used to describe features of the psychological and behavioral attributes of the patient who abuses prescription opioids. These phenomena are clearly of great concern to practitioners, who recognize the individual and social harm associated with opioid abuse. Given the dire consequences of abuse, the risk of this outcome would have to be extremely small to justify the long-term use of opioid drugs in patients with chronic nonmalignant pain. The data relating to this risk are discussed at length below.

The term "addiction" may be too replete with negative connotations, and too often confused with physical dependence, to be useful clinically without further definition. While physical dependence is accepted as a component of "addiction" by the World Health Organization (79), major pharmacology text defines the term in a way that fully distinguishes "addiction" from physical dependence (75). In the latter view, addiction can be defined as a "behavioral pattern of drug use, characterized by overwhelming involvement with the use of a drug (compulsive use), the securing of its supply, and a high tendency to relapse after withdrawal" (75). In a similar way, the AMA Task Force concluded that "addiction" is a chronic disorder characterized by "the compulsive use of a substance resulting in physical, psychological or social harm to the user and continued use despite that harm" (76). Oddly, and in a manner likely to confuse the issue, the AMA Task Force defined the "addict" as a person who is "physically dependent. . . , whose long-term use has produced tolerance, who has lost control over his intake, and would manifest withdrawal . . ." (76). Even the latter definition, however, includes reference to loss of control, and thereby distinguishes the addict from the patient who is merely physically dependent.

Other terms are commonly used and also must be defined. "Drug dependence" is a generic term that can refer to either physical or psychological dependence or both, and therefore should not be used clinically without further elaboration. "Psychological dependence" has been used interchangeably with the term "addiction," as defined above (42). "Drug abuse" has variably been viewed as the use of an agent outside socially and medically approved patterns of use in a given culture (75) or as a pattern of use that results in physical, psychological, economic, legal, or social harm to the individual or others affected by his/her use (76).

It is apparent that these variations in the use of the terminology applied to the aberrant behavior of some individuals who consume opioid drugs may result in the mislabeling of observed phenomena, which in turn may have ill effects on either the treatment of the individual or the assessment of a therapy. Moreover, it should be recognized that the terminology discussed above has been developed by those whose primary population of reference is the drug abuser without a chronic painful disorder. There have been no efforts to determine if the taxonomies or terminology of drug abuse should vary in discussions of this subgroup of patients with pain. For example, the "relapse" after drug withdrawal that is posited as a cardinal feature of addiction by one author (75) may be seen as appropriate reinstitution of therapy for pain exacerbation in some patients with chronic painful disease. Similarly, the pathologic nature of opioid craving may come into question in some patients with pain, for whom it may represent an appropriate search for relief. Clinical experience suggests that there may be a spectrum of responses, which range from appropriate and acceptable "drug-seeking" behaviors to a group of clearly pathologic behaviors, even in those with substantial pain.

There thus remain serious inconsistencies in the terminology used to define phenomena that are critical in the evaluation of the safety and utility of chronic opioid therapy. Since the term "addiction" is used commonly in clinical practice, it is important to agree on a reasonable definition and to use this consistently in evaluating the risk of this outcome in patients with nonmalignant pain. It is likewise useful to underscore the differences between this definition and the manner in which the term is used by others evaluating the role of these drugs in patients.

A clinically useful definition of "addiction" within the context of medical treatment can be derived from the above discussion: This outcome is a psychological and behavioral syndrome in which there is a psychological state characterized by intense desire for the drug (psychological dependence) and overwhelming interest in securing its supply, and an associated group of aberrant behaviors, including compulsive drug use (characterized, for example, by unsanctioned dose escalation or increased frequency of dosing, or continued dosing despite significant side effects), manipulation of the treating medical system for the purposes of obtaining additional drug supply, acquisition of drugs from other medical sources or from a nonmedical source, use of drug to treat other than target symptoms or unapproved use during periods of no symptoms, drug hoarding or sales, or unapproved use of other drugs (particularly alcohol or other sedative/hynotics) during opioid therapy. It is the risk of these phenomena, and not those associated with physical dependence, specifically withdrawal, that constitutes the major issue in chronic opioid therapy for nonmalignant pain.

Physical Dependence

The occurrence of an abstinence syndrome is undoubtedly a noxious experience, and the potential for this phenomenon must be taken into account in the clinical management of pain. Studies of physical dependence have demonstrated that the physiologic changes indicative of physical dependence are produced by very little opioid exposure and that these changes can persist for prolonged periods following cessation of dosing (77, 78). For example, abstinence phenomena can be elicited by administration of an opioid antagonist after only hours of opioid intake (80). These changes, however, are subclinical, and it is generally accepted that days to weeks are required to fully establish physical dependence. The prolonged abstinence syndrome, which is associated with persistent physiologic changes and a period of relatively high drug craving in street addicts (78), has not been reported to cause a manifest problem in pain patients treated chronically with opioids.

The degree of dependence (i.e., the severity of the abstinence syndrome on drug withdrawal) is directly proportionate to the duration and dose of opioid consumption (75). Although, as noted, the doses typically employed by practitioners administering chronic opioid therapy to patients with nonmalignant pain are relatively low, the lowest dose and duration of opioid use associated with a significant abstinence syndrome in patients is unknown, and the potential for withdrawal is prudently assumed to exist in all such patients. In practical terms, the possibility of an abstinence syndrome is obviated by avoidance of sudden discontinuation of the drug or administration of an opioid antagonist. This approach can be likened to the management of a variety of other drug classes, including antihypertensives and cardiotonic agents, the use of which is associated with the same concerns about morbidity from sudden discontinuation. Furthermore, physical dependence does not appear to preclude the rapid and uncomplicated tapering and cessation of dosing, as indicated by the ease of detoxification reported by pain clinic programs that utilize this maneuver as a first step in management (70). Taken together, these observations suggest that physical dependence per se, a phenomenon that compromises neither the function of the individual nor the efficacy of treatment, is not problematic in the analgesic management of the patient as long as the abstinence syndrome is avoided through appropriate measures.

Opioid Addiction

The far more compelling issue, of course, is the potential for psychological dependence and addictive behaviors in patients treated with opioid drugs. As discussed previously, these phenomena are accepted as evidence of an aberrant psychological reaction to opioid drugs. The critical question for the practitioner considering a trial of opioid therapy in a patient with chronic pain is thus the following: What is the risk that the typical patient with chronic pain will develop drug addiction when chronically exposed to opioid drugs for medical purposes? As a related question, it is useful to consider whether the impetus for addiction resides in factors endogenous to the patient or in the properties of opioid drugs themselves, such as their capacity to cause physical dependence (and produce drug seeking to avoid withdrawal) or act as a reinforcer (perhaps through the production of euphoria). Epidemiologic data and information related to the differential effects of these drugs in addicts and patients can be adduced to address this issue.

Opioid Drugs and Addicts

It is widely believed that opioids produce euphoria and that this affective change reinforces the use of the drug. This perception represents an extrapolation of the well-known "rush" or "high"

of the street addict to the medical patient administered opioids for the treatment of pain. Both clinical experience and substantial data contradict this view. Cancer patients do not report euphoria after opioids are instituted (1–3, 5)). In a study that assessed the mood of patients given opioids for postoperative pain, elation was not demonstrated and dysphoria was common, especially in those who received meperidine (81). Similarly, a study in which normal subjects were given morphine reported increased dysphoria following drug administration (82). In contrast to the reactions of the addict, the nonabusing subject does not appear to experience reinforcing affective changes following opioid administration.

The lack of euphoria does not exclude the possibility that other powerful reinforcements inhere in the pharmacologic properties of the opioids. For example, the aversive experience of abstinence may be the substrate for drug-seeking behavior. This consideration has played a central role in the development of classical conditioning hypotheses to explain the development of addiction (83, 84). In this conceptualization, pharmacologic abstinence is viewed as an unconditioned response that determines a conditioned abstinence syndrome, which is identical to the abstinence produced by opioid withdrawal but does not need the opioid for expression. The relief of these abstinence symptoms (both unconditioned and conditioned) is reinforcing and perpetuates addictive behaviors.

Opioids have also been found to be highly reinforcing drugs in animals, even in those not yet physically dependent (85), and conditioned responses that perpetuate opioid consumption and increase the likelihood of use after detoxification have been well demonstrated in nonhuman experimentation (83). The high recidivism rate in treated street addicts (86, 87) can be viewed as the human correlate of these data, and may suggest that drug exposure produces changes that increase the likelihood of future abuse. The implication that the reinforcing properties of opioid drugs, which result in part from the potential for physical dependence, may produce long-lasting changes that predispose to addiction is troubling, and, if true, would certainly contraindicate the long-term use of these agents in pain patients.

Studies in animals and the addict population, however, may have limited relevance to the medical patient with chronic nonmalignant pain. While it is true that there is, with the exception of euphoria, no direct evidence that the reinforcing properties of these drugs that result in operant and classical conditioning do not operate in the otherwise normal patient who receives opioid drugs for the treatment of pain, there are, adequate data to infer that these processes are insufficient in themselves to produce psychological dependence and addictive behaviors in the vast majority of pain patients. The importance of physical dependence itself as a primary motivator of drug-seeking behavior can be contested by studies in which this effect can be produced by opioids that are not abused; withdrawal from these drugs is not associated with drug-seeking behavior (88). More important, a psychological aberration rare in the general community of medical patients, psychopathy, appears to be a predominating characteristic of the street addict (89, 90) and of drug-addicted soldiers in Vietnam (91). Additionally, situational and social factors never experienced by the typical medical patient appear to play a significant role in the development and perpetuation of addictive behaviors, and there is suggestive evidence that a genetic factor may also be important (92, 93). The latter has been convincingly demonstrated in alcoholism (94), and it has been postulated that the development of alcoholism in a small minority of those who imbibe is a parallel process to that determining opioid addiction in a small proportion of those administered these drugs (95).

Epidemiologic Data

Epidemiologic surveys have been invoked for many years as evidence for the contention that the medical exposure to opioid drugs carries a substantial risk of subsequent abuse. Support for this view originated in several older surveys of the addict population. In 1925, Kolb noted that 9% of addicts undergoing treatment reported that their addiction began with the medical prescription of opioid drugs (96). A similar survey of the same population more than a decade later revealed this history in less than 4%, still a substantial proportion (97). Finally, in what became a particularly influential survey, Rayport reported that 27% of white male addicts and 1.2% of black male addicts began opioid abuse as medical patients given these drugs for the treatment of painful disorders (98). These data imply that a substantial risk of abuse is associated with the medical use of opioid drugs.

A different view emerges, however, from surveys in which medical patients were assessed for the development of psychological dependence following the administration of opioids. For example, of 11,882 patients surveyed in the Boston Collaborative Drug Surveillance Project, only four cases of well-documented psychological dependence occurred in patients without a prior history of drug abuse (99). A national survey of burn centers could find no cases of addiction from a sample of over 10,000 patients without prior drug abuse history who were given opioids for pain (100). Similarly, a survey of a large headache treatment center observed that only three of 2369 patients admitted for treatment, most of whom had access to opioids, abused these drugs (101). In contrast to data obtained from surveys of addicts, therefore, these data suggest that patients without a prior history of substance abuse are at extremely small risk of abuse behaviors following the short-term administration of opioid drugs.

Other data also contradict the notion that exposure to opioid drugs reliably leads to escalating use, recidivism after detoxification, and addictive behaviors. The existence of so-called "chippers," individuals who use heroin recreationally on a periodic basis, belies the inevitability of the full addiction syndrome, even in those who consume the drugs for purposes other than pain control (102) More interesting perhaps are data that indicate that a large proportion of soldiers who abused heroin in Vietnam stopped this activity abruptly on return to the United States and demonstrated a low rate of relapse subsequently (91, 103). Although the likelihood of drug abuse among these soldiers was increased in those with a prior history of drug use and sociopathic behavior (91), addictive behaviors in most ceased with a return to a more normal living situation. The prompt cessation of addictive behaviors in these soldiers is somewhat analogous to the experience of the two patients reported above, who developed abuse behaviors while receiving opioid maintenance therapy for nonmalignant pain but promptly returned to controlled dosing after the behavior was checked by the prescribing physician.

Taken together, these data contradict the widely held perception that opioid exposure for the medical treatment of pain carries a substantial liability for the development of psychological dependence. Implied is the important notion that there is a fundamental difference between the street addict, or the person predisposed to become one, and the typical patient who is a candidate for chronic opioid therapy. The assumption that the risk of addictive behaviors resides solely in the substance is not supported by the available evidence. A reasonable alternative hypothesis can be expressed as follows: Although patients who become physically dependent (an unknown proportion of those receiving opioid maintenance therapy) may be subject to the same negative reinforcements induced by the occurrence of withdrawal phenomena as the street addict, the lack of other reinforcers (e.g., euphoria on drug administration or a social environment supportive of drug abuse) and other predisposing psychologic and genetic factors (e.g., psychopathy or the experience of euphoria on opioid intake) in the great majority of patients prefigures an extremely low risk of psychological dependence and addiction in this population. Although the data described above support this hypothesis, there is currently little direct evidence. Research in the population of pain patients is badly needed to evaluate this speculation and determine the factors that may be important in identifying patients who will develop aberrant reactions to opioid drugs.

CONCLUSIONS AND GUIDELINES

Notwithstanding its controversial nature, it has been the thesis of this chapter that a selected subgroup of patients with chronic nonmalignant pain syndromes, including low back pain, can obtain sustained improvement in comfort from opioid drugs without the development of significant toxicity or evidence of psychological dependence or addictive behaviors. It is undeniable that the direct evidence in favor of this proposition is meager, but it is also true that the data in support of the more accepted opposing view are weak as well. At the least, the information extant suggests that the emphatic rejection of chronic opioid therapy in all patients with nonmalignant pain is overstated. Scientific discourse and valid investigations should replace the doctrinaire pronouncements that have characterized discussion of the issue in the past.

Based on a review of the evidence, it is possible that thoughtful physicians who know their patients well, and who are willing to be subjected to the scrutiny that the adoption of this approach often produces, may come to the conclusion that chronic opioid therapy is worthy of a trial in some patients. Selection criteria are entirely empirical at the present time. The surveys reported herein suggest that the only clinical evidence predictive of problems with the approach is a recent or remote history of substance abuse. Interestingly, psychological distress, and even a diagnosis of psychogenic pain, has not presaged the occurrence of management problems in these patients.

Of the concepts suggested by the aforementioned survey data, as well as several other lines of evidence, one in particular has great implications for the clinical management of patients with chronic pain. Although confirmatory studies are needed, it appears likely that the typical pain patient, an individual without history of drug abuse, can have opioid therapy stopped after it has been started and doses lowered after they have been raised. If true, it would be feasible for a patient to undergo a trial of opioid treatment, with the decision to continue it contingent on outcome. Data are inadequate at the present time to accept this proposition as true, however, and the implementation of chronic opioid therapy should still be undertaken only after careful consideration and with due respect for the potential problems that the development of psychological dependence would cause. Nonetheless, the possibility that a trial of opioids could be instituted with extremely low risk to the patient or practitioner remains and can only be clarified with additional research.

The importance of the practitioner must also be emphasized. All surveys of patients successfully managed with opioids imply the existence of one identified practitioner, or a discrete group, who agrees to a long-term commitment to the patient. It is impossible to deny the possibility at the present time that the viability of therapy relates primarily to the concern, experience, and availability of these individuals. Given current evidence this consideration suggests that chronic opioid therapy should only be implemented by practitioners who understand the issues involved and are willing to invest the necessary time and energy into the management of these challenging patients.

This presentation in no way implies that opioid maintenance therapy is better than any of the currently accepted approaches. There are no data to suggest this. While it may be reasonable, albeit unproven, to suggest that a trial of opioids is safer than an invasive neurolytic procedure for pain control in a patient with a chronic nonmalignant pain syndrome, and thus should be considered first, there is no evidence to support the use of this therapy in lieu of other methods.

Currently, multidisciplinary treatment reliant on physical therapy and cognitive and behavioral interventions is generally viewed as the state of the art for the treatment of chronic low back pain. This approach need not be viewed as antagonistic to chronic opioid therapy, and the following points should be considered:

1. The predominating goal of most multidisciplinary pain programs is return of function, and improvement in function without relief of pain is a common outcome (104–106). Although the data suggest that opioids may not yield improvement in function, comfort is enhanced

and it may therefore be reasonable to view the approaches as complementary (40).

2. Although many patients improve with the therapies offered in multidisciplinary pain programs, there is a substantial failure and dropout rate, and many programs offer short-term therapy, after which patients return to practitioners in the community for continuing care. Given the enormous personal and social cost of chronic pain, it is reasonable to speculate that opioid maintenance therapy may be useful in some of these patients.

3. In many countries, and in some regions of this country, the expertise required for multidisciplinary pain management programs is not available, and additionally, many patients are unable to afford this expensive approach. Again, it is reasonable to conjecture that chronic opioid therapy, carefully monitored by single practitioners, may be beneficial to some of these patients who have failed other affordable approaches.

As a final consideration, it must be acknowledged that current data do not exclude the possibility, suggested repeatedly in the literature, that the use of opioids worsens the clinical condition of some patients with chronic pain. This is an extremely important concept, which should not—like the potential for benefit—be obscured by exclusive focus on the risk of psychological dependence and addiction. Additional research is needed to determine the incidence and mechanism of augmented pain and deteriorated function related to the use of opioids. It is likely, given the evidence presented above, that this outcome derives from pathologic processes endogenous to the patient or clinical environment, rather that the drug per se. Just as clinical predictors of drug abuse in pain patients must be identified through further research in this population, potential predictors of clinical decline must also be evaluated.

GUIDELINES FOR USE

Given current information about opioid maintenance therapy for nonmalignant pain, it is possible that concerned and knowledgeable clinicians charged with the long-term care of these challenging patients may choose to embark on such a course. For these cases, the experience of those who have managed similar patients can be used to generate a series of guidelines (Table 13.4). These can be annotated as follows.

1. Chronic opioid therapy should be considered only after all reasonable nonopioid therapies

Table 13.4
Proposed Guidelines for the Management of Opioid Maintenance Therapy

1. Consider only after all reasonable nonopioid therapies are exhausted.
2. Consent discussion required, including possibilities of side effects, minimal risk of psychological dependence and addictive behaviors, and implications of physical dependence; this should be noted in the chart.
3. Agreed-upon period of titration, aiming for at least partial relief of pain.
4. After titratioin, agreed-upon monthly quantity of drug, with some leeway in daily dose but return to maintenance dose by month's end. Flexibility in dosing can be arranged as follows:
   a. An increase in dose by 20% allowed on any day, but must be followed by equal decrease, so that monthly quantity is fixed; or
   b. A number of extra doses ("rescue doses") can be offered per week, which the patient can take as needed, as long as the usual maintenance dose is continued at month's end.
5. Monthly visits.
6. Improvement in physical, psychological, and social function should continue to be a major emphasis of therapy, and other therapeutic interventions should be instituted or continued as appropriate.
7. Manipulation of the system to obtain additional drug, drug hoarding or diversion, or acquisition of the drug elsewhere should not be tolerated; discontinuation of therapy must be strongly considered if this occurs.
8. Escalating pain, progressively impaired function, rapid dose escalation (with medical approval), or escalation without subsequent decrement suggests need for hospitalization.

are exhausted. Clinical experience suggests that the approach is safer and more likely to yield analgesia in many patients than additional operations and neurolytic procedures. Use of the approach is not contrary to the simultaneous application of any of the usual therapies employed in multidisciplinary treatment, and indeed, may be complementary in many patients.

2. A consent discussion with the patient is required. Similar to the use of other drugs, patients should be warned about potential short-term and persistent side effects, particularly the potential for additive sedation to that produced by alcohol and other drugs. Women of childbearing years should be informed of the risk to the fetus should pregnancy occur during opioid maintenance therapy, specifically that the child may be born physically dependent on opioids. Finally, the patient must be told that current information is inadequate to exclude the possibility that the use of opioids will eventuate in the development of psychological dependence.

3. There should be an agreed-upon period of dose titration, which is directed toward at least partial relief of pain. This period is clearly delicate and requires the exercise of considerable clinical judgment. Patients who experience partial relief of pain may request continued upward dose titration in the desire to be pain free. The clinician must balance the risk of short-term toxicity, predictions of the potential for greater analgesia, and concerns about the controversial nature of a therapy that is monitored by government and medical oversight committees. The therapy becomes too problematic should the clinician feel great discomfort in administering it. These issues must be explained in a way that reveals the nonmedical considerations, but continues to express the clinician's primary interest in the well-being of the patient. Although sometimes difficult, a dose must be chosen that may provide less analgesia than possible, at least in the short-term, but can be continued comfortably by clinician and patient. Clinical experience strongly suggests that the oral route of administration is best in this situation.

4. After titration, a monthly quantity of drug should be set. Given the common observation of great day-to-day variability in the experience of chronic pain, there should be some leeway in the daily dose, although the maintenance dose should be retained at month's end. This flexibility can be accomplished in several ways. Patients can be allowed to take an additional quantity, for example 20% of the daily dose, on any day, but are told that a reduction in dose subsequently must be accomplished so that the monthly quantity remains fixed. Alternatively, patients can be offered several extra doses, so-called rescue doses, each week, to use at their discretion. An accounting of these doses must be made at each visit.

5. Monthly visits are strongly recommended. More frequent visits during periods of pain exacerbation may be necessary.

6. Although the occurrence of analgesia is used to determine the viability of therapy and the dose, continued emphasis must be placed on the total rehabilitation of the patient. Every effort should be made to capitalize on enhanced comfort with improved physical and social functioning. The use of other interventions should be considered at all times.

7. Evidence of psychological dependence or addictive behaviors should be sought and managed aggressively. Manipulation of the system to obtain additional drugs, drug hoarding or sales, or acquisition of drugs from other practitioners cannot be

tolerated. Discontinuation of therapy must be strongly considered should these behaviors occur.

8. Temporary pain exacerbation is common in nonmalignant pain syndromes, and clinicians may choose to allow a transient increase in dosage to manage these. Clinical experience suggests, however, that rapidly escalating pain or need for rapid dose increments, or dose escalation without reduction, may be difficult to manage and may warrant hospitalization of the patient. During hospitalization, doses can be transiently increased in a controlled setting. When pain is controlled, doses can usually be decreased to the baseline maintenance level.

The risks and benefits of chronic opioid therapy for nonmalignant pain will only be determined by dispassionate scientific evaluation of the relevant data available and continued investigation of patients with pain. This process is complicated by the great concern about substance abuse in our society. Societal reaction to the drug abuse subculture has exercised great influence on the way in which opioid drugs are viewed within the medical context. It is incumbent on pain specialists to define the medical issues involved, investigate the many questions remaining, and educate the public and policymakers about the needs of the pain patient.

REFERENCES

1. Saunders CM: *The Management of Terminal Malignant Disease,* ed 2. London, Edward Arnold, 1984.
2. Ventafridda V, Tamburini M, De Conno F: Comprehensive treatment in cancer pain. In Fields HL, Dubner R, Cervero F (eds): *Advances in Pain Research and Therapy.* New York, Raven Press, 1985, vol 9, pp 617–628.
3. Houde RW: Systemic analgesics and related drugs: narcotic analgesics. In Bonica JJ, Ventafridda V (eds): *Advances in Pain Research and Therapy.* New York, Raven Press, 1979, vol 2, pp 263–273.
4. Cleeland CS, Rotondi A, Brechner T, Levin A, MacDonald N, Portenoy RK, Schutta H, McEniry M: A model for the treatment of cancer pain. *J Pain Symp Manag* 1:209–215, 1986.
5. Twycross RG, Lack SA: *Symptom Control in Far Advanced Cancer: Pain Relief.* London, Pitman Books, 1983.
6. Foley KM: The treatment of cancer pain. *N Engl J Med* 313:84–95, 1985.
7. Beaver WT: Management of cancer pain with parenteral medication. *JAMA* 244:2653–2657, 1980.
8. Portenoy RK: Optimal pain control in elderly cancer patients. *Geriatrics* 42:33–40, 1987.

9. Health and Public Policy Committee, American College of Physicians: Drug therapy for severe chronic pain in terminal illness. *Ann Intern Med* 99:870–873, 1983.

10. McGivney WT, Crooks GM: The care of patients with severe chronic pain in terminal illness. *JAMA* 251:1182–1188, 1984.

11. Cancer Pain Relief Program, World Health Organization: *Cancer Pain Relief.* Geneva, World Health Organization, 1986.

12. National Institutes of Health Consensus Development Conference: The integrated approach to the management of pain. *J Pain Symp Manag* 2:35–44, 1987.

13. Swerdlow M, Stjernsward J: Cancer pain relief—an urgent problem. *World Health Forum* 3:325–330, 1982.

14. Stjernsward J: Cancer pain relief: an important global public health issue. In Fields HL, Dubner R, Cervero F (eds): *Advances in Pain Research and Therapy.* New York, Raven Press, 1985, vol 9, pp 555–558.

15. Hening WA, Walthers A, Kavey N, Gidro-Frank S, Cote L, Fahn S: Dyskinesias while awake and periodic movements in sleep in restless legs syndrome: treatment with opioids. *Neurology* 36:1363–1366, 1986.

16. Walters A, Hening W, Chokroverty S, Fahn S: Opioid responsiveness in patients with neuroleptic-induced akathisia. *Movement Disorders* 1:119–127, 1986.

17. Sandyk R, Bamford CR: Efficacy of an opiate-benzodiazepine combination in the restless legs syndrome. *Neurology* 37 (suppl 1):105, 1987.

18. Robin ED, Burke CM: Single-patient randomized clinical trial: opiates for intractable dyspnea. *Chest* 90:888–892, 1986.

19. Bar-or D, Marx JA, Good J: Breathlessness, alcohol, and opiates (letter). *N Engl J Med* 306:1363–1364, 1982.

20. Donovan M, Dillon P, McGuire L: Incidence and characteristics of pain in a sample of medical-surgical inpatients. *Pain* 30:69–78, 1987.

21. Cohen F: Postsurgical pain relief: patients' status and nurses' medication choices. *Pain* 9:265–274, 1980.

22. White PF: Use of a patient-controlled analgesia infuser for the management of postoperative pain. In Harmer M, Rosen MA, Vickers MD (eds): *Patient-Controlled Analgesia.* London, Blackwell Scientific Publ, 1985, pp 140–148.

23. Bonica JJ: Treatment of cancer pain: current status and future needs. In Fields HL, Dubner R, Cervero F (eds): *Advances in Pain Research and Therapy.* New York, Raven Press, 1985, vol 9, pp 589–616.

24. Portenoy RK: Cancer pain: epidemiology and syndromes. *Cancer* (in press).

25. Ventafridda V, Tamburini M, Caraceni A, De Conno F, Naldi F: A validation study of the WHO method for cancer pain relief. *Cancer* 59:850–856, 1987.

26. Saunders CM: Current views of pain relief and terminal care. In Swerdlow M (ed): *The Therapy of Pain.* Lancaster, England, MTP Press Ltd, 1981, pp 215–241.

27. Marks RM, Sachar EJ: Undertreatment of medical inpatients with narcotic analgesics. *Ann Intern Med* 78:173–181, 1973.

28. Charap AD: The knowledge, attitudes and experience of medical personnel treating pain in the terminally ill. *Mt Sinai J Med* 45:561–580, 1978.

29. Shine D, Demas P: Knowledge of medical students, residents and attending physicians about opiate abuse. *J Med Educ* 59:501–507, 1984.

30. Sriwatanakul K, Weiss OF, Alloza JL, Kelvie W, Weintraub M, Lasagna L: Analysis of narcotic analgesic usage in the treatment of postoperative pain. *JAMA* 250:926–929, 1983.

31. Caraceni A: Availability and use of opioids for cancer pain patients in Italy. *J Pain Symp Manag* 2:127–128, 1987.

32. Wenk R: Availability of analgesics in Argentina. *J Pain Symp Manag* 2:191–192, 1987.

33. Kanner RM, Portenoy RK: Unavailability of narcotic analgesic for ambulatory cancer patients in New York City. *J Pain Symp Manag* 1:87–90, 1986.

34. Sigler KA, Guernsey BG, Ingrim MB, et al: Effects of a triplicate prescription law on prescribing of Schedule II drugs. *Am J Hosp Pharm* 41:108–111, 1984.

35. Tennant FS, Uelman GF: Narcotic maintenance for chronic pain: medical and legal guidelines. *Postgrad Med* 73:81–94, 1983.

36. Rose HL: Letter to the editor. *Pain* 29:261–262, 1987.

37. Morgan JP: American opiophobia: customary underutilization of opioid analgesics. *Adv Alcohol Subst Abuse* 5 (Fall-Winter):163–173, 1985–1986.

38. Berina LF, Guernsey BG, Hokanson JA, Doutre WH, Fuller LE: Physician perception of a triplicate prescription law. *Am J Hosp Pharm* 42:857–859, 1985.

39. Taub A: Opioid analgesics in the treatment of chronic intractable pain of non-neoplastic origin. In Kitahata LM, Collins D (eds): *Narcotic Analgesics in Anesthesiology.* Baltimore, Williams & Wilkins, 1982, pp 199–208.

40. France RD, Urban BJ, Keefe FJ: Long-term use of narcotic analgesics in chronic pain. *Soc Sci Med* 19:1379–1382, 1984.

41. Urban BJ, France RD, Steinberger DL, Scott DL, Maltbie AA: Long-term use of narcotic/antidepressant medication in the management of phantom limb pain. *Pain* 24:191–197. 1986.

42. Portenoy RK, Foley KM: Chronic use of opioid analgesics in non-malignant pain: report of 38 cases. *Pain* 25:171–186, 1986.

43. Portenoy RK, Kanner RM, Berger M: Opioid maintenance therapy in chronic non-malignant pain. *Proc Comm Prob Drug Depend* (in press).

44. Tasker RR: Deafferentation. In Wall PD, Melzack R (eds): *Textbook of Pain.* New York, Churchhill Livingstone, 1984, pp 119–132.

45. Portenoy RK, Moulin DE, Rogers A, Inturrisi CE, Foley KM: IV infusion of opioids for cancer pain: clinical review and guidelines for use. *Cancer Treat Rep* 70:575–581, 1986.

46. Dole VP: Narcotic addiction, physical dependence and relapse. *N Engl J Med* 286:988–992, 1972.
47. Twycross RG: Clinical experience with diamorphine in advanced malignant disease. *Int J Clin Pharmacol* 9:184–198, 1974.
48. Kanner RM, Foley KM: patterns of narcotic drug use in a cancer pain clinic. *Ann NY Acad Sci* 362:161–172, 1981.
49. Ventafridda V, Oliveri E, Caraceni A, et al: A retrospective study on the use of oral morphine in cancer pain. *J Pain Symp Manag* 2:77–82, 1987.
50. Gildenberg PL, DeVaul RA: *The Chronic Pain Patient.* New York, Karger, 1985.
51. Black RG: The clinical syndrome of chronic pain. In Ng LKY, Bonica JJ (eds): *Pain, Discomfort and Humanitarian Care.* New York, Elsevier, 1980, pp 207–209.
52. Maruta T, Swanson DW: Problems with the use of oxycodone compound in patients with chronic pain. *Pain* 11:389–396, 1981.
53. Maruta T, Swanson DW, Finlayson RE: Drug abuse and dependency in patients with chronic pain. *Mayo Clin Proc* 54:241–244, 1979.
54. Ready LB, Sarkis E, Turner JA; Self-reported vs. actual use of medications in chronic pain patients. *Pain* 12:285–294, 1982.
55. Turner JA, Calsyn DA, Fordyce WE, Ready LB: Drug utilization pattern in chronic pain patients. *Pain* 12:357–363, 1982.
56. Aronoff GM, Evans WO, Enders PL: A review of follow-up studies of multidisciplinary pain units. *Pain* 16:1–11, 1983.
57. Turner JA, Romano JM: Evaluating psychologic interventions for chronic pain: issues and recent developments. In Benedetti C, Chapman CR, Moricca G (eds): *Advances in Pain Research and Therapy.* New York, Raven Press, 1984, vol 7, pp 257–298.
58. Jaffe JH, Martin WR: Opioid analgesics and antagonists. In Gilman AG, Goodman LS, Rall TW, Murad F (eds): *The Pharmacological Basis of Therapeutics,* ed 7. New York, Macmillan, 1985, pp 491–531.
59. Kreek MJ: Tolerance and dependence: implications for the pharmacological treatment of addiction. In Harris LS (ed): *Problems of Drug Dependence, 1986* (NIDA Research Monograph 76). Rockville, MD, National Institute on Drug Abuse, 1987, pp 53–62.
60. Kreek MJ: Medical safety and side effects of methadone in tolerant individuals. *JAMA* 223:665–668, 1973.
61. Kreek MJ: Medical complications in methadone patients. *Ann NY Acad Sci* 311:110–134, 1978.
62. Kreek MJ, Dodes S, Kne S, et al: Long-term methadone maintenance therapy: effects on liver function. *Ann Intern Med* 77:598–602, 1972.
63. Maruta T: Prescription drug-induced organic brain syndrome. *Am J Psychiatry* 135:376–377, 1978.
64. McNairy SL, Maruta T, Ivnik RJ, Swanson DW, Ilstrup DM: Prescription medication dependence and neuropsychologic function. *Pain* 18:169–177, 1984.
65. Rounsaville BH, Novelly RA, Kleber HD, Jones C: Neuropsychological impairment in opiate addicts: risk factors. *Ann NY Acad Sci* 362:79–90, 1981.
66. Martin WR, Jasinski DR, Haertzen CA, et al: Methadone—a reevaluation. *Arch Gen Psychiatry* 28:286–295, 1973.
67. Fritz ER, Shiffman SM, Jarvik ME, et al: Physiological and psychological effects of methadone in man. *Arch Gen Psychiatry* 32:237–242, 1975.
68. Haertzen CA, Hooks NT: Changes in personality and subjective experience associated with the chronic administration and withdrawal of opiates. *J Nerv Ment Dis* 148:606–614, 1969.
69. Lombardo WK, Lombardo B, Goldstein A: Cognitive functioning under moderate and low dose methadone maintenance. *Int J Addict* 11:389–401, 1976.
70. Halpern LM, Robinson J: Prescribing practices for pain in drug dependence: a lesson in ignorance. *Adv Alcohol Subst Abuse* 5(Fall-Winter):184–197, 1985.
71. Hendler N, Cimini C, Ma T, Long D: A comparison of cognitive impairment due to benzodiazepines and to narcotics. *Am J Psychiatry* 137:828–830, 1980.
72. Kozel NJ, Adams EH: Epidemiology of drug abuse: an overview. *Science* 234:970–974, 1986.
73. WHO Expert Committee on Drugs Liable to Produce Addiction: *Technical Report Series, 3rd Report,* No. 57, Geneva, World Health Organization, 1952.
74. WHO Expert Committee on Addiction Producing Drugs: *Technical Report Series, 13th Report,* No. 273. Geneva, World Health Organization, 1964.
75. Jaffe JH: Drug addiction and drug abuse. In Gilman AG, Goodman LS, Rall TW, Murad F (eds): *The Pharmacological Basis of Therapeutics,* ed 7. New York, Macmillan, 1985, pp 532–581.
76. Rinaldi RC, Steindler EM, Wilford BB, Goodwin D: Clarification and standardization of substance abuse terminology. *JAMA* 259:555–557, 1988.
77. Martin WR, Jasinski DR: Physiological parameters of morphine dependence in man—tolerance, early abstinence, protracted abstinence. *J Psychiatr Res* 7:9–17, 1969.
78. Redmond DE, Krystal JH: Multiple mechanisms of withdrawal from opioid drugs. *Annu Rev Neurosci* 7:443–478, 1984.
79. World Health Organization: *Technical Report No. 516, Youth and Drugs.* Geneva, World Health Organization, 1973.
80. Martin WR, EAdes CG, Thompson WO, Thompson JA, Flanary HG: Morphine physical dependence in the dog. *J Pharmacol Exp Ther* 189:759–771, 1974.
81. Kaiko RF, Foley KM, Grabinski PY, et al: Central nervous system excitatory effects of meperidine in cancer patients. *Ann Neurol* 13:180–185, 1983.
82. Jarvik LF, Simpson JH, Guthrie D, Liston EH: Morphine, experimental pain and psychological reactions. *Psychopharmacology* 75:124–131, 1981.
83. Lynch JJ, Stein EA, Fertziger AP: An analysis of 70 years of morphine classical conditioning: implications for clinical treatment of narcotic addiction. *J Nerv Ment Dis* 163:47–58, 1976.

84. Wikler A: *Opioid Dependence: Mechanisms and Treatment.* New York, Plenum, 1980.

85. Koob GF: Neural substrates of opioid tolerance and dependence. In Harris LS (ed): *Problems of Drug Dependence, 1986* (NIDA Research Monograph 76). Rockville, MD, National Institute on Drug Abuse, 1987, pp 46–52.

86. Simpson DD, Savage LJ, Lloyd MR: Follow-up evaluation of treatment of drug abuse during 1969 to 1972. *Arch Gen Psychiatry* 36:772–780, 1979.

87. Valliant GE: A 20-year follow-up of New York narcotic addicts. *Arch Gen Psychiatry* 29:237–241, 1973.

88. Martin WR, Gorodetsky CW: Demonstration of toleranace to and physical dependence on *N*-allylnormorphine (nalorphine). *J Pharmacol Exp Ther* 150:437–442, 1965.

89. Hill HE, Haertzen CA, Davis H: An MMPI factor analytic study of alcoholics, narcotic addicts and criminals. *Q J Stud Alcohol* 23:411–431, 1962.

90. Hill HE, Haertzen CA, Glaser R: Personality characteristics of narcotic addicts as indicated by the MMPI. *J Gen Psychol* 62:127–139, 1960.

91. Robbins LN: *Final Report, September 1973, Special Action Office Monograph, Series A, No 2: The Vietnam Drug User Returns.* Washington, DC, Special Action Office for Drug Abuse Prevention, 1974.

92. Alksne H: The social basis of substance abuse. In Lowinson JH, Ruiz P (eds): *Substance Abuse: Clinical Problems and Perspectives.* Baltimore, Williams & Wilkins, 1981.

93. Martin WR: General problems of drug abuse and drug dependence. In Martin WR (ed): *Drug Addiction I.* New York, Springer-Verlag, 1977, pp 3–40.

94. Goodwin DW, Schulsinger F, Moller N, Hermansen L, Winokur G, Guze SB: Drinking problems in adopted and nonadopted sons of alcoholics. *Arch Gen Psychiatry* 31:164–169, 1974.

95. Newman RG; The need to redefine addiction. *N Engl J Med* 18:1096–1098, 1983.

96. Kolb L: Types and characteristics of drug addicts. *Ment Hyg* 9:300, 1925.

97. Pescor MJ: The Kolb classification of drug addicts. *Publ Health Rep* 155, suppl, 1939.

98. Rayport M: Experience in the management of patients medically addicted to narcotics. *JAMA* 156:684–691, 1954.

99. Porter J, Jick H: Addiction rare in patients treated with narcotics. *N Engl J Med* 302:123, 1980.

100. Perry S, Heidrich G: Management of pain during debridement: a survey of U.S. burn units. *Pain* 13:267–280, 1982.

101. Medina JL, Diamond S: Drug dependency in patients with chronic hedache. *Headache* 17:12–14, 1977.

102. Graeven DB, Folmer W: Experimental heroin users: an epidemiologic and psychosocial approach. *Am J Drug Alcohol Abuse* 4:365–375, 1977.

103. Robins LN, Davis DH, Nurco DN: How permanent was Vietnam drug addiction? *Am J Publ Health* 64:38–43, 1974.

104. Parris WCV, Jamison RN, Vasterling JJ: Follow-up study of a multidisciplinary pain center. *J Pain Symp Manag* 2:145–154, 1987.

105. Duckro PN, Margolis RB, Tait RC, Korytnyk N: Long-term follow-up of chronic pain patients: a preliminary study. *Int J Psychol Med* 15:283–292, 1985.

106. Newman R, Seres J, Yospe L, Garlington B: Multidisciplinary treatment of chronic pain: long-term follow-up of low back pain patients. *Pain* 4:283–292, 1978.

Chapter 14

NONSTEROIDAL ANTI-INFLAMMATORY MEDICATIONS

THOMAS G. KANTOR, MD

Nonsteroidal anti-inflammatory drugs (NSAID) are important therapeutic adjuncts in three specific areas in the treatment of low back pain. First, they have potent analgesic effect that can be sustained over long periods of time without concerns for tachyphylaxis or dependence liability. Second, they have almost specific effects in reducing the pain and inflammation of inflammatory spondyloarthropathies. Third, by their anti-inflammatory and analgesic activity, they promote the initiation and maintenance of rehabilitation efforts that might otherwise be impossible. Low back pain patients must be managed, since most of the etiologies of these conditions are unknown and therefore "cure" may be an unreasonable goal.

Although pain is one of the cardinal signs of inflammation as established by Celsum in antiquity (1), pain need not be associated with obvious inflammation. This chapter first describes the activation of the peripheral pain signal and then demonstrates how NSAIDs reduce pain. The individual drugs are then discussed in chemical classes. I describe how the NSAIDs influence pain and inflammation, why there are so many of them, and the adverse effects and contraindications to their use.

PAIN PATHWAYS

The pain signal is initiated at specialized nociceptive pain endings in the periphery. It is then carried through unmyelinated nerves called C fibers or lightly myelinated fibers through cell bodies in the dorsal ganglia alongside the spine into the dorsal grey matter of the spinal cord. There the pain signal is amplified, modulated, or suppressed by arrays of cells that interact with the incoming pain signal and send nerve fibers across the spinal cord that ascend on the contralateral side of the cord through the spinothalamic tracts to the central nervous system. The degree and significance of the pain is processed in the limbic systems of the brain, and the location of the pain is perceived through connecting nerves to the cortex.

PERIPHERAL PAIN RECEPTOR MEDIATORS

The chemical trigger for the initiation of the pain signal in the periphery is an 11-amino-acid polypeptide named Substance P. This polypeptide is produced in the cell bodies of the nociceptive nerves and moves to the periphery through microtubules in these nerves. There it serves at least two functions: (a) the initiation of the electrical impulse for the nerve at the periphery and (b) triggering the connective tissue–fixed mast cell to produce histamine (2). Histamine is one of the initiating chemical mediators of the inflammatory process but is also an initiator of the pain and itch sensations at the periphery and acts as a vasodilator. Substance P also has receptor sites on the cell walls of the macrophage and lymphocyte that are stimulatory in function, and thus impinges on the immune system, which may also be involved in inflammation (3).

In addition to the chemical mediators there are peripheral nerve mechanoreceptors and polymodal receptors as well, the latter responding to a variety of pain-producing stimuli (4). The mechanoreceptors are mostly activated by stretch or vigorous motion. In the context of this chapter, it is of interest that most of the pain-producing nerves in and around joints, and almost exclusively those in the joint capsules, tendons, and the periosteum of the bones, are mechanoreceptors (5).

INFLAMMATION

The early cellular events of inflammation include the recruitment of white blood cells that stick to the endothelial lining of the vessel walls. By a process of diapedesis, these cells progress through openings between the endothelial cells into the interstitium of the connective tissue. The granulocytes and macrophages then ingest the initiator of the insult or the detritus of the inflammation and in doing so regurgitate enzymes that act on plasma constituents that have leaked into the interstitium (6). Among the products of this enzyme action is the 9-amino-acid compound bradykinin.

When the inflammatory process is initiated by a nociceptive agent, cell wall breakdown also occurs and lipid material in the cell wall is made available to the enzyme phospholipase A. This enzyme transforms the fatty acids of the cell walls into arachidonic acid, the basic chemical for the formation of prostaglandins. Two enzyme groups are known to affect arachidonic acid. One, cyclo-oxygenase, produces prostaglandin end products, including some that mediate inflammation (7) and even one that modifies inflammation (8). In addition, prostaglandins (PGs) E_2 and I_2 (prostacycline) are produced. These are known to sensitize the peripheral pain nerves, although they do not directly stimulate these nerves. Bradykinin is known to directly stim-

ulate pain nerve endings in the peritoneum but not in other locations (9). It has been shown that PGE_2 and/or PGI_2 sensitize the peripheral pain nerves to the further action of bradykinin and/or histamine, which somehow interact with substance P to stimulate the peripheral nerve endings (10).

Thus bradykinin does not need prostaglandin sensitization in the peritoneum but does in all other parts of the body.

A second group of enzymes, lipoxygenases, which act on arachidonic acid, produce leukotrienes and various eicosatetraenoic acids. One of these, leukotriene B_4, enters our story later.

NSAIDs

All of the NSAIDs, including the salicylates, inhibit the enzyme cyclo-oxygenase and therefore prevent the further production of PGE_2 and PGI_2. These drugs have little if any effect on lipoxygenase. Our paradigm for the analgesic effect of NSAIDs, then, is that they reduce or eliminate the production of the sensitizers for peripheral nerve endings associated with pain (11) (Fig. 14.1). There are two aspects of this that are worth further comment. In clinical analgesic trials, including back pain as a pain model, there seems to be a ceiling for the analgesic produced by NSAIDs beyond which further increments in dosage do not lead to increased analgesia. One explanation for this is recent work done by Levine and his coworkers, who have found that leukotriene B_4 can substitute for PGE_2 and PGI_2 as a sensitizer (12). Since the enzyme lipoxygenase, which produces this leukotriene, is relatively unaffected by the NSAIDs there is thus a

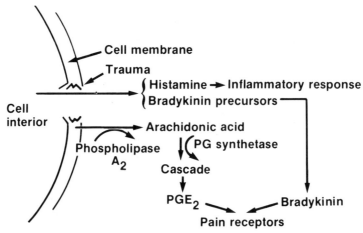

Figure 14.1. Proposed peripheral mechanism of pain.

component of sensitization that is unaffected by the NSAIDs, and this mechanism may account for the ceiling effect of analgesia.

Another feature worth noting is the effect of the acetyl moiety of aspirin. There is evidence that this is donated to the enzyme cyclo-oxygenase and destroys the enzyme (13). All of the other nonacetylated salicylates and the other NSAIDs only inhibit the enzyme and, when metabolized by the liver and excreted by the kidney, leave the enzyme intact. In the case of aspirin, this is primarily of interest for the platelet. Since the platelet is an organelle, having no manufacturing capacity after its extrusion from the megakaryocyte, any damage done to it is irreparable over the 7–10-day residence of the platelet in the plasma. With its cyclo-oxygenase destroyed, the platelet cannot produce thromboxane, which is the mediator of secondary aggregation of the platelet, the first step in blood clotting. This is a very sensitive system, and bleeding times in patients subjected to as little as one dose of 80 mg aspirin are likely to be prolonged for the better part of a week (14). This is obviously disturbing to surgeons, who regularly ban aspirin for patients at least 1 week before elective surgery. However, they not infrequently use small doses of aspirin postoperatively to avoid phlebothrombotic complications. On the other hand, there is recent good evidence that small doses of aspirin daily or every other day can prevent myocardial infarction and/or cerebrovascular accidents due to clots by the same mechanism (15).

ADVERSE EFFECTS OF NSAIDs

Prostaglandins produced by cyclo-oxygenase are physiologic substances with many roles in the body. In the stomach, they modulate mucosal function by reducing acid formation and increasing mucus production and mucosal blood supply. These are primarily mucosa-protective effects. If NSAIDs reduce their production, acid increases, mucus decreases, and mucosal blood supply is lessened—conditions suitable for gastric irritation or ulcer formation.

In the kidney, prostaglandins are produced near the juxtaglomerular apparatus and the tubular mucosa, particularly when a pressor influence is presented to the kidney, such as the renin or angiotensin response to reduced blood volume. Under such conditions, prostaglandins have a vasodilatory effect, assuring that the pressor response does not go too far. In their absence, the pressor substances act unopposed, which leads to the retention of salt and water and possible kidney damage as a result

of prolonged reduced blood flow. Hypertension and opposition to diuretic effect may also result.

Prostaglandins also are active in the uterine mucosa and cause uterine contraction. They help evacuate the detritus of menses and, at the proper time, cause the contractions responsible for parturition. Severe contractions during menses cause dysmenorrhea, and the NSAIDs are a great boon to women so afflicted. However, by the same mechanism, they may prolong labor.

Other known effects of prostaglandins include action in the temperature-regulating centers of the central nervous system (CNS), where they can cause fever. All of the NSAIDs are excellent fever reducers.

It can be seen from the above that the major pharmacologic effect of the NSAIDs, cyclo-oxygenase inhibition and thus prostaglandin production reduction, is responsible for the major adverse effects of these drugs. In addition to reduction of prostaglandins in the gastric mucosa, uncoated aspirin tablets have a direct mucolytic and mucosa-damaging effect, which is why enteric-coated tablets are suggested for long-term use. Enteric coating of aspirin puts aspirin on a par with the other NSAIDs with respect to gastric irritation by eliminating one of the ways aspirin irritates the stomach. However the NSAIDs as a group have an incidence of peptic ulcer production of between 1 and 3% and unacceptable gastric toxicity of up to 20%. Worse, gastroscopic examination reveals incidences of peptic ulcer without symptoms that are not trivial. Totally unexpected hemorrhages may result, which seem to be more prevalent in elderly females.

The renal problems are much more rare and are seen particularly under conditions of reduced blood volume due to dehydration. Summer is a time for increased vigilance on the part of the physician for these complications.

NSAIDs are contraindicated in the last trimester of pregnancy for the reasons noted above. Children and patients with systemic lupus erythematosus seem to be somewhat more in danger of hepatic toxicity of NSAIDs, which is a rare complication.

In general, careful monitoring with occasional determinations of blood urea nitrogen and creatinine values, liver function tests, and testing of the stool for blood are useful in managing patients on chronic NSAID therapy.

THE INDIVIDUAL NSAIDs

The first NSAIDs, salicylates, were essentially infusions of willow bark, a remedy known from ancient times. When these were made into powders and eventually tablets, an industry for relief of pain by ingested medications was born. The mechanism for the analgesic effect remained a mystery until Ferriera in John Vane's laboratory demonstrated the inhibitory effect of aspirin on the enzyme cyclo-oxygenase (11). This so-called Vane Hypothesis is accepted as the major mechanism by which NSAIDs reduce pain and inflammation. Recently, however, several investigators have pointed out inhibitory effects of NSAIDs on immune cell function and the adhesion of granulocytes to endothelial cells (16, 17). These may be of at least equal importance to the modulation of inflammation by NSAIDs as the cyclo-oxygenase inhibition mechanism.

ASPIRIN AND THE SALICYLATES

Aspirin's presumed mode of action in pain has been described above. However, a variety of non-acetylated salicylates, both organic and inorganic, are also analgesic. Recently Vane and his associates have shown that the salicylate moeity itself has the capacity to inhibit cyclo-oxygenase, which explains the analgesic effect of salicylates (18). Those other than aspirin are somewhat weaker in analgesic effect (19). For chronic usage, aspirin in an enteric-coated form is suggested. There are low-dose enteric-coated forms available without prescription (Ecotrin, etc.) and high-dose (925 mg/tablet) forms that must be prescribed (Easprin). Aspirin and the other salicylates have an elimination half-life in the plasma that varies with the dose, in contrast to the other NSAIDs, which are first-order drugs (Table 14.1). Aspirin in high doses has a much longer half-life than in low doses. The total residence time of a compound in the plasma is generally 6–7 times the half-life, and the NSAIDs vary widely in this regard (Table 14.1).

Nonacetylated salicylates, organic and inorganic, do not have the acetyl radical to destroy cyclo-oxygenase and simply inhibit the enzyme as noted above. In addition, they do not have the antiplatelet aggregating effect of aspirin and may therefore be useful in patients with coagulation defects, whether provoked by drug or disease (20). Those available include choline magnesium salicylate (Trilisate), salsalate (Disalcid), and magnesium, aluminum, and sodium salts of salicylate. All seem somewhat weaker than aspirin on a milligram-for-milligram basis, both for analgesic and for anti-inflammatory effect. However, the gastrointestinal toxicity also seems to be less. They are useful in special circumstances where aspirin is either unacceptably toxic or otherwise contraindicated.

PYRAZOLES

Phenylbutazone (Butazolidin) is the only member of this group available at present. It is considered so toxic that several countries have banned it from their formularies. It is a very strong cyclo-oxygenase inhibitor and may inhibit enzymes responsible for the further metabolism of arachidonic acid as well (21) (Fig. 14.1). Phenylbutazone is still available in this country because rheumatologists perceive it to have a certain specificity for spondyloarthritides (22). For example, ankylosing spondylitis and the spondylitic components of juvenile arthritis, Reiter's syndrome, and psoriatic arthritis may be successfully treated only with phenylbutazone, which works well when all other NSAIDs may not.

Unfortunately, idiosyncratic bone marrow suppression, which may lead to aplastic anemia, is a rare but potentially fatal adverse effect, more common with this drug than the other NSAIDs. Through a mechanism to be explained later, phenylbutazone is the most potent salt and water retainer of all NSAIDs, which may lead to initiation or aggravation of congestive heart failure and hypertension (23). In addition, it has all of the adverse effects common to all the NSAIDs (see below).

However, in doses as low as 100–200 mg/day, it has sustained patients with ankylosing spondylitis for years. Some of its toxicity may be related to its 96-hour elimination half-life (Table 14.1), which means that any single dose may not clear the body for a month. In chronic usage, however, phenylbutazone induces the hepatic enzymes responsible for its metabolism, bringing the half-life down into the 50-hour range (24). These metabolites are excreted by the kidney, so that severe hepatocellular disease or significant renal insufficiency are contraindications for the use of phenylbutazone.

INDOLEACETIC ACIDS

Indomethacin

Indomethacin (Indocin) was the first of this chemical group to be passed by the Food and Drug Administration (FDA), and the drug is the standard potent cyclo-oxygenase inhibitor against which all others are compared. Its half-life of 3–4.5 hours suggests a 3- or 4-times-a-day dosing schedule, although recent sustained-release (SR) and suppository forms have allowed dosage every 12 hours. It is metabolized in the liver and excreted by the kidney, as are all other NSAIDs.

Indomethacin has certain unique adverse effects that include a poorly characterized headache after the first dose in the morning. Many patients com-

Table 14.1

Overview of Available Nonsteroidal Anti-inflammatory Drugs (NSAIDs) in the United States

DRUG	DOSAGE SCHEDULE (CAPSULE OR TABLET SIZE)	ELIMINATION HALF-LIFE (HOURS)
Salicylate series		
Acetylsalicylic acid (aspirin)	2.6 g or more (variable)	3–16
Choline magnesium trisalicylate (Trilisate)	1500–2500 mg given in two or three divided doses (500 mg, 750 mg)	7–18
Magnesium salicylate (Magan, Mobidin)	Two 545-mg tablets three times per day	2–2.5
Salsalate (Disalcid)	3000 mg daily in two or three divided doses (500 mg, 750 mg)	8
Salicylate-like series		
Diflunisal (Dolobid)	500–1000 mg daily in two divided doses (250 mg, 500 mg)	8
Indole-like series		
Indomethacin (Indocin)	25–200 mg one to four times daily in divided doses (25 mg, 50 mg, 75 mg sustained release)	3–4.5
Sulindac (Clinoril)	300–400 mg twice daily in divided doses	13
Tolmetin sodium (Tolectin)	1200–1800 mg three to four times daily in divided doses (200 mg, 400 mg)	1
Pyrazole series		
Phenylbutazone (Azolid, Butazolidin etc.)	100–400 mg two to three times daily in divided doses (100 mg)	84–96
Propionic acid series		
Ibuprofen (Motrin, Rufen)	900–2400 mg three to four times daily in divided doses (300 mg, 400 mg, 600 mg, 800 mg)	2–3
Fenoprofen calcium (Nalfon)	900–2400 three to four times in divided doses (300 mg, 600 mg)	3
Naproxen (Naprosyn)	250–1000 mg two to three times daily in divided doses (250 mg, 375 mg, 500 mg)	13
Ketoprofen (Orudis)	150–300 mg three to four times daily in divided doses (50 mg, 75 mg)	2–3
Anthranilic acid series		
Meclofenamate sodium (Meclomen)	200–400 mg/day in divided doses (50 mg, 100 mg)	2–5
Benzothiazine series		
Piroxicam (Feldene)	20 mg once a day (10 mg, 20 mg)	44

plain of a sensation of "spaciness" or a drugged effect with indomethacin that may be severe enough to preclude its use (see Table 14.1 for dosing details).

There is some feeling among rheumatologists that indomethacin also has some specificity in the treatment of the spondyloarthritides (22).

Tolmetin

Tolmetin (Tolectin) has the shortest elimination half-life of all the NSAIDs. For this reason, it has been approved for use in children, who may not have developed the adult enzyme systems that would safely metabolize other drugs. For the same reason, it is a useful drug in the very elderly, whose total available nephrons may be inadequate to safely excrete longer acting NSAIDs.

In addition to the usual adverse effects, tolmetin has a slightly greater incidence of anaphylactic reactions than other NSAIDs (P. Stewart, McNeil Laboratories, personal communication). This may be related to its close chemical relation to zomepirac (Zomax), which was withdrawn from the market for anaphylactic reactions.

Sulindac

Sulindac (Clinoril) is the third available indole-acetic acid derivative. In addition to the usual enzymatic conjugation in the liver, it is also excreted in the bile in an oxygenated form, which may be responsible for its higher incidence of diarrhea than other NSAIDs.

Sulindac itself is a pro-drug, meaning that the parent drug has no pharmacologic activity of its own but must be metabolized to a reduced sulfide form that is the active drug. Since this metabolism takes place in the liver, severe hepatocellular disease such as hepatitis will lead to much-reduced activity of cyclo-oxygenase inhibition. The sulfide circulates in equilibrium with the inactive parent drug. However, there is evidence that this equilibrium shifts to the inactive form on circulation through the kidney (25). It is perhaps for this reason that sulindac is considered to have fewer renal adverse effects than other NSAIDs (26) (see below).

The sulfide has a half-life of 13 hours, which suggests twice-daily dosing. Sulindac is approved for use in ankylosing spondylitis.

PROPIONIC ACIDS
Ibuprofen

Ibuprofen (Rufen, Motrin, Advil, Nuprin, etc.) has had a constant increment in its suggested dose pattern. After its introduction in England in 1967 at a suggested dose of 600 mg daily, it was introduced in the United States in 1974 at a suggested dose of 1200–1600 mg daily. Since then, there are reported uses as high as 4800 mg daily (27), and there is a recent introduction of an 800-mg tablet. Ibuprofen's overall record has shown sufficient safety to allow its over-the-counter (OTC) sale in a 200-mg tablet size with an indication for headache, dysmenorrhea, and mild musculoskeletal pain (28). Other NSAIDs will presumably follow soon as OTC drugs.

Ibuprofen's half-life of 2–3 hours suggests a 3- or 4-times-a-day dosage schedule, although some have claimed success with twice-daily schedules.

Fenoprofen

Fenoprofen (Nalfon) is another propionic acid derivative with a short half-life requiring dosage 3 or 4 times daily. As with other NSAIDs, it is conjugated to glucuronides and sulfides in the liver and excreted as such, and also as unchanged drug, by the kidney.

Fenoprofen is considered to be more nephrotoxic than other NSAIDs, although the reason for this is unclear (29). Its other toxicities are in line with other NSAIDs.

Ketoprofen

Ketoprofen (Orudis) is as of this writing the latest NSAID introduced into the United States. The drug has a long experience in England and many other countries, which allows us to assume that any strange adverse effects have already been ruled out (30). If it follows the track of other short half-life propionic acids, ketoprofen's dose schedule will probably be increased from the suggested top dose of 300 mg in 24 hours. It is available now in 50- and 75-mg tablets, and a 3- or 4-times-a-day schedule is also suggested by its half-life. It is metabolized and excreted similarly to other NSAIDs, and its adverse effect incidence and pattern are similar as well.

Naproxen

Naproxen (Naprosyn) is available in three formulations: the parent drug as a tablet, a sodium salt of the parent drug named Anaprox, and a liquid suspension of the parent drug. Its excellent safety record and pharmacologic effectiveness have propelled it into the number one position in prescription NSAID sales in the United States. The sodium salt is more readily absorbed from the gastrointestinal tract and is presumably a faster analgetic, but evidence for this is meager. The liquid suspension is a boon to pediatric patients for whom the drug is approved and for patients unwilling or unable to swallow tablets.

Naproxen's half-life of 12 hours allows twice-daily dosing. There has been uncertainty as to its total daily dosage. A 250-, 375-, and 500-mg tablet of the parent drug are available, and dosage up to 1500 mg daily has been reported. In my experience, there is a small but definite increment in adverse effects of the general NSAID type with increasing dosage.

FENAMIC ACIDS

Meclofenamic acid (Meclomen) is the only drug in this group approved for chronic use. In addition to the usual NSAIDs metabolism and excretion, there is an extensive enterohepatic circulation accounting for a high incidence of diarrhea.

Meclomen is said to not only inhibit cyclo-oxygenase but inhibit prostaglandins from binding to their receptor sites. Evidence for this latter effect is indirect (31).

Meclomen's short half-life allows a suggested 3-times-daily dose schedule, and its adverse effects are the same as those of other NSAIDs except for the higher incidence of diarrhea.

OXICAMS

Piroxicam (Feldene) is the only oxicam available in the United States. In addition to the usual cyclo-oxygenase inhibition, it is said to interfere with leukocyte function as a further reason for its potent anti-inflammatory effect. Piroxicam has a 44-hour half-life, which allows a once-daily dose of 20 mg that is helpful to compliance. (For a discussion of compliance related to half-life, see below.) Doses of over 20 mg/day are associated with an alarming increment in peptic ulcer incidence (32). A 10-mg tablet is available for possible reduction in dose in the very elderly and in those with possible hepatic and renal defects that may further prolong the half-life. Another possible protection is an every-other-day dose schedule.

Other adverse effects, metabolism, and excretion are similar to those of other NSAIDs.

A recent admonition by consumer groups to the FDA to restrict usage was based on data in the United States and England for the first 2 years after approval that suggested that piroxicam was more ulcerogenic than other NSAIDs. However, the so-called Weber curve shows that in its first 2 years after approval, any drug has a large amount of adverse effects reported. After that, as clinicians become more skilled in prescribing a drug and are more aware of its contraindications, the adverse effect reports settle down to a much lower incidence. The consumer groups noted above were comparing piroxicam in its first 2 years to other established NSAIDs after much longer usage. When the data were corrected for this, piroxicam was no more toxic than all other NSAIDs.

CONTRAINDICATIONS TO NSAID THERAPY

NSAIDs are all acidic in function and over 90% of the total serum concentration is bound to serum albumin. Their avidity for albumin is stronger than that of most drugs and they can replace less strongly bound substances. The free as opposed to bound component of a drug's serum concentration is the pharmacologically active component. If a weakly bound drug is pushed away from albumin by an NSAID, the weak drug may become pharmacologically more active. This is especially true in the case of oral hypoglycemic agents and coumarin derivatives. This is not an absolute contraindication for using NSAIDs and hypoglycemics together, but dose adjustments may be necessary. However, there is an absolute contraindication for using NSAIDs concomitantly with coumarin derivatives or other anticoagulants and in patients with blood clotting deficiencies. Prostaglandins are also responsible for aggregation of platelets, the first step in blood clotting, and their elimination leads to prolonged blood clotting times.

When high-dose methotrexate is used in chemotherapy, NSAIDs should not be used since an augmentation, possibly fatal, of the effect of methotrexate may occur (34). Otherwise NSAIDs are good starting therapy for the pain of metastatic disease in bone, particularly the spine. The enlargement and spread of bony metastases is under prostaglandin control in that prostaglandins aid in leeching out the calcium of the bone containing the metastasis. Suppressing this prostaglandin effect with NSAIDs is often rewarding to the patient (34).

As already noted, NSAIDs are absolutely contraindicated in patients with active peptic ulcers and relatively contraindicated in those with a history of peptic or esophageal ulceration. With caution, some of these patients may be simultaneously treated with antacids, histamine-2 blockers, or sucralfate. However, antacids may interfere with NSAID absorption and promote excretion. Histamine-2 blockers do not seem to work well for the dyspepsia NSAIDs cause. Sucralfate or pharmacologic prostaglandins seem to suppress symptoms best, but their effect on ulcer formation by NSAIDs is uncertain (35).

Compliance in drug taking is a problem, especially in those such as the elderly, who may be taking as many as eight or nine drugs daily. The addition of an NSAID with a short half-life requiring dosage 3 or 4 times daily may overburden the drug management ability of some patients (36). It is tempting, then, to use an NSAID requiring dosage only once or twice a day. However, the elderly, who are by far the greatest users of NSAIDs, have reduced nephron capacity, and a long half-life drug may have an even longer half-life with toxic consequences. This is essentially what happened with benoxaprofen (Oraflex), which had to be removed from the market because of deaths in older patients. Faced with this dilemma, the physician will have to judge his/her patients well and be sure of achieving their own or a significant other's cooperation with the decided-upon dosing schedule. In general, the older the patient the shorter half-life drug should be used.

Another feature of NSAID therapy in the elderly should be noted. In some patients over the age of 70, memory loss, confusion, and depression may be adverse effects and are reversible on stopping the offending drug (37).

THE FUTURE

Because of the capriciousness of individual response to these drugs, many more have been presented to the FDA for approval. However, the FDA is under no pressure to approve others simply because they inhibit cyclo-oxygenase, considering the large number already available. A substantiated claim for an additional pharmacologic action or lesser toxicity will probably by demanded.

Of those awaiting approval, diclofenac (Voltaren), a somewhat different chemical entity with an additional feature of an injected formulation, and proquazone (Biarson), because it is nonacidic in chemical function, may be among the next to be approved.

REFERENCES

1. Celsum AC: *De Mediana* (translated from L. Targa's edition by Alex Smith). London, E. Cox, 1831, p 182.
2. Fields HL: Central nervous system mechanisms for control of pain transmission. In Fields HL: *Pain*. New York, McGraw-Hill, 1987 pp 99–133.
3. Payan DG, Levine JD, Goetzl EJ: Modulation of immunity and hypersensitivity by sensory neuropeptides. *J Immunol* 132:1601–1603, 1984.
4. Torebjork HE: Afferent C units responding to mechanical, thermal and chemical stimuli in human non-glabrous skin. *Acta Physiol Scand* 92:374–390, 1974.
5. Guilband G, Iggo A: The effect of aspirin on the mechanical sensitivity of joint-capsule sensory receptors in the arthritic rat. *Exp Brain Res* 61:164–168, 1985.
6. Weissmann G, Smolen JE, Korchak HM: Release of inflammatory mediators from stimulated neutrophils. *N Engl J Med* 303:27–34, 1980.
7. Vane JR: Prostaglandins and the aspirin-like drugs. *Hosp Prac* 7:61–71, 1972.
8. Zurier RB, Quagliata F: Effect of prostaglandin E on adjuvant arthritis. *Nature* 243:309–310, 1971.
9. Kantor TG, Jarvik ME, Wolff BB: Bradykinin as a mediator of human pain. *Proc Soc Exp Biol Med* 126:505–506, 1967.
10. Fields, HL: The peripheral pain sensory system. In Fields HL: *Pain*. New York, McGraw-Hill, 1987, pp 13–40.
11. Ferreira SH: Prostaglandins, aspirin-like drugs and analgesia. *Nature* 240:200–203, 1972.
12. Levine JD, Lau W, Kwiat G, Goetzl EJ: Leukotriene B4 produces hyperalgesia that is dependent on polymorphonuclear leukocytes. *Science* 225:225–233, 1984.
13. Roth GJ, Stanford N, Majerus PN: Acetylation of prostaglandin synthetase by aspirin. *Proc Natll Acad Sci (USA)* 72:3073–3076, 1975.
14. Fitzgerald GA, Oates JA, Hawiger J, et al: Endogenous biosynthesis of prostacyclin and thromboxane and platelet function during chronic administration of aspirin in man. *J Clin Invest* 71:676–688, 1983.
15. The Steering Committee of the Physician's Health Study Research Group: Special Report. *N Engl J Med* 318:262–264, 1988.
16. Abramson SE, Kochak M, Ludewig R, Weissman G: Modes of action of aspirin-like drugs. *Proc Natl Acad Sci (USA)* 82:7227–7231, 1985.
17. Goodwin JS: Immunologic effects of non-steroidal anti-inflammatory drugs. *Am J Med* (Suppl) 74(4B):7–11, 1984.
18. Higgs GA, Salmon JA, Henderson B, Vane JR: Pharmacokinetics of aspirin and salicylate in relation to inhibition of arachidonate cyclooxygenase and anti-inflammatory activity. *Proc Natl Acad Sci (USA)* 84:1417–1420, 1987.
19. Beaver WT: Mild analgesics. A review of their clinical pharmacology. *Am J Med Sci* 252:576–599, 1966.
20. Zucker MD, Rothwell KG: Differential influence of salicylate compounds on platelet aggregation and serotonin release. *Curr Ther Res* 23:194–199, 1978.
21. Kuehl FA Jr, Humes JL, Egan RW: Role of prostaglandin endoperoxide PGG2 in anti-inflammatory processes. *Nature* 265:170–173, 1977.
22. Katz WA: Ankylosing spondylitis. In Katz WA (ed): *Rheumatic Diseases*. Philadelphia, JB Lippincott, 1977, pp 520–539.
23. Simon S, Mills JA: Drug therapy: non-steroidal anti-inflammatory drugs. *N Engl J Med* 302:1179–1186, 1980.
24. Domenjoz R: The pharmacology of phenylbutazone. *Ann NY Acad Sci* 86:263–291, 1960.
25. Miller MJS, Bednar MM, McGiff JC: Renal metabolism of sulindac: functional implications. *J Pharmacol Exp Ther* 231:449–456, 1984.
26. Ciabattoni G, Cinotti GA, Pierucci A, et al: Effects on sulindac and ibuprofen in patients with chronic glomerular disease. Evidence for the dependence of renal function on prostacyclin. *N Engl J Med* 310:279–283, 1984.
27. Kantor TG: Ibuprofen. *Ann Inter Med* 91:877–883, 1979.
28. Kantor TG: Availability of nonsteroidal anti-inflammatory drugs as over-the-counter drugs: the case in favor. In Willkens RF, Dahl SL (eds): *Therapeutic Controversies in the Rheumatic Diseases*. San Francisco, Grune & Stratton, 1987.
29. Feinfield DA, Olesnicky L, Pirani CL, et al: Nephrotic syndrome associated with the use of non-steroidal anti-inflammatory drugs. *Nephron* 37:174–179, 1984.
30. Kantor TG: Ketoprofen: a review of its pharmacologic and clinical properties. *Pharmacotherapy* 6:93–103, 1986.
31. Tolman EL, Partridge R: Multiple sites of interaction between prostaglandins and non-steroidal anti-inflammatory agents. *Prostaglindens* 9:349–359, 1975.
32. Semble E, Metcalf D, Turner R, et al: Genetic predictors of patient response and side effects in the treatment of rheumatoid arthritis with a high dose NSAID drug regimen. *Arthritis Rheum* 25:370–375, 1982.
33. Daly H, Boyle J, Roberts C, Scott G, et al: Interaction

between methotrexate and non-steroidal anti-inflammatory drugs (letter). *Lancet* 1:557, 1986.

34. Kantor TG: Nonsteroidal anti-inflammatory analgesic agents in management of cancer pain. In: Symposium on The Management of Pain, (William Beaver, Chairman). *Hosp Pract* (Suppl) Summer 1984.

35. Caldwell JR, Roth SH, Heller MD, et al: Sucralfate therapy of non-steroidal anti-inflammatory drug-induced gastritis. *Clin Pharmacol Ther* 37:186–191, 1985.

36. Belcon MC, Haynes RB, Tugwell P: A critical review of compliance studies in rheumatoid arthritis. *Arthritis Rheum* 27:1227–1231, 1984.

37. Goodwin JS, Regan M: Cognitive dysfunction associated with naproxen and ibuprofen in the elderly. *Arthritis Rheum* 25:1013–1015, 1982.

Chapter 15

PSYCHOPHARMACOLOGIC AGENTS

J. HAMPTON ATKINSON, Jr, MD
MARK A. SLATER, PhD

This chapter reviews the therapeutic efficacy of psychiatric medications (the antidepressant agents, neuroleptics, antianxiety drugs, and psychostimulants) in the rehabilitation of patients with chronic low back pain (CLBP), and provides guidelines for their use. Psychotropic drugs have been used as (a) analgesics, (b) adjunctive agents to enhance pain relief offered by conventional analgesics, and (c) as primary treatment for psychological symptoms or psychiatric disorders associated with pain. Because anxiety, depression, insomnia, fatigue, and similar symptoms so commonly complicate the course of CLBP, virtually every clinician treating CLBP should have some knowledge of the advantages and limitations of psychiatric medications in this population.

Despite the prevalence of CLBP, and the abundant literature on psychotropic drugs and pain, few of the available studies can be considered scientifically complete. The ideal clinical trial of a psychotropic drug's efficacy in CLBP would include: (a) a reliable method to measure the intensity of pain and functional impairment; (b) a placebo control or reference analgesic to compare with the experimental drug; (c) a measurement of mood, side effect, and patient expectations; (d) a measure of the biologic activity or of serum levels of the psychotropic agent employed; (e) a double-blind or crossover design; and (f) adequate follow-up. Since pain is a phenomenon with both sensory and emotional components, the ideal study would determine which of these domains responded to the experimental drug, how treatment affected behavior and impairment (e.g., hours of daily activity, analgesic intake), and how long treatment should be maintained. Obviously few studies describe rigorously diagnosed CLBP samples in such rich detail.

This chapter is in two parts. The first section critically assesses evidence of efficacy, generally from controlled studies, for each major class of psychopharmacologic agent. We follow the principle that accurate medical and psychiatric characterization is as essential to evaluating clinical and research reports of drug treatment outcomes as it is to formulating successful therapy for individual patients. Therefore, we differentiate experimentally induced and clinical acute pain from their chronic pain counterparts, and we discriminate between studies of back pain patients and studies involving pain at other sites (e.g., headache). We realize that CLBP is a heterogeneous disorder whose pathophysiology is imperfectly understood, but where possible, drug efficacy is discussed in relation to presumed etiology of the CLBP syndrome. When psychiatric disorders complicate or overlap the course of CLBP, we discuss their diagnosis and response to treatment also.

The second section offers some clinical guidelines for using psychoactive drugs. It describes selecting a drug, preparing and evaluating patients for treatment, and conducting initial and longer term pharmacotherapy. Thus, the clinician considering a particular psychopharmacologic strategy for a patient with CLBP can review selected examples of evidence for efficacy in the text and tables of part one. The practitioner then can refer to the next section for specifics on treatment approaches.

STUDIES OF EFFICACY
ANTIDEPRESSANT AGENTS

Each of the three major classes of antidepressant drugs, the tricyclic antidepressants (TCAs), monoamine oxidase inhibitors (MAOIs), and lithium car-

169

bonate, have been used as primary or adjunctive agents in pain management. There are four major clinical questions with regard to antidepressants in acute and chronic pain:

1. Are some antidepressants analgesic, and if so, in which pain disorders?
2. Is this analgesia independent of an antidepressant effect?
3. Do antidepressants potentiate narcotic or non-narcotic analgesics in a clinically relevant manner?
4. Do antidepressants relieve depression associates with CLBP?

Crucial to evaluating the role of antidepressant medication is defining what is meant by "depression." The term can be used to describe a mood, a symptom, and a syndrome or disorder. Fluctuations in mood, or unhappiness as a reaction to life events or physical limitations, is not a disorder. Indeed, the symptom of depressed mood may not be present even in patients diagnosed as having a depressive disorder. A diagnosis of a major depressive disorder, as described by the third edition of the *Diagnostic and Statistical Manual of Mental Disorders* (DSM-III) (1), requires an inability to experience pleasure, reduced interest in the environment, and reduced energy. A major depressive episode is thus defined as a period lasting at least 2 weeks that may be marked by a dysphoric mood, and is often accompanied by a disorder of sleep and appetite, loss of energy, loss of interest, self-reproach, difficulty concentrating, and thoughts of death or suicide. Major depression differs from depressive symptoms in that the above problems are persistent, *interfere with function,* and are not explained better by other illness (1). Dysthymic disorder is defined as a chronically depressed mood for most of each day, on more days than not, for at least 2 years. This disturbance of mood must be associated with some symptoms of alteration either in appetite, sleep, energy, self-esteem, or ability to concentrate. Interference in everyday functioning generally is related to chronicity rather than severity of symptoms. Chronic pain can be associated with intermittent or persistent fatigue, withdrawal, insomnia, or other depressive symptoms, which do not amount to a diagnosis of major depression. Nevertheless, perhaps 25% of CLBP patients suffer a major depressive episode at some point in their pain career (2), and its detection is extremely important.

Tricyclic Antidepressants

Tricyclic antidepressants have been tested in numerous intractable pain syndromes. The agents tested include amitriptyline (Elavil), desipramine (Norpramin), imipramine (Tofranil), and doxepin (Sinequan). The data most clearly support their efficacy for neurologic (deafferentation) pain and headache syndromes. Their effectiveness in other chronic pain syndromes, arthritic disorders, and low back pain—which may well represent the diagnosis for which the drugs are most commonly employed—varies by diagnosis of the underlying disorder impeding rehabilitation. Results from treatment studies are summarized in Table 15.1.

Low Back Pain

Two basic groups of CLBP patients have been studied. The first includes those with rigorously diagnosed major affective disorders (unipolar depression or dysthymic disorder) that either precede or are secondary to pain. The second includes patients with depressive symptoms, but who do not meet criteria for a diagnosable depressive disorder. Efficacy of antidepressants depends on the diagnostic group considered.

Several studies report that CLBP complicated by a major affective disorder (major depression or dysthymic disorder) responds well to TCAs. For example, in a series of investigations (3, 4) Ward and coworkers noted that both doxepin and desipramine significantly reduced self-reported and objective ratings of depression and anxiety, pain severity, and percentage of day in pain. Over half of the patients achieved 30% or greater reduction in pain intensity and 40% reduction in severity of depressive symptoms (4). Clinical pain relief and clinical depression relief were significantly related. The doses achieved were within the usual antidepressant range (3 mg/kg, or at least 150 mg daily for either agent), and the onset of maximum therapeutic response occurred after 3–4 weeks. These factors argued for a primary antidepressant effect. The best clinical predictor of response was a shorter duration of pain complaint; age, number of surgeries, employment status, and orthopaedic ratings of the amount of physical impairment did not predict outcome (4).

Mixed effects are reported in CLBP patients having depressive symptoms, but without diagnosed major affective disorder. Alcoff et al. (5) described a sample of CLBP patients, 10% of whom had documented depressive symptoms. After 6 weeks of treatment, the group given imipramine (150 mg

Table 15.1
Tricyclic Antidepressants: Populations, Experimental Design, and Treatment Outcome

AUTHORS	POPULATION	N	INTERVENTIONS	DESIGN	CONTROL	DEPENDENT MEASURES	FOLLOW-UP	RESULTS
				CHRONIC LOW BACK PAIN				
Alcoff & coworkers, 1982 (5)	Chronic low back pain	41	Compared imipramine 150 mg with placebo	Double blind, group outcome	Placebo medication	Beck depression scores, activity level, work function, pain severity, analgesic use	8 wk	Imipramine significantly improved activity and work function, but not pain severity, analgesic use, or level of depression
Jenkins & coworkers, 1976 (10)	Chronic low back pain	44	Compared imipramine with placebo	Double blind, group outcome	Placebo medication	Standardized personality inventory, Beck despression inventory, self-report of pain and stiffness	4 wk	Imipramine no different from placebo
Sternbach & coworkers, 1976 (9)	Chronic low back pain	9	Compared chlorimipramine, amitriptyline, and placebo	Double blind, counterbalanced	Placebo medication	Self-report of pain, pain tolerance on tourniquet test	2 wk	Chlorimipramine reduced pain estimate and increased pain tolerance. Amitriptyline ineffective
Ward & coworkers, 1979 (3)	Low back pain with major depression	16	Doxepin 150 mg	Single blind, group outcome	None	Rigorous (Research Diagnostic Criteria) diagnosis of depression, retrospective self-report of pain before and after treatment, Hamilton depression score	4 wk	Pain "diminished" as depression remitted
Ward, 1986 (4)	Low back pain with major depression	35	Compared doxepin (3 mg/kg) with desipramine (3 mg/kg)	Double blind, group outcome	Placebo respondors eliminated from study pool	Hamilton depression, Spielberger anxiety, Profile of Moods, McGill Pain Inventory, Illness Behavior, EMG recording, ice-water pain tolerance	4 wk	Doxepin and desipramine equally reduced pain intensity and frequency, depression, and anxiety. Ice-water pain tolerance unaffected

continued

Table 15.1 (continued)

AUTHORS	POPULATION	N	INTERVENTIONS	DESIGN	CONTROL	DEPENDENT MEASURES	FOLLOW-UP	RESULTS
Gringas, 1976 (13)	Mixed arthritic disorders	55	Compared imipramine 75 mg with placebo	Double blind, counterbalanced crossover	Placebo medication	Self-report of pain and stiffness, objectively assessed grip strength, observer-assessed function and stiffness	4 wk	Treatment group showed significantly less subjective pain and stiffness and improved observer ratings of function and stiffness. Objective grip strength unchanged
McDonald-Scott, 1969 (14)	Mixed arthritic disorders	22	Compared imipramine 75 mg added to anti-inflammatory regimen with placebo	Double blind, crossover	Placebo medication	Patient "preference" of interventions	3 wk	Patients "preferred" imipramine to placebo
MacNeill & Dick, 1976 (12)	Mixed arthritic disorders	29	Compared imipramine with placebo	Double blind, group outcome	Placebo medication	Pain self-report, objectively determined grip strength, Beck depression inventory	10 wk	No between-group differences in pain report on grip strength; results potentially confounded because imipramine group significantly more depressed at baseline
Pilowsky & coworkers, 1982 (7)	Mixed chronic pain without organic findings	52	Compared amitriptyline with placebo	Double blind, crossover	Placebo medication	Illness Behavior Questionnaire, Zung and Levine-Pilowsky depression, Spielberger anxiety, Sickness Impact Profile	6 wk on each treatment	Amitriptyline superior to placebo at 2 and 4 weeks. No group differences at 6 weeks. High dropout (40%) and variability of scores may have obscured treatment effect
	NEUROPATHIC STATES							
Kvinesdal & coworkers, 1984 (23)	Diabetic neuropathy	12	Compared imipramine 100 mg with placebo	Crossover, double blind	Placebo medication	Clinical assessment of neuropathy & global improvement	5 wk for each treatment	Imipramine superior for global improvement

Study	Condition	N	Comparison	Design	Comparator	Outcome measures	Duration	Results
Turkington, 1980 (25)	Diabetic neuropathy with depression and depressive symptoms	59	Compared amitriptyline 100 mg, imipramine 100 mg, and diazepam 15 mg	Randomized, double blind	Diazepam	Kufer-Detre depression inventory, unspecified pain estimates	3 mo	Antidepressants superior to diazepam for relief of pain and mood disorder
Langohr & coworkers, 1982 (29)	Mixed mono- and polyneuropathy	48	Compared clomipramine 100 mg with aspirin	Open label & double blind, crossover	Aspirin	Rated degree of relief and overall function	5 wk	Clomipramine superior to aspirin. On 14-mo follow-up 41% maintained good relief
Watson & coworkers, 1982 (24)	Postherpetic neuralgia	24	Compared amitriptyline 75 mg with placebo	Double blind, crossover	Placebo medication	MMPI, Beck, pain self-report, sleep self-report	Up to 19 mo	Pain reduced in two-thirds of patients, to at least "mild" level; 6/9 with depressive symptoms had mood improvement and pain relief and others had pain relief alone. 50% had pain return on follow-up

OTHER SYNDROMES

Study	Condition	N	Comparison	Design	Comparator	Outcome measures	Duration	Results
Carette & coworkers, 1985 (19)	Fibromyalgia	59	Compared amitriptyline with placebo	Double blind	Placebo medication	Self-report of pain and sleep, physician global assessment	9 wk	Duration of morning-only stiffness significantly reduced at 9 wk
Caruso & coworkers, 1987 (21)	Fibromyalgia	52	Compared dothiepin with placebo	Double blind	Placebo medication	Self-report of pain, tender points elicited	8 wk	Pain severity and number of tender points significantly reduced on dothiepin
Dinerman & coworkers, 1985 (20)	Fibromyalgia	35	Compared naproxen with and without amitriptyline	Double blind	Placebo medication	Self-report of pain and sleep, patient global assessment	6 wk	Addition of amitriptyline significantly improved pain and global assessment compared to naproxen

daily) showed significantly higher activity levels and work capacity, but did not differ from those on placebo in pain severity, analgesic use, or degree of change in Beck depression scores. This study is particularly informative because the groups were well matched for pain chronicity, prior surgery, and depressive symptoms. Plasma antidepressant concentrations did not correlate with change in depressive symptoms or pain intensity in the subgroup of patients with higher depression scores.

In another controlled study of back pain patients with documented depressive symptoms, Hameroff et al. (6) reported that doxepin (2.5 mg/kg daily) was clearly superior to placebo for improving mood and sleep and reducing muscle tension and the percentage of time patients reported being in pain. Pain intensity, level of activity, and analgesic consumption did not respond to the antidepressant.

In a crossover study of amitriptyline, Pilowsky et al. (7) used a pain clinic sample comprised mostly of CLBP patients without significant organic pathology. They reported the treated group had significantly less pain than the placebo group at weeks 2 and 4, but that pain ratings became equivalent to those in placebo treatment after 6 weeks of drug therapy. While amitriptyline generally did not improve daily functioning or symptoms of anxiety and depression, the authors concluded that patients showing clear-cut major depression were quite responsive.

Finally, Pheasant et al. (8) reported a controlled, crossover trial of amitriptyline (50–150 mg daily) in CLBP patients with depressive symptoms. Analgesic consumption significantly decreased (by 46%) during treatment with amitriptyline, but mood and activity level were unaltered. A related finding from another controlled trial (9) was that chlorimipramine (Anafranil) (150 mg), an analogue of imipramine, signficantly decreased verbal pain estimates in low back pain patients and increased tolerance to experimentally induced pain after 2 weeks of therapy. The same study showed, however, that the efficacy of amitriptyline (150 mg) did not differ from placebo. Studies using lower dosages of imipramine (75 mg) reported no significant differences between treatment and control groups in objective or self-reported mood, pain, or stiffness in patients with and without documented depressive symptoms (10). One major problem in evaluating these studies is that questionnaires were used to rate depressive symptoms, but patients were not examined clinically for psychiatric diagnosis. It is possible that some of those patients had an undiagnosed major depression. A second problem is that follow-up is

generally limited to 2–6 weeks, whereas the effect of these agents often may not appear within 6 weeks.

In summary, it would appear that TCAs are especially effective in CLBP with associated major depression, and that dosages customarily used in treatment of major affective disorders (2.5–3.0 mg/kg) are indicated. In patients not having major depression, symptoms such as insomnia or subjective muscle tension may be improved, but an increase in functional activity and a reduction in analgesic consumption may not occur. Imipramine and desipramine may reduce pain intensity in CLBP uncomplicated by depression, but this is not thoroughly documented. The data, then, do not support chronic use of these agents in the absence of major affective disorder.

Arthritic Disorders with Associated Back Pain

Intriguing new evidence indicates that TCAs may have anti-inflammatory effects in chronic adjuvant-induced arthritis in rats. These effects reduce the physical signs of arthritis itself, increase mobility, and reduce pain-associated behaviors (11).

Three placebo-controlled trials of imipramine have evaluated its use as an adjunct in samples of patients with arthritic disorders (rheumatoid arthritis, osteoarthritis, ankylosing spondylitis) that are often associated with complaints of back pain. In each study imipramine (75 mg) was added to a nonsteroidal anti-inflammatory drug (NSAID) regimen. One study (12) noted no significant drug effect, whereas another (13) showed significant improvement in pain, stiffness, and activity. In the third study (14) patients "preferred" the antidepressant to placebo, but specific dependent variables (mood, pain, grip strength, and physical function) were not assessed. Thus, imipramine may have therapeutic effects, but more rigorous controlled studies are needed to establish its role in these arthritic disorders.

Other Chronic Pain Syndromes

These are heterogeneous groups of patients who have chronic back pain as only one of several sites of pain. One example is primary fibromyalgia syndrome. This condition is characterized by generalized musculoskeletal aching, multiple tender points, fatigue, morning stiffness, and disturbed sleep (15). Mechanical stress in the neck and low back, psychiatric illness, a primary disorder of sleep, and other disturbances are proposed as etiologies (16). While the clinical validity of this syndrome is under scrutiny (17), some investigators consider it the undiagnosed etiology of pain in many patients with

CLBP (18). Controlled studies examining the efficacy of tricyclic agents in treating fibrositis provide mixed results, reminiscent of those described above for CLBP patients without major depression. Carette et al. (19) noted that patients treated with amitriptyline (50 mg daily) reported significantly better sleep at 9 weeks' follow-up, but compared to placebo did not differ in pain, morning stiffness, or physician's rating of overall functioning. Dinerman et al. (20) observed that amitriptyline (25 mg daily) added to a nonsteroidal analgesic was associated with improved observer ratings of global functioning and reduced pain intensity. Caruso et al. (21) reported that dothiepin (75 mg daily), an analogue of doxepin, significantly reduced pain severity and number of tender points at 8 weeks. Again, patients were not examined for major depression.

Too few trials have been conducted in these patients to provide definitive assessment of the role of TCAs. As yet there appears to be little evidence indicating that these agents should be employed in fibromyalgia, unless the patient has a coexisting major depression.

Neurologic Disorders

Arachnoiditis, thought to be due to surgical injury or to an inflammatory response to radiopaque material used during myelography, may be responsible for persistent pain in a small proportion of patients with CLBP. Such neuropathic or deafferentation pain etiologically is thought to arise from spontaneous neuronal hyperactivity or disturbed inhibition following injury to the central nervous system or to peripheral nerves. Neuropathic syndromes reported to respond to TCAs include postherpetic neuralgia (22), diabetic peripheral neuropathy (23–25), persistent postoperative scar pain (26), trigeminal neuralgia (27), thalamic pain (28), and neuralgias from lesions of plexus or peripheral nerves (e.g., postamputation stump pain) (29).

Treatment is effective in depressed or nondepressed patients, and improvement appears to be independent of a primary antidepressant effect. Therapeutic serum tricyclic levels are reported to be below those usually associated with antidepressant activity (24); dosage regimens generally are less than one-half those used in major depression, and relief of pain generally occurs within 1–2 weeks (23, 24). Some authors reported that higher dosages produced increased pain in some patients, suggesting that there was a "therapeutic window" for dosage. In patients with some syndromes (e.g., postherpetic neuralgia) there was a later decay of drug efficacy, casting doubts on the long-term ben-

efits of treatment (24). Nevertheless, some patients discontinued therapy but maintained their improvement beyond 12 months.

We are not aware of controlled drug trials involving patients selected for arachnoiditis and CLBP. Yet to the extent that this disorder resembles neuropathic or deafferentation syndromes known to respond to tricyclic agents, then it may represent another indication for these antidepressants.

Tricyclics as Adjuncts to Analgesics

Amitriptyline (30), nortriptyline (Aventyl, Pamelor) (30), chlorimipramine (31), desipramine (32), and doxepin (33) are all reported to potentiate opiate analgesia acutely in animal models, but not necessarily after chronic administration (34). In human acute clinical pain, chronic administration of desipramine (25–75 mg), but not amitriptyline, potentiates and prolongs morphine analgesia, resulting in 10–20% lower verbal estimates of pain intensity (35).

In chronic back pain France et al. (36, 37) reported that the combination of either doxepin or amitriptyline (25–75 mg daily) with a narcotic analgesic reduced pain intensity more than either an antidepressant or a narcotic agent alone. Narcotic dose escalation and narcotic abuse did not occur, and no patient required more than the equivalent of methadone (Dolophin) 20 mg daily. Since these patients also were enrolled in a comprehensive pain management program, the authors speculate that both the program itself and the tricyclics may have contributed to the low maintenance dosages of narcotic.

The combination of TCAs with conventional analgesics may be a promising approach, but it remains unproven. Controlled trials assessing the efficacy of combination versus single-drug therapy on pain intensity, functional status (e.g., employment, exercise tolerance), and emotional state are needed to clarify the adjunctive use of TCAs.

Mechanisms of Action

Tricyclic antidepressants have several postulated actions, including (a) antidepressant effects, (b) "anticonvulsant" properties, (c) anti-inflammatory–like properties, (d) serotonergic and noradrenergic activity with augmentation of endogenous pain-inhibitory mechanisms, and (e) central skeletal muscle relaxation. It is possible to speculate that the major therapeutic action depends upon the etiology or etiologies of the back pain syndrome. An antidepressant effect would be paramount in pain patients with coexisting major depressive illness. Improved mood is generally followed by increased activity and by more available psychological resources to cope with pain. In arachnoiditis, stabilizing aberrantly conducting neurons or inhibiting their afferent transmission at the level of the spinal cord may be therapeutic. An anticonvulsant mechanism (38, 39) is possible, given the evidence of epileptiform activity in deafferentated neurons, the structural similarity of tricyclics to traditional anticonvulsants like carbamazepine, and their ability to suppress firing in polysynaptic neurons (27, 38, 39). Peripheral anti-inflammatory–like properties may be prominent in other pathologic states. Here, possible sites of action include (a) altering the transport or activity of substances involved in inflammation, such as serotonin; (b) inhibiting prostaglandin synthetase, an enzyme crucial to inflammation and to activation of primary afferent nociceptors; and (c) modifying of protein binding capacity, another property tricyclic agents share with conventional anti-inflammatory drugs (11). Finally, amitriptyline has a chemical structure almost identical to cyclobenzaprine (Flexeril), a centrally acting skeletal muscle relaxant. The centrally acting skeletal muscle relaxants are sedatives and preferentially depress polysynaptic reflexes, without directly relaxing skeletal muscle or depressing neuronal conduction or muscle excitability. Amitriptyline potentially could act by sedative or neuronal mechanisms to provide symptomatic relief in selected low back disorders. Of course, an augmentation of serotonergic or other endogenous pain-inhibitory neurotransmitter systems may be a fundamental therapeutic effect common to many of these sites of action.

Monamine Oxidase Inhibitors and Lithium Carbonate

Monoamine oxidase (MAO) is a term for intra-mitochondrial enzymes widely distributed throughout the body. Intraneuronal MAO deactivates biologically active amines potentially important in pain perception, including norepinephrine, 5-hydroxytryptamine (serotonin), and dopamine. Monoamine oxidase inhibitors (MAOIs) increase intraneuronal pools of these neurotransmitters by inhibiting their degradation. Phenelzine (Nardil) and tranylcypromine (Parnate) are the most commonly prescribed MAOIs.

Monoamine oxidase inhibitors do not appear to have analgesic properties in acute pain. While MAOIs show promise for treatment of migraine headache (40), atypical facial pain (41), and major depression

with secondary pain, no known trials evaluate their efficacy in patients with primary CLBP.

Raft et al. (42) reported a significant antidepressant effect of phenelzine (1.5 mg/kg) in a controlled study of psychiatric patients with definite primary depression in whom pain was symptomatic of depression and did not precede it. The effect of phenelzine on pain was not reported, but the patients' daily functioning improved. Interestingly, the authors observed that pain clinic populations may contain a high proportion of patients with "atypical" depression. Such patients exhibit "reverse" vegetative symptoms of depression (e.g., increased sleep and appetite) and may be specifically responsive to MAOIs. The available data suggest that MAOIs would benefit CLBP patients with major depression, although TCAs would remain the drugs of first choice. There is no evidence recommending the use of MAOIs in prolonged back pain unless there coexists a major affective disorder that has not responded to TCAs.

Lithium is widely used in psychiatric disorders and has been employed for numerous medical and neurologic conditions (43). The rationale for its use in pain syndromes derives from its postulated effects on central nervous system (CNS) dopaminergic and serotonergic systems, and its demonstrated efficacy in treating cyclic or recurrent disorders (e.g., bipolar affective disease). Trials employing lithium for chronic pain have been confined to recurrent headache syndromes (e.g., refs. 44–46), and the drug has not been used systematically in the treatment of back pain. In CLBP patients with major depression, the tricyclic agents are again agents of first choice, with the possible exception that patients with a cyclical major depression might be candidates for lithium.

Mechanisms of Action

The therapeutic mechanism of action of MAOIs and lithium in headache syndrome is unknown, but probably is not simply a primary antidepressant effect. Their widespread effects on serotonergic and noradrenergic neurotransmission may interact with endogenous pain-modulating systems.

Summary

In summary, studies involving TCAs, and to some extent the MAOIs, identify promising approaches to the restoration of function in some patients with back pain. Unfortunately, there are as yet no clinical or biologic markers to predict drug responders and nonresponders, beyond our knowledge that patients with definite major depression are likely to benefit. It can be hoped that improved clinical and laboratory methods for demarcating homogeneous syndromes within CLBP and for detecting major depression will permit more specific application of these drugs.

NEUROLEPTIC DRUGS

Neuroleptics include the various classes of phenothiazines, butyrophenones, and other compounds used primarily as antipsychotic drugs or "major tranquilizers." Like opiates they inhibit gross motor activity, and act at higher centers to produce affective indifference and emotional quieting. Neuroleptics are used widely in combination with narcotics to treat postoperative pain and have been employed for chronic pain syndromes. Recently, however, it has been recognized that there is very little evidence that neuroleptics have analgesic effects or that they potentiate opiate analgesia, and a reassessment of their use is in order. Results from clinical trials are summarized in Table 15.2.

Phenothiazines and Related Drugs
Experimentally Induced and Clinical Acute Pain

The extensive work of Dundee et al. (47–50), assessed the effect of 14 different phenothiazines on pain experimentally induced by pressure on the anterior surface of the tibia, using healthy patients admitted for minor surgical procedures. All phenothiazines tested increased sensitivity to pain at 20 min after injection. By 60 min, however, two distinct response patterns emerged. First, some agents demonstrated mild analgesic activity [e.g., chlorpromazine (Thorazine), promazine (Sparine), and propiomazine (Largon)] (47). Next, some agents moderately amplified pain reports [e.g., prochlorpromazine (Compazine), perphenazine (Trilafon), and trifluoperazine (Stelazine)], and one agent [promethazine (Phenergan)] markedly increased pain report over baseline (47). Further observations suggested that the action of certain phenothiazines was biphasic—initially antianalgesic and hours later analgesic (47–50). Only one neuroleptic, methotrimeprazine (Levoprome), has clinically reliable analgesic properties in acute pain (51, 52). The agent is roughly equipotent with morphine on a milligram-for-milligram basis.

The Dundee group (48) also explored the ability of phenothiazines to potentiate a narcotic analgesic, meperidine (Demerol). Promazine slightly but significantly increased the analgesic activity of meperidine at 60–90 min after injection. Other phenothiazine derivatives (propiomazine, trifluoperazine) had no effect on meperidine analgesia. An important finding was that perphenazine and promethazine were strongly antianalgesic and diminished the therapeutic effect of meperidine when given in combination with the narcotic.

Chronic Low Back Pain

Investigations of neuroleptic medications for chronic pain syndromes focus on chronic headaches and neuropathic disorders, rather than upon CLBP. Further, the risk of tardive dyskinesia must be considered before employing antipsychotic agents to treat any chronic pain syndrome. While the daily dosages of antipsychotic medications indicated in chronic pain use are small, the cumulative amounts pose some risk, and lasting dyskinesias may appear even after brief treatment (53). This problem is discussed in detail later (see "Clinical Guidelines").

Neurologic Disorders

Several anecdotal reports suggest that phenothiazine or butyrophenone antipsychotic agents, when used in combination with TCAs, are effective for neuropathic or deafferentation syndromes (e.g., diabetic peripheral neuropathy, postherpetic neuralgia) (54, 55) when treatment with a tricyclic agent alone was ineffective (54, 56). Suggested combinations include amitriptyline 25–75 mg plus fluphenazine (Prolixin) 1–3 mg (54), or imipramine 25–75 mg with haloperidol (Haldol) 1–3 mg (28). The use of an antipsychotic agent alone is less likely to be helpful in these conditions. Arachnoiditis not responsive to a tricyclic agent may be a CLBP syndrome suitable for a trial of combination therapy.

Neuroleptics as Adjuncts to Analgesics

Data regarding the chronic use of neuroleptics to augment conventional narcotic and nonnarcotic analgesics come mainly from cancer populations rather than from CLBP patients. In well-designed trials, neither outpatients with mild to moderate pain treated with aspirin (57), nor hospitalized patients with severe pain treated with morphine (58) have had improved analgesia when a neuroleptic was added. It appears that these drugs have little use as meaningful adjuncts to the analgesic regimen of most CLBP patients.

Mechanisms of Action

The therapeutic mechanism of action of neuroleptic medications for pain syndromes is unclear.

Table 15.2
Antipsychotic Drugs: Populations, Experimental Design, and Treatment Outcome

AUTHORS	POPULATION	N	INTERVENTIONS	DESIGN	CONTROL	DEPENDENT MEASURES	FOLLOW-UP	RESULTS
				ACUTE PAIN				
Dundee & coworkers, 1960, 1961, 1963 (47–50)	Patients awaiting minor surgery, experimentally induced pain sensitivity	20–140	Compared effect of 14 different phenothiazines on sensitivity to experimentally induced pain	Group outcome, open label	No treatment	Self-report of sensitivity to experimentally induced pain	3 hr	All phenothiazines increased sensitivity to pain at 20 min. Methotrimeprazine, chlorpromazine, promazine, and propiomazine slightly analgesic 60 min after injection
Moore & Dundee, 1961 (47)	Patients awaiting minor surgery, experimentally induced pain sensitivity	42–60	Compared ability of 5 phenothiazines to enhance meperidine	Group outcome, open label	No treatment	Self-report of sensitivity to experimentally induced pain	3 hr	Promethazine and perphenazine antagonized meperidine analgesia. Promazine slightly enhanced meperidine. Propiomazine and trifluoperazine ineffective
Lasagna & DeKornfeld, 1961 (51)	Postoperative, postpartum pain	37–66	Compared methotrimeprazine with morphine; methotrimeprazine with placebo	Double blind, case control	Placebo, reference analgesic (morphine)	Self-report of pain improvement	Hours	Methotrimeprazine 15 mg equivalent to morphine 10 mg
Minuck, 1972 (52)	Postoperative pain	197	Compared methotrimeprazine, meperidine, and placebo	Double blind, group outcome	Placebo medication	Observer rating of analgesia as excellent, good, fair, poor	Hours	Methotrimeprazine 5–10 mg equal to meperidine 25–50 mg; both superior to placebo for analgesia

ADJUNCT TO NARCOTICS

Houde & Wallenstein, 1955 (58)	Severe cancer pain	34	Compared chlorpromazine, morphine, and their combination	Case control, double blind	Placebo medication, reference analgesic (morphine)	Self-report of pain intensity	Hours	Chlorpromazine had no analgesic effect and did not potentiate morphine analgesia
Moertl & coworkers, 1974 (57)	Cancer pain	100	Compared promazine 50 mg, aspirin, and other non-narcotic oral analgesics	Case control, double blind	Placebo medication	Self-rated % pain relief for 6 hr after each drug	6 hr	Promazine 50 mg orally had no analgesic activity and did not potentiate aspirin

Table 15.3
Antianxiety Agents: Populations, Experimental Design, and Treatment Outcome

AUTHORS	POPULATION	N	INTERVENTIONS	DESIGN	CONTROL	DEPENDENT MEASURES	FOLLOW-UP	RESULTS
				ACUTE PAIN				
Chapman & Feather, 1973 (62)	Experimentally induced pain in nonpatients	30	Diazepam compared to aspirin & placebo	Double blind, group outcome	Placebo and reference analgesic	Self-report of pain (0–4 scale), pain tolerance	Hours	Diazepam 10 mg orally prolongs tolerance to pain, diminishes pain-associated anxiety; does not alter sensory sensitivity
Gracely & coworkers, 1978 (63)	Experimentally induced pain in dental patients	16	Compared pain intensity and quality before and after diazepam	Group outcome, within subject	Within subject, no treatment	Verbal descriptions of affective and sensory quality of pain, match handgrip force to pain intensity	Hours	Diazepam reduced affective response to pain without altering sensory perception
Beaver & Feise, 1976 (66)	Postoperative patients	96	Single dose of hydroxyzine alone and in combination with morphine	Double blind, group outcome	Placebo medication	Self-report and observer ratings of pain	Hours	Hydroxyzine 100 mg intramuscularly was superior to placebo and equivalent to morphine 8 mg; hydroxyzine analgesia additive to morphine analgesia
Hupert & coworkers, 1980 (67)	Postoperative patients	82	Compared hydroxyzine 100 mg in combination with morphine to morphine alone	Double blind, group control	Morphine	Self-report of pain intensity (0–3) and pain relief (0–4)	Hours	Hydroxyzine 100 mg intramuscularly with morphine gave significantly greater analgesia than morphine alone; combination did not increase percentage of patients reporting > 50% pain reduction; increased drowsiness with hydroxyzine confounded analgesia

Kantor & Steinberg, 1976 (64)	Postoperative patients	135	Compared oral hydroxyzine 100 mg with meperidine, and placebo	Double blind, group outcome	Placebo medication	Self-report of pain intensity	Hours	Hydroxyzine 100 mg orally equivalent to placebo
				CHRONIC PAIN				
Yosselson-Superstine & coworkers, 1985 (69)	Mixed chronic cancer and noncancer patients	9	Compared chlordiazepoxide, hydroxyzine, prochlorperazine	Double blind, group outcome	Placebo	Self-report of pain (0–5), Multiple Adjective Affect Checklist (MAACL)	8 wk	No overall differences between study drugs and placebo on any dependent measure; individual comparisons reveal anxiety and depression lower with chlordiazepoxide vs. placebo

Antidopaminergic activity may explain the analgesic effects of methotrimeprazine in acute pain, although other neuroleptic agents with similar ability to block dopamine neurotransmission are not analgesics. The membrane-stabilizing properties of antipsychotic drugs may account for their therapeutic effects in some neuropathic or deafferentation syndromes (38, 39). Alternatively, the neuroleptic may simply increase serum concentrations of the tricyclic to a therapeutic range.

ANTIANXIETY AND SEDATIVE AGENTS

Three classes of antianxiety drugs are used in pain syndromes. The most frequently used are the benzodiazepines [chlordiazepoxide (Librium), diazepam (Valium), clonazepam (Clonopin), and others]; less often employed are the diphenylmethane derivatives [hydroxyzine (Vistaril)], and the barbiturates (phenobarbital, secobarbital, and others). Indeed, the benzodiazepines have generally replaced the barbiturates in routine clinical care. The rationale for antianxiety agents is to treat anxiety secondary to pain, or to alleviate low back skeletal muscle spasm and contraction associated with pain, emotional arousal, or anxiety. The benzodiazepines also show promise in the treatment of neuralgias, perhaps by reducing neuron firing rates. An overview of outcome studies is given in Table 15.3.

Benzodiazepines and Hydroxyzine
Experimentally Induced and Clinical Acute Pain

Diazepam has neither primary antinociceptive effects nor the ability to potentiate the antinociceptive activity of narcotic analgesics in animal models (59, 60). Nevertheless, diazepam decreases the affective emotional response to pain and potentiates this property of opiates in animal paradigms (61) and in experimentally induced pain in humans (62, 63). Chapman and Feather (62) noted that diazepam (10 mg orally) prolonged tolerance to experimentally induced pain significantly more than did placebo and aspirin, and diminished pain-associated anxiety better than did placebo. Gracely et al. (63) confirmed that diazepam reduced the affective response to experimentally induced pain without altering sensory sensitivity. The use of benzodiazepines as adjuvants for reducing the affective response to acute clinical (e.g., postoperative) pain, however, has not been widely investigated. Clinical experience indicates that benzodiazepines are often useful in anxious postoperative patients, and that reduction of anxiety helps diminish pain complaints.

Hydroxyzine is a diphenylmethane derivative having antihistaminic, antiemetic, spasmolytic, and anxiolytic activity. Hydroxyzine, like the benzodiazepines, has minimal analgesic activity and an inconsistent ability to enhance opiate analgesia in animal models of pain, but it potentiates opiate reduction of the affective component of pain (61).

Results of studies in clinical pain indicate that hydroxyzine has a limited role in postoperative care of patients with CLBP. Hydroxyzine 100 mg orally has not been shown to be superior to placebo in relieving postoperative pain, and does not potentiate oral meperidine (64) or alter meperidine pharmacokinetics or metabolism (65). Hydroxyzine 100 mg parenterally is reported to be superior to placebo and equivalent to very low-dose morphine (8 mg) in patients suffering severe pain (66). Two studies indicate hydroxyzine 100 mg intramuscularly combined with morphine produced greater pain relief than morphine alone (66, 67). Nevertheless, in these studies the addition of hydroxyzine to morphine did not increase the percentage of patients who reported better than 50% reduction in pain. The combination did produce, however, significantly greater drowsiness, which may have confounded pain reports.

Thus, hydroxyzine (75–100 mg parenterally) may have an analgesic effect equivalent to 8–10 mg of morphine. Hydroxyzine administration causes sedation and marked discomfort at the injection sites, and subcutaneous administration can produce sever tissue damage. Because of these liabilities and the limited data for therapeutic efficacy, the routine use of hydroxyzine to potentiate opiate analgesia in postoperative care cannot by recommended.

Musculoskeletal Chronic Low Back Pain

Musculoskeletal CLBP is an unsatisfactory diagnostic term, but is often employed to describe pain thought to derive from chronic skeletal muscle contraction, resulting from injury or chronic anxiety. Given the extensive use of benzodiazepines in the care of patients with chronic back pain it is surprising that there are so few rigorous studies of their efficacy, indications, and interactions with other treatments. While there is some evidence that benzodiazepines are useful in short-term management of tension headaches, their role in CLBP remains largely unexplored. Hollister et al. (68) suggested that diazepam produces extended relief in chronic pain from musculoskeletal disorders and is rarely associated with abuse. Others (69, 70) argue that conventional measures like heat, rest, and nonnarcotic analgesics are as effective as diazepam, and that even high doses of this drug do not produce clinically detectable skeletal muscle relaxation (69). Furthermore, Hendler et al. (71) reported evidence of significantly more cognitive impairment in chronic pain patients receiving diazepam than in those receiving nonnarcotic or narcotic analgesics. The clinical impact and reversibility of benzodiazepine-associated deficits in cognitive functioning, memory, and motor-perceptual performance deserves much further investigation. This is especially important since many chronic pain management programs emphasize behavioral approaches that require intact cognitive skills.

As discussed more fully below in the section on treatment approaches, benzodiazepines appear to be vastly overused in CLBP, and there are only a few instances in which chronic anxiety and "tension" should be treated with these drugs.

Neuralgia

A substantial number of uncontrolled trials support the effectiveness of clonazepam for treatment of chronic neuropathic pain, particularly cranial neuralgias (72–74). Responsive syndromes include trigeminal neuralgia, sphenopalatine ganglion neuralgia, and diverse neuropathies (75). These preliminary reports might encourage their use in CLBP patients with arachnoiditis. Nevertheless, limitations of these data include open-study designs, the difficulty in assessing the magnitude of functional improvement, and the limited follow-up (76).

The relative efficacy of benzodiazepines compared to other drugs for treatment of neuropathic pain syndromes is an important therapeutic issue. For example, one controlled report indicated that both imipramine and amitriptyline 100 mg outperformed diazepam 15 mg in relieving painful diabetic peripheral neuropathy (23). Additional studies are needed to fully assess the role of benzodiazepines in treating arachnoiditis and other neuropathic pain states.

Mechanism of Action

Benzodiazepines increase the ability of γ-aminobutyric acid (GABA) to inhibit brain and spinal cord neurotransmission; they also inhibit cholinergic and monoaminergic pathways (77). The anxiolytic effects may be mediated by GABAergic inhibitory effects on the limbic system. Since GABA is thought to mediate presynaptic and postsynaptic inhibition and facilitate recurrent inhibition (78), benzodiazepines might decrease the central transmission of ascending noxious stimuli, or inhibit firing peripherally in aberrant neurons. This may explain their putative efficacy in neuropathic syndromes.

CNS STIMULANTS

The most common stimulants now in medical use are the amphetamines [*d,*1-amphetamine (Benzedrine), *d*-amphetamine (Dexedrine), and methamphetamine (Methedrine)]; the related compound methylphenidate (Ritalin); cocaine; and caffeine. The amphetamines and methylphenidate are used primarily for attention-deficit disorders and hyperactivity associated with minimal brain dysfunction in children, and in narcolepsy. Cocaine has traditional use as a local anesthetic, and caffeine appears in numerous combinations with analgesics. Evidence with regard to efficacy is given in Table 15.4.

Amphetamines, Cocaine, and Caffeine
Experimentally Induced and Clinical Acute Pain

Psychostimulants lack primary analgesic properties (79). Amphetamines potentiate narcotic and nonnarcotic analgesia in animals (80, 81) and in man (82–84), presumably by catecholaminergic mechanisms (80). Several laboratories (82, 83) have demonstrated that dextroamphetamine enhances the analgesic effect of morphine in experimentally induced pain in man. With regard to clinical pain, a single-dose study of postoperative patients concluded that the combination of dextroamphetamine 10 mg parenterally and morphine 10 mg was twice as potent as morphine alone, and a combination with dextroamphetamine 5 mg was 1.5 times as potent as a given dosage of morphine (84). There were minimal effects on blood pressure, pulse, and respiratory rate. Because of the study design, the effects of longer term use of amphetamine on mood, appetite, sensorium, and other aspects of postoperative convalescence could not be addressed.

Caffeine may be a useful addition to nonsteroidal anti-inflammatory analgesics. A review of the results of single-dose trials in over 10,000 patients suffering from episiotomy pain indicated that caffeine (100–200 mg orally) increased the analgesic potency of aspirin and acetaminophen by 40% (85). Oral dosages up to 600 mg/day of caffeine cause few side effects. Although caffeine may have some usefulness as an adjunct to analgesics used in the acute rehabilitation of CLBP patients who have undergone surgery, it is rarely used in practice.

Chronic Pain

The two possible uses of potent stimulants in chronic back pain are as an adjunct of analgesia, and as treatment for depression. While very few

Table 15.4
Psychostimulants: Populations, Experimental Design, and Treatment Outcome

AUTHORS	POPULATION	N	INTERVENTIONS	DESIGN	CONTROL	DEPENDENT MEASURES	FOLLOW-UP	RESULTS
				ACUTE PAIN				
Ivy & coworkers, 1944 (82)	Experimentally induced pain in nonpatients	30	Dextroamphetamine added to morphine	Double blind, group outcome	Morphine	Self-report of pain intensity	Hours	Dextroamphetamine improved morphine analgesia
Evans, 1962 (83)	Experimentally induced pain in nonpatients	24	Dextroamphetamine 10 mg added to morphine	Double blind	Morphine	Self-report of pain intensity	Hours	Dextroamphetamine improved morphine analgesia
Forest & coworkers, 1977 (84)	Postoperative patients	450	Single dose of dextroamphetamine 5–10 mg added to morphine	Double blind, group outcome	Morphine	Observer and self-rated pain intensity	Hours	Dextroamphetamine 10 mg doubled analgesic activity of morphine 10 mg
Laska & coworkers, 1984 (85)	Postpartum pain	>10,000	Caffeine added to aspirin, acetaminophen, or salicylamide	Double blind, group outcome	Aspirin, acetaminophen, salicylamide	Self-rated pain (0–3 scale)	Hours	Caffeine 100–200 mg orally increased relative potency of analgesic by 40%
Kaufman & coworkers, 1982 (89)	Hospitalized medically ill patients with major depression secondary to illness, with and without pain	5	Dextroamphetamine or methylphenidate given daily	Open label, case studies	None	Unspecified assessment of mood, activity, pain	4 wk	Dextroamphetamine 2–20 mg/daily and methylphenidate 10–20 mg/daily improved mood, increased activity, and reduced pain report
Woods & coworkers, 1986 (90)	Hospitalized medically ill patients with major depression secondary to illness, with and without pain	66	Dextroamphetamine or methylphenidate given daily	Retrospective chart review	None	Clinical response of depression	1–87 d	Dextroamphetamine 2–20 mg/daily and methylphenidate improved mood, increased activity, and reduced pain report

CHRONIC PAIN

Reference	N	Intervention	Design	Control	Outcome measures	Duration	Results
Bruera & coworkers, 1987 (86)	32	Outpatients and inpatients with advanced cancer and chronic cancer pain	Methylphenidate added to narcotic analgesics	Randomized, double blind, crossover	Placebo medication	Self-rated pain intensity; narcotic intake, self-estimate of anxiety, depression, activity	3 d	Methylphenidate 15 mg daily significantly improved analgesia and activity, decreased extra doses of narcotic, decreased sedation

patients with CLBP require long-term management with narcotic analgesics, there is preliminary evidence that psychostimulants potentiate opioids in chronic pain.

A recent placebo-controlled study in cancer patients with persistent pain demonstrated that methylphenidate 15 mg daily added to a regimen of narcotic analgesia decreased pain intensity by an additional 20% (86). This study evaluated patients only during a 3-day trial. A recommendation for use of stimulants as adjuvants in treatment of chronic pain of nonneoplastic origin must await more rigorous studies assessing longer term side effects and benefits. Given the hazards of psychostimulants, the more rational approach would be to increase maintenance doses of the narcotic rather than adding an additional drug.

There is some evidence that psychostimulants are effective antidepressants in depressed medically ill subjects (87). Recent anecdotal reports (88–90) suggest that dextroamphetamine (2–20 mg/day) and methylphenidate (up to 20 mg/day) may be effective antidepressants in hospitalized medically ill patients both with depressive symptoms as well as with major depression related to medical illness. Improved mood, reduced focus on pain, and renewed interest in rehabilitation occurred in about 50% of patients within 2–7 days. The major side effect was confusion, which developed in demented patients. Most patients were successfully treated in about 1 week, although some required several months of treatment. Whether these agents might be used in the rehabilitation of hospitalized and demoralized CLBP patients is speculative and controversial. In any event, use of psychostimulants should only be undertaken in consultation with a psychiatrist experienced in their use.

Mechanism of Action

The mechanism of action of psychostimulants is unclear. The therapeutic effects probably result from activation of monoamine systems important in pain suppression. Amphetamines exert their effects directly by stimulating adrenergic receptors, and indirectly by releasing catecholamines and inhibiting their degradation by the enzyme monoamine oxidase. Caffeine has direct and indirect effects similar in kind to those of the amphetamines, but obviously less potent.

SUMMARY

This review has been conservative, and may well underestimate therapeutic effects of psychotropic agents in CLBP syndromes. Indeed, several experimental factors may mask actual therapeutic action of these drugs. First, given the limits of present diagnostic methods, drug-responsive and nonresponsive subtypes of CLBP disorders may be lumped in a single group in clinical trials. When overall group outcome is determined, benefits for responsive subtypes could be overpowered. Second, problems such as extreme variability of outcome scores, small sample size, or pretreatment between-group differences plague many studies and may obscure significant effects. In addition, some psychotropic drugs may produce a therapeutic effect only after 6 weeks or more of treatment. Patients not followed longitudinally appear to be treatment failures. Also, these agents may affect a variable that is not being assessed (e.g., activity level) while not altering a measured variable (e.g., mood or pain intensity).

Given the available evidence, the TCAs have the most clearly documented efficacy in the rehabilitation of patients with CLBP. Their primary indication is in patients with concurrent major affective disorder and CLBP, although they may be helpful in pain associated with arachnoiditis. Other classes of antidepressants (MAOIs and lithium) may be employed if the affective illness is unresponsive to TCAs.

By contrast the antipsychotic agents should be considered only as adjunctive to TCAs in the management of patients with neuropathic pain. The benzodiazepines are overprescribed in CLBP, and little documentation exists for their efficacy in treatment of chronic skeletal muscle contraction or chronic anxiety. Clonazepam may have use in neuropathic pain. The potent psychostimulants—the amphetamines and methylphenidate—have no established role as primary or adjunctive agents in rehabilitation of patients with CLBP. Their short-term role in activating depressed or demoralized patients toward fruitful participation in rehabilitation awaits controlled investigation.

In the next section we emphasize psychopharmacologic treatments that have solid support in controlled studies, but also describes less proven alternatives worth considering.

CLINICAL GUIDELINES FOR USE OF PSYCHOTROPIC AGENTS IN CLBP

TRICYCLIC ANTIDEPRESSANT AGENTS

The indications for tricyclic antidepressants are described in Table 15.5, and the compounds and dosages in Table 15.6.

Table 15.5
Diagnostic Indications for Psychotropic Drug Treatment in Chronic Low Back Pain

TREATMENT	DIAGNOSIS AND CLINICAL EFFICACY	
	RELATIVELY WELL-ESTABLISHED CLINICAL EFFICACY[a]	POSSIBLE CLINICAL EFFICACY[b]
Tricyclic antidepressants	*Chronic Pain* Primary major depression with secondary pain Major depression secondary to chronic pain	Neuropathic pain (arachnoiditis) Augment narcotics
MAO inhibitors	Primary major depression with secondary pain Major depression secondary to chronic pain	
Lithium carbonate	Primary major depression with secondary pain	
Neuroleptics		Neuropathic pain (arachnoiditis)
Antianxiety agents		Chronic anxiety, neuropathic syndromes
Stimulants		Depression-pain syndromes

[a]Effectiveness established in controlled trials.
[b]Effectiveness reported in open-label studies.

Table 15.6
Commonly Used Antidepressants

TRICYCLIC	USUAL DAILY ORAL DOSE IN NEUROPATHIC PAIN (MG)[a]	USUAL DAILY ANTIDEPRESSANT DOSE (MG)
Tertiary amines		
Imipramine (Tofranil)	10–75	150–250
Amitriptyline (Elavil)	10–75	150–250
Doxepin (Sinequan)	10–75	150–250
Secondary amines		
Desipramine (Norpramin)	10–75	100–250
Nortriptyline (Aventyl)	10–75	100–150
Maprotiline (Ludiomil)	b	150–200
Atypical		
Trazodone (Desyrel)	b	
Monoamine oxidase inhibitors		
Tranylcypromine (Parnate)	10–30	10–30
Phenelzine (Nardil)	15–90	45–90
Lithium carbonate	300–1200	900–2400

[a]Usual neuropathic syndrome in low back pain is arachnoiditis.
[b]Experience insufficient to determine usage. Probably below usual antidepressant dose.

Properties and Side Effects

Tricyclic antidepressants were derived from neuroleptics: imipramine, the first TCA introduced, represents a modification of chlorpromazine, and amitriptyline was derived from imipramine. More recently available drugs such as maprotiline (Ludiomil) and amoxapine (Ascendin) are variations on the basic tricyclic structure and are pharmacologically and clinically similar to imipramine (91). Tricyclic antidepressants increase serotonergic and/or noradrenergic tone by blockade of serotonin and norepinephrine reuptake at presynaptic nerve endings, may increase norepinephrine or serotonin receptor density or sensitivity, and may reduce β-adrenergic receptor sensitivity (92). The tricyclics also have strong anticholinergic properties, producing autonomic, cardiac, and CNS side effects. Autonomic effects include dry mouth, blurred vision, constipation, ileus, and urinary retention. Cardiovascular effects include orthostatic hypotension, increased heart rate, and repolarization abnormalities on the electrocardiogram (Q-T interval prolongation and T wave inversion or flattening). Atrial and ventricular arrhythmias, as well as conduction delay with bundle-branch block, may occur. This results from prolongation of the H-V interval, the time from activation of the bundle of His to activation of ventricular myocardium. These effects resemble the properties of type I cardiac antiarrhythmics, such as quinidine and procainamide (93). The tricyclics also can depress myocardial contractility. Central nervous system effects can include agitated states (not uncommon in elderly patients, perhaps because there is less protein plasma binding of the drug in the elderly and higher plasma concentrations), and deliria caused by an anticholinergic brain syndrome. Other common side effects are weight gain, delayed ejaculation, and impotence. Extrapyramidal symptoms are rare.

Selected Drug Interactions

Sympathomimetic Amines

Tricyclics potentiate the pressor response of direct-acting amines such as norepinephrine, epinephrine, and phenylephrine (94), with possible hypertensive crisis characterized by hypothermia, sweating, severe headache, and cerebrovascular accident.

Neuroleptics

Since tricyclics and neuroleptics compete for the same hepatic metabolic pathways their anticholinergic and hypotensive properties may be additive or potentiated (95).

Sedative-Hypnotics

Tricyclics increase the CNS and respiratory depressant activity of barbituates and related sedatives (95, 96) and increase the toxicity and potential lethality of these agents.

Propranolol

Tricyclic antidepressants may potentiate propranolol-induced depression of myocardial contractility and hypotension from central vasomotor regulatory centers (97), and patients with migraine headaches treated with these combinations should be monitored closely.

Opiates

Tricyclics potentiate meperidine-induced respiratory depression in animals (96), and increase anticholinergic activity of opiates.

Pretreatment Evaluation

Patients over the age of 50 or who have a history of cardiovascular disease (stroke, myocardial infarction, angina, congestive heart failure, syncope, or arrhythmias) should have an electrocardiogram (ECG) and measurement of standing and supine blood pressures before treatment. Careful assessment of the risk-benefit ratio and cardiology consultation are indicated in the presence of bradyarrhythmias, heart block, or very long Q-T intervals. Orthostatic blood pressure changes of over 10 mm Hg before drug treatment may be associated with pronounced postural changes during treatment, and these patients should be carefully observed (98). A careful drug history should be obtained, not only to assess possible drug interactions, but to determine past response and reactions to TCAs. Additional laboratory investigation should include a complete blood count with differential and liver function tests.

Drug Selection

Amitriptyline, nortriptyline, imipramine, and desipramine all have approximately equivalent antidepressant efficacy. Additionally, these agents are probably equally effective in the back pain syndromes for which they are indicated. Drug selection therefore depends on side effects. In general, anticholinergic, cardiac, and CNS side effects are more common with tertiary amines (amitriptyline, imipramine, and doxepin) than with demethylated secondary amines (nortriptyline, desipramine, and others). Thus, desipramine is the least anticholinergic and sedating of the tricyclic drugs. Patients with agitation or insomnia may benefit more from sedating drugs. There is some evidence that nortriptyline is less likely to depress H-V conduction and less likely to produce orthostatic hypotension (at the serum concentrations usually employed to treat depression) than other tricyclics (98). Nortriptyline may thus be preferred in patients with bradyarrhythmias, heart block, or prolonged Q-T interval. Doxepin is also thought to be relatively noncardiotoxic, but that is now well documented. All tricyclics will increase heart rate secondary to adrenergic and anticholinergic effects. Furthermore, imipramine suppresses ventricular arrhythmias (ectopy) and patients on quinidine may need their dosage of that agent revised.

Some second-generation antidepressants [e.g., trazodone (Desyrel)] are structurally unrelated to exert their action through mechanisms different from tricyclic drugs. The efficacy of these agents for neuropathic syndromes has not been adequately assessed, but their antidepressant efficacy approached that of the first-generation agents (amitriptyline and imipramine). Most patients with responsive neuropathic syndromes or depression should be treated initially with a first-generation drug. Claims of an improved safety record for second-generation antidepressants await documentation. Indeed, two antidepressants with novel structures, nomifensine (Merital) and buproprion (Wellbutrin), have been withdrawn recently because of serious side effects. Newly available agents with more specific and potent serotonergic effects [e.g., fluoxetine (Prozac)] may hold additional promise for management of chronic pain and associated depression.

Treatment Technique for Chronic Pain
Initial Treatment of the Nondepressed
Pain Patient

In the absence of major depression the primary indication is likely to be that of arachnoiditis with associated pain. Patients without evidence of complicating medical or psychiatric disorders are generally started on nortriptyline or imipramine at 10–25 mg at night, with 10–25-mg increases every 3 days to a maximum of 75 mg daily. The drug is usually given at bedtime to take advantage of any sedating effects, although doses initially may be divided if a single dose produces excessive side effects. Elderly patients or those with cardiovascular disease should receive a 10–25 mg test dose and have orthostatic blood pressure determinations taken 1 hour later.

A therapeutic response usually ensues within 2 weeks, often within 5–7 days. The physician should schedule follow-up appointments at least every week during the initial month of treatment, with orthostatic blood pressure determinations or ECGs as warranted. Every-other-week appointments are useful in the next month of therapy to ensure compliance and monitor progress.

If no benefit appears within 3–4 weeks, or if side effects are unusually severe, a determination of the plasma concentration of the antidepressant is warranted. Plasma concentrations may be used to check compliance, improve efficacy, diminish toxicity, and detect unsuspected drug interactions (99). This allows the clinician to assess whether an alternative therapy is indicated, or if an increase or decrease in dose is necessary. The practitioner should have his/her own history of interpreting results from any particular laboratory.

The most effective plasma concentrations of antidepressants for pain syndromes generally are thought to be below those usually therapeutic for depression. Therapeutic levels for treating depression with amitriptyline are 200 ng/ml total tricyclic (amitriptyline plus nortriptyline); for nortriptyline there may be a therapeutic window of efficacy between 50 and 150 ng/ml. Concentrations below or above this interval may be ineffective for an antidepressant response. With imipramine, concentrations exceeding 225 ng/ml are therapeutic in depression; doxepin therapeutic concentrations are uncertain, but perhaps in the range of 150–250 ng/ml.

Blood samples drawn for plasma concentrations of antidepressants should reflect steady state levels, and a patient's dosage should have been stabilized for at least 1 week. Samples are obtained 10–16 hours after a single dose, or 2–5 hours after the morning dose if a divided-dosage regimen is employed.

Other indications for a plasma concentration measurement include patients with cardiovascular disease, who may warrant routine plasma monitoring because of being at increased risk for toxicity.

Maintenance Treatment

A positive response warrants treatment for about 5–6 months. The maintenance dose should be the minimum effective level after control is established. Attempts to discontinue the tricyclic should be made at least every 6 months. The TCA should be discontinued over a 2–3-week period, to avoid an abstinence syndrome.

Treatment Nonresponse

An inadequate response is defined at less than 50% reduction in pain after a 3–4-week trial, providing there is clinical or laboratory evidence of adequate dosage. Several approaches are then possible. The antidepressant can be changed to a tricyclic affecting a different neurotransmitter system (i.e., if a serotonergic agent was used first, then the switch would be to a noradrenergic drug) for another 3–4-week trial. Alternatively, an adjunctive neuroleptic drug may be added to the initial tricyclic regimen. This technique is described in the section on neuroleptics. The usual neuroleptics chosen are haloperidol 0.5–3 mg daily or fluphenazine 0.5–3 mg daily. Results of adjunctive therapy should be evident within 2 weeks. If combination therapy is unacceptable because of side effects or concerns about tardive dyskinesia, and if alternative tricyclics have not been helpful, a regimen of clonazepam is indicated. The usual regimen is clonazepam 1–3 mg daily. Conventional anticonvulsants [diphenylhydantoin (Dilantin), carbamazepine (Tegretol)] are the drugs of third choice for most practitioners because of unfamiliarity with the drug used and need for closer monitoring of plasma drug concentrations. Other combinations reported to be successful in neuropathic syndromes are nortriptyline with carbamazepine (Tegretol) or diphenylhydantoin (Dilantin) (28).

Initial Treatment of the Depressed Back
Pain Patient

All depressed patients should be evaluated for suicidality and the need for hospitalization, and psychiatric consultation is warranted. If a diagnosis of major depression is made, treatment with a tricyclic agent is indicated. Additionally, there is some evidence that CLBP patients with dysthymic disorder respond to tricyclics (4). These agents are not indicated for patients having a depressed mood, but who do not qualify for a diagnosis of major depression or marked dysthymic disorder. Prescriptions for tricyclics should be monitored closely according to the concern about suicide, and hospitalization may be indicated. Tricyclic antidepressant overdoses amounting to 1000 mg produce serious side effects and those of 2000 mg of any tricyclic commonly are lethal. If major depression is present then full antidepressant dosages should be commenced. We usually begin at a lower initial dosage (e.g., imipramine 25 mg) with increases of 25–50 mg every 3 days to a final dose of 150–300 mg daily. Hospitalized patients may receive higher initial dosage with 50-mg increases daily up to the full amount.

An antidepressant effect is evidenced by improved activity, energy, and mood, and should appear within

3–8 weeks. Patients should be informed that these agents take time to exert their full effect, and not to expect immediate relief. Reduction of pain intensity may lag behind improvement in activity and mood by several weeks, and is not a target symptom. As above, plasma antidepressant concentrations would be indicated for a poor response after 6 weeks or if severe side effects intervene.

Maintenance Treatment of the Depressed
Pain Patient

A maintenance dose of a TCA is usually about 25% lower than the acute antidepressant dosage (91). Treatment is maintained for about 5–6 months (the usual length of an affective episode), and the antidepressant may then be discontinued (100). Again, tapering the tricyclic regimen over several weeks is indicated to avoid an abstinence syndrome. Continuing vigilance is important, however, since over 40% of those hospitalized for major depression may experience chronic fluctuating depressive symptoms on 2-year follow-up (101, 102) and almost 25% may relapse within 3 months after full recovery from the index episode (102).

Treatment Nonresponse in the Depressed
Pain Patient

Further treatment of the depressed pain patient who does not respond to initial therapy is a complex topic beyond the scope of this chapter. Such treatment nonresponse indicates a need for consultation by an experienced psychiatrist to reevaluate the diagnosis and treatment regimen. If the treatment of depression is still required, the choices include adding L-triiodothyronine (Cytomel) 25–50 μg to the TCA; switching to another antidepressant of a different class, with or without adding L-triiodothyronine; considering electroconvulsive therapy; switching to a MAOI; or attempting combination therapy using lithium or a MAOI with a TCA (91).

A Note on the Dexamethasone Suppression Test

The dexamethasone suppression test (DST) was developed as a laboratory aid to assist in the diagnosis of depression, based on finding that approximately 50% of patients with major depression do not suppress plasma cortisol concentrations below 5 μg/dl after receiving dexamethasone 1 mg orally (103). The procedure involves administering dexamethasone 1 mg at 11 P.M. and obtaining blood samples for cortisol concentration at 8 AM, 4 PM, and 11 PM the following day. Any one concentration above 5 μg/dl is regarded as abnormal or positive. The test has a high sensitivity (the percentage of patients with major depression who have a positive test), but it has lower specificity (the percentage of patients without major depression who also have a positive test). Thus, the proportion of patients with dementia who have an abnormal DST is 40%; agoraphobia, 15–30%; alcohol use and abstinence, 20–30%; and acute psychological stress, up to 30%. Medications and medical illness also confound interpretations of test results. False-positive tests may result from barbiturates, anticonvulsants, fever, other acute medical illness, diabetes mellitus, and discontinuation of tricyclic antidepressants. False-negative tests may occur with indomethacin (Indocin) (104). Chronic pain by itself does not appear to affect the DST (105).

About 40–50% of CLBP patients with major depression will have a positive DST, if confounding psychiatric and medical illnesses or medications are excluded (106, 107). The clinical utility of the DST is limited because of these confounding factors. Theoretical but unestablished uses of the test are to confirm a diagnosis of major depression in pain patients in whom other psychiatric or medical causes have been excluded, or to follow the response of depressed patients being treated with antidepressants. As the patient begins to respond clinically to treatment, the DST should revert to normal. A partial clinical response, but failure of the DST to become normal, may indicate a higher risk of relapse. Few clinicians actually employ the DST in this fashion, and clinical judgment should supercede data from neuroendocrine markers for the evaluation and management of depressed patients. The DST does not predict which patients are most likely to respond to treatment.

MONOAMINE OXIDASE INHIBITORS

The indications for MAOIs are described in Table 15.5, and the compounds and doses in Table 15.6.

Properties and Side Effects

Monoamine oxidase inhibitors, like the TCAs, enhance the availability of norepinephrine and serotonin in the brain by inhibiting their catabolism. Antidepressant activity may also be related to effects on norepinephrine and serotonin postsynaptic receptor function or sensitivity.

In psychiatric populations the major indications for MAOIs are (a) agoraphobia with or without panic attacks; (b) the so-called atypical depressive disorders with "reversed" vegetative symptoms (increased sleep, weight gain, reactive mood); and (c) major depression that has not responded to trials of TCAs.

The MAOI side effect profile is similar to that of the TCAs but of a lesser degree, and includes postural hypotension, agitation, confusion, and mild anticholinergic symptoms: blurred vision, dry mouth, constipation, ileus, and urinary retention. The major issue in using these agents is the need to instruct patients to avoid foods or medications containing pressor amines. Because the MAOIs block metabolism of tyramine and other pressor amines, a hypertensive crisis may ensue after their ingestion, manifested by abrupt and severe hypertension and possible subarachnoid hemorrhage. Proscribed foods include cheeses (except cottage cheese and cream cheese), pickled foods, beer and red wines, and fava beans (108).

Selected Drug Interactions
Sympathomimetic Agents

All medication with sympathomimetic activity, including phenylephrine and ephedrine (found in cold tablets), can produce a hypertensive crisis.

Narcotic Analgesics

The so-called type I interaction is a potentiation of primary narcotic effects (including analgesia, hypotension, respiratory depression, and coma) as a result of MAOI inhibition of hepatic metabolism of narcotics (93, 109). Naloxone (Narcan) reverses this response. Phenelzine may be safer in this regard than other MAOIs.

The type II interaction is similar to that resulting from administration of sympathomimetic amines or tyramine to patients on MAOIs. The concurrent use of MAOIs and meperidine (110, 111) or dextromethorphan (112) produces agitation, excitement, restlessness, hypertension, headache, rigidity, and convulsions. The mechanism of this response is unknown, but it may be mediated by increased brain serotonin release (113).

Codeine may be used safely in patients on MAOIs who require moderate analgesia (108). If other narcotics are mandatory only 20–25% of the usual therapeutic narcotic dose should be used and vital signs and level of consciousness should be observed carefully (108). Meperidine should never be used since its interaction with MAOIs is too unpredictable and life-threatening complications can occur rapidly.

Sedative-Hypnotics

Monoamine oxidase inhibition of microsomal enzymes prolongs the effects of sedative-hypnotics, including barbiturates and chloral hydrate (114).

Lower doses of sedative-hypnotics and close monitoring are advised.

Pretreatment Evaluation

The physical and laboratory evaluation is similar to that used for TCAs, with a special emphasis on drug and dietary history, the patient's ability to comply with the complex dietary restrictions, and cardiovascular status.

Drug Selection

Phenelzine and tranylcypromine are the most commonly prescribed agents. Tranylcypromine is sometimes preferred because it is much shorter acting and will be out of a patient's system within a day. Phenelzine continues to inhibit MAO for over a week after it is discontinued.

Treatment Technique for Chronic Pain
Initial Treatment

The principal use in CLBP is in patients with coexisting major affective disorder. Monoamine oxidase inhibitors are not the drug of first choice for CLBP patients with major depression. They are most often used in complex cases that have failed first-line (tricyclic) treatment. Again, it is recommended that psychiatric consultations be obtained to reevaluate the patient's diagnosis before commencing treatment. Serious side effects from use of MAOIs are relatively rare, and their danger has probably been overstated, but relatively few clinicians are experienced in their use.

Most treatment failures with MAOIs are secondary to inadequate dosage. The clinical end point for correct dosage is mild postural hypotension and muscle fasiculations after the second week of treatment. The usual dosage of phenelzine for initial treatment is up to 90 mg/day. Treatment begins with phenelzine 15 mg on day 1, 30 mg on day 2, and 15 mg in the morning and 30 mg in the evening on day 3, if the patient is asymptomatic. Phenelzine 45 mg daily is maintained until day 14 if there are no side effects, and then the dosage is increased to 30 mg each morning and 30 mg in the evening; on day 21 the dosage can be increased to 30 mg in the morning, 15 mg in the afternoon, and 30 mg in the evening; on day 28 the dosage can be increased to 30 mg three times daily if there are no side effects. After adequate or maximum dosage is achieved, the patient should be monitored weekly for another 4–6 weeks (108).

Maintenance Treatment

There are few data regarding proper maintenance dosages for CLBP patients with major depression, but little reason to believe that guidelines should differ from those established for psychiatric patients. Psychiatric patients with major depression may experience a relapse of symptoms at dosages below the initial optimal regimen (108). As with TCAs, an attempt should be made after approximately 6 months of therapy to discontinue the medication, cutting back by 15 mg every 1–3 weeks until the patient is off the drug.

Treatment Nonresponse

Again, experienced psychiatric consultation is indicated, and the alternatives are the same as described above for TCAs. Another MAOI may be used. Monoamine oxidase inhibitors have been combined with various medications, including TCAs and L-tryptophan. It is difficult to evaluate the efficacy of these combinations, and both tricyclics and tryptophan may provoke a hypertensive crisis.

While lithium has been employed in recurrent headache syndromes (e.g., cluster headache) there are no apparent applications documented for CLBP disorders, and its use for such patients is restricted to treatment of patients with major depression who have failed first-line therapies or who have concurrent specialized psychiatric illness (e.g., bipolar affective disorder). For these reasons we refer the interested reader to standard sources for discussion of the properties of this drug (see ref. 91).

NEUROLEPTIC AGENTS

The neuroleptic drugs are described in Table 15.5, and the compounds and dosages in Table 15.7. Their use in CLBP is adjunctive and limited.

Properties and Side Effects

Neuroleptics increase the central arousal threshold by suppressing afferent sensory transmission from the periphery. The most important pharmacologic effects are widespread inhibition of dopaminergic transmission in the CNS. Blockade of the nigrostriatal system produces extrapyramidal symptoms (tremor, rigidity, bradykinesia, akathisia, and dystonia). Blockade of the tuberoinfundibular system produces hyperprolactinemia with gynecomastia and lactation, and inhibition of pituitary gonadotrophins. Blockade at the chemorceptor trigger zone of the hypothalamus produces antiemetic properties. Blockade in the limbic system and associated cortex produces antianxiety and antipsychotic effects (115).

Neuroleptics also have anti-α-adrenergic and anticholinergic effects. These properties are most prominent with the aliphatic agents (e.g., chlorpromazine) and less so with piperadine and piper-

Table 15.7
Commonly Used Neuroleptics

CLASS	RELATIVE POTENCY	USUAL DAILY ORAL DOSE IN PAIN TREATMENT (MG)
Phenothiazines		
Chlorpromazine		
(Thorazine)	Low	10–50
Methotrimeprazine		
(Levoprome)	Low	10–50
Thioridazine		
(Mellaril)	Low	10–75
Perphenazine		
(Trilafon)	High	1–5
Trifluoperazine		
(Stelazine)	High	1–5
Fluphenazine		
(Prolixin)	High	1–3
Butyrophenones		
Haloperidol		
(Haldol)	High	1–3

azine agents and the butyrophenones—the agents most likely to be used in CLBP patients. Cardiovascular effects include increased heart rate, and dose-related postural hypertension. Repolarization abnormalities of the ECG include T wave abnormalities, prolonged PQ-T intervals, and ST segment depression. Direct myocardial depressant effects result in diminished myocardial contractility in patients with preexisting cardiovascular disease. Neuroleptic agents may alter conduction times and induce potentially fatal ventricular arrhythmias. Cognitive defects on timed tasks include diminished performance on tests of speed, reaction time, and accuracy.

Idiosyncratic allergic responses can occur, with suppression of the hematopoietic system (leukopenia, anemia, or thrombocytopenia). These reactions usually occur within the first 6 weeks of treatment, and their clinical hallmark is the sudden onset of painful pharnygitis and fever. Similarly, an allergic hepatotoxicity with mild increases in liver function test results can occur, and cholestatic jaundice is reported.

The most commonly encountered clinical side effects are the extrapyramidal symptoms, the dystonias, and tardive dyskinesia. Extrapyramidal symptoms can be managed with antiparkinsonian agents [benztropine mesylate (Cogentin), trihexphenidyl (Artane), diphenhydramine (Benadryl), or amatadine (Symmetrel)]. The antiparkinsonian drug should not be given prophylactically. Extrapyramidal symptoms often do not occur, especially at the low doses of neuroleptics prescribed in CLBP pa-

tients, and the antiparkinsonian agent can produce adverse anticholinergic effects (toxic megacolon, toxic psychosis). If these agents are used, the usual daily dose is benztropine mesylate 1–6 mg daily or trihexphenidyl 2–10 mg daily. Because of anticholinergic toxicity, some clinicians prefer treating extrapyramidal symptoms with diphenhydramine 10–25 mg 3 times daily or amantadine 100 mg 1–3 times daily, reserving the antiparkinsonian drugs for symptoms not responsive to less toxic agents (115). If such symptoms are treated, it is recommended that these drugs be tapered or discontinued after 3 months.

Dystonia (tonic contraction of muscles, especially involving the head and neck with grimaces, posturing, and torticollis) rarely occurs in the low dosages used in pain patients, but can be treated with diphenhydramine 25–50 mg intramuscularly. Akathisia, the sensation of an inability to sit still, responds best to dose reduction of the offending drug (115), and would be rare at the low dosages employed for pain patients.

Tardive dyskinesia is a syndrome of involuntary choreiform movements that commence after prolonged treatment with neuroleptics and persist up to years after the neuroleptics are withdrawn. Symptoms can include periodic tongue protrusions, lip smacking, chewing movements of the mouth, athetoid movements of the fingers, and restless shifting from leg to leg. In their severe form such movements can be disabling. The mechanism for tardive dyskinesia is unknown but may involve dopaminergic receptor supersensitivity or excessive dopaminergic activity in the basal ganglia. Treatment with various agents has been only sporadically effective. The best approach is prevention (115). Elderly patients appear to be at higher risk for this disorder. Dosages for the neuroleptics should be kept below 5 mg daily of the high-potency agents or the equivalent in the low-potency agents. Treatment should be limited to months rather than years.

Selected Drug Interactions
Nonnarcotic Analgesics

There are no apparent adverse drug interactions between nonnarcotic analgesics and neuroleptics, although acetaminophen inhibits metabolism of some neuroleptics (e.g., chlorpromazine) and therefore augments its effects.

Narcotic Analgesics

Phenothiazines enhance and prolong the hypotensive and respiratory-depressant effect of narcotics. Chlorpromazine also increases serum levels of the neurotoxic and cardiotoxic *N*-demethylated metabolites of meperidine, which are associated with neuromuscular irritability, seizures, bradycardia, and hypotension.

Pretreatment Evaluation

The medical evaluation is the same as that for candidates for TCAs, including an ECG for patients over age 50 or those with preexisting heart disease, and genitourinary assessment for benign prostatic hypertrophy. These drugs are metabolized by the liver, and patients with hepatic disease will need lower dosages. Laboratory assessment should include baseline complete blood count with differential, and liver function tests.

Drug Selection

Generally CLBP patients with neuropathic syndromes will be treated with a high-potency, low-dose agent, such as haloperidol or fluphenazine. The side effect profile and therapeutic efficacy of these agents are equivalent, and the clinician need select only one or two neuroleptics in this classification and become thoroughly familiar with their properties and usage.

Treatment Techniques for Chronic Pain
Initial and Maintenance Treatment

The neuroleptics are not first-line treatment for any CLBP syndrome, and are employed simply as adjuncts to TCAs in treatment of neuropathic conditions. The risk of tardive dyskinesia always must be kept in mind. One can employ neuroleptics if a trial of one or two different classes of TCAs (e.g., desipramine and nortriptyline) has produced unsatisfactory relief. We add a high-potency neuroleptic, generally fluphenazine or haloperidol, to the chosen TCA. The starting dose is fluphenazine or haloperidol 0.5–1 mg at night, with an increase to 1 mg twice daily after 3–5 days, or to 1 mg 3 times daily if there is no improvement after 10 days. Once the maximum dose of 3 mg daily is reached, this is given as a one-time dose at bedtime. There should be a response within 2–3 weeks. If there is no response with a neuroleptic from one drug class (e.g., fluphenazine) the clinician may switch to an agent from a different class (e.g., haloperidol). Some authorities employ low-potency/high-dose aliphatic agents such as methotrimeprazine, a congener of chlorpromazine. The usual dosage is 50 mg or less, given once daily at bedtime (116). At present, the value of assessing neuroleptic plasma drug concentration is not known for this use.

The patient should be carefully monitored for symptoms of tardive dyskinesia. After 3 months, the drug should be tapered to the lowest therapeutic dosage. At no more than 6 months we taper the patient off the neuroleptic and observe for an increase in pain. If continued treatment is needed the maintenance dosage should be at the lowest possible amounts, with periodic attempts to discontinue the neuroleptic.

Treatment Nonresponse

Some clinicians would prefer to use clonazepam if tricyclics fail, and avoid tricyclic-neuroleptic combinations. The usual dosage range is 1–3 mg daily. A response should occur within 3 weeks. If no response occurs, then a trial of a conventional anticonvulsant (e.g., diphenylhydantoin or carbamazepine) is indicated.

ANTIANXIETY DRUGS

The indications for anxiolytic drugs are described in Table 15.5, and the compounds and dosages in Table 15.8.

Benzodiazepines
Properties and Side Effects

The benzodiazepines have a broad spectrum of pharmacologic activity. Their primary effect is to enhance GABA-mediated presynaptic and postsynaptic inhibition. This action occurs in the spinal cord, brainstem, cerebellar cortex, cerebral cortex, and other structures. The major properties of these drugs are their antianxiety, anticonvulsant, and sedative effects, along with an ability to produce centrally induced muscle relaxation. Like other sedatives, all benzodiazepines have the potential to produce tolerance, psychological as well as physical dependence, and an abstinence syndrome upon withdrawal. Their effects are additive with those of other CNS depressants, and cross-tolerance and cross-dependence develop.

Sudden discontinuation of benzodiazepines after prolonged, uninterrupted use can produce an abstinence syndrome. The syndrome consists of insomnia, nausea, myalgia, muscle twitching, diaphoresis, and potentially major motor seizure. The probability of developing a withdrawal syndrome appears to vary with the length of treatment: patients treated for less than 4 months at the usual therapeutic dosage are unlikely to develop symptoms; about 5% of those treated for up to 1 year may develop symptoms, and those treated for over 1 year run a much higher risk (117).

The most common side effects are sedation, ataxia, and dysarthria. In the elderly these agents may

Table 15.8
Commonly Used Antianxiety Agents

BENZODIAZEPINE	USUAL DAILY ORAL ANTIANXIETY DOSE IN PAIN TREATMENT (MG)	USUAL ORAL HYPNOTIC DOSE (MG)
Long half-life		
Clorazepate (Tranxene)	3–15	15–30
Flurazepam (Dalmane)	—	15–30
Intermediate half-life		
Chlordiazepoxide (Librium)	15–30	50
Diazepam (Valium)	2.5–15	15–30
Short half-life		
Alprazolam (Xanax)	0.5–3.0	—
Lorazepam (Ativan)[a]	2–5	—
Oxazepam (Serax)[a]	10–50	30–60
Other		
Hydroxyzine	100–400	—

[a] No active metabolites.

produce confusion and paradoxical excitement. Teratogenic effects (i.e., cleft palate) during pregnancy are postulated but are not thoroughly documented. There are few autonomic side effects, although bradycardia and hypotension can occur. Allergic phenomena are also reported, and include neutropenia and jaundice.

Drug Interactions
The most important interactions involve additive effects with other CNS depressants. Cimetidine (Tagamet), disulfiram (Antabuse), and oral contraceptives can increase the half-life of benzodiazepines.

Pretreatment Evaluation
In patients for whom benzodiazepines are acutely indicated the major concern is for the patient's ability to tolerate the CNS-depressive effects of the drug. The primary concern in candidates for prolonged treatment is misuse or abuse. Elderly patients are particularly at risk for falls as a result of intoxication and ataxia as well as acute confusional episodes. Such side effects may occur at relatively low dosages because of the elderly's reduced rate of drug metabolism and reduced protein binding. A cardiovascular history and ECG should be obtained as indicated: benzodiazepine withdrawal can precipitate angina, elevated blood pressure, or cardiac arrhythmias. Liver function tests should be obtained, and patients with liver disease may require a diminished dose.

Drug Selection
All benzodiazepines have similar anxiolytic properties, side effect profiles, and potential for dependency and abuse. They differ mainly in their elimination half-life and presence of active metabolites. Those with the longest half-life are chlorazepate (Tranxene), prazepam (Centrax), and halazepam (Paxipam). Moderately long-acting agents are diazepam (Valium) and chlordiazepoxide (Librium). The shortest acting are oxazepam (Serax), lorazepam (Ativan), and alprazolam (Xanax). All these drugs have clinically important active metabolites except for oxazepam and lorazepam. The duration of action reflects the presence of active metabolites. Cumulative clinical effects occur with repeated dosage. If drug accumulation or prolonged effects are problems (as in elderly patients or those with hepatic disease), short-acting agents with no active metabolites may be preferred. The problems of drug accumulation also can be met by reducing the dosage of longer acting drugs. Again, the best clinical practice is to choose one or two agents and learn to employ them effectively. Overall the benzodiazepines have a good margin of safety. By themselves they are unlikely to be lethal in overdoses. Nevertheless their depressant effects are dangerous if they are taken with alcohol, barbiturates, or other drugs that depress the CNS, and potentially suicidal or depressed patients should not have access to these medications

Treatment Techniques for Chronic Pain
Initial and Maintenance Treatment. Patients with neuropathic conditions are candidates for chronic benzodiazepines, and some clinicians believe that patients with chronic low back skeletal muscle spasm also may benefit from these drugs. Neuro-

pathic syndromes may be responsive to clonazepam. The usual dosage is 1–3 mg daily. A therapeutic effect may be evident within 2 weeks. A major problem for many patients, particularly the elderly, has been oversedation at the dosage required for a therapeutic effect (74). Maintenance treatment is not well described, but probably should follow guidelines offered for other therapy of neuropathic pain. The lowest therapeutic dose should be maintained for 3–6 months, then an attempt to slowly discontinue the drug may be entertained.

Given the relative lack of documented efficacy we do not recommend or employ benzodiazepines chronically for simple complaints of skeletal muscle spasm. Instead we prefer treatment with a graduated physical reconditioning program, education about the nature and effects of chronic pain, and specialized instruction in back anatomy and function (i.e., a "back school" program). Biofeedback training is also useful for some patients.

Anxiety as a Special Problem. Many patients with CLBP appear to be acutely or chronically anxious and complain additionally of chronic tension headaches and neck pain, presumably related to painful muscular contraction. We rarely employ antianxiety agents for these patients in the absence of psychiatric assessment documenting the severity of anxiety. If anxiety if believed to be the major etiology of functional disability or of pain, then benzodiazepines may be indicated. If the clinician decides to institute treatment, therapy should follow the principles outlined by Hollister (118) and others (119) for the proper use of benzodiazepines. Seven guidelines have been described (118):

1. Use benzodiazepines only when indicated
2. Use nondrug methods when possible
3. Drug treatment should be brief and intermittent
4. Doses should be titrated individually
5. Efficacy should be assessed early
6. Avoid benzodiazepines if a history of drug abuse is known
7. Gradually discontinue the drug after chronic treatment

This approach allows the physician to avoid the pitfall of overprescribing these agents.

Treatment with benzodiazepines may be useful when anxiety interferes with the patient's performing his/her usual life activities. Nonpharmacologic measures for managing anxiety include psychotherapy, exercise programs, relaxation training, and biofeedback. These methods are often components of a comprehensive pain management program, and can help reduce reliance on anxiolytics and prevent relapse.

Ideal drug treatment is intermitten and brief. Most anxiety related to life stress is resolved within 1 month. Chronic anxiety, like chronic pain, waxes and wanes in intensity. Anxiolytics would be used only during exacerbations of the patient's chronic disorder. In any event, chronically anxious patients should not be treated indefinitely without assessing the need for continuous treatment. If prolonged therapy is needed the lowest possible dosage consistent with efficacy should be used. In both acutely and chronically anxious individuals a drug response generally occurs within the first 2–3 weeks of treatment, since state anxiety is usually more responsive that trait anxiety (119). Therefore, if there is no improvement after several weeks on a proper regimen, then benefit is unlikely with prolonged therapy and other avenues should be explored. If anxiety is relieved the physician can propose that the drug be discontinued, and reinstituted if symptoms return. Thus tolerance and/or dependence are avoided (118).

Dose titration involves determining the minimum amount of drug necessary to produce mild sedation. Hollister (118) recommended initiating treatment at night, 2–3 hours before normal bedtime. The minimum effective dose is determined as the amount required to produce restful sleep when taken 2–3 hours before bedtime. If the initial dose does not produce effective hypnosis the first night, twice the dose is given the second night, four times the dose is given the third night, and eight times the dose is given the fourth night. The patient can commence with diazepam 2.5 mg and then increase to 5 mg, 10 mg, or 20 mg. The usual minimum effective hypnotic dose is 10 mg or less. As a result, the patient achieves a good night rest, unwanted oversedation is avoided during the daytime, and the anxiolytic effect is retained. If additional amounts are required during the day usually one-half or one-third of the nighttime dose will suffice. This approach works best for long-acting benzodiazepines and is not suited for short-acting agents.

Treatment efficacy should be assessed within 3 weeks. Failure to respond may indicate an inadequate dosage regimen, or a misdiagnosis. For example, anxiety frequently accompanies depressive syndromes and an antidepressant would be required to successfully treat this disorder. Alcohol abuse may also be present, and treatment with benzodiazepines may be undermined by the patient's tolerance to CNS depressants (118).

Patients with a past history of abuse of alcohol

or other CNS depressants generally are not good candidates for benzodiazepines. Some authorities recommend short-term treatment with agents less likely to be abused, such as hydroxyxine.

Maintenance Treatment for Anxiety. Occasionally chronically anxious patients may benefit from long-term treatment, although there is no documentation of this notion. Again the minimum effective dose should be used; reevaluation of the regimen should occur at least every 6 months. Tolerance to anxiolytic effects may not occur. The clinician therefore should be alert that requests for escalating the dose may indicate misuse of the agent rather than tolerance.

Patients who have been treated for more than 4 months with diazepam 20–40 mg daily (or the equivalent) should be withdrawn slowly, usually over 4–6 weeks.

Buspirone

Buspirone (BuSpar) is a new anxiolytic chemically and pharmacologically unrelated to the benzodiazepines. Since maximum benefit emerges only after 3–4 weeks of treatment, it has been advocated for treatment of chronic anxiety. Preliminary data indicate it has few CNS side effects. Its abuse potential is unknown.

CNS STIMULANTS

Indications for psychostimulants are described in Table 15.5, and the compounds and dosages in Table 15.9.

Properties and Side Effects

Central nervous system stimulants include *d,1*-amphetamine (Dexedrine), methylphenidate (Ritalin), and pemoline (Cyclert). They are rapidly absorbed orally. For example, methylphenidate has a half-life of 2–7 hours and dextroamphetamine 4–21 hours. Central nervous system stimulants are metabolized by hepatic oxidation and conjugating enzyme systems and also are excreted unchanged

Table 15.9
Commonly Used Psychostimulants

	USUAL DAILY ANTIDEPRESSANT AND PAIN MANAGEMENT DOSE (MG)
d-Amphetamine (Dexedrine)	10–20
Methylphenidate (Ritalin)	15–20

in the urine. They produce cerebral stimulation and arousal by decreasing neuronal reuptake and deactivation of norepinephrine and dopamine. Physiologic dependence does not seem to occur in the same sense as with CNS depressants, although a withdrawal syndrome of inertia and depressed mood appears upon sudden withdrawal after high intake. Tolerance to euphoriant effects occurs rapidly (91). Side effects are those of anorexia, plus sympathomimetic actions. Other untoward effects include catatonia (mute and bizarre behavior), paranoid reactions, and confusion (120). These agents generally are thought to have fewer cardiovascular side effects (e.g., bundle-branch block) than TCAs.

Drug Interactions

The ability of psychostimulants to compete for hepatic enzymes reduces the metabolism of TCAs, neuroleptics, antianxiety agents, and many other drugs. There are additive effects with other sympathomimetic drugs.

Pretreatment Evaluation

Patients over age 50 years and those with a history of hypertension or cardiovascular disease are at increased risk for the drug's sympathomimetic effects, and risk-benefit ratios must be carefully appraised. The elderly are particularly vulnerable to acute agitation or confusion. History of substance abuse must be elicited.

Drug Selection

There are few data available to help distinguish among the psychostimulants. Methylphenidate and pemoline may be less subject to abuse than are amphetamines (91). Because of its short half-life methylphenidate may be preferred in the elderly to reduce duration of any toxic effects.

Initial and Maintenance Treatment in Acute and Chronic Pain

The CNS stimulants have limited use in management of acute or chronic pain. While they augment narcotic analgesia acutely, there really seems to be little advantage to these drugs since simply increasing the dose of analgesic accomplishes the desired goal.

These agents are not recommended for first-line, routine use in depressed pain patients because of their limited efficacy and risk of increasing agitation (91). If a TCA is contraindicated in a pain patient with a major depression, then a CNS stimulant may be employed. For pain control or depression the initial dose of dextroamphetamine or methylphen-idate is usually 5–10 mg each morning. With its longer half-life dextroamphetamine may be given once daily, whereas methylphenidate is adminis-tered in two divided doses at 8 AM and noon. If no response occurs after 2 days, the dose is increased, but more than 20 mg daily is rarely required (90). A response should ensue by 7–10 days.

Maintenance treatment is not well described, and rarely extends beyond several weeks. Reports usu-ally indicate that the agent is discontinued a few days after the patient becomes asymptomatic (90). Given the controversial nature of treatment with CNS stimulants the physician should carefully doc-ument his/her reasons for employing these drugs and his/her explanation to the patient of side effects and risk-benefit ratio. Treatment should be brief, prescription quantities limited in size, and follow-up frequent.

GENERAL COMMENTS AND CONCLUSIONS

Pain is a multidimensional phenomenon. We know little about the basic mechanisms that pro-duce or perpetuate the sensory component of pain following tissue damage, or of mechanisms relevant to the affective or behavioral response to the pain experience. Our knowledge of basic mechanisms is particularly limited for chronic pain. A better un-derstanding of these mechanisms is necessary to design specific and more effective psychopharma-cological treatments.

Four issues must be addressed to ensure appro-priate use of psychotropic agents. First, as clear an understanding as is possible of the etiology of pain must be established to identify drug-responsive pain syndromes. Psychiatric disorders contributing to pain or disability must also be accurately diagnosed so that appropriate psychiatric target symptoms can be selected for treatment. Second, detoxification from excessive regimens of analgesics or sedative-hypnotic medications is essential for evaluating perceived pain, functional capacity, and treatment outcome. Third, psychopharmacologic medications are adjunctive treatment, and are not a substitute for a comprehensive treatment plan agreed upon with the patient, involving education, physical re-conditioning, behavioral assessment, and evalua-tion of family and occupational roles. Fourth, me-ticulous follow-up is necessary to detect recurrent symptoms or discontinue ineffective treatments. Few studies reporting initial therapeutic gains fol-low patients beyond the first weeks of treatment. Psychopharmacologic treatment is effective only if it leads directly to observable improvement in daily

function and psychological symptoms, or dimin-ished use of analgesics or other medical resources.

Chronic low back pain is a complex problem with biologic, psychological, and social aspects. By the time back pain has become chronic it may signifi-cantly disrupt multiple areas of the patient's life (e.g., work and household responsibilities, social and recreational pursuits, interpersonal relation-ships, moods and thoughts, sexual function, fi-nances, and self-perception). Therefore, patients typically present not with back pain in isolation, but rather with a constellation of symptoms, com-plaints, and complicating factors, such as functional impairment, emotional distress, medication misuse or abuse, and family problems. It is unlikely that psychopharmacologic approaches alone will be sufficient to ameliorate the numerous problems presented in complicated cases. Thus, we believe psychoactive medications are best used as one component of a comprehensive program of pain management and rehabilitation.

Given the chronic nature of the pain, and the multiple treatment objectives, careful cost-benefit analyses and assessment of side effects should be standard procedure in the administration of psy-chopharmacologic agents. As discussed above, these drugs have multiple effects that may hinder as well as facilitate rehabilitation. Decisions regarding the appropriate use of a particular medication should be based on the individual patient's symptom con-stellation, age, general health, prognosis, and treat-ment goals. For some patients the increased com-fort provided by psychoactive medications may not be worth the trade-off in inhibition of full functional capacity.

Physicians also are advised to consider the special needs of chronic pain patients when prescribing and scheduling medications for pain. Medication usage should be scheduled to (a) derive maximum benefit from the pharmacologic properties of the agent, (b) encourage compliance with the overall treatment regimen, and (c) minimize the risk of medication misuse or abuse. Patients must be ed-ucated that fixed-interval medication schedules are essential to the therapeutic efficacy of the agents, and that *pro re nata* (PRN) usage is contraindicated. Regularly scheduled physician contact should be maintained to encourage patients to function in-dependently and to avoid making physician contact and medication prescription contingent upon com-plaints of pain. With these conditions in mind, psychopharmacologic agents can be useful adjuncts to the comprehensive care of patients with chronic low back pain.

ACKNOWLEDGMENT

This work was supported in part by the Veterans Administration.

REFERENCES

1. American Psychiatric Association: *Diagnostic and Statistical Manual,* ed 3. Washington, DC, American Psychiatric Association Press, 1978.
2. Sternbach RA: *Pain Patients: Traits and Treatment.* New York, Academic Press, 1974.
3. Ward NG, Bloom VL, Friedel RC: The effectiveness of tricyclic antidepressants in the treatment of coexisting pain and depression. *Pain* 7:331–341, 1979.
4. Ward NG: Tricyclic antidepressants for chronic low back pain. *Spine* 11:661–665, 1986.
5. Alcoff J, Jones E, Rust P, Newman R: Controlled trial of imipramine for chronic low back pain. *J Family Prac* 14:841–846, 1982.
6. Hameroff SR, Cork RC, Scherer K, Crago BR, Neuman C, Womble JK, Davis TP: Doxepin effects on chronic pain, depression and plasma opioids. *J Clin Psychiatry* 43:22–27, 1982.
7. Pilowsky I, Hallett EC, Bassett DL, Thomas PG, Penhall RK: A controlled study of amitriptyline in the treatment of chronic pain. *Pain* 14:169–179, 1982.
8. Pheasant H, Bursk A, Goldfarb J, Azen SP, Weiss JN, Borelli L: Amitriptyline and chronic low back pain. *Spine* 8:552–557, 1983.
9. Sternbach RA, Janowsky DS, Huey LY, Segal DS: Effects of altering brain serotonin activity on human chronic pain. In Bonica JJ, Albe-Fessard D (eds): *Advances in Pain Research and Therapy,* New York, Raven Press, 1976, vol 1, pp 601–606.
10. Jenkins DG, Ebbutt AF, Evans CD: Tofranil in the treatment of low back pain. *J Int Med Res* 4(Suppl 2):28–40, 1976.
11. Butler SH, Weil-Fugazza J, Godefoy F, Besson J-M: Reduction of arthritis and pain behavior following chronic administration of amitriptyline or imipramine in rats with adjuvant-induced arthritis. *Pain* 23:159–175, 1985.
12. MacNeill AL, Dick WC: Imipramine and rheumatoid factor. *J Int Med Res* 4(Suppl 2):23–27, 1976.
13. Gringas M: A clinical trial of Tofranil in rheumatic pain in general practice. *J Int Med Res* 4(Suppl 2):41–45, 1976.
14. McDonald Scott WA: The relief of pain with an antidepressant in arthritis. *Practitioner* 202:802–805, 1969.
15. Smythe HA: Fibrositis and other diffuse musculoskeletal syndromes. In Kelly WN, Harris ED, Ruddy S (eds): *Textbook of Rheumatology.* Philadelphia, WB Saunders, 1980, pp 485–493.
16. McCain GA, Scrudds RA: The concept of primary fibromyalgia (fibrositis): clinical value, relation and significance to other chronic musculoskeletal pain syndrome. *Pain* 33:273–287, 1988.
17. Wolfe F, Cathey MA: The epidemiology of tender points, a prospective study of 1520 patients. *J Rheumatol* 1216:1164–1168, 1985.
18. Simons DG, Travell JG: Myofascial origins of low back pain. I. Principles of diagnosis and treatment. *Postgrad Med* 73:68–77, 1983.
19. Carette S, McCain GA, Bell DA: A double-blind study of amitriptyline versus placebo in patients with primary fibrositis (abstract). *Arthritis Rheum* 158 (Suppl):28, 1985.
20. Dinerman H, Felson D, Goldenberg D: A randomized clinical trial of naproxen and amitriptyline in primary fibromyalgia (abstract). *Arthritis Rheum* 159(Suppl):28, 1985.
21. Caruso I, Puttini PCS, Boccassini L, Santandrea S, Locati M, Volpato R, Montrone F, Benevenuti C, Beretta A: Double-blind study of dothiepin versus placebo in the treatment of primary fibromyalgia syndrome. *J Int Medical Res* 15:154–159, 1987.
22. Woodforde JM, Dwyer B, McEwen BW, DeWilde FW, Bleasel K, Connelley TJ, Ho CY: Treatment of postherpetic neuralgia. *Med J Aust* 2:869–872, 1965.
23. Kvinesdal B, Molin J, Froland A, Gram LF: Imipramine treatment of painful diabetic neuropathy. *JAMA* 251:1727–1730, 1984.
24. Watson CP, Evans RJ, Reed K, Merskey H, Goldsmith L, Warsh J: Amitriptyline versus placebo in postherpetic neuralgia. *Neurology* 32:671–673, 1982.
25. Turkington RW: Depression masquerading as diabetic neuropathy. *JAMA* 243:1147–1150, 1980.
26. Clark IMC: Amitriptyline and perphenizine (Triptafen DA) in chronic pain. *Anaesthesia* 36:210–212, 1981.
27. Dalessio DJ: Chronic pain syndromes and disordered cortical inhibition: effects of tricyclic compounds. *Dis Nerv System* 28:325–328, 1967.
28. Kocher R: Use of psychotropic drugs for treatment of chronic severe pain. In Bonica JJ, Albe-Fessard D (eds): *Advances in Pain Research and Therapy.* New York, Raven Press, 1976, vol 1, 579–582.
29. Langohr HD, Stohr M, Petruch F: An open and double-blind cross-over study on the efficacy of clomipramine (Anafranil) in patients with painful mono- and polyneuropathies. *Eur Neurol* 21:309–317, 1982.
30. Malseed R, Goldstein FJ: Enhancement of morphine analgesia by tricyclic antidepressants. *Neuropharmacology* 18:827–829, 1979.
31. Lee RL, Spencer PSJ: The effect of clomipramine and other amine-uptake inhibitors on morphine analgesia in laboratory animals. *Postgrad Med J* 53:53–60, 1977.
32. Liu SJ, Wang RIH: Increased analgesia and alterations in distribution and metabolism of methadone by desipramine in rats. *J Pharmacol Exp Ther* 195:94–104, 1975.
33. Gonzalez JP, Sewell RDE, Spencer PSJ: Antinociceptive activity of opiates in the presence of the antidepressant agent nomifensine. *Neuropharmacology* 19:613–618, 1980.
34. Kellstein DE, Malseed R, Goldstein FJ: Contrasting effects of acute vs. chronic tricyclic antidepressant

treatment on central morphine analgesia. *Pain* 20:323–334, 1984.

35. Levine JD, Gordon NC, Smith R, McBryde R: Desipramine enhances opiate postoperative analgesia. *Pain* 27:45–49, 1986.

36. France RD, Urban BJ, Keefe FJ: Long-term use of narcotic analgesics in chronic pain. *Soc Sci Med* 19:1379–1382, 1984.

37. Urban BJ, France RD, Steinberger EK, Scott DL, Maltbie AA: Long-term use of narcotic/antidepressant medication in the management of phantom limb pain. *Pain* 24:191–196, 1986.

38. Anderson LS, Black RG, Abraham J, Ward AA: Neuronal hyperactivity in experimental trigeminal deafferentation. *J Neurosurg* 35:444–452, 1971.

39. Loeser JD, Ward AA, White LE: Chronic deafferentation of human spinal cord neurons. *J Neurosurg* 29:48–50, 1968.

40. Anthony M, Lance JW: Monoamine oxidase inhibitors in the treatment of migraine. *Arch Neurol* 21:263–268, 1969.

41. Lascelles RG: Atypical facial pain and depression. *Br J Psychiatry* 112:651–659, 1966.

42. Raft D, Davidson J, Wasik J, Mattox A: Relationship between response to phenelzine and MAO inhibition in a clinical trial of phenelzine, amitriptyline and placebo. *Neuropsychobiology* 7:122–126, 1981.

43. Yung CY: A review of clinical trials of lithium in neurology. *Pharmacol Biochem Behav* 21(Suppl 1):57–64, 1984.

44. Medina JL, Diamond S: Cyclical migraine. *Arch Neurol* 38:343–344, 1981.

45. Chazot G, Chauplannaz G, Biron A, Schott B: Migraines: treatment per lithium. *Nouv Presse Med* 8:2836–2837, 1979.

46. Kudrow L: Lithium prophylaxis for chronic cluster headache. *Headache* 17:15–18, 1977.

47. Moore J, Dundee JW: Alterations in response to somatic pain associated with anaesthesia, Part VII: the effects of nine phenothiazine derivatives. *Br J Anaesth* 33:422–431, 1961.

48. Dundee JW, Love WJ, Moore J: Alterations in response to somatic pain associated with anaesthesia, Part XV: further studies with phenothiazine derivatives and similar drugs. *Br J Anaesth* 35:597–609, 1963.

49. Moore J, Dundee JW: Alterations in response to somatic pain associated with anaesthesia, V: the effect of promethazine. *Br J Anaesth* 33:3–8, 1961.

50. Dundee JW, Moore J: Alterations in response to somatic pain associated with anaesthesia, I: an evaluation of a method of analgesimetry. *Br J Anaesth* 32:396–406, 1960.

51. Lasagna L, DeKornfeld TJ: Methotrimeprazine—a new phenothiazine derivative with analgesic properties. *JAMA* 178:887–890, 1961.

52. Minuck R: Postoperative analgesia—comparison of methotrimeprazine and meperidine as postoperative analgesia agents. *Can Anaesth Soc J* 19:87–96, 1972.

53. Baldessarini RJ: Drugs in the treatment of psychiatric disorders. In Gilman AG, Goodman LS, Rall TW, Murad F (eds): *The Pharmacological Basis of Therapeutics,* ed 7. New York, Macmillan, 1985, pp 387–445.

54. Taub A: Relief of post-herpetic neuralgia with psychotropic drugs. *J Neurosurg* 39:235–239, 1973.

55. Merskey H, Hester RA: The treatment of chronic pain with psychotropic drugs. *Postgrad Med J* 48:594–598, 1972.

56. Davis JL, Lewis SB, Gerich JE, Kaplan RA, Schultz TA, Wallen JD: Peripheral diabetic neuropathy treated with amitriptyline and fluphenozine. *JAMA* 238:2291–2292, 1977.

57. Moertel CG, Ahmann DL, Taylor WF, Schwartau N: Relief of pain by oral medications. *JAMA* 229:55–59, 1974.

58. Houde RW, Wallenstein SL: Analgetic power of chlorpromazine alone and in combination with morphine. *Fed Proc* 14:353, 1955.

59. Shannon HE, Holtzman SG, Davis DC: Interaction between narcotic analgesics and benzodiazepine derivatives on behavior in the mouse. *J Pharmacol Exp Ther* 199:387–399, 1976.

60. Weis J: Morphine antagonistic effect of chlordiazepoxide (Librium). *Experientia* 25:381, 1969.

61. Morichi R, Pepeu G: A study of the influence of hydroxyzine and diazepam on morphine antinociception in the rat. *Pain* 7:173–180, 1979.

62. Chapman CR, Feather BW: Effects of diazepam on human pain tolerance and pain sensitivity. *Psychosom Med* 35:330–340, 1973.

63. Gracely RH, McGrath P, Dubner R: Validity and sensitivity of sensory and affective verbal pain descriptors: manipulation of affect by diazepam. *Pain* 5:19–29, 1978.

64. Kantor TG, Steinburg FP: Studies of tranquillizing agents (hydroxyzine and meprobamate) and meperidine in clinical pain. In Bonica JJ, Albe-Fessard D (eds): *Advances in Pain Research and Therapy*. New York, Raven Press, 1976, vol 1, pp 567–572.

65. Stambaugh JE, Wainer IW: Metabolic studies of the interaction of meperidine and hydroxyzine in human subjects. In Bonica JJ, Albe-Fessard D (eds): *Advances in Pain Research and Therapy*. New York, Raven Press, 1976, vol 1, pp 559–565.

66. Beaver WT, Feise G: A comparison of the analgesic effects of morphine, hydroxyzine and their combination in patients with post-operative pain. In Bonica JJ, Albe-Fessard D (eds): *Advances in Pain Research and Therapy*. New York, Raven Press, 1976, vol 1, pp 553–557.

67. Hupert C, Yacoub M, Turgeon LR: Effect of hydroxyzine on morphine analgesia for the treatment of postoperative pain. *Anesth Analg* 59:690–696, 1980.

68. Hollister LE, Conley FK, Britt RH, Shuer L: Long-term use of diazepam. *JAMA* 246:1568–1570, 1981.

69. Yosselson-Superstine S, Lipman AG, Sanders SH: Adjunctive anti-anxiety agents in the management of chronic pain. *Isr J Med Sci* 21:113–117, 1985.

70. Greenblatt DJ, Shader RI, Abernathy DR: Current status of benzodiazepines. *N Engl J Med* 309:410–416, 1983.

71. Hendler N, Cimi C, Terence MA, Long D: A comparison of congitive impairment due to benzodiazepines and to narcotics. *Am J Psychiatry* 137:828–830, 1980.

72. Caccia MR: Clonazepam in facial neuralgia and cluster headache. Clinical and electrophysiological study. *Eur Neurol* 13:560–563, 1975.

73. Smirne S, Scarlato G: Clonazepam in cranial neuralgias. *Med J Aust* 1:93–94, 1977.

74. Swerdlow M, Cundill JG: Anticonvulsant drugs used in the treatment of lancinating pain. A comparison. *Anaesthesia* 36:1129–1132, 1981.

75. Martin G: Recurrent pain of a pseudotabetic variety after laminectomy for lumbar disc lesion. *J Neurol Neurosurg Psychiatry* 43:283–286, 1980.

76. Maciewicz R, Bouckoms A, Martin JB: Drug therapy of neuropathic pain. *Clin J Pain* 1:39–49, 1985.

77. Haefely WE: Behavioral and neuropharmacological aspects of drugs used in anxiety and related states. In Lipton MA, DiMascio A, Killam KF (eds): *Psychopharmacology: A Generation of Progress*. New York, Raven Press, 1978, pp 1359–1374.

78. Game CJA, Lodge D: The pharmacology of inhibition of dorsal horn neurones by impulses in myelinated cutaneous afferents in the cat. *Exp Brain Res* 23:75–84, 1975.

79. Goetzl FR, Burrill DY, Ivy AC: The analgesic effect of morphine alone and in combination with dextroamphetamines. *Proc Soc Exp Biol Med* 55:248–250, 1944.

80. Notl MW: Potentiation of morphine analgesia by cocaine in mice. *Eur J Pharmacol* 5:93–99, 1968.

81. Sigg EB, Capriob A, Schneider JA: Synergism of amines and antagonism of reserpine to morphine analgesia. *Proc Soc Exp Biol Med* 97:97–100, 1958.

82. Ivy AC, Goetzl FR, Burril DY: Morphine-dextroamphetamine analgesia. *War Med* 6:67–71, 1944.

83. Evans WO: The synergism of autonomic drugs on opiate or opioid-induced analgesia: a discussion of its potential utility. *Milit Med* 127:1000–1003, 1962.

84. Forest WH, Brown BW, Brown CR, Defalque R, Gold M, Gordon HE, James KE, Katz J, Mahler DL, Schraff P, Teutsch G: Dextroamphetamine with morphine for the treatment of post-operative pain. *N Engl J Med* 296:712–715, 1977.

85. Laska EM, Sunshine A, Mueller F, Elvers WB, Siegel C, Rubin A: Caffeine as an analgesic ajuvant. *JAMA* 251:1711–1718, 1984.

86. Bruera E, Chadwick S, Brenneis C, Hanson J, MacDonald RN: Methylphenidate associated with narcotics for the treatment of cancer pain. *Cancer Treat Rep* 71:67–70, 1987.

87. Silverman EK, Reus VI, Jimerson DC: Heterogeneity of amphetamine response in depressed patients. *Am J Psychiatry* 138:1302–1306, 1981.

88. Katon W. Raskind M: Treatment of depression in the medically ill elderly with methylphenidate. *Am J Psychiatry* 137:963–965, 1980.

89. Kaufman MW, Murray GB, Cassem NH: Use of psychostimulants in medically ill depressed patients. *Psychosomatics* 23:817–819, 1982.

90. Woods SW, Tesar GE, Murray GB, Cassem NH: Psychostimulant treatment of depressive disorders secondary to medical illness. *J Clin Psychiatry* 47:12–15, 1986.

91. Baldessarini RJ: *Chemotherapy in Psychiatry: Principles and Practice*. Cambridge, MA, Harvard University Press, 1985.

92. Charney DS, Menkes DB, Heninger GR: Receptor sensitivity and the mechanism of action of antidepressant treatment: implications for the etiology and therapy of depression. *Arch Gen Psychiatry* 38:1160–1179, 1981.

93. Risch SC, Groom GP, Janowsky DS: Interfaces of psychoparmacology and cardiology, Part I and II. *J Clin Psychiatry* 42:23–34, 47–59, 1981.

94. Boakes AJ, Laurence DR, Teoh PC, Barar FSK, Benedikter LT, Prichard BNC: Interactions between sympathomimetic amines and antidepressant agents in man. *Br Med J* 1:311–315, 1973.

95. Thornton WE, Pray RJ: Combination drug therapy in psychopharmacology. *J Clin Pharmacol* 15:511–517, 1975.

96. Griffin JP, O'Arcy PF (eds): *A Manual of Adverse Drug Interactions*. Bristol, England, John Wright and Sons Ltd, 1975.

97. Bigger JT, Kantor SJ, Glassman AH, Perel JM: Cardiovascular effects of tricyclic antidepressant drugs. In Lipton MA, DeMascio A, Killam KF (eds): *Psychopharmacology: A Generation of Progress*. New York, Raven Press, 1978.

98. Roose SP, Glassman AH, Giardina EG, Walsh TB, Woodring S, Bigger JT: Tricyclic antidepressants in depressed patients with cardiac conducion disease. *Arch Gen Psychiatry* 44:273–275, 1987.

99. Risch SC, Kalin NH, Janowsky DS, Huey LY: Indications and guidelines for plasma tricyclic antidepressant concentration monitoring. *J Clin Psychopharmacol* 1:59–63, 1981.

100. Prien RF, Kupfer DJ: Continuation drug therapy for major depressive episode: how long should it be maintained? *Am J Psychiatry* 143:18–23, 1986.

101. Weissman MM, Prusoff BA, Klerman GL: Personality and the prediction of long term outcome of depression. *Am J Psychiatry* 135:797–800, 1978.

102. Keller MB, Klerman GL, Lavori PW, Coryell W, Endicott J, Taylor J: Long-term outcome of episodes of major depression. Clinical and public health significance. *JAMA* 252:788–792, 1984.

103. Carroll BJ, Feinberg M, Greden JF, Tarika J, Albala AA, Haskett RFMcL, James N, Kronfol Z, Lohr N, Steiner M, deVigne JP, Young E: A specific laboratory test for the diagnosis of melancholia: standarization, validation, and clinical utility. *Arch Gen Psychiatry* 44:273–275, 1987.

104. Arana G, Baldessarini RJ, Ornsteen M: the dexame-thasone suppression test for diagnosis and prognosis in psychiatry. *Arch Gen Psychiatry* 42:1193–1204, 1985.
105. Atkinson JH, Kremer EF, Risch SC, Ward HW, Hopper B, Yen SSC: Pre- and post-dexamethasone saliva cortisol determinations in chronic pain patients. *Biol Psychiatry* 19:1155–1159, 1984.
106. France RD, Krishnan KRR: The dexamethasone suppression test as a biologic marker of depression in chronic pain. *Pain* 21:49–55, 1985.
107. Atkinson JH, Kremer EF, Risch SC, Janowsky DS: Pre- and post-dexamethasone cortisol and prolactin concentrations in patients with chronic pain syndromes. *Pain* 25:23–34, 1986.
108. Sheehan DV, Claycomb JB, Kouretas N: Monoamine oxidase inhibitors: Prescription and patient management. *Int J Psychiatr Med* 10:99–121, 1981.
109. Yeh SY, Mitchell CL: Potentiation and reduction of the analgesia of morphine in the rat by pargyline. *J Pharmacol Exp Ther* 179:642–651, 1971.
110. Palmer H: Potentiation of pethidine. *Br Med J* 2:944, 1960.
111. Shee JC: Dangerous potentiation of pethidine by iproniazid and its treatment. *Br Med J* 2:507–509, 1960.
112. Rivers N, Hornes P: Possible lethal reaction between

nardil and dextromorphan. *Can Med Assoc J* 103:85, 1970.
113. Roger KJ: Role of brain monoamines in the interaction between pethidine and tranylcypromine. *Eur J Pharmacol* 14:86–88, 1971.
114. Domino E, Sullivan TS, Luby ED: Barbiturate intoxication in a patient treated with a MAO inhibitor. *Am J Psychiatry* 118:941–943, 1962.
115. Taylor MA, Sierles FS, Abrams R: *General Hospital Psychiatry*. New York, The Free Press, 1985.
116. Monks R, Merskey H: Psychotropic drugs. In Wall PD, Melzack RD (eds): *Textbook of Pain*. London, Churchill Livingstone, 1984, pp 526–537.
117. Marks J: Benzodiazepines—for good or evil. *Neuropsychobiology* 10:115–126, 1983.
118. Hollister LE: Principles of therapeutic applications of benzodiazepines. In Smith DE, Wesson DR (eds): *The Benzodiazepines. Current Standards for Medical Practice*. Lancaster, England, MTP Press Limited, 1985, pp 87–96.
119. Rickels K, Case WG, Diamond L: Issues in long-term treatment with diazepam therapy. *Psychopharmacol Bull* 18:38–41, 1982.
120. Johnstone M: The effects of methylphenidate on postoperative pain and vasoconstriction. *Br J Anaesth* 46:778–783, 1974.

Section 5
PSYCHOLOGICAL THERAPIES

Chapter 16

BEHAVIORAL MANAGEMENT

DANIEL M. DOLEYS, PhD
KIMBERLY S. GOCHNEAUR, BA

This chapter attempts to trace the "natural history" of the development of chronic low back pain from a behavioral perspective. Emphasis is given to identifying the key situations and factors that may directly influence the development and rehabilitation of functional disability. The term "functional disability," in this case, relates to alterations in normal life-style and behavioral patterns that cannot be accounted for on the basis of the physical pathology present, or is disproportionate to what would be expected. Such patterns as chronic use of narcotics, nonparticipation in gainful employment and/or activities of daily living, disrupted interpersonal relationships, excessive use of the medical community, and dependency upon treatment and assistive devices are included.

The essence of the behavioral approach to chronic pain has been described by Fordyce (1). The term "behavioral" refers to a reliance on experimentally derived principles of conditioning and learning to account for and alter human behavior. It also refers to a philosophy committed to a functional analysis of behavior using scientific methodology. Behavior is assumed to be lawfully related to identifiable antecedents and consequences, whether overt or covert, rather than presumed "psychic structures" or unconscious mechanisms. In many ways a behavioral approach focuses on acceptance of the possibility of iatrogenic pain; that is, the activity of the treating professional can be functionally related to the development and maintenance of chronic pain behavior. Therefore, any analysis of the chronic low back pain syndrome must include the treatment community and not just the patient. Too often, the patient is held totally accountable for his/her behavior, whether we appeal to conscious or unconscious motivation, while those in the position of

influence, such as professionals, family, and insurance companies, are exonerated from responsibility.

In this chapter we attempt to look at the etiology of chronic low back pain syndrome or behavior by examining the critical periods when the patient's behavior is most susceptible to modification (Fig. 16.1). Various principles likely to be involved are discussed. Obviously, the biggest source of data is naturalistic observation, and to some degree animal modes of behavior.

PREINJURY

Much to do has been made about the "pain-prone personality" (c.f. refs. 2, 3). It is quite apparent that not everyone who is injured develops chronic pain. In fact, about 85% of patients with back injuries return to normal functioning within weeks (4). Almost by definition, the problem is not the injury per se, but the patient's "reaction" to the injury. It is frequently noted that the "pain behavior is out of proportion to the physical finding." Why? It must be kept in mind that injury happens to people with a given behavioral and biologic history. This history may set the occasion for the response. Some have encountered pain in the past, such as athletes, and then shaped to cope and conquer. Such statements as "no pain, no gain" abound in sports. Peer pressure and reinforcement to play while hurt can force the development of cognitive coping strategies for managing pain. On the other hand, some persons have received a good deal of attention or time-out from undesirable tasks because of pain. Cultural differences (5, 6) have been documented in response to pain. Work in the area of childhood pain (7) will certainly help to elucidate the role of early experi-

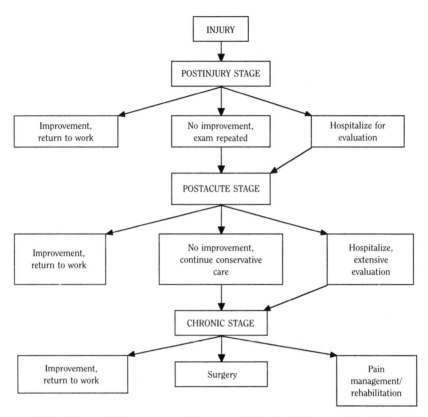

Figure 16.1. The possible outcomes of the stages following injury resulting in low back pain.

ence. The psychological literature often refers to the "meaning of the pain" to the patient. This meaning may well be established in the patient's reinforcement history.

The work of Melzack and Wall (8) has given us an appreciation for the biologic complexity of pain. Certainly, as with many biologic mechanisms, some people have a lower threshold of nociception. Their own genetic makeup renders them more hypersensitive. Therefore, the initial stimulus event (the nociceptive input following injury) may be quantitatively different, resulting in what would appear to be an abnormal response to the injury.

To label individuals with such behavioral or genetic histories as "pain prone" all but implies conscious control over such factors. Almost instantly such patients have the authenticity of their pain questioned and are held up to be "crocks" or malingerers. These terms have no diagnostic or treatment value. They do, however, form the basis for how others will respond to the patient and the patient's attitude toward his/her problem and rehabilitation.

POSTINJURY STAGE

It has been said that the largest problem faced is the overtreatment of chronic pain, and that the most frequent cause is the undertreatment of acute pain. The initial management of the injured patient may set the stage for the development of chronic low back pain syndrome. A caring attitude and thorough examination can be reassuring to the patient. Many chronic pain patients, in discussing their initial interactions, are quick to note how brief the exam was, that it was carried out by a "company doctor" and in a rather unprofessional manner. On the surface, it is easy to discount these comments by appealing to the patient's personality. Yet, we must be careful about exonerating ourselves from all responsibility and thereby ignoring an opportunity to prevent a potential problem from occurring.

Chronic pain obviously begins with some injury or acute pain. This results in the patient receiving some type of examination. The examination presents the first choice point at which the patient can be treated in a fashion that will either resolve the problem or encourage the development of chronic pain. Addison (9) has very eloquently outlined various procedures and considerations in examining the patient with low back pain. The use of as-needed medications and time-contingent rest and activity, along with such rule-governed behavior as "if it hurts, don't do it," promotes the development 56 behavioral patterns inextricably tied to the person's experience of pain and the necessity of moment-to-moment assessment of pain. The alternative strategy is fixed-time treatment, which emphasizes fixed-time delivery of medications, rest, and exercise. Medications, rest, and exercise are not based on the patient's experience of pain but upon our knowledge of the pharmacology of the medication and the natural healing process of the injury. A thorough explanation of the problem, along with reassurance as to the expected time course of recovery and acknowledgment that there may be some continuation of pain but activity will not produce any harm, helps to establish more positive expectations for the ultimate outcome.

A paper by Fordyce and coworkers (10) examined the effects of these two different approaches to the treatment of recent-onset back pain. In a random design, patients in treatment A received the traditional approach consisting of as-needed medications, with medication refills left open and/or based upon negotiation between the patient and physician. The medications for group B were prescribed to be taken at a fixed time of day and for a predetermined number of days based upon the estimated healing time. Activity limits for the two groups were also handled differently. Group A patients were placed on bed rest except to go to the bathroom, and they were told to let their pain dictate how much they did or did not do. Group B was given a specific period of time for limitation of their activities and told to then resume general day-to-day activity. Instructions for exercise were similar; group A was not given a specific time to begin exercising. Furthermore, the number of repetitions and rate of increase was left up to the patient based upon his/her subjective tolerance level and pain. Group B, however, was given a specific time to begin exercising. The number of repetitions and rate of increase was prescribed by the physician. In essence, the patients in group A were allowed, and indeed forced, to make their own determination of healing time and progress. The patients in group B had this ambiguity and uncertainty removed by virtue of the manner in which their medications, general activity level, and exercise level were prescribed.

The dependent measures included scores on a sick/well scale, vocational status, health care utilization, claimed impairment, and pain. The results indicated that the two groups were comparable in level of functioning at 6 weeks after their initial visit. However, at 9–12 months follow-up group A consistently showed more sickness and pain-oriented scores than did group B. Of particular interest are the data related to "claimed impairment." The patients in group A endorsed many more items indicating the presence of impairment due to their injury at the 9–12-month follow-up than did those in group B. Because the two groups were comparable regarding such characteristics as severity of injury, this outcome would seem to be a result of the type of intervention. These results appear to mimic an all-too-common observation, that is, patients with similar injuries reporting dramatically different outcomes. This project by Fordyce et al. clearly implicates the initial intervention for acute pain as a significant factor in the development of chronic low back pain syndrome.

This picture is further complicated by the negative effects of prolonged rest on various body systems (11) and the development of pain behavior (12). Sustained bed rest for even a few days can bring about physiologic changes significant enough to make activity more difficult and painful. Unless patients are made aware of this and placed on a fixed activity and exercise schedule, they may well interpret the physiologic cues associated with rest and muscular misuse as symptoms related to their recent injury, and continue to limit their activity until healing is complete. This preoccupation with nociception affects the patient's activity and perceived pain. Sustained use of various medications and uncertainty as to the course of recovery are present. This is the stuff of which chronic pain behavior is made.

The initial physical examination can be followed by one of three outcomes. The first is that the patient gets better and returns to work without sequelae. The second outcome is that the patient's problem does not resolve as expected and the examination process is repeated. The difficulties here are generated by the implication that the problem is "more serious than what was first thought," creating the notion in the patient's mind that the initial assessment was inadequate and that continuation of pain can be a signal for some unidentified pathology. The opportunity for positively reinforcing and therefore encouraging pain behaviors is also present here. Continuation of pain-contingent activities, medications, and the like in the absence of any identifiable pathology to account for this helps to establish the onset of chronic pain syndrome. Every attempt should be made to explain why the expected course of recovery was not observed. If the patient was initially on as-needed treatment, this should be modified to a fixed-time protocol.

The third outcome following the initial examination is hospitalization for evaluation. This presents many messages to the patient. The first is that he/she cannot trust the physician's initial examination or the physician who initially examined him/her. It implies that something has been missed. It also sets the occasion for pain behavior such as bed rest, inactivity, and medication seeking to be reinforced. If hospitalization is necessary, a complete and thorough evaluation should be undertaken so that no stones will remain unturned. This might include a bone scan, electromyogram, x-ray, computed tomography scan, myelogram, and/or magnetic resonance imaging. If a nonsurgical lesion, such as a bulging disk, is identified, the patient should be given a complete explanation of what this means and that it might be a contributing factor to the problem but is not a surgical problem. All too often the patient is told that nothing can be found, only to have someone else later notify the patient that in fact there is a bulging disk. Whether or not the bulge is relevant to the patient's complaint is immaterial. The fact remains that the patient perceives that information has been withheld. This is often the time when legal and clinical judgments may be at cross-purposes. Perhaps, from a clinical perspective, extensive invasive study need not be carried out, yet for the purpose of clarifying the problem and minimizing legal entanglements, either through the patient's feeling the need to get legal representation or concerns on the physician's part of mismanagement of the patient, studies may need to be carried out.

If a repeat of the examination process is carried out on an outpatient basis and/or the patient is hospitalized, detailed feedback should be provided not only to the patient but to the spouse, significant others, lawyer, workers' compensation representative, and others. Discriminatory distribution of information only leads to confusion and mistrust that may trigger the onset of more pain behaviors. A reasonable course of action should be identified. For example, if there are muscular or mechanical contributions to the pain, therapy or rehabilitation should be recommended so that the patient has a sense that something positive is being done rather than merely distributing medications and being sent back home. If organic pathology is identified,

but is not surgical in nature, this should be explained carefully. If surgery is indicated, it should be described to the patient and the projected course of recovery outlined. Personality testing may be helpful here to identify those candidates who are at risk for continued pain and disability because of their personality styles. The need for this should be explained by the attending physician, rather than simply having a psychological consultant appear without any forewarning given to the patient.

The next level of decision making where problems can emerge is the choice between return to work, rehabilitation program, or surgery. Return to work should be preceded by some reconditioning, while recognizing the fact that even 3–5 days of bed rest for a person whose job is their main source of physical conditioning can result in deterioration of endurance and strength (11), thereby predisposing the patient to "reinjury." A gradual reintroduction to the work force involving a short work week or half-days for a brief period of time is preferable. Clear communication is required as to what can be expected from the patient. The employer should make every effort to clear the way for return to employment and discourage supervisors from "hassling" the patient regarding time off or the nature of the injury.

The inescapable conclusion is that our response in the treatment of acute pain may in fact be the difference between the injured individual returning to a full productive life or developing a chronic pain syndrome. The use of time-contingent rest, exercise, and medications, along with a thorough examination, explanation, and reassurance, is preferable to an "as-needed" approach to acute pain.

POSTACUTE STAGE

The postacute stage is the period of time after the initial treatment regimen for the acute trauma has expired. In general, one of three tracks is taken. In the first, the individual has recovered from the injury and returns to work and normal day-to-day duties. In the second, the pain and/or underlying organic pathology persist and the patient continues to be treated in a conservative fashion. In the third, the patient is admitted to the hospital for more extensive studies.

The first alternative, of course, poses no problems. This in fact appears to happen to the vast majority of injured individuals. Unfortunately, it is not attended to in many cases by the employer and insurance company. It is the authors' belief that some type of bonus should be provided for those individuals who undergo a rather significant work-related injury and who, by virtue of their own motivation and energy, overcome the effects of the injury and return to work in a reasonable period of time. An example is that of a female patient seen by the first author who, after working for some 20 years in a clothing factory, had her hands caught in a cutting device. This accident resulted in the amputation of part or all of seven fingers. This remarkable lady, in spite of what appeared to be minimal follow-up care after the initial surgeries, rehabilitated herself through extensive exercise at home and was back on the job within 4 months. She was working in spite of her rather significant pain, which turned out to be a reflex sympathetic dystrophy relieved by sympathectomy. Following return to work she missed no days because of pain. She denied any consideration of disability either from the company or social security and never once contacted a lawyer. Her single goal was to resume to as normal functioning as possible and return to work. It seems as though this is the type of behavior that needs to be strongly reinforced. This lady easily could have sought damages and probably obtained permanent disability. Her own approach to the problem saved the company untold thousands of dollars. It might have been an appropriate response for the company to provide this worker with a substantial bonus for her rapid recovery and return to productive work. Instead, it appears to have gone unnoticed.

A second track in the postacute stage is continued conservative treatment. This may engender the production of chronic pain syndrome via the patient beginning to believe that the problem was more serious than was initially indicated. Health care professionals must be specific in explaining the continuation of conservative treatment and why the patient's recovery has not proceeded as initially expected. Patients become highly anxious and concerned at this point as to the "real nature" of their problem and the competence of the people treating them. An abrupt and cavalier attitude by the practitioners further reinforces this concern and may stimulate the patient to engage in maladaptive alternatives in the treatment regimen. These alternatives can be observed as inappropriate use of medication, self-initiation of the use of assistive devices, "doctor shopping," and the like. Oftentimes it is during this stage, and in the presence of an uncertain attitude, that legal consultation is sought, which may further reinforce the chronic pain pattern. The health care community must commit the

necessary time to communicating an effective explanation for the nature of the problem and, if conservative treatment is continued, be sure that the above-mentioned fixed-time regimen is employed.

The third track, admission to the hospital for further diagnostic study, needs to be introduced to the patient carefully. Some patients interpret this as an indication that the initial evaluation was not extensive and thorough and that the physician cannot be trusted. They may also see this as an indication that something has been missed. Hospitalizing patients can, for some, reinforce their pain behaviors and afford them the opportunity to have time-out from undesirable activities, and to obtain narcotic medication. A complete explanation as to the rationale for hospitalization, what will be done, why it will be done, and the expected outcome should be given. If medications, especially narcotics, are to be utilized they should be presented on a time-contingent basis rather than as needed and be given because the condition appears to warrant it rather than merely based upon the patient's complaints. The workup should be comprehensive so that all questions regarding the organic pathology of the problem can be answered. All attempts should be made to avoid doing only the minimal studies and therefore running the risk of having to rehospitalize the patient for additional workups at a later point.

Again, inadequate explanation of findings and how they may or may not relate to the patient's complaints can foster suspiciousness, insecurity, anxiety, and other emotional/behavioral states associated with the chronic pain syndrome. If, by this time, rehabilitation specialists, workers' compensation representatives, and lawyers are involved they should be included as much as possible in the feedback. Presenting the information to everyone at one time can substantially reduce misunderstanding and misinterpretation. Taking the time to obtain psychosocial data and psychometric testing can be of value. It can be presented to the patient as a mechanism for assessing the effects of their pain or their coping ability rather than a means of trying to determine if their pain is "real" or as a mechanism of claiming it all to be mental or psychiatric.

All too often patients are merely advised that they have "no surgical lesion" and are discharged. A review of the report and an explanation as to the possible nonsurgical components, including muscular/mechanical deviations or ligament irritation, can be helpful. A prescribed regiment of outpatient therapy utilizing the principles of fixed-time scheduling should be outlined to the patient. An exploration of the physical demands of the job and how, if in any way, the problem could interfere with job performance is vital.

During the hospital stay confinement to the room may significantly reduce the amount of stimulation the patient is accustomed to and can be a factor in the perception of pain and demand for narcotics (13). If the patient's condition allows, he/she should be involved in as many activities as would be appropriate during the stay in the hospital. It is often the case that the initial hospital visit, incorporating as-needed injectable narcotics, stimulates drug-seeking behavior. Patients are maintained on powerful narcotics during their hospital stay and then upon discharge these drugs are abruptly discontinued and the patient sent home to cope on his/her own. A gradual reduction of drugs would seem to be preferable. This would prolong a hospital stay by a few days but may well avoid the additional expense of medications and rehospitalization.

CHRONIC STAGE

One of three outcomes will be present at this time. First, the problem will have resolved and the patient returned to work or preinjury activities. Second, an identifiable organic lesion will lead to the patient having surgery. Third, the patient will enter some type of pain management/rehabilitation program.

If the patient returns to daily activities and the problem appears to have resolved, consideration should be given to the patient participating in preventative activities. Recurrent pain, especially if there has been some history of problems, may signal a need to adjust the demands of the patient's job or to improve the patient's overall physical conditioning. Job site visits by trained individuals may identify activities that place the patient in danger of reinjury. Many patients have little or no exercise other than their jobs, and with advancing age become vulnerable to reinjury. Enrollment in an exercise program or "back school" may eliminate future problems and give the patient the confidence needed to return to normal activities without fear of reinjury. Without this approach, patients may begin to anticipate reinjury and become overly cautious, engaging in muscle splinting and guarding that could, in fact, lead to reinjury. Depending upon how long the patient has been out of work, a

gradual return combined with a "work hardening" program may be appropriate.

For those patients who ultimately go to surgery, a complete explanation as to the nature of the surgery and expected outcome should be provided. Patients need to understand the difference between operating on a physical defect versus operating on pain. Patients oftentimes expect that the surgery will totally relieve their pain and are disheartened when it does not. Explanation of expected postoperative recovery and the use of fixed-time treatment protocols can be beneficial. Screening the patient for behavioral/psychological dysfunction may alert the treatment team to the presence of a potential problem. There appear to be certain personality types that may not respond to treatment, including surgery (c.f. ref. 2).

Many patients have a distorted view of what gets done in surgery. The use of terms such as "laminectomy," "hemilaminectomy," "discectomy," and "fusion" may conjure up all types of exaggerated responses. The use of diagrams, pictures, and plastic models to demonstrate what is being done and why may substantially improve the response to surgery. Providing adequate postoperative pain relief with a predetermined adjustment schedule will help to avoid the development of drug dependency. Activity avoidance and anticipatory pain are less likely to happen if the patient can be started in a program of gradually increasing activity as soon as possible following the immediate postoperative recovery. Simply allowing patients to identify their own physical recovery through "as-needed" activities and medications can result in many of the problems identified above.

Once reasonable medical assessments and treatments have been carried out for resolution of the problem, prompt referral to a pain management/ rehabilitation program should be considered. The longer a patient lingers in pain the more recalcitrant the problem becomes. Patients who have experienced their problems for 6 months or more are less likely to return to work than those who are effectively managed in the first 6 months. Prolonged inactivity becomes reinforcing, and develops into the mainstay of the person's life-style. Reinforcement of disability behaviors such as prolonged "down-time" becomes inevitable. Lack of improvement in the absence of any identifiable organic pathology can lead to argumentative situations between the patient and the treating physician. It is often at this point that the patient may experience the need to validate the authenticity of his/her complaints and begin seeking unconventional treatment or overusing medications.

Oftentimes referral to a pain management or rehabilitation program is delayed until all other options have failed. Unfortunately, repeated treatment failures serve only to reinforce the patient's notion that the problem is untreatable. Patients then become willing to take part in almost any therapy recommended but do not anticipate benefit. Early referral may substantially increase the likelihood of success.

Pain management and rehabilitation programs should be interdisciplinary in nature. This is considerably different from a multidisciplinary approach where many disciplines are involved but there is no orchestration of treatment, and communication between the disciplines may be marginal at best (14). No single behavioral treatment model has emerged as being the most efficacious. Treatment times seem to vary from 3 to 6 weeks or longer. Some facilities use an inpatient setting while others are strictly outpatient and still others have motel facilities. Some programs, especially those generally labeled as work hardening, only emphasize the physical conditioning aspects of treatment without attending to the overall issue of the pain problem.

PAIN MANAGEMENT AND REHABILITATION THERAPY

Although there is considerable variability among behaviorally oriented pain management and treatment rehabilitation programs, there are some common features. The early work of Fordyce (1) and the extensive investigation of Keefe and his colleagues (15, 16) has pointed out the importance of modifying "pain behavior." These pain behaviors may include such activities as bracing, posturing, limping, sighing, and the reliance upon unnecessary assistive devices. The use of an exercise quota system emphasizing a gradual increase in activity (17) is well accepted. This model seems to effect changes through a gradual desensitization to activity. It also encourages the patient to focus attention on what he/she is doing rather than on nociceptive input. The work of Turk and Rudy (18) pointed out the importance of modifying cognitive behavior. The emphasis is on altering self-talk, attitudes, expectancies, and attributions (19). The use of relaxation/meditation/biofeedback therapies is commonly incorporated. These techniques may provide a means of pain control, reduction of muscular hyperreactivity, and anxiety management. A specific mechanism by which the effects are obtained is unclear, but patients do report procedures to be beneficial (20).

Medications are managed by the use of a fixed-time schedule and may be masked in some type of cocktail. This type of scheduling helps to avoid medication-seeking behavior and can be an effective procedure for detoxification. Education of the patient and significant others as to the biologic, psychological, and sociologic components of pain and disability is undertaken. Treatment is initiated by a thorough evaluation of the patient's situation and most effectively carried out within an interdisciplinary model. When possible, work stimulation can be used to help promote generalization of treatment effects. The chronic low back pain patient entering a pain management/rehabilitation setting often poses significant management problems.

Issues of secondary gain, medication dependence, physical condition and disability, marital conflict, and somatic preoccupation are constantly present. Effective management of these difficulties requires a dedicated and knowledgeable staff. Many chronic pain patients are quite resistant to treatment. The rate of reinforcement to staff members is therefore very low. Burnout can manifest itself in complacency and ambivalence, which further antagonizes the situation. Program directors must focus as much on use of behavioral principles to maintain staff motivation and satisfaction with work as on providing an efficient program for the patients.

Generalization of treatment effects beyond the treatment setting has caused great concern. Our own experience has indicated increased probability of patients relapsing to pretreatment behavioral patterns between 3 and 6 months after discharge. There is some suggestion that the expectations of the patient as to ability to function at an improved level and how or to what he/she attributes this improvement may correlate highly with long-term outcome (19). Those patients who, even though they are functioning at a much-improved level, report continued fear, worry, and concern about the future do not do as well after treatment. Similarly, patients who tend to attribute their success to the treatment environment rather than to their own initiative and skill acquisition, tend to have a poor prognosis. It is obvious that the level of positive reinforcement for appropriate behavior will be substantially higher in the treatment setting than in the natural environment. This fact alone may account for the changes. This further emphasizes the need to involve significant others in the treatment program and to utilize work simulation and outings in the natural environment as much as possible.

BEHAVIORAL CONCEPTS

There are a number of key behavioral concepts and principles frequently invoked in the management of chronic low back pain patients. These include positive reinforcement, extinction, extinction burst, stimulus control, differential reinforcement of other behaviors, desensitization, and contingency contracting.

The principle of *positive reinforcement* specifies that any behavior followed by a desirable consequence will increase in frequency. An aspect of this principle that is often overlooked is that the consequence must be positive to the patient and not simply something that is thought to be positive by the careful observer. Without being able to systematically manipulate consequences and observe the effects upon the individual's behavior, it is oftentimes hard to determine if a particular consequence may in fact be positive or not. Unfortunately, many chronic pain patients receiving workers' compensation are assumed to be manifesting their disability behavior for the purpose of financial gain. There are, undoubtedly, cases where this has occurred, and once financial compensation has been resolved the patient improves. It is inappropriate, however, to generalize from a limited number of cases to the population at large. In fact, there are data that show that patients who are receiving compensation do not necessarily respond differentially to treatment (21). In addition, there may be many other characteristics of the workers' compensation patient that can account for his/her behavior that have nothing to do with financial gain. To automatically discount all other possibilities and to label these patients as having "compensation neurosis" intensifies the already adversarial environment.

If chronic pain behavior is maintained by attention and positive reinforcement, it seems logical that withdrawing such reinforcement will eliminate the behavior. This process of removal of positive reinforcement from a specific class of behaviors is referred to as *extinction*. There are two difficulties in attempting to implement this approach to the patient. First, there frequently are multiple sources of reinforcement, including family, friends, peers, avoidance of unpleasurable activities, and the like.

For extinction to work, most, if not all of these sources of reinforcement must be removed. Otherwise, the individual's behavior will merely come under the control of those remaining sources of reinforcement. Therefore, what the patient actually learns is not a new set of behaviors, but where to go to obtain the desirable consequences. A second aspect of extinction that is not frequently attended to is what is referred to as *extinction bursts*. Withdrawal of positive reinforcement for a particular behavior is often associated with a temporary increase in that behavior. This increase may also be associated with various maladaptive behaviors and acting out. This is easily observed in animals and children, who demonstrate a variety of maladaptive behaviors when a frequently reinforced event is suddenly placed on extinction. It may be for this reason that patients in a controlled environment pose such a management problem if pain behavior is no longer reinforced.

One possible solution to the above difficulties is the application of *differential reinforcement*. If the intent of therapy is to replace one set of behaviors with another, individuals must be taught and reinforced for demonstrating the appropriate behaviors. All too often, unfortunately, appropriate behavior on the part of the pain patient is ignored. Treatment programs unwittingly adopt a policy of "let sleeping dogs lie" or "don't rock the boat." Others look upon this change of behavior as the pain patient finally behaving in a way that he/she should and therefore do not provide any particular reinforcement. In fact, when patients with chronic back pain begin to demonstrate appropriate behavior, such as increased activity tolerance or reduction in complaining behavior, at this point the staff is obliged to provide positive feedback and help to reestablish these more adaptive behaviors as part of the patient's repertoire.

It is obvious that many chronic low back pain patients engage in "anticipatory pain" and activity avoidance. An article by Fordyce and colleagues (22) demonstrated a case study showing the procedures for reducing activity avoidance. There appear to be a number of parallels between the behaviors shown by chronic pain patients and those of patients with anxiety or phobic disorders. In both cases, there is a good deal of anticipation of and apprehension about negative consequences. Undesirable outcomes are expected long before the behaviors are even demonstrated (23). Certain situations become associated with pain or anxiety and, through the process of conditioning, also become associated with undesirable physical and psychological symptoms. Patients engage in a variety of behaviors in an attempt to avoid the anxiety-provoking, or in this case pain-provoking, circumstances. The anticipation of pain may be associated with increased perception and responsiveness to nociceptive input and heightened muscular activity that may make general activity more difficult and painful.

Many phobic and anxiety states can be effectively treated through a process of systematic *desensitization* and graduated in vivo exposure. In this model, situations are ranked in terms of the degree to which they are associated with anxiety. The patient is then exposed to those that are least anxiety provoking and gradually advanced to those more anxiety provoking. It is possible that the use of this system accomplishes a similar purpose for the pain patient. The model would suggest that patients' rehabilitation should be initiated by jointly establishing physical goals that are easily achievable. The demand should then be gradually accelerated, with success being followed by positive reinforcement. *Contingency contracting* can be a mechanism for orchestrating these treatment goals and outcomes. A contingency contract is an agreement arrived at through negotiations between the treatment staff and patient. It specifies what behavior will be required to produce a given consequence. Too often health care professionals dictate therapy goals, failing to realize that unless the goals are relevant or important to the patient, commitment to treatment will be minimal.

LONG-TERM MEDICATION USE

The controversy over long-term medications for chronic noncancer low back pain patients continues. Portenoy and Foley (24) described 38 patients who had been maintained on a constant level of narcotic intake for several years without apparent indication of tolerance. Others would argue that providing narcotic medications serves only to reinforce the pain and disability pattern and may encourage the patient not to utilize other pain-control strategies. The issue seems somewhat more complicated when considering the broad variety of medical conditions encountered in the chronic low back pain patient. Some patients have a virgin back and little or no evidence of any pathology, including musculoskeletal dysfunction. Others have had multiple surgeries, which may include multilevel fusions and neurodestructive procedures. Scarring and arachnoiditis may be in evidence. While the

specific contribution that these abnormalities make to the experience of pain may be in question, the presence of the pathology is clearly evident.

The problem becomes even more clouded by realizing that the patients may turn to other substitutes. Abuse of over-the-counter preparations, prescription narcotics, and alcohol are found with regularity in our population. For example, one patient reported taking four to five Robaxin at a time, up to 30 per day. Another was consuming three to five Extra-Strength Tylenol at one time with a total of 30 per day. Yet anther patient who had no history of drug or alcohol abuse was regularly consuming one-half or more of a fifth of liquor per night in an attempt to quell the pain and obtain a few hours of rest. While the possibility of misuse of prescription or nonprescription drugs should not be the determining factor for providing prescription narcotics, the awareness of this possibility and potential for harm to the patient must be acknowledged.

In our view, it may be possible to approach the issue of long-term prescription drug use from a behavioral perspective. Setting up criteria that ensure improved functioning and nonabuse of a substance seems to merit consideration. We have employed three specific criteria with patients who are receiving medications on a chronic basis. First, the medications must in fact be associated with a reduction in self-reported pain. Second, the medication used must be associated with improved functioning and allow the patient to carry out more normal daily activities and work activities. Third, medications must be taken as prescribed, and there should be no evidence of physical tolerance as might be suggested by increased drug-seeking behavior, presence of withdrawal symptoms upon discontinuation of the drug, and/or reduced effectiveness.

SUMMARY

It is hoped that this chapter has met its initial goals and objectives: to help to identify stages in the management of the injured patient that can set the occasion for the development of the chronic pain syndrome. There are obviously a number of individuals who, for a variety of reasons, are more likely to develop chronic pain and are more susceptible to the nuances of early management than others. Our options seem to be limited: (a) accept the notion that a given percentage of injured patients will go on to develop chronic problems, and

(b) take whatever steps are necessary in the management of these patients to help reduce the frequency and severity of the problem. Following through with the various recommendations may in fact be time consuming. However, the potential long-term savings would seem to warrant the effort.

REFERENCES

1. Fordyce WE: *Behavioral Methods for Chronic Pain and Illness*. St. Louis, CV Mosby, 1976.
2. Bradley LA: Assessing the psychological profile of the chronic pain patient. In Dubner R, Gebhart GF, Bond MR (eds): *Proceedings of the Vth World Congress on Pain: Pain Research and Clinical Management*. New York, Elsevier, 1988, vol 3, pp 251–262.
3. Love AW, Peck CL: The MMPI and psychological factors in chronic low back pain: a review. *Pain* 28:1–12, 1987.
4. Andersson G, Svensson H, Anders O: The intensity of work recovery in low back pain. *Spine* 8:880–885, 1983.
5. Sternbach RA, Tursky B: Ethnic differences among housewives in psychophysical and skin potential responses to electric shock. *Psychophysiology* 1:241–246, 1965.
6. Tursky B, Sternbach RA: Further physiological correlates of ethnic differences in responses to shock. *Psychophysiology* 4:67–74, 1967.
7. Elliott CH, Jay SM: Chronic pain in children. *Behav Res Ther* 25:263–271, 1987.
8. Melzack R, Wall PD: *The Challenge of Pain*. New York, Basic Books, 1973.
9. Addison RG: Chronic low back pain (CLO-BAP). *Clin J Pain* 1:50–59, 1985.
10. Fordyce WE, Brockway J, Bergman J, Spengler D: A control group comparison of behavioral vs. traditional management methods in acute low back pain. 5:127–140, 1986.
11. Bortz W: The disuse syndrome (commentary). *West J Med* 141:691–694, 1984.
12. Fordyce WE: Pain and suffering: a reappraisal. *Am Psychol* 43:276–283, 1988.
13. Dolce JJ, Doleys DM, Raczynski JM, Crocker M: Narcotic utilization for back pain patients housed in private and semi-private rooms. *Addict Behav* 10:91–95, 1985.
14. Turk DC, Stieg RL: Chronic pain: the necessity of interdisciplinary communication. *Clin J Pain* 3:163–167, 1987.
15. Keefe FJ, Bradley LA: Behavioral and psychological approaches to the assessment and treatment of chronic pain. *Gen Hosp Psychiatry* 6:49–54, 1984.
16. Keefe FJ, Wilkins RH, Cook WA Jr, Crisson, J.E. Muhlbaier LH: Depression, pain and pain behavior. *J Consult Clin Psychol* 54:665–669, 1986.
17. Doleys DM, Crocker MF, Patton D: Response of patients with chronic pain to exercise quotas. *Phys Ther* 62:1111–1114, 1982.
18. Turk DC, Rudy TE: Assessment of cognitive factors in chronic pain: a worthwhile enterprise? *J Consult Clin Psychol* 54:760–768, 1986.
19. Dolce JJ: Self-efficacy and disability beliefs in behavioral treatment of pain. *Behav Res Ther* 25:289–299, 1987.
20. Mizes JS, Doleys DM, Dolce JJ: The psychophysiological effects of the relaxation component of a comprehensive pain program: a clinical descriptive study. *Clin J Pain* 2:87–92, 1986.
21. Jamison RN, Matt DA, Parris WCV: Effects of time limited versus unlimited compensation on pain behavior and treatment outcome in low back pain patients. *J Psychosom Res* (in press).
22. Fordyce WE, Shelton JL, Dundore DE: The modification of avoidance learning pain behaviors. *J Behav Med* 5:405–414, 1982.
23. Philips HC: Avoidance behaviour and its role in sustaining chronic pain. *Behav Res Ther* 25:273–279, 1987.
24. Portenoy RK, Foley KM: Chronic use of opioid analgesics in non-malignant pain: report of 38 cases. *Pain* 25:171–186, 1986.

Chapter 17

GROUP THERAPY

W. DOYLE GENTRY, PhD
W. DAVID CREWS, Jr, MS

While a variety of individual therapies, such as relaxation training, biofeedback, operant conditioning, hypnosis, and cognitive restructuring, have been applied to persons suffering with chronic back pain and have been well researched as regards their relative efficacy in ameliorating pain and accompanying emotional distress (1, 2), little systematic attention has been given to the role of group therapy in helping chronic pain patients make a healthier adaptation to their burdensome pain experience. In fact, the introduction of group therapy as a "treatment of choice" with such patients, along with the similar use of family therapy (3; see Chapter 18), suggests a beginning shift away from a model of "psychological individualism" (4) toward a more "social context" model of understanding and treating patients in chronic pain.

In this chapter, we will review the existing literature dealing with the use of pain groups, as well as recap our own experience over the past 5 years using this technique (5). In so doing, we will address such issues as: (a) rationale for choosing group therapy as a primary treatment modality; (b) so-called how-to-do-it mechanics of pain groups; (c) our thoughts about the therapist role(s) in group therapy, especially as it differs from that typically perceived in more individual therapies; (d) therapeutic themes and "point(s) of focus" addressed within the pain groups; and (e) outcome.

RATIONALE

There are two broad categories of rationale for viewing group therapy as a treatment of choice for persons suffering from intractable pain and disability: (a) economic use of therapeutic resources and (b) patient need and perspective.

Because chronic pain patients tend to present a spectrum of all-too-common problems (e.g., mood disturbance, addiction, conflict over dependency-independency issues), despite their rather individualized efforts to cope with their pain experience they tend to require similar advice, education, counseling, and therapeutic confrontation. Pain groups thus, to a large extent, eliminate therapist redundancy and provide for a more economical use of therapeutic resources (therapist time and energy). In effect, while the pain patients themselves are viewed as a heterogeneous population, the problems they present are seen as homogeneous. As Sternbach (6) noted, the so-called pain games in which these patients unwittingly become involved are indeed few in number compared to the large and growing number of persons playing them. Particularly in an outpatient, private practice setting, where typically the therapist functions solo or without large numbers of support staff, pain groups would allow for a greater degree of ongoing therapeutic contact, in terms of either number of patients seen or amount of time with any given patient, than would be possible with most individual treatment strategies. Since chronic pain, especially back pain, is epidemic in our society (7), we believe this is an important consideration.

Pain groups also provide the therapist with a somewhat different diagnostic perspective, apart from the standard psychometric approach (Minnesota Multiphasic Personality Inventory; MMPI) and historical review common to individual treatment strategies, that is, an opportunity to witness the chronic pain patient's behavior within the real-life social context of the group. This, of course, provides much needed validation of the patient's self-reported coping patterns and offers new "grist for the mill" for individual therapy with these same patients. We have frequently found that involvement in a pain group often decreases patient resistance in individual psychotherapy and thereby accelerates progress in the latter; for example, patients are more willing to open up and identify painful feelings and areas of concern previously hidden beneath their "pain talk."

From the standpoint of patient need and perspective, there are a number of important considerations. First, and perhaps most important, chronic pain patients tend to perceive their struggle with pain as an individual one rather than one common to millions of other Americans (7), a perspective than goes basically unchallenged if they are treated as individuals. This, of course, largely accounts for their abiding sense of social alienation, noted earlier by Timmermans and Sternbach (8) as one of the core psychological characteristics of persons suffering from chronic pain. Pain groups obviously provide a new, rich source of social support that competes with this sense of isolation and alienation. Involvement in group therapy also allows patients an opportunity to define a new reference group (other pain patients) and engage in what we have referred to as lateral versus vertical conformity (5), the second major reason for utilizing pain groups. That is, chronic pain patients are exposed to social pressures from other group members to conform to certain shared (hence the term "lateral") realities regarding their pain experience and rules about living within the limitations established by traumatic injury and disease, rather than conforming to advice and/or behavioral prescriptions espoused by caregivers who are seen as being on a higher (hence the term "vertical") plane of health. Simply put, pain patients are more apt to receive what they themselves perceive as "credible" feedback in pain groups and less likely to resist efforts to alter their maladaptive attitudes and coping patterns by virtue of the fact that they cannot as easily (or at all) counter with the all-too-familiar, defensive admonition: "You don't understand what it's like to live with pain 24 hours a day. You'd be a bitch too!" As Greenhoot and Sternbach (9, p. 599) observed: "Patients may deceive themselves or the staff, but they do not long deceive other patients. . . ." Third, group therapy allows the therapist and patient alike to avoid the dependency trap, whereby both look to the therapist to assume primary responsibility for "fixing" the patient's myriad of psychological

problems. In group therapy, this responsibility is to a large extent shared by other group members, with the therapist in fact (as we shall see later) assuming more the role of facilitator and/or observer.

MECHANICS

At this point, it would perhaps be helpful to share the collective wisdom of those who have specifically employed group therapy with chronic pain patients (5, 10–18) as regards the "nuts and bolts" or mechanics of this treatment modality.

FORMAT

There is at this stage no consensus about whether pain groups should be open or closed ended. Patients' attendance in our pain groups may often be sporadic because of the ebb and flow of their back condition, which at times is severe enough to prevent them from coming during periods of "flare-ups," interruptive surgical procedures, and/or resistance on the part of family members who fail to appreciate the potential benefit of such treatment. This causes them to exit and reenter at various intervals; however, they still maintain a reasonably cohesive relationship with the group. As we (5) have noted, once group cohesion is firmly established, it is often difficult to introduce new members without disrupting the group process. In effect, it can destroy the pain group's sense of "continuity both in terms of issues discussed and group interaction," if new patients are constantly being added (11, p. 95). On the other hand, with open-ended groups, newly admitted patients can learn much from veteran participants, who have graduated to a higher level of adaptation and who may "streamline the newcomer's journey toward awareness of key issues in pain management" (14, p. 224). These veteran patients can also feel good about themselves (self-reinforced) for the obvious progress they have made vis-à-vis the new participants.

Similarly, there seems to be no consensus on how structured or unstructured the group therapy experience should be. McLaughlin (14), for example, advocated a high degree of structure throughout the group experience, including: theme-specific didactic discussions, regularly occurring functional tasks (e.g., preparing meals) to be carried out by the group as a whole, goal-setting, family nights, films, handouts, and forced exposure to "What The Experts Say," the latter consisting of a series of fairly negative appraisals of chronic pain patients by professionals. Others advocate what might be termed a semi-structured format, whereby "Each session is a mixture of educational and free-interaction group therapy . . . , but the content depends upon many variables" (13, p. 337). Still others (5) argue for a general minimization of structure altogether in an effort to (a) enable the therapist to shift away from the more active role of individual therapist to that of facilitator/observer and (b) encourage chronic pain patients to take greater responsibility for what actually transpires in each session in terms of both content (issues) and nature/extent of interaction among participants (dynamics).

SIZE

All those who have commented on the size of their pain groups have essentially agreed that an average of 8 to 10 participants is ideal. If one has fewer than five participants at a given session, one for all intents and purposes loses "the effect of a group per se" (13, p. 337). On the other hand, if one tries to work with more than 10 at one time, one is almost by definition forced into a highly structured, educational, didactic format. The general intensity of group interaction, in essence, tends to be watered down greatly or lost altogether, because the therapist is more likely to retreat into a question-and-answer and/or individual therapy style of relating to patients. The more highly structured therapy groups (14) can more easily accommodate a slightly larger number of patients at any one time (e.g., 12).

From a practical standpoint, it is generally wise to "overenroll" patients in the pain group, because our experience suggests that few chronic pain patients, no matter how motivated, attend every session (at least 25–30% of patients enrolled fail to show for any given session) and there is a significant attrition or shrinkage in group membership over time. For example, Hendler et al. (13) and Gamsa et al. (11) reported dropout rates of 27% and 30%, respectively, over a 3-month period.

FREQUENCY AND DURATION

Inpatient pain groups typically meet daily. Outpatient pain groups, on the other hand, vary from meeting twice weekly to every 2 weeks. We (5) have chosen to have our patients attend less frequently (every 2 weeks) primarily because we view the adjustment problems associated with chronic pain as ongoing, recurring, and not subject to dramatic change in any short period of time; the scheduling of our groups at less frequent intervals, we believe,

helps communicate the message that "There is no quick fix for your problems here!" Patients, therapists, family, physicians, and insurance carriers, all eager to see quick results in terms of diminished pain and suffering, often prefer treatment programs that meet frequently and for a set number of sessions, implying that one will graduate "pain free" and/or "back like I used to be" in short order. We believe that such programs are misleading and potentially harmful to the chronic patient in that they create false rather than realistic hope/expectations. I was delighted recently to attend the grand opening of a new business started by one of our patients who had attended a total of 94 group therapy sessions over the past 5 years. This young woman, who had suffered for years with debilitating lower back pain, unfortunately not corrected by four successive back operations, had initially presented herself as markedly depressed, alienated (feeling that her life was "dull, boring, frustrating, and painful"), and virtually housebound 90% of the time. With the help of the group, she began a systematic progression of healthy, prosocial behaviors (e.g., playing bingo, volunteer work, and eventual part-time employment at a variety of jobs). All of this "experimentation" took time, several years, before culminating in her courageous new career. All along the way, there were skeptics, quite honestly including myself at times, who essentially underestimated both the resolve of the patient and the power of the group therapy experience, and wondered "What could she possibly be getting out of the group after such a long time?" Interestingly, the total cost of these 94 sessions ($4,230) pales by comparison with the expense of repetitive back surgery or inpatient pain management programs.

Typically, group therapy sessions last from 1 to 2 hours each. Little can be accomplished in less than an hour, and chronic pain patients have difficulty sitting for longer than 1½ to 2 hours without experiencing a noticeable exacerbation in their pain experience. In our own groups, we generally take a short break midway through the session to allow patients a much needed opportunity to walk about, stretch, and informally socialize. We find that this break both (a) lessens the possibility that they will shift their attention away from the group discussion to their now increased pain in the second half of the session (pain interferes with concentration after it reaches a certain intensity, such that patients begin to "listen to but not hear" what is being said in group); and (b) ensures that pain per se will not suddenly become the primary topic of discussion. As we discuss later, we make every effort possible to keep the focus on "learning to live with" chronic pain and not the pain experience itself.

Whether pain groups should be time limited or not, and, if so, how long they should last, is an issue of some importance not only to patients and therapists, but also to what I collectively refer to as "all other interested parties," ranging from immediate family to referring physicians, therapist colleagues, and third-party carriers who largely finance the treatment. For our part, we have so far chosen not to set time limits (i.e., specific number of sessions) on our pain groups since by definition chronic pain itself has no time limits. As we repeatedly remind our patients: "It is a problem that has a beginning, a middle, but no end . . . !" Thus, while some of our patients choose to attend only for a few sessions and others remain in the group for several years, the group itself is ongoing. A few of our patients have terminated group therapy after only one session, while our longest attending patient came for a total of 94 sessions before deciding that she had learned and relearned all she could from her fellow chronic pain sufferers. A recent review of our past 5 years of work with pain groups shows that our average chronic pain patient attends the group 17.25 times. Unfortunately, almost half (46%) of these individuals attended for five or fewer sessions. Hendler et al. (13) have advocated this same open-ended approach for up to 2 years after discharge from an inpatient pain treatment program. McLaughlin (14) also advocated the use of open-ended group therapy.

Still others using pain groups have tended to put a time limit on their treatment efforts, ranging anywhere from a one-shot "Wellness Weekend" (10) to a 10-week program (11), whereupon presumably patients are "graduated," that is, left on their own to apply the principles of chronic pain management learned in the group.

GROUP COMPOSITION AND EXCLUSION CRITERIA

There seems to be fairly good consensus among persons using group therapy with chronic pain patients that such groups should be kept relatively "pure" with respect to diagnosed chronic pain disorders (e.g., arthritis, low back pain, cervical pain, injuries of the extremities such as hand and knee) rather than mixing pain and nonpain patients within the same therapy group. Many also believe that certain subgroups of pain disorder differ sufficiently from others (e.g., low back pain vs. headache) both in terms of their self-reported pain experience and

the nature/extent of their associated disability to justify separate groups for these individuals.

Otherwise, group therapy seems an appropriate intervention strategy for most persons suffering from chronic benign pain. Certainly, there is no evidence to suggest using sociodemographic characteristics (age, gender, race, ethnicity, marital status, education level, social class) or severity of impairment/disability as a basis for selecting or excluding patients for participation in pain groups. On the contrary, we have found chronic pain to be a very democratic phenomenon, affecting virtually all categories of persons with no regard for age, skin color, intelligence, ethnic heritage, or material wealth. Because of this, as we have noted before (5), pain groups in fact do represent a "microcosm" of the real world.

Suggested exclusion criteria include: alcoholism (12); being actively suicidal (16); seeking a "pain cure" (14); pending litigation (16); not ambulatory without a walker or wheelchair (16); evidence of gross personality disorganization (e.g., active or borderline psychosis) (5, 12, 16); elevated score on the MMPI Pd scale (5); and general lack of motivation to actively participate (14, 16). McLaughlin (14), as far as we are aware, is the only one to specify to what extent patient exclusion is a major consideration, as she noted that 40% of patients screened for participation in her highly structured ADAPT groups are not accepted.

It is a well-known fact that men generally are more resistant to self-disclosure than are women, and this tends to be even more the case with group therapy, which requires more public disclosure of feelings and actions than is true of individual therapies. Thus, our experience suggests that it is more difficult to enroll men than women to begin with, and men may be less open and interactive within the group once enrolled. Their attitude most often seems to be "every man for himself" when it comes to adapting to chronic pain (5). Similarly, some of us have found that patients who have been in chronic pain a shorter period of time and/or have not yet had elective surgery to presumably correct their back problems are less likely to actively involve themselves in the group process, preferring instead to remain somewhat detached from the "war stories" of those who have had one or more unsuccessful surgeries and who have suffered with pain for much longer periods of time (5, 18). Repeated treatment failure ("I've tried everything—biofeedback, surgery, pain medication, physical therapy—and nothing works to get rid of this damned

Table 17.1
Summary of Therapeutic Approaches Utilized in Group Therapy for Chronic Pain Patients

STUDIES CITED	TYPES OF APPROACHES USED			
	EDUCATIONAL	INSTRUCTIONAL	INSPIRATIONAL	INTERACTIONAL
Azariah et al. (10)	X	X		X
Gamsa et al. (11)			X	X
Gentry & Owens (5)	X		X	X
Heffron (12)			X	
Hendler et al (13)	X			X
McLaughlin (14)	X	X		X
Miller (15)	X	X		
Pinsky (16)	X		X	X
Rosen et al. (17)	X	X		X
Schwartz et al. (18)		X		X

pain!") and increasing frustration may, in fact, be required before most patients become "psychologically minded" and open to the possible benefits of either structured or unstructured group therapy, that is, if they haven't already reached a point of demoralization and learned helplessness where they are resigned to the belief that nothing will help.

Heffron (12) suggested creating a balance in each group between so-called habitual talkers and habitual listeners, lest the group become overly quiet (leaving it up to the therapist to take a more active role) or overly distracting and competitive, where all participants are fighting to have their say at the same time (forcing the therapist to serve as a referee or gatekeeper).

THERAPEUTIC APPROACHES

As can be seen in Table 17.1, a variety of therapeutic approaches have been utilized under the general rubric of "group therapy" with chronic pain patients. For the most part, pain groups have tended to be multimodal in their approach to these patients, using some combination of strategies and techniques that can be categorized as: educational, instructional, inspirational, and/or interactional. Education is for the most part didactic and consists of providing information about pain and stress management, the psychophysiology of pain, and myths about pain and its treatment (e.g., that elective back surgery is curative). The instructional approaches involve teaching patients pain and stress management skills such as hypnosis, relaxation, cognitive-restructuring, and assertiveness. Inspirational strategies refer to peer-modeling and sharing experiences, whereby other chronic pain patients become "a stimulus to and a reinforcer of adaptive change" (11, p. 93) among group members, resulting in a "contagion effect" (5). Finally, the interactional approach, or what is typically regarded as the "group process" or "dynamic" approach, stresses the importance of such things as confrontational feedback, group "coercive" behavior, affect evocation, emotional catharsis, and directive interpretation. Starting with the nonprocess approaches (educational-instructional) and moving toward the process approaches (inspirational-interactional) is generally recommended (5, 14).

Psychodrama (12, 13) and videotaping (11, 14) appear to be useful therapeutic aids both in instructing pain patients about adaptive coping skills (e.g., alternative ways of coping with anger) and in providing "noninterpretive, direct feedback which is difficult to dismiss" (14, p. 224.)

Because these widely differing approaches are used in pain groups, it is easy to see why some are simply referred to as "classes" (15) or "courses" (10) and still others as "therapeutic social clubs" (12).

OTHER ISSUES

Two other issues that should be considered have to do with (a) the formation of "after-group groups" and (b) the involvement of patient spouses/families in pain groups. As hendler et al. (13) have suggested, the former are a natural by-product of group therapy, reflecting a greater degree of cohesion among group participants, and should be encouraged. In fact, one clinical marker of how well the group process is working is the extent to which patients "come early and stay late" to engage in healthy interaction when they attend group sessions.

As regards involvement of nonpatient "significant others" in group therapy per se, this has for the most part not been done. Most likely, it would serve as a barrier to group identification and sharing of true feelings, especially toward those individuals closest to the patients, on whom they increasingly depend yet at whom they are often angry for "being well" and "not having to deal with pain all the time." McLaughlin (14) suggested the use of Family Night, which is held separately from group therapy every 6–8 weeks, as an alternative strategy for involving significant others without hampering the group process. Periodic involvement of patient spouses/families in ongoing group therapy, on the other hand, should not be confused with or substituted for either marital or family therapy (see Chapter 18).

GROUP THERAPIST ROLE(S)

It should at this point be clear that the role of the therapist in pain groups varies considerably depending on the particular therapeutic approach(es) used. Because the majority of pain groups heavily emphasize education and instruction as regards specific skills, one obvious role played by group therapists is that of educator/instructor. A second role is that of group facilitator; that is, the therapist either directly or indirectly works toward developing greater sharing among group members and movement away from leader-centered discussion (11, 18). For example, as a rule, I (WDG) am not present when the group enters the therapy room and begins its discussion; rather, I have found it helpful to take coffee orders and be conveniently absent for the first few minutes, thus allowing the group to set its own agenda, mood, and so on rather than waiting for me to take the initiative. Also, I always fill out any paper-and-pencil psychological instruments (e.g., the Beck Depression Inventory) that are given to group participants, share my own responses/scores, and essentially model for them what appropriate, desired group behavior consists of. Finally, when my own back "acts up" with occasional disk-related pain, I use it as a therapeutic tool both for (a) sharing their "universal" pain experience and (b) again modeling adaptive coping behavior(s).

A third and final role of the therapist is that of observer (5, 18), in which the therapist "remains in the background" (12), takes "an overview of the group dynamics" (18), and feeds his/her impressions/feelings back to the group as a whole.

To illustrate the observer role more fully, it may be helpful to consider the following group vignette.

After a group therapy session in which the therapist had sat quietly for about 45 minutes, the following exchange took place.

Patient: Well, Dr. _____, what'd you think about today's session? You've been awfully quiet this morning.

Therapist: Actually, I haven't been thinking so much as I have been feeling, feeling sad, that is. For the first time, maybe ever, I found myself watching you folks interact with one another, pain and all, and it suddenly hit me that as hard as I might try I can't make any of you well, pain free. I guess I've known that all along, but this is the first time I've felt it! I guess doctors have denial just like patients do about chronic pain, and it hurts when something breaks through that denial. I like you folks and it really makes me sad to realize that your pain is here to stay, not a good feeling at all.

Patient: (tearful) Now you know how we feel a whole lot of the time.

Therapist: Yes, I do, _____. And, I also know now why all of you work so hard to deny that your pain is chronic, that it has a beginning, a middle, but no end. . . . I guess this is something we're all going to have to work at, accepting your pain, aren't we?

Group: (all affirmative responses . . .)

Obviously in a closed-ended group format, it is easier to naturally evolve or progress from the more active, information-giving, didactic role of educator to the more passive, commentator role of observer. In open-ended groups, where new patients are entering at irregular intervals, the group therapist must be more flexible, shifting from one role to the other within any given session. Hendler et al. (13) suggested that the role of the group therapist differs depending on the context in which the group is operating. They noted, for example, that "Inpatient groups rarely, if ever, evolve to the point at which the therapist need not serve as leader" (p. 338), whereas in an outpatient setting the therapist can take a much less active role.

Some pain groups have multiple cotherapists representing different professional specialties. Schwartz et al. (18), for example, described a multidisciplinary group therapy experience for rheumatoid arthritis patients that includes a rheumatologist, a psychiatrist, and a physiatrist, all of whom play different roles (e.g., educator/resource person vs. observer/commentator). Similarly, McLaughlin (14) described a group jointly led by an occupational therapist and a psychologist, who complement one another in giving patients "an important message about the need to simultaneously address physical and social-emotional aspects of their injuries" (p. 221). She argued rather convincingly that the "leadership alliance" between these two cotherapists provide chronic pain patients with a much more balanced or "integrated" perspective as regards their pain and/or distressful life circumstances, which is especially helpful to skeptical, resistant, and/or borderline (all-or-nothing) patients.

POINT OF FOCUS AND THERAPEUTIC AGENDA

Unlike many of the reported efforts to treat chronic pain patients individually (1, 2), group therapy has perhaps a unique focus on the social context in which patients both begin to appreciate the burdensome nature of their chronic pain experience and, more importantly, begin to develop more adaptive ways of coping with it in the everyday social world. The general focus is clearly on the emotional and interpersonal correlates of the patient's chronic pain experience, not on the experience itself. Chronic pain patients, we have found, come into treatment "totally" preoccupied with their pain, unable for the most part to see or act beyond it. They have, as we say, "their eyeballs turned inward," unable to focus on life outside of their own immediate sensory-emotional pain experience. All they talk or think about is their pain! Our task is to shift this focus away from how much they hurt (since we don't really believe that this is subject to much change or, for that matter, control) and reorient them toward a discussion of life *with* rather than *without* pain. As one rather chagrined nurse observed: "I'm confused. I thought this was a pain group. I didn't hear that many people talking about their pain the last hour or so. Even more surprising, they were laughing, talking about things they were doing, like normal people. How are they going to learn to deal with their pain if they don't talk about it?"

More specifically, the focus of group therapy is on promoting a sense of "universality," where patients can for the first time be exposed to "kindred souls" struggling more or less successfully with the same problem (5); on providing a basis for new or renewed hope that they can once again find effective, fulfilling ways of acting on the social environment to meet their own needs, pain or no pain (5);

on developing new, meaningful social ties (19); and on validating their own adaptive/maladaptive perceptions and feelings about their ability to "learn to live with it" against others (16).

There are obvious interpersonal differences in life circumstances, intellect, and personality that characterize this patient population both before and after the onset of chronic pain. However, we have found that virtually all such patients sooner or later find themselves struggling with the following recurring therapeutic agenda, which makes up the "meat" of our group discussions:

Issues of legitimacy ("No one believes me!").

Denial of the harsh reality of the chronic, endless pain experience, which often serves as a primary motivating factor behind "pain games," including addiction, "doctor shopping," excessive disability, litigation, and questionable polysurgery (20).

The need to distinguish between pain versus suffering as distinct, yet interrelated psychological parameters of the patient's self-perception.

Conflict over forced, albeit much needed dependency and the failure to properly utilize available resources (psychosocial, economic, vocational, educational).

Greatly altered role(s) and function(s) within marriage, family, and community systems.

Fear and negative anticipation as regards possible worsening of one's physical condition (e.g., degenerative disease).

The absolute need for identity resolution; the "identity confusion which pain patients experience is reminiscent of adolescence" (14, p. 221).

The importance of grieving over lost identity, function, and relationships, ". . . the stuff that dreams are made of. . . ."

The ever-present ability of mood disturbance (depression, anger, agitation). We have a saying in our group that "depression is always right around the corner," reflecting our belief that mood disturbances, albeit at times mild and short lived, will occur intermittently throughout the course of one's chronic pain experience. This suggests that one should anticipate bouts of moodiness and prepare a plan for coping with them when they do, in fact, occur.

Avoidance of pleasure-giving activities in the pursuit of a pain-free existence.

Self- and other-imposed alienation, isolation, and rejection.

THERAPEUTIC OUTCOME

As we noted from the outset, little systematic attention has been given to group therapy as a treatment modality for ameliorating pain and accompanying emotional distress compared to various individual pain intervention strategies (1, 2). Therefore, we have little beyond clinical anecdotes and descriptive statistics to indicate the possible nature and extent of benefit of chronic pain sufferers participating in such groups. However, what we do know is quite encouraging.

Azariah et al. (10) Gamsa et al. (11), for example, suggested that between 67 and 86% of patients who participate in pain groups demonstrate "significant improvement" and feel that the group has been helpful to them. Rosen et al. (17) similarly found that 80% of group participants reported a significant reduction in their pain experience, anxiety, and tendency to exaggerate somatic complaints and/or be preoccupied with bodily symptoms (somatization). McLaughlin (14) noted that 68% of group members returned to some type of gainful employment and remained there for at least 1 year. Finally, Hendler et al. (13) found that about 88% of patients who remained in group therapy for at least 3 months had abstained from narcotic and hypnotic drug use, as compared to only 42% of similar patients seen individually by a psychiatrist. This latter report, which includes a reference to a paper by Hall et al. (21), as far we we know is the only one to discuss the possible relative efficacy of group therapy versus other nongroup therapies; it suggests that group therapy is more effective in alleviating depression in chronic pain patients, for example, than is "supportive individual psychotherapy, analytically oriented therapy, and management by a surgical specialist" (p. 340).

Pinsky (16) summarized the hoped-for general outcome for patients suffering from what he refers to as the Chronic Intractable Benign Pain Syndrome (CIBPS) who are treated with group therapy: "At its worst, the CIBPS shifts to chronic pain without the full-blown syndrome. At its best, pain and suffering are significantly diminished and the quality of the patient's life is palpably enhanced" (p. 21).

In more specific terms, the variety of expected therapeutic benefits derived from pain groups include: pain reduction per se, decreased use and misuse of pain narcotics, increased optimism and self-confidence, increased self-reliance and accompanying self-esteem, increased ability to appropriately ask for and use available supportive resources, decreased social isolation and alienation, and a renewed sense of hope that "I'm OK, I'm going to be OK!" (5, p. 111).

In a recent survey of patients participating in our pain group, we asked them to rank seven possible benefits of group therapy based on their own needs and experience. Their responses suggest the following order of importance from the patient's perspective:

1. The pain group gave me a chance to hear and see how others deal with their pain. (mean rank = 2.6)
2. The pain group gave me the feeling that someone actually understands what I am going through. (mean rank = 2.8)
3. The pain group made me feel less alone with my pain problem. (mean rank = 3.3)
4. The pain group gave me a chance to get rid of some of my frustration/anger over being in chronic pain. (mean rank = 4.2)
5. The pain group gave me an opportunity to form relationships with others who also had chronic pain. (mean rank = 4.9)
6. The pain group gave me a chance to talk about my pain. (mean rank = 4.9)
7. The pain group helped me shift the focus away from my pain condition. (mean rank = 6.0)

REFERENCES

1. Turner JA, Chapman CR: Psychological interventions for chronic pain: a critical review. I. Relaxation training and biofeedback. *Pain* 12:1–21, 1982.
2. Turner JA, Chapman CR: Psychological interventions for chronic pain: a critical review. II. Operant conditioning, hypnosis, and cognitive-behavioral therapy. *Pain* 12:23–46, 1982.
3. Roy R: A problem-centered family systems approach in treating chronic pain. In Holzman AD, Turk DC (eds): *Pain Management.* New York, Pergamon Press, 1986, pp 113–130.
4. Alonzo AA: Illness behavior during acute episodes of coronary heart disease (dissertation). Berkeley, CA, University of California, 1973.
5. Gentry WD, Owens D: Pain groups. In Holzman AD, Turk DC (eds): *Pain Management.* New York, Pergamon Press, 1986, pp 100–112.
6. Sternbach RA: *Pain Patients: Traits and Treatment.* New York, Academic Press, 1974.
7. Turk DC, Meichenbaum D, Genest M: *Pain and Be-*

havioral Medicine: A Cognitive-Behavioral Perspective. New York, Guilford Press, 1983.

8. Timmermans G, Sternbach RA: Factors of human chronic pain: an analysis of personality and pain reaction variables. *Science* 184:806–807, 1974.

9. Greenhoot JH, Sternbach RA: Conjoint treatment of chronic pain. *Adv Neurol* 4:595–603, 1974.

10. Azariah R, Beautrais P, Azariah M: Brief psychosocial intervention for chronic pain: an evaluation of group therapy (abstract).

11. Gamsa A, Braha RED, Catchlove RFH: The use of structured group therapy in the treatment of chronic pain patients. *Pain* 22:91–96, 1985.

12. Heffron WA: Group therapy in family practice. *Am Fam Physician* 10:176–180, 1974.

13. Hendler N, Viernstein M, Shallenberger C, Long D: Group therapy with chronic pain patients. *Psychosomatics* 22:333–340, 1981.

14. McLaughlin AM: Coping in context: adaptation groups for chronic pain patients. In Keller PA, Heyman SR (eds): *Innovations in Clinical Practice: A Source Book.* Sarasota, FL, Professional Resource Exchange, 1987, vol. 6, pp 219–229.

15. Miller RS: Pain management classes for medical patients: evaluating a psychological treatment program for in-patients (abstract).

16. Pinsky JJ: Chronic, intractable, benign pain: a syndrome and its treatment with intensive short-term group psychotherapy. *J Human Stress* 172:17–21, 1978.

17. Rosen G, Kvale A, Husebo S: Multimodal group-treatment of chronic pain patients (abstract).

18. Schwartz LH, Marcus R, Condon R: Multidisciplinary group therapy for rheumatoid arthritis. *Psychosomatics* 19:289–293, 1978.

19. Syme SL: Sociocultural factors and disease etiology. In Gentry WD (ed): *Handbook of Behavioral Medicine.* New York, Guilford Press, 1984, pp 13–37.

20. Gentry WD: Does elective surgery benefit chronic back pain patients with evidence of psychological disturbance? *South Med J* 75:1169–1170, 1982.

21. Hall RC, Hall AK, Gardner ER, et al: A comparison of tricyclic antidepressants and analgesics in the management of chronic postoperative surgical pain. Paper presented at the annual meeting of the Academy of Psychosomatic Medicine, San Francisco, 1979.

Chapter 18

COUPLE THERAPY

RANJAN ROY, ADV, DIPSW

Literature on family therapy to treat medical and psychosomatic disorders is scanty. The reasons for this are not self-evident. Given the magnitude of change that a chronic illness is capable of producing within a family system, it stands to reason that an effective family approach to address the negative consequences of illness may be desirable and the reasons for such intervention readily comprehensible. Nevertheless, a quick glance at the literature reveals that over the past 10 years there has been a concerted effort, at least at the clinical level, to develop a rationale for and demonstrate efficacy of family intervention with medically ill patients and their families (1).

Before an exploration of literature, perhaps the reasons for family involvement in the assessment and treatment of psychosomatic disorders, including chronic back pain, should be briefly reviewed. Many authors have articulated reasons for a family approach as an adjunct to the treatment of medical illnesses (2–5). Three principal reasons have been offered as a rationale for intervention with medical illness: (a) the role of family dynamics in the genesis of disease (6); (b) the role of family members in the perpetuation of disability and disease (7, 8); and (c) the impact of disease on the well-being of the family members (9, 10). The etiologic significance of the family has not proven to be a particularly fruitful area from the point of view of research, and to date much of the data, which are very limited, remain basically unconvincing. The role of family members in the perpetuation of disease-related behaviors, on the other hand, has received considerable currency and is recognized as a critical area of exploration and understanding by family therapists (11, 12). Clinical evidence suggests that illness in a family member has a variety of meanings for the family, and family dynamics can contribute to not

only the perpetuation of the problem but even the worsening of it (13, 14). The last area, impact of illness on the family, is perhaps most readily understandable and to date has received considerable support both clinically and empirically (15, 16). It is a matter of common sense that chronic illness in a family member has a significant effect on his/her role functioning, which in turn engenders, indeed necessitates, changes in the entire system. Literature on the family and chronic pain, as well as chronic disorders, on the whole concentrated more on this area than on any of the others.

In the rest of this chapter, first, there is a review of the application of family therapy for medical and psychosomatic illnesses; second, a brief review of the problem-centered systems family therapy (PCSFT) is provided; and third, the relevance of PCSFT in the case of a chronic pain patient and his wife is demonstrated, followed by a general discussion.

FAMILY THERAPY FOR MEDICAL ILLNESSES

Family therapy for physical illnesses can be divided into two broad categories. The first is family-oriented therapy, which promotes involving family members in some form of therapeutic venture in the overall treatment of the patient (17–20). The second category involves treatment of the family as a whole. This literature review concentrates on the latter category. The majority of the reports on family therapy with families of the physically ill concentrate on the disruptive effects of the illness on the family system, and only a handful are concerned with the etiologic aspects of family interaction on the development and maintenance of disease. Family therapy, or therapy with members of a family with a physically ill person, has been used with a wide variety of medical problems (1). Two distinct subcategories of literature can be discerned in the category of family therapy for medical illness: (a) family therapy programs not clearly predicated on theoretical models (21–24); and (b) programs in which the therapy is clearly based on clinical theories for family therapy practice (25–27). A wide range of disorders are reported in the first category, and the rationale for family therapy is solely predicated on its efficacy to counteract the negative consequences of serious illness on family functioning. These reports make a strong case for family therapy and at least clinically attempt to demonstrate the beneficial effects of such an intervention. A major criticism of most of these reports is the lack of empirical evidence derived from controlled studies.

Studies of family therapy for psychosomatic or physical illness based on well-defined family therapy methods are few. These studies also tend to be uncontrolled. Much of the theoretical underpinning for family therapy with physically ill patients and their families has emerged from two principal schools, structural family therapy and strategic family therapy.

Structural family therapy in the treatment of childhood asthma, diabetes, and anorexia nervosa has been reported by Minuchin and his colleagues (6, 28). They have reported an extraordinary level of success in treating these three conditions. Unfortunately, much of their work, although empirically based, was uncontrolled. Nevertheless, Gustaffson and his colleagues (29), in a controlled study of treatment of severe childhood asthma using the structural family therapy approach, have demonstrated its efficacy as an adjunct treatment. Unfortunately, much of the research raises serious questions about the psychosomatogenic model as well as about structural family therapy as an efficacious way of conceptualizing and treating psychosomatic disorders. Parker and Lipscomb (30), in a controlled study, found that overprotection toward a very sick child was a reaction to the illness. This particular study cast serious doubt on the etiologic significance of overprotection in childhood asthma. Burbeck (31) failed to find support for the psychosomatogenic model in a study of asthmatic children. Despite the lack of evidence in support of structural family therapy as an effective form of treatment for psychosomatic disorders, at a clinical level its utility has been noted by several authors. Lask (2), for example, has described at length the application of

structural family therapy in the treatment of a variety of disorders both in children and in adults.

Strategic family therapy, the principal proponent of which is Haley, has had extremely limited application in the treatment of physical illness. Palazzoli (32) used this method in the treatment of anorexia nervosa, brittle diabetes, and childhood asthma in a series of uncontrolled studies and claimed an extraordinary level of success in treatment outcome. In a unique study, Hobel (33) used the strategic approach to reduce risk factors in patients with myocardial infarction by involving the family members in the treatment. There are a few clinical reports on the efficacy of this method in the treatment of psychogenic pain, and they are discussed in the next section.

FAMILY THERAPY AND CHRONIC PAIN

REASONS FOR FAMILY THERAPY

Before proceeding to a review of the literature on family treatment for chronic pain, a brief exploration of the reasons for family therapy for such a complex condition may be meritorious. There is substantial evidence that chronic pain has serious repercussions on the well-being of the spouse (34–36). In particular, spouses appear to be vulnerable to depression and other psychosomatic disorders. Additionally, there is mounting evidence that the presence of a person with chronic pin within a family system may produce undesirable changes in the functioning of the family. Using the McMaster model of family functioning (which is described later), Roy (37, 38) demonstrated that not a single aspect of family functioning remains unaffected by chronic pain. In an earlier study, Hudgens (39) also made similar observations. In short, chronic pain and healthy family functioning appear to be mutually exclusive. Rowat and Knafl (40), in an elegant study, demonstrated the far-reaching consequences of chronic pain in various aspects of spousal functioning. One of the most striking findings of that study was the hazard of having to live with the uncertainty of the pain condition from day to day and year to year, which proved to be a source of great strain on the well-being of the spouse. Admittedly, many of these studies have methodologic shortcomings such as being uncontrolled and having highly selected subjects. Nevertheless, taken together, they are indicative of the considerable strain and stress that the presence of a chronic pain patient exerts on other members of the family. In this context it is curious to observe that to date there are no studies addressing the question of impact of parental chronic pain on children. This is an inexplicable and major omission.

REVIEW OF STUDIES ON FAMILY THERAPY

Given the magnitude of negative consequences produced by chronic pain on various aspects of family functioning and on the spouse, reports of family therapy with this population are limited (41). It should also be stated that use of the family therapy approach with this population is a relatively recent innovation and, as with any recent development, the focus is primarily on clinical application rather than on research to determine the efficacy of family therapy. In other words, the clinical evidence clearly suggests the need for family intervention, but whether or not such intervention makes any lasting difference to the well-being of the patient and the family awaits empirical validation. Two broad categories of family therapy have been applied in the treatment of chronic pain: behaviorally oriented therapies and systems-based therapies. Fordyce (7) produced convincing evidence of the efficacy of behavior therapy in replacing pain-reinforcing behaviors in spouses with healthy behaviors. Hudgens (39) combined operant treatment and systems theory with 24 families with a member with chronic pain and reported considerable success with the patient's resumption of occupational roles as well as general improvement in the level of satisfaction with family life. Moore and Chaney (42), in a behaviorally based treatment program for chronic low back pain patients with and without involvement of the spouses, found that spousal involvement did not significantly alter the outcome of treatment. However, Flor and her colleagues (43) observed that "the spouse involvement in this study was minimal." They were critical of the fact that the behavioral and cognitive-behavioral approaches were almost exclusively focused on the spouse's influence on the patient, with virtually no attention being given to either the impact of the patient's pain on the spouse or on the overall family functioning.

TYPES OF FAMILY THERAPY

A variety of approaches are included in the category of family systems therapy. Among them are: (a) the strategic approach, (b) the structural approach, (c) the "cognitive" approach, and (d) the problem-centered systems approach. Application of the first two approaches to the treatment of chronic

pain are very few (41). The reasons for the relative lack of popularity of the strategic approach in the treatment of chronic pain have been described elsewhere (44), but the most important reason is that the etiology of chronic pain cannot be solely attributed to ineffective or dysfunctional communication patterns within the family system. This last point is at the very heart of the strategic approach.

The structural approach has somewhat of a checkered history in terms of its application to treat chronic pain. There are two reports of family treatment of abdominal pain in children (45, 46). Both studies were uncontrolled. They reported a remarkable rate of success in the amelioration of the pain problem in their young subjects. Lask (2) has successfully used a structural family approach in treating chronic pain problems in adults as well as in children. His reports are exclusively clinical in nature.

The central feature of "cognitive" family therapy is self-disclosure, which in turn facilitates marital intimacy (47). Waring observed that many chronic pain patients with a history of obscure etiology presented with a history of marital disharmony (47). These marital relationships were characterized by lack of intimacy. The therapy was to increase feelings of intimacy.

Problem-Centered Systems Family Therapy

The problem-centered systems family therapy (PCSFT) has a history that dates back over a quarter-century. Preliminary research for this model was conducted by Westly and Epstein (48) at McGill University in the 1960s. Their original task was to ascertain the nature of healthy family functioning. Early research led to the development of the Family Category Schema, which was later developed into the McMaster Model of Family Functioning (49, 50). A substantial number of research studies have been reported on the development of the model, the teaching of this method, and actual assessments of various kinds of problematic families (51, 55). Very few studies or even clinical reports are available on the therapeutic approach (PCSFT) that emerged from the research on family functioning (41).

The PCSFT is predicated on some of the assumptions of systems theory (55): (a) that the parts of the family are interrelated, (b) that one part of the family cannot be understood in isolation from the rest of the system, (c) that family functioning cannot be fully explained or comprehended by simply understanding each of its parts, (d) that the family structure and organization are important factors in determining the behavior of family members, and (e) that the transactional patterns of the family system shape the behavior of family members. These assumptions are central to the understanding of PCSFT. Families are complex organizations with intricate relationships within, as well as with external systems. Individual members interact and thereby determine as well as influence each other's behavior, and they in turn are individually and collectively affected by society's morals, value systems, and the like.

The PCSFT has four clearly defined "macro-stages": assessment, contracting, treatment, and closure. These are discrete stages and therefore, by definition, invariant. Each stage has a distinct beginning and ending, and to ensure clear separation between the stages every stage commences with an orientation phase. This ensures that the therapist, as well as the family, clearly recognize the termination of one phase and the beginning of the next.

The actual role of the family therapist is not clearly defined within this model. Nevertheless, the family therapist performs a whole range of roles that include a mediator, a catalyst, a "conductor," and a clarifier. His/her actions with the family are defined by the PCSFT as "micro"-moves. These micro-moves constitute the skills component that enables the therapist to conduct an effective assessment and enter and complete the therapeutic process.

Assessment Stage

The assessment (diagnostic) stage is critical to any therapeutic venture. Perhaps it is for this reason that the success of PCSFT is totally independent upon a thorough and comprehensive assessment of the family along several dimensions. The orientation aspect of the assessment phase is critical. It is during the orientation that a sense of the need for family therapy is sought from each family member, as well as their individual expectations of what they hope to achieve from therapy. It is also during this phase that the therapist emphasizes the need for each family member to assume responsibility for the success of family therapy.

An important departure from Epstein and Bishop's (55) approach to orientation during the assessment phase is that very few of the chronic pain patients voluntarily seek family or couple therapy. In this author's experience, despite routine requests of patients to bring their spouses to the pain clinic at the point of inception, very few comply. It is somewhat of a rarity if a patient is accompanied by his/her spouse at that point. This changes the nature of the orientation to a significant degree. The onus is on the therapist to explain to the patient and other family members the need for their collective involvement, and the rationale is of necessity a simple one. It is explained to them that no one in the family remains unaffected by the chronic and refractory nature of the patient's problems, and agreement is sought on this point. A vast majority of the families seem to have the capacity to develop a consensus that individually and collectively they have been adversely affected by the patient's condition.

Following the completion of the orientation phase, a careful exploration is conducted of the presenting problem. It is not uncommon for family members to have extremely varied views of the presenting problem(s) and equally varied interpretations as to their causes and effects. When the presenting problem happens to be a rather mystifying one such as chronic pain, family confusion is frequently profound. There is, first, an inclination to attribute their difficulties to the pain itself, and amelioration and elimination of the pain is seen as the only solution. It must be emphasized that despite a semblance of agreement, or even acquiescence, that the problem of chronic pain has a negative impact on the family, family members, including the patient, frequently demonstrate a level of commitment to finding a medical cure that makes any kind of psychological intervention virtually impossible.

Therefore the therapist requires a high level of skill to help the family disengage from their preoccupation with a medical cure and shift their focus to intrafamilial problems. The therapist has to acknowledge that a medical cure may not be at hand in view of the fact that the patient has had extensive evaluation and treatment, but in the meantime the family relationships have deteriorated and require urgent attention. In addition, the therapist may choose to offer an explanation about the very nature of chronic pain, which does not remain unaffected by psychological and psychosocial factors. As is evident in the case example that follows, a spouse may remain thoroughly dubious about any beneficial outcome of couple or family therapy and merely acquiesce to engage in that process. However, as results become evident, and improvements both in the level of the patient's functioning and in family relationships are recognized, such early skepticism frequently melts away. Through this very complex process, presenting problems are identified and the central task of reframing the problem of chronic pain into interpersonal and family problems is thus begun. The process of reframing is a continuous one with families of patients with chronic pain and chronic illness. This is so for the simple reason that their primary goal at all times remains that of obtaining a permanent cure, and any other activity is seen as peripheral.

Following the exploration of presenting problems, the overall functioning of the family is assessed on six dimensions of family functioning using the McMaster Model of Family Functioning (MMFF) (50). The MMFF may be regarded as the heart of the assessment process, and (as is demonstrated below) a thorough and comprehensive assessment utilizing the MMFF is an essential ingredient for successful outcome of family therapy. The MMFF purports to examine family functioning in the following areas: problem-solving, communication, roles, affective responsiveness, affective involvement, and behavior control. Within each dimension the affective and instrumental issues are separately addressed and guidelines are used to establish effective functioning within each area of family functioning.

According to the MMFF the *problem-solving* process consists of seven substances (they are described below in the case analysis). Effective *communication* is clear and direct, as opposed to ineffective communication, which is indirect and masked. The directness of communication is concerned with the clarity with which the person for whom the message is intended is identified, and clear communication consists of the clarity of the message itself.

The complexity that surrounds the concept of *role functioning* is clearly identified by Epstein and his colleagues. Some roles are absolutely necessary for the survival of the family and others are not. Roles can also be subdivided into instrumental and affective areas. It is the performance of roles that allows family members to fulfill their functions. There are five essential areas of role functioning: (a) provision of resources, (b) nurturance and support, (c) adult sexual gratification, (d) personal development, and (e) maintenance and management of the family system. In addition, role allocation (the task involved in the assignment of roles to individual members of the family) and role accountability (which ensures that functions are fulfilled) are two critical aspects of role.

The dimension of *affective responsiveness* addresses the family members' ability to express a whole range of emotions. Emotions are divided into two distinct categories, welfare emotions and emergency emotions. Welfare emotions consist of positive feelings such as joy, happiness, love, and affec-

tion. Emergency emotions represent negative emotions such as anger, fear and sadness. A healthy family is capable of expressing the full range of emotions.

Affective involvement is concerned with the extent to which the family shows interest in the particular activities of individual family members. Six types of affective involvements are noted: (a) lack of involvement, (b) involvement devoid of feelings, (c) narcissistic involvement, (d) empathic involvement, (e) overinvolvement, and (f) symbiotic involvement. Empathic involvement is the most desirable form of family relationship and symbiotic the least desirable.

Finally, *behavior control* is concerned with the rules by which families live. There rules are divided into four categories: (a) rigid behavior control, (b) flexible behavior control, (c) laissez-faire behavior control, and (d) chaotic behavior control. The most desirable form of behavior control is flexible and the least is chaotic, although the other two are considered undesirable as well.

Contracting Stage

During the last stage of the assessment process, families are oriented to the need for a well thought out and clear contract. Epstein and Bishop (55) suggested that a written contract be drawn up and signed by the family members and the therapist. This is an excellent suggestion for beginning therapists. The essential ingredients of the contracting stage should consist of very clearly defined problems that family members expect to resolve during therapy and also a clear statement about their expectations. During this phase the therapist may help the family to formulate some of the problems, and there are occasions when the family members and the therapist may have to enter into negotiation to agree on inclusion of certain kinds of problems. This problem is evident in the course of the case discussion that follows. It may also be advisable to have a time limit for the duration of therapy. Minimally, a review process should be built into the contract to examine progress of therapy or lack thereof.

Treatment and Closure Stages

The next macrostage of PCSFT is the actual intervention (treatment). This process is examined in some depth in a subsequent section. The final stage is closure, which is concerned with termination of therapy.

CHRONIC PAIN AND PCSFT

Application of PCSFT to the problem of chronic pain remains extremely limited to date. Much of the work in this area has been conducted by this author, and over the years I have reported on the efficacy of this model in both assessment and treatment of chronic pain. Roy (56) assessed 20 patients with problems of chronic head pain and their spouses on the basis of the MMFF. Problems were found to be pervasive in virtually every dimension of family functioning. In a subsequent report, Roy (38) compared the family functioning of 20 headache sufferers with 12 patients with chronic back pain. All 20 subjects and their spouses encountered difficulties in the affective domain as far as problem solving was concerned. Nine patients with back pain and their spouses demonstrated similar difficulties with the problem-solving dimensions. Fifty percent of the back pain subjects and their spouses engaged in masked and indirect forms of communication as compared to 75% of headache patients and their spouses. In terms of role performance 100% of the headache couples and 75% of the back pain couples demonstrated pervasive difficulties in relation to nurturance and support in their marital relationships.

Seventy-five percent of the back pain sufferers and 60% of the headache sufferers and their spouses reported absence of sexual enjoyment in their marriage. In terms of occupational role 90% of the headache subjects had jobs, but only 50% of the back pain patients were employed. Headache patients were also more efficient in performing their household roles (75%) as opposed to their back pain counterparts (50%). The performance of both pain groups in the area of affective responsiveness was seriously impaired. Two-thirds of the back pain couples and 65% of the headache couples had difficulty in expressing the whole range of emotions and revealed an inability to express welfare emotions. In relation to affective involvement, only 17% of the back pain couples demonstrated an ability to engage in affective involvement, as opposed to 40% of the headache couples. Finally, in the area of behavior control, 93% and 80% of the back pain and headache couples, respectively, engaged in unhealthy behavior control that ranged from rigid to chaotic. Overall the headache couples were somewhat better functioning, especially in the area of roles, than their back pain counterparts.

Accounts of the application of PCSFT to treat chronic pain are very limited and mostly clinical in nature. Again, those accounts are almost entirely confined to this author. Roy has provided accounts of treating couples and families with problems of chronic pain using the PCFST (41). He has demonstrated the efficacy at least at a clinical level, and has argued that the success of this model can be attributed to the level of motivation that the couples often bring into the treatment situation. By definition, couples who agree to enter into this method of treatment are highly motivated and are anxious to change their situation. Second, this type of intervention makes eminent sense to the couples. The approach is practical; problems and solutions are worked out by themselves and they recognize from the very outset that it is their "ballgame." They remain in charge of the therapeutic process at all times. Third, because treatment is of a short-term and active nature, many couples experience also immediate benefits and do have some sort of ending of treatment and at least some resolution of their problem in sight.

Roy (41), in an uncontrolled study, reported that 15 of 20 couples in whom one partner had a history of chronic headache agreed to engage in couple therapy. Fourteen couples demonstrated improvement in their marital relationship and 11 patients also experienced some improvement in their headaches. A retrospective analysis of successful versus unsuccessful outcome of PCSFT with chronic headache patients and spouses is underway. The data suggest that a major determinant of successful outcome in treatment could very well be absence of emotional investment in the symptom either on the part of the patient or the spouse or both. Emotional investment in the symptom on the part of both spouses inevitably predicts the poorest outcome. The actual efficacy of PCSFT or other forms of family treatment will remain moot until such time as controlled studies are conducted.

RATIONALE FOR PCSFT

Not only is there an absence of controlled studies of family therapy with chronic pain, comparison or relative merit of different methods of family therapy to treat this complicated condition is virtually unknown. In truth, there is as yet no clear evidence to claim one method of family therapy as the choice of intervention over any other. The problem of research with family therapy is well known, and several scholars have addressed the nightmarish proportion of methodologic difficulties in this field of research. Poorly defined concepts, therapist variables, vague descriptions of the therapeutic processes, and other equally complex factors mitigate against family therapy outcome research.

Under those circumstances, a major consideration for the selection of a particular method or approach of family therapy is predicated on its ability to clearly delineate the problems. The McMaster Model of Family Functioning provides one of the clearest expositions of problems in various dimensions of family functioning. Other modalities of family therapy, such as structural or strategic, simply do not see the need to understand the disruptive effect of problems such as chronic illness on various aspects of family functioning. Strategic family therapy derives its strength from communication theory and is quite narrowly based. Structural family therapy does not concern itself directly with the question of family functioning and is more preoccupied with identifying faulty subsystems within the family structure. It explains family dysfunction entirely on the basis of such faults.

The PCSFT does not directly concern itself with the question of etiology. Most of the other methods of family therapy do. It will be difficult to explain chronic pain simply on the basis of faulty communication or flawed subsystems. The major preoccupation of the PCFST, with the MMFF at the center, is to ascertain the degree of dysfunction that problems such as chronic pain may cause to the various aspects of family functioning. To that extent, the PCSFT is a powerful tool. The Family Assessment Device (FAD) is the research instrument that has evolved from the MMFF and has become useful in assessing outcome of family intervention. The process of PCSFT is clearly delineated. It is a remarkably simple process, as is evident in the following section. The method can be learned easily. It is a behavioral-interactional mode of intervention and lends itself easily to common sense. Once the areas of family dysfunction are established, tasks are developed to ameliorate those deficiencies, and treatment consists mainly of ensuring that family members remain engaged in performing those tasks. It is through the performance of tasks that families begin to rectify the pathological aspects of family functioning.

Finally, as Roy (37) has acknowledged before, to date selection of one method of family therapy over another remains a function of one's training. In spite of all the arguments that have been offered in the preceding paragraphs, until such time that studies comparing various modalities of family treatment are available, preference for any method of family intervention remains truly a matter of one's bias. Claims of superiority of one method over another at this point in history must be tempered with caution.

CASE STUDY: MR. AND MRS. JOHNSON

Mr. Johnson, a 67-year-old retired civil servant, was referred to the pain clinic with a long list of complaints, at the top of which was his chronic back pain and herpes zoster. He also had a lifelong history of emphysema and a past history of clinical depression. He was leading the life of a semi-invalid, and the concern at the pain clinic was that his level of disability could not be wholly accounted for on the basis of his pain conditions. His emphysema was under reasonable control. His mood was chronically low.

The marriage had always been a difficult one, reported Mrs. Johnson. There was really one main reason for that—Mr. Johnson had never been a well man. Despite his poor health, he held a senior position in the civil service. The youngest daughter had Down's syndrome and continued to live at home with them. She was in her mid-20s and both parents were understandably very concerned about her future. The task of obtaining a succinct history of the marriage and its current status proved extremely hazardous. Mrs. Johnson was reticent and defensive and Mr. Johnson seemed content to leave all matters to his wife. He occasionally volunteered some information, only to be contradicted by Mrs. Johnson. The history of the marriage revealed, albeit very slowly, that this marriage had not been devoid of conflicts. Both parents shared some guilt over the birth of their retarded child, but underneath that there was also some element of recrimination. During the early years of their marriage Mrs. Johnson received very little help from him in caring for a growing family and she still had residual feelings of resentment. Mr. Johnson's involvement with the children was nominal and he was seen by almost all members of the family not only as peripheral, but also as unwell.

Mr. Johnson's self-concept, as well as others' perceptions of him, was that of a sick man. Over the years, this perception of him as not being well had a profound effect on his role and responsibility within the family. Exacerbation of his emphysema complicated by back pain and herpes zoster brought to an end whatever limited role he had within the family. He was catered to by his wife for virtually all his needs, and the relationship between these two individuals had basically turned into that of a nurse and patient. It would be more appropriate to describe Mrs. Johnson's role as the nurse-cum-homemaker plus any other role that was necessary for her to keep this family together.

Mrs. Johnson was somewhat baffled by the need for a couple interview and questioned the wisdom of engaging in such a process.

In the orientation phase of the assessment, it was explained to them that Mr. Johnson's prolonged illness and his more recent difficulties with chronic pain must have created an extraordinary level of pressure on Mrs. Johnson, and it was suggested that perhaps the impact of all of this on their marital relationship should be explored. There was very little hope at this point that Mrs. Johnson would agree to remain engaged in this process. Quite surprisingly, she began to express her feelings of frustration or anger, mostly at the medical profession for their inability to help her husband. The problem of reframing Mr. Johnson's pain problems and herpes zoster into the context of family issues was very difficult. Both of them needed reassurance that perhaps certain aspects of their family life could be changed for the better. Surprisingly, Mr. Johnson was quite enthusiastic, but the source of the enthusiasm was unclear. Mrs. Johnson really did not truly agree, she merely acquiesced to attend the conjoint session, and remained quite skeptical.

Assessment

Some areas of family functioning proved more difficult to explore than others. For example, in relation to *problem solving*, both these individuals were quite bashful in providing information. They did not have too many problems to solve; their life was quite settled and their needs were limited. But how did they go about solving their problems and their differences? Basically, what emerged was that Mrs. Johnson took all the major initiatives in resolving family difficulties, and that pattern had evolved over very many years. While they were concerned about the future of their retarded child, they had not had any serious discussion about her future care. (One point needs to be made about the life stage of this couple. This couple had undoubtedly made all the major decisions that they had to and they were at the point where, other than day-to-day decisions, they did not have any major problems confronting them other than the future of their daughter. The point is made to illustrate that life stage of a family is a critical factor in ascertaining the kind of decision making a family is required to undertake.) As far as the Johnsons were concerned, they functioned quite well at an instrumental level.

Mrs. Johnson appeared to make all the day-to-day decisions, so affective issues basically remained unidentified and therefore never were resolved. The most important aspect of problem solving for Mr. and Mrs. Johnson was that while problems were not solved together, there was no dissension between them.

Mrs. Johnson made all the decisions she had to make for her husband, for her daughter, and for herself. Mr. Johnson was not only resigned to the current state of affairs, he was in some ways even relieved that he didn't have to concern himself. He was firmly entrenched in the chronic sick role, and people around him had little or no expectations of him or from him. Given Mr. Johnson's chronic sick role, it was difficult to clearly ascertain the effectiveness of this family's capacity to engage in problem solving. There was no expectation for Mr. Johnson to participate in the problem-solving process. This lack of participation did not prevent the family from functioning adequately at the instrumental level. In terms of the seven steps of problem solving (identifying the problem, communicating with appropriate people about the problem, developing a list of alternative solutions, deciding on one of the alternatives, carrying out actions required with the alternative, monitoring to ensure that the action is carried out, and evaluating the effectiveness of the problem-solving process), it was evident that Mr. and Mrs. Johnson as a couple did not participate in the process, simply because Mrs. Johnson had assumed almost total responsibility for the running of this family. It is important to note that they themselves did not view problem solving as a problematic area. This case provided an extreme example of one of the more pronounced consequences of chronic illness and pain: the shifting of responsibilities from the patient to the well partner.

Communication is defined as "exchange of information in a family." Communication is subdivided into instrumental and affective areas. Clear communication means that the message has clarity and direct communication means that the message is received by the person for whom it is intended. Four styles of communication patterns arise from these two independent attributes: clear and direct, clear and indirect, masked and direct, and masked and indirect. Clear and direct is the most effective form of communication, and masked and indirect the least effective.

Illness in a family has discernible impact on the patterns of communication. Roy (57) argued that in the face of illness in a spouse, communication cannot remain clear and direct as expressions of true emotions become increasingly difficult between two individuals, one of whom is unwell. Generally speaking, the well partner tends to lose his/her freedom to express, especially negative emotions, and the patient, by the virtue of becoming more dependent, also has a sense of loss of freedom to give expression to his/her true feelings. Given the scenario, communication that might have been clear and direct at the premorbid level tends to become pathologic. For Mr. and Mrs. Johnson, there was a very major issue with communication: the lack of it. They said very little to each other in the course of the day, and most of their communication centered on mundane daily chores such as Mr. Johnson's enquiring if his wife were planning anything that day. Mrs. Johnson did not discuss her concerns and worries about their daughter with Mr. Johnson lest he should become more upset. It was interesting to note that what little communication they had tended to be direct and clear. On the other hand, what they left unsaid was significant. In short, communication on instrumental issues was clear and direct and on affective issues there was no communication. The actual amount of communication was very low.

The next dimension of family functioning, *roles*, was very distorted with the Johnsons. Roles are divided into (a) instrumental roles such as provision of resources and (b) affective roles such as nurturance and support, sexual gratification, and marital fondness. For Mr. and Mrs. Johnson, the issue of roles was really quite uncomplicated. Mr. Johnson's predominant role was that of a patient and he was more than adequately fulfilling his obligations in that regard. He was seeking expert help and maintaining his hope to recover. Mrs. Johnson, in effect, had assumed all the necessary roles to keep this family together. This relationship was not devoid of nurturing and support. Mrs. Johnson was very supportive of Mr. Johnson's sick role and she did provide a great deal of nurturance in the way of looking after him. There was no evidence of sexual gratification or overt marital fondness. Nevertheless, they explained that they cared for each other, but their caring rarely found any external expression. The family was secure financially because Mr. Johnson had a substantial pension as well as savings. The finances were managed by Mrs. Johnson. Mr. Johnson had little or no interest in the day-to-day affairs of the family. It is noteworthy that obtaining their premorbid marital history from this couple proved to be virtually impossible. Mr. Johnson claimed that he did not remember and Mrs.

Johnson did not care. For that reason it was impossible to ascertain the degree to which their roles had altered due to Mr. Johnson's illness.

Affective responsiveness, according to the MMFF, consists of (a) welfare emotions such as love, happiness, and other positive feelings; and (b) the emergency emotions such as anger, fear, and mainly negative feelings. Effective families are capable of expressing wide ranges of emotions and they respond to a given stimulus with appropriate quantity and quality of feelings. It was hard to ascertain precisely what kind of emotions Mr. and Mrs. Johnson displayed toward each other. It was clear that Mrs. Johnson had very positive feelings toward her daughter and Mr. Johnson shared some of her feelings, although he rarely expressed them. It seemed as though these two individuals lived in an emotional vacuum. They claimed, and it was very evident during the interviews, that they rarely expressed any strong emotions. Their lives were highly routinized and predictable and they seemed to feel that they simply did not have the need to express emotions. Long years of illness seemed to have had a retarding effect on their capacity to express any kind of emotions. Over time, they had become emotionally handicapped. One interesting observation during an interviewing session was that Mr. Johnson was somewhat more expressive of his feelings, but Mrs. Johnson remained very constrained and gave no evidence of her inner feelings. The only time she gave vent to any emotion was in relation to the physicians who had failed to cure her husband. She was visibly angry with them.

In the area of *affective involvement,* this couple seemed to be quite distant from each other. There was some suggestions that Mrs. Johnson's involvement bordered on overinvolvement, which was unquestionably due to Mr. Johnson's disabilities and her daughter's retardation. It was very difficult to get a clear picture of Mr. Johnson's involvement with Mrs. Johnson. He needed her, he definitely had some feelings for her, but at the same time he was unable to do anything for her. Neither did he express his appreciation for her concern or for all that she did for him. His involvement could be described as almost bordering on lack of involvement, but this early assessment proved to be erroneous. As will become evident, in the course of therapy he was able to demonstrate empathic involvement with his wife.

A point should be made regarding the context of affective involvement between Mr. and Mrs. Johnson; given the chronicity of Mr. Johnson's illness and the level of his disability, which invariably induced a high level of dependency on Mrs. Johnson, the likelihood of empathic relationship being the predominant pattern of affective involvement would be highly improbable. In many ways, the relationship very much had the appearance of a caring and even doting mother and that of somewhat of a spoiled child who took everything that was being done for him for granted. Since there was no outward expression of how they felt for each other it was hard to ascertain the quality of their relationship.

The final dimension of the MMFF is *behavior control*, which is defined as the standard or rules adopted by a family for handling behavior in the following areas: (a) physically dangerous situations; (b) situations involving meeting and expressing psychobiological needs and drives; and (c) situations involving interpersonal socializing behavior.

With the Johnsons the behavior control was very definitely rigid. Mrs. Johnson made all the decisions; she made the rules and given the fact that she had a chronically ill husband and a retarded daughter, the rules were somewhat inflexible. She was almost like a nurse to these individuals, and one of her major functions was to ensure that the daily routine was maintained, medications were taken, the safety of the daughter was ensured, and the basic needs of the family members were met. Exploration of this dimension established the above facts, and this pattern was confirmed by both Mr. and Mrs. Johnson. Mr. Johnson almost seemed to be grateful that he did not have to take any responsibilities and very willing to follow his wife's dictum. The face that he was somewhat resentful about that was revealed later.

The above assessment led to some interesting observations about this family. According to the MMFF, there was no question that they seemed to be performing in the ineffective range on almost every dimension of family functioning. On the other hand, the situation was vastly complicated by chronic illness and retardation in family members. Under those circumstances, it seemed that the pattern of behavior that the family had adopted for managing their daily lives, while less than satisfactory, was not altogether ineffective. Mrs. Johnson had the singular responsibility for keeping this family together. She was the principal decision maker, manager for day-to-day affairs, and a nurse and a parent to her husband and daughter, respectively. Nevertheless, there were one or two areas where the family functioning could be definitely improved if the couple chose to do so.

Contracting

Given the history of this family, and the visible reluctance of Mrs. Johnson to participate in the process, it was somewhat of a surprise when they agreed to return for the contracting stage. This stage consists of two separate steps: problem description and contracting. The purpose of problem description is to engage the family in deciding upon the issues and problems they might like to address during the course of the therapy. This is also an opportunity for the therapist to identify some central issues that might have emerged during the course of the assessment. One of the key features of the assessment was Mr. Johnson's almost total dependency on Mrs. Johnson. It was also evident that Mrs. Johnson fed into this overdependent behavior, or in other words, perpetuated his pain behaviors. The question was raised rather cautiously about Mr. Johnson's ability to perhaps do a little more, and, quite out of character, he jumped at this opportunity. He stated that he would indeed like to go out to the corner shop to get his newspaper in the morning, perhaps occasionally make a cup of tea for himself and his wife, go out for longer drives on warm days, and perhaps even have a little more conversation with his wife about various things around the house and especially about his retarded daughter. Mrs. Johnson was visibly surprised and felt accused by her husband as though she was preventing him from doing any of those things. She was carefully steered into considering whether his proposition seemed reasonable. After further explanation, she either acquiesced or agreed; it was hard to tell the difference.

A contract was arrived at that consisted of the following tasks:

1. Mr. Johnson would engage in doing simple household chores such as dusting, making their midmorning tea, and taking more responsibility for banking. The last task was a surprise because it was suggested by Mrs. Johnson. She expressed rather strongly her feeling that she was tired of managing the money affairs of this family.

2. Mr. Johnson would engage in activities that gave him pleasure, such as going for walks and taking long drives with his wife, and he would like to make those decisions without Mrs. Johnson's being overly concerned.

3. Mr. Johnson would like to be more involved in discussion about their daughter's future.

It would be an exaggeration to state that Mr. and Mrs. Johnson engaged in active negotiation over these issues, but she sat somewhat passively and appeared to be in general agreement with his propositions. She herself did not enter into any kind of active negotiations to change this relationship. By and large, both of them seemed to be unwilling to address their affective issues such as intimacy and absence of sexual relationship. It was the therapist's decision not to pursue those matters, and that decision was based on the very chronic nature of marital relationships, which was discussed earlier, and perhaps a more important fact that Mrs. Johnson, in all probability, would refuse to participate in therapy if such matters were pursued with any degree of vigor. As far as their affective life was concerned both these individuals either did not recognize the deficiencies, or, if they did, accepted them quite fully.

In any event the modest tasks listed above were agreed upon and a plan was worked out to implement some of those tasks almost immediately. Agreement was also reached that Mr. and Mrs. Johnson would participate in the 1-hour sessions as and when they were needed, but still, over a limited period of time. The first few sessions were held at weekly intervals and then farther apart.

Treatment

The first treatment session was an enormous surprise. Mrs. Johnson came in looking somewhat animated for the first time and reported that her husband was doing things that he had not done in a very long time. He had gone out every single morning for walks and sometimes they lasted over an hour. Instead of going to a corner shop, he walked further and went to a mall to buy his newspaper. His mood was better and he seemed to be enjoying "pottering about the house." Mr. Johnson reported that not only had he felt better but he and his wife had talked more than they had done in a very long time. The rest of the session focused on some of Mrs. Johnson's lingering concerns and her generally cautious and protective attitude toward Mr. Johnson. Mr. Johnson tried to be reassuring to his wife, but she still felt that perhaps he should do less. It should be added that the dialogue between these two individuals during the first session and in all the subsequent sessions was very halting and intermittent with long pauses. It was very evident during the treatment sessions that these two individuals had a hard time talking to each other.

In the subsequent sessions Mr. Johnson continued to report some improvement. In broad terms he maintained the activities that he had embarked

upon; however, he and Mrs. Johnson still had a great deal of difficulty discussing day-to-day matters, especially issues surrounding their daughter. The central issue about their daughter was what might happen to her, because they themselves were getting older and it was imperative to make some kind of a long-term plan for her. Mrs. Johnson explained that she had fallen out of habit of discussing emotional matters and was having a hard time engaging in that process. On the other hand, they were able to sit together and review their finances (which was not a problem) and Mr. Johnson had tentatively agreed to look after the banking affairs. The first four sessions went along in this vein at weekly intervals.

During the fifth session the patient reported that he had experienced a setback. He had more pain and also a mild attack of emphysema and consequently had not done much in the preceding week. Mrs. Johnson's attitude was extremely protective and she almost suggested that this could be the result of Mr. Johnson's overactivity. Mr. Johnson was very disappointed with the setback, especially, as he put it, when he was beginning to feel "on the up and up." The fact that Mr. Johnson had several chronic problems had to be carefully explained by the therapist. It was also imperative to point out that these ups and downs would be part and parcel of his daily living, but that during his periods of relative health, it was important for him to pursue his goals with the help of his wife. It was not clear by the end of the session whether they had been reassured to any degree.

Arrangement was made to hold the sixth session after a 2-week interval to give Mr. and Mrs. Johnson time to try out their tasks. Fortunately, there was some improvement in Mr. Johnson's health and he was able to resume his pleasurable activities as well as his domestic chores. The therapy was terminated after two more sessions, which were held at 3-week intervals, and there was further evidence of Mr. Johnson's ability to engage in the tasks with increasing support from his wife.

Closure

During the final session a complete review of the treatment was carried out and there was consensus among all three parties that Mr. Johnson seemed to be quite capable of carrying out the tasks with the help of his wife. They had some more work to do in the area of discussing their daughter, which was proving to be most intractable. Nevertheless, they expressed optimism that even in that regard there had been some nominal movement. Arrangements were made for a 3-month and a 6-month review. At the time of the 3-month review the couple reported that Mr. Johnson had had several ups and downs with his health problems, but always returned to doing the things he had agreed on, and, most encouragingly, Mrs. Johnson had lost a great deal of her fear about Mr. Johnson's frailty. The situation remained basically unaltered at the 6-month review.

Discussion

This case was selected for the specific purpose of demonstrating that even in most intractable and chronic situations some minor improvement can be effected through couple therapy. In discussing the efficacy of PCSFT, Roy (37) reported on its effectiveness in treating less serious problems than those of Mr. and Mrs. Johnson with very favorable outcome. The central purpose of this paper has been to show that the goal of therapy is a function of several factors, the most important of which are: (1) the functional capacity of the patient given the nature of the illness and degree of disability; and (2) attitude of the spouse toward the patient and the degree to which he/she may be consciously or unconsciously invested in maintaining the patient's sick role. The first point was obvious in relation to Mr. Johnson; as for the second, the issues were very complex. In view of the length of Mr. Johnson's illness it could be argued that Mrs. Johnson had no option but to assume more and more responsibility and became a nurse as well as a caretaker rather than a marriage partner.

One of the key issues that should be addressed in the effectiveness of MMFF to assess a family such as the Johnsons. They clearly had deficits in almost every dimension of family functioning. The question is, given the multiplicity of problems that this family faced, namely, chronic illness in the husband and retardation in the child, could they have functioned at a higher level of effectiveness? In some dimensions there clearly was room for improvement. For example, the empathic relationship between Mr. and Mrs. Johnson and the level of nurturance and support could have been present at a somewhat higher level. It is the opinion of this author that this couple never truly enjoyed a genuine empathic and loving relationship, and the onset of early illness in Mr. Johnson and the birth of a retarded child further enhanced the distance between the two. It is in the area of role functioning that one may adopt a somewhat critical view of the MMFF. Arguably, Mrs. Johnson alone kept this family together; but for her assumption of some of the central family maintenance roles, this family

could not have continued to function as a viable unit. She also was forced into assuming a very high level of responsibility for problem solving and again, given the limitations, she did a very effective job.

In order to assess the effectiveness of a family's functioning, it is imperative that allowance be made for special circumstances. A family harboring a chronically ill spouse and a dependent and retarded daughter cannot in all probability function at the effective range of all the dimensions of family functioning. Perhaps a case can be made that any attempts to do so would be deleterious for the family. For example, it would be unreasonable to expect Mr. Johnson to share equal amounts of responsibility in the running of the family affairs. It would be equally unreasonable to expect him to engage in adult sexual gratification activities given his deficits. The chronic sick role imposes certain major limitations. A question of major clinical impact is to ascertain clearly the functional level of the patient. It is in that context that the family functioning has to be assessed for its effectiveness. In many ways the Johnsons remained a viable family unit fulfilling most of its instrumental tasks. The fact that they fell considerably short in terms of effectiveness in accordance with the MMFF may not in itself be sufficient grounds to make a negative judgment about the family's adaptability.

Mr. and Mrs. Johnson, with their daughter, had functioned in a certain way for a very long time. Mrs. Johnson was firmly committed to doing things in her own way and only grudgingly agreed to making some minor changes. She had been most resistant to bringing about any major changes in the prevailing homeostasis of the family for the simple reason that in her mind the family was functioning quite effectively. She did not see any choice but to carry the major burden of responsibility, and indeed she had done so for very many years. There was also some indication of her resistance to any suggestion of change in the family arrangements. The circumstances were such for the Johnsons that if they were not functioning optimally, the family seemed to be functioning efficiently. There was no evidence that either Mr. or Mrs. Johnson was particularly dissatisfied with the family situation.

Therefore, it remains somewhat of a surprise that Mr. and Mrs. Johnson agreed to enter into couple therapy and participated with a certain amount of enthusiasm—enthusiasm was certainly more apparent in Mr. Johnson than Mrs. Johnson. Modest goals were established and successfully achieved. It is hoped that this case study has demonstrated that even with a system that was as firmly entrenched as this one, problem-centered systems family therapy can still be effective in making minor but significant modifications.

REFERENCES

1. Roy R: Physical illness, chronic pain and family therapy. In Tunks E, Bellissimo A, Roy R (eds): *Chronic Pain: Psychosocial Factors in Rehabilitation,* ed 2. Melbourne, Fl. Krieger Publishing Co. (in press).
2. Lask B: Illness in the family: a conceptual model. In Walrond S (ed): *Developments in Family Therapy: Theories and Application since 1948.* London, Routledge and Kegan Paul, 1981.
3. Livsey CG: Physical illness and family dynamics. *Adv Psychosom Med* 8:237, 1972.
4. Minuchin S, Baker L, Rosman B, Liebman R, Milman L, Todd T: A conceptual model for illness in children: family organization and family therapy. *Arch Gen Psychiatry* 18:76, 1975.
5. Turk D, Rudy T, Flor H: Why a family perspective for pain? *Int J Fam Ther* 7:223, 1985.
6. Minuchin S, Rosman B, Baker L: *Psychosomatic Families.* Cambridge, MA, Harvard University Press, 1978.
7. Fordyce E: *Behavioral Methods for Chronic Pain and Illness.* St. Louis, CV Mosby, 1976.
8. Waring E: The role of the family in symptom selection and perpetuation of psychosomatic illness. *Psychother Psychosomat* 28:253, 1977.
9. Anderson K, Bradley L, Young L, McDaniel L: Rheumatoid arthritis: review of psychological factors related to etiology, effects and treatment. *Psychol Bull* 96:358, 1985.
10. Anthony E: The impact of mental and physical illness on family life. *Am J Psychiatry* 127:138, 1970.
11. Block A, Kremer E, Gaylor M: Behavioral treatment of chronic pain: the wife as a discriminative case for pain behavior. *Pain* 9:243, 1980.
12. Kremer E, Sieber W, Atkinson J: Spousal perpetuation of chronic pain behavior. *Int J Fam Ther* 7:258, 1985.
13. Roy R: "I have a headache tonight: functions of pain in marriage." *Int J Fam Ther* 6:165, 1984.
14. Roy R: The international perspective of pain behavior in marriage. *Int J Fam Ther* 7:271, 1985.
15. Croog S, Levine S: *The Heart Patient Recovers.* New York, Human Science Press, 1977.
16. Leventhal H, Levanthal E, Van Nguyen T: Reactions of families to illness: theoretical models and perspectives. In Turk D, Herns D (eds): *Health Illness and Families: A Life-Span Perspective.* New York, John Loxley & Sons, 1985.
17. Cunningham C, Betsa N, Gross S: Sibling groups. *Am J Pediatr Hematol Oncol* 3:135, 1980.
18. Huberty D: Adapting to illness through family groups. *Int J Psychiatry Med* 5:231, 1974.
19. Shambaugh P, Kanter S: Spouses under stress: group meetings with spouses of patients on hemodialysis. *Am J Psychiatry* 125:931, 1969.
20. Spiegel D: Psychological support for women with metastatic carcinoma. *Psychosomatics* 20:780, 1979.
21. Binger C: Psychosocial intervention with child cancer patient and family. *Psychosomatics* 25:899, 1984.
22. Bodie U: "Caring" oncology: a unified treatment program for the total care of cancer patient and family. *J SC Med Assoc* 76:563, 1980.
23. Sandler N: Working with families of chronic asthmatics. *J Asthma Res* 15:15, 1977.
24. Simon R: Hemophilia and the family system. *Psychosomatics* 25:845, 1984.
25. Hanrahan G: Beginning work with families of hospitalized adolescents. *Fam Process* 23:391, 1986.
26. Lask B, Matthew D: Childhood asthma: a controlled trial of family psychotherapy. *Arch Dis Child* 54:116, 1979.
27. Tomm K, McArthur R, Leahey M: Psychologic management of children with diabetes mellitus. *Clin Pediatr (Phila)* 16:1151, 1977.
28. Liebman R, Minuchin S, Baker L: The use of structural family therapy in the treatment of intractable asthma. *Am J Psychiatry* 131:535, 1974.
29. Gustaffson P, Kjellman H, Cedarblad M: Family therapy in the treatment of severe childhood asthma. *J Psychosom Res* 30:369, 1986.
30. Parker G, Lipscombe P: Parental overprotection and asthma. *J Psychosom Res* 23:295, 1979.
31. Burbeck T: An empirical investigation of the psychosomatogenic model. *J Psychosom Res* 23:295, 1979.
32. Palazzoli M: *Self-Observation: From the Intrapsychic to the Transpersonal Approach to Anorexia Nervosa.* London, Chaucer Publishing, 1974.
33. Hoebel F: Coronary artery disease and family intervention. A study of risk factor modification. In Watzlawick P, Weakland J (eds): *The Interactional View.* New York, WW Norton, 1977.
34. Mohamed S, Weisz G, Waring E: The relationship of chronic pain to depression, marital and family dynamics. *Pain* 5:282, 1978.
35. Shanfield S, Heiman E, Cope N, Jones J: Pain and marital relationships: psychiatric distress. *Pain* 7:343, 1979.
36. Ahern D, Follick M: Distress in spouses of chronic pain patients. *Int J Fam Ther* 7:247, 1985.
37. Roy R: Problem-centered systems family therapy in treating chronic pain. In Holzman A, Turk D (eds): *Chronic Pain: A Handbook of Treatment Strategies.* Elmsford, NJ, Pergamon Press, 1986.
38. Roy R: Impact of chronic pain on marriage: systems perspective. In: *Advances in Pain Research and Clinical Management.* Amsterdam, Elsevier, 1988.
39. Hudgens A: Family-oriented treatment of chronic pain. *J Marriage Fam Ther* 5:67, 1979.
40. Rowat K, Knafl K: Living with chronic pain: the spouses' perspective. 1985, 23:259, *Pain.*
41. Roy R: Family treatment for chronic pain: state of the art. *Int J Fam Ther* 7:297, 1985.
42. Moore J, Chaney E: Outpatient group treatment of chronic pain: effects of spouse involvement. *J Consult Clin Psychol* 53:326, 1985.

43. Flor H, Turk D, Rudy T: Pain and families. II. Assessment and treatment. *Pain* 30:29, 1987.

44. Roy R: Family etiology of psychogenic pain: the systems perspective. *Contemp Fam Ther* 9:263, 1987.

45. Berger H, Honig P, Liebman R: Recurrent abdominal pain: gaining control of the symptom. *Am J Dis Child* 131:1340, 1977.

46. Liebman R, Honig P, Berger H: An integrated treatment program for psychogenic pain. *Fam Process* 15:397, 1976.

47. Waring E: Conjoint and marital therapy. In Roy R, Tunks E (eds): *Chronic Pain: Psychosocial Factors in Rehabilitation.* Baltimore, Williams & Wilkins, 1982.

48. Westley A, Epstein N: *The Silent Majority.* San Francisco, Jossey-Bass, 1970.

49. Epstein N, Rakoff V: *Family Categories Schema.* Montreal, Jewish General Hospital, 1963.

50. Epstein N, Bishop D, Baldwin L: McMaster model of family functioning. A view of the normal family. In Walsh F (ed): *Normal Family Process.* New York, Guilford Press, 1982.

51. Bishop D, Byles J, Horn D: Family therapy training methods: minimal contact with an agency. *J Fam Ther* 6:323, 1984.

52. Bishop D, Epstein N, Keitner G, Miller I, Srinivasan S: Stroke: morale, family functioning, health status & functional capacity. *Arch Phys Med Rehabil* 67:84, 1986.

53. Epstein N, Baldwin L, Bishop D: The McMaster family assessment device. *J Marriage Fam Ther* 9:171, 1983.

54. Miller I, Kabacoff R, Keitner G, Epstein M, Bishop D: Family functioning in the families of psychiatric patients. *Compr Psychiatry* 27:302, 1986.

55. Epstein N, Bishop D: Problem-centered systems therapy of the family. In Gurman A, Kniskern D (eds): *Handbook of Family Therapy.* New York, Brunner/Mazel, 1981.

56. Roy R: Family dynamics of headache sufferers. A clinical report. *J Pain Manage* 1:9, 1987.

57. Roy R: Chronic pain and marriage difficulties. *Health Social Work* 10:199, 1985.

Chapter 19

HYPNOSIS

FREDERICK J. EVANS, PhD

HYPNOSIS AND PAIN: THEORY AND RESEARCH FINDINGS

Dramatic demonstrations of the use of hypnosis as an anesthetic in surgery, childbirth, and dentistry, and as an analgesic for controlling pain, may promote interest in professionals about hypnosis as a clinical technique. The interest is often fleeting because it is soon discovered that, occasional claims notwithstanding, hypnosis does not provide the instant "magic wand" quality that many patients, and some professionals, are seeking. Hypnosis certainly has an established role in medicine in the management of pain (1). Its successful use is predicated on a careful understanding of the nature of hypnosis and the professional skills of the therapist within his/her discipline, as well as the characteristics and expectations of the patient who will use it.

The aim of this chapter is to provide a background for understanding hypnosis within the context of pain management, especially focusing on clinical techniques relevant to the control of chronic pain such as low back pain. The discussion will be general, because there are relatively few reports of the use of hypnosis in low back pain patients. This may seem surprising because of the number of anecdotal reports of success from clinicians. It is not especially surprising when the difficulty of treating back pain and other chronic pain syndromes is noted. Consideration of psychodynamic issues involved in the chronic pain syndrome indicates that, while the successful application of hypnotic techniques will not be simple, there is a promise of success that may not be possible with other approaches.

Although clinical reports document that hypnosis has been used as an effective technique to control chronic pain (2), and in the management of pain in the terminally ill patient (3), there are relatively few well-controlled empirical studies of the clinical efficacy of hypnosis in pain management (4). About 50% of terminal cancer patients (5) and 95% of dental patients (6) can be helped to gain some pain control by the adjunctive use of hypnotic techniques. Crasilneck (7) found that 69% of 29 consecutive referrals for low back pain reported an average of 80% subjective pain relief during mostly outpatient treatment. Only four patients were considered treatment failures, although five others were eliminated from the program for psychological reasons. These patients were initially seen daily, then irregularly for a mean of 31 sessions over 9 months. The successful patients were withdrawn from medication during the course of the study. Another study (8) found little difference between the use of hypnosis and relaxation in the treatment of back pain. In a well-controlled study of chronic pain, hypnosis and biofeedback (9) did not produce differences in outcome: there were only a few back pain patients in this sample.

HYPNOSIS AND PAIN: THEORETICAL BACKGROUND

The modern history of hypnosis dates back to the late 18th century with Mesmer. However, it was the Scottish physician Esdaile (10) who most dramatically documented the early use of hypnosis in the control of pain. Just prior to the development of chemical anesthesia, Esdaile was using hypnosis widely in India as the only form of anesthesia for amputations, tumor removals, and complex surgical procedures. Overlooked in Esdaile's reports was the fact that most of his patients survived surgery: this was especially compelling because at that time most surgical patients died because of hemorrhage, shock, and postsurgical infection. Hypnosis may have had autonomic and/or immunologic effects that minimized the usual complications of the surgical techniques of the time, an issue that is only now beginning to attract research interest. Currently, when hypnosis is used in surgical procedures, it is usually used with markedly reduced dosages of analgesic drugs. Except for some evidence from hemophiliac patients (11), there is little scientific, but abundant clinical, evidence that the use of hypnosis preoperatively or during surgical techniques reduces bleeding volume and time, and facilitates various physiologic postoperative recovery measures, as well as reducing pain and postoperative medication (1).

There is controversy concerning the nature of hypnosis. One's theoretical stance may influence research design and strategies used in hypnotic treatment programs. There is not a consensus definition of hypnosis, but most investigators emphasize one of four aspects: suggestibility; expectations (and the hypnotist-subject interaction); cognitive distortions, including imagery and attentional processes; and dissociation (12).

The popular notion that hypnosis is a form of suggestibility is certainly an oversimplification (13), even though this "definition" dominated the otherwise impressive research on hypnotic phenomena from the 1930s (14) through the late 1950s (15). Although it is agreed that response to suggestion is an important aspect of what happens during hypnosis, it is also generally agreed that hypnosis is a more complex phenomenon.

Some authors emphasize expectations, motivation, and the social psychological interaction between hypnotist and subject as the main component of hypnotic behavior. Hypnosis involves motivated striving to play the role of the good hypnotic subject. The experience of hypnosis is operationally defined as a response to the induction process (16–19). For such theories, pain reduction involves interpersonal processes or self-generated cognitive and motivational strategies, such as the reallocation of attention away from the pain, focusing of attention, distraction, verbal relabeling, imagery, and possibly anxiety reduction, attribution, denial, or convincing oneself that the pain isn't really that severe. These cognitively based strategies are presumably facilitated by the hypnotic relationship (although it is not always clear how this is done). These strategies have been statistically shown to be successful in research studies (18). Results are usually not related to individual differences in hypnotizability, which are often not even measured.

Another dominant view of hypnosis is that it reflects a special state or stable capacity of the individual. The hypnotic experience may involve an ability to readily change states of awareness or levels of consciousness. These changes may be either interpersonally or self-induced (12, 20–22). This view is supported by data showing very stable individual differences in hypnotic ability over many years (22). From this approach, an important research strategy is to show how differences in pain-control strategies relate to individual differences in hypnotic ability.

Significant contributions to understanding the nature of acute pain have been made in the hypnosis literature, particularly the meticulous psychophysical studies of experimental pain conducted by Ernest H. Hilgard (5, 21, 22). Under controlled experimental conditions, Hilgard and his colleagues have shown that the relationship between the intensity of the noxious stimulation and the subjective experience of transient, acute pain follows standard psychophysical curves. This relationship has been shown to be legitimate both for normal conditions and for the reduction of pain following hypnotic analgesia in subjects differing in hypnotic susceptibility (5).

Experimental studies of acute pain have been conducted in situations in which the significance of the stimulation is not psychologically meaningful beyond the confines of the transient noxious stimulation. Anxiety about the meaning of the painful stimulation has been minimized or eliminated in these studies. It is doubtful whether such studies are particularly helpful to the clinician confronted with patients in pain, although they are important for understanding pain mechanisms. In his later work Hilgard (22) elaborated on pain control within the context of neodissociation theory, particularly using the method of the "hidden observer." This procedure helped document that pain perception may take place at several different levels of awareness. Multiple cognitive pathways are readily accessible to the hypnotized subject. This enables him/her to experience minimal pain at a conscious level, even though at another cognitive level (or an observing ego), he/she is able to report the actual intensity of the painful stimulation. Complex and subtle techniques have been developed to study pain control that capitalize on the highly hypnotizable subject's ability to maintain this dissociative control: remaining comfortable with suggestions of hypnotic analgesia while experiencing pain at another level. The multiple cognitive controls implicit in the "hidden observer" procedures are not especially different from our own subjective experiences under dental analgesia, for example, when we experience that the drill does not hurt, even though we maintain awareness of the level of pain stimulation that we would be experiencing without the chemical intervention.

Hilgard formulated this approach in terms of neodissociation or multiple cognitive pathways. Evans (12) viewed hypnosis as a manifestation of a more general ability involving cognitive flexibility, or a switching mechanism that allows one to change physiologic, psychological, or cognitive processes, or readily access different levels of consciousness. Hypnotizability correlates with such variables as the ability to utilize imagery effectively, the ability to become absorbed in other engaging experiences such as becoming "lost" in a movie or novel and experiencing some of the emotions of the characters, napping and the ease of falling asleep, occasional lateness for appointments, and the ease with which patients gave up psychiatric (and possibly medical) symptoms (12).

In relation to pain, if empirical data confirmed that measured hypnotizability correlates highly with pain control, or if situational and/or relationship variables were found to be better predictors of pain control, then the controversy would be readily resolved. However, the correlation between measured hypnotizability and pain control in a variety of experimental situations is only a moderate .5 (5). This is significantly less than the joint reliabilities of the pain reports (measured by subjective analogue scales or by behavioral methods) and the hypnotizability measures. When data consistently fall somewhere between two extreme sets of predictions, the most likely conclusion is that both views have some degree of validity. The ambiguity of this basic piece of data—the modest relationship between hypnotic and analgesia and hypnotic depth—highlights the fundamental paradox in hypnotic pain control: Clinicians claim that most of their patients can benefit from hypnotic intervention techniques, whereas the empirical data suggest that only relatively few people have sufficient (dissociative) capacity to experience the profound sensory and cognitive skills that eliminate pain The resolution of this paradox, discussed below, has important implications for the application of hypnotic techniques in chronic pain management.

METHODOLOGIC ISSUES IN HYPNOTIC ANALGESIA RESEARCH

Although the clinical reports of hypnotic analgesia and pain control have been impressive, the effects of hypnotic intervention on experimental pain tasks have only been shown over the last two decades. Unfortunately, most earlier studies failed to show convincing hypnotic analgesia (9, 22–24). These early, well-controlled studies probably failed to show hypnotic effects because they used transient painful stimulation such as electric shock and radiant heat. These stimuli share neither the enduring qualities of chronic pain nor the debilitating anxiety of acute pain. The deliberate attempt to minimize anxiety in early experiments obscured the problem that these methods of pain stimulation are not affected by standard analgesic drugs, such as morphine, and therefore may not be useful analogues of clinical pain.

Partly for reasons of subject welfare, many of these early studies were restricted to measuring pain threshold, or the point at which pain first becomes noticeable. Clinically, patients do not report that they have a problem with their pain threshold! Recent meaningful studies have used protracted measures of pain approaching pain tolerance and endurance levels. For the most part, the only viable experimental pain induction methods satisfying adequate clinical pain criteria are the cold pressor and ischemic pain tasks. Both tasks measure severe, protracted pain, and are sensitive to analgesic medications, and therefore reflect some of the qualities of chronic pain.

A second important methodologic issue is the measurement of hypnotic responsiveness. If there are individual differences in hypnotizability it is clearly inadequate to define hypnosis in terms of an induction procedure. Screening for hypnotizability must be done carefully in studies of hypnotic pain control. Many studies do not carefully select extreme high- and low-hypnotizable subjects. If hypnosis involves a unique set of skills, then subjects who have been selected for high hypnotizability will have the best opportunity to experience hypnotic analgesia. Even in an experimental setting, it is difficult to get stable measures of hypnotizability without using two or three scales because the initial session tends to be contaminated by preconceptions, curiosities, and anxieties about the meaning of hypnosis. This is even more complicated in the clinic because a hypnotized patient may respond well to hypnosis during a screening session, but may refuse to experience hypnosis in a subsequent therapeutic context because of an unreadiness to give up the pain symptom. Therefore it is critically important to evaluate hypnosis in the clinic independently of the treatment session so that hypnotic ability will not be confounded with the desire to be helpful, or the impact of an unreadiness to get better (25).

REPRESENTATIVE STUDIES OF HYPNOTIC ANALGESIA

A few key studies illustrating the methodologic and conceptual issues involved in the clinical application of hypnosis in pain control are reviewed here briefly. Comprehensive reviews are available (5, 18, 22, 26).

In a marked deviation from the methods used in prior hypnotic analgesia studies, McGlashan and coworkers (27–30) tested 12 extremely high- and 12 extremely low-hypnotizable male subjects. Hypnotizability had been carefully assessed during several earlier sessions. The ischemic pain task was used to measure pain tolerance during three separate sessions: (a) highly motivated baseline conditions, (b) following the careful induction of hypnotic analgesia, and (c) after ingesting a placebo capsule. The capsule was legitimized as an experimental pain-killing drug serving as a control procedure against which to evaluate the effects of hypnosis. The experimenter believed subjects were randomly given placebo or Darvon compound in order to maintain proper double-blind conditions. In fact, all subjects received placebo.

The logic of this study was to maximize variables that could produce nonspecific placebo treatment effects, such as is done in the clinic, rather than to control or eliminate nuisance factors, as is done in traditional experimental studies. No attempt was made to control variables (demand characteristics, 30) such as expectations, anxieties, and order effects that might affect the results. Instead, a deliberate choice was made to maximize the effect of confounding variables that might influence changes in (ischemic) pain tolerance. Thus, a conservative test was set up to evaluate whether the hypnotic analgesia achieved by deeply hypnotized subjects would exceed the pain relief produced in hypnotically unresponsive subjects who were set up to respond to nonspecific aspects of the hypnotic treatment context (the induction procedure, prior expectations, and other accoutrements of the hypnotic context) and to placebo medication. A similar test of the effects of hypnotic analgesia was conducted, using the subject as his own control, after he ingested what was thought to be a powerful pain-killing medication.

It is difficult to motivate low-hypnotizable subjects to participate in a hypnotic procedure because they are convinced hypnosis will not work with them. A simple but compelling deception was used

with the low-hypnotizable subjects to legitimize an expectancy of analgesia. Prior to the experimental hypnosis session, an independent experimenter induced a glove analgesia (numb hand that was insensitive to touch), using a hypnotic relaxation induction geared to each subject's description of his/her prior minimal hypnotic experiences. This was tested by administering a brief electric shock to the fingers. To their surprise, low-hypnotizable subjects experienced the analgesia—because the experimenter surreptitiously turned down the shock intensity from the preanalgesic test level!

Measures of pain tolerance involved time to maximum tolerance (quit point), volume of water displaced as the subject pumped to induce rapid ischemia in the occluded arm, and a subjective 1-to-10 rating of pain severity at the quit point. The improved ability to tolerate excruciating ischemic muscle pain for these extremely high- and/or low-hypnotizable subjects after suggestions of hypnotic analgesia, and subsequently after ingesting a placebo, is shown in Figure 19.1. This figure shows changes in time from baseline, indicating (increased) ability to tolerate ischemic pain under hypnotic or placebo conditions. In each of the high and low groups some subjects rated their pain based on a 1-to-10 subjective rating as decreasing (+) under hypnosis or "drug," whereas some found no change or even a slight increase (−) in pain in either of the two treatment sessions. Results for the subjective change subgroups are also presented. Three aspects of the results should be noted.

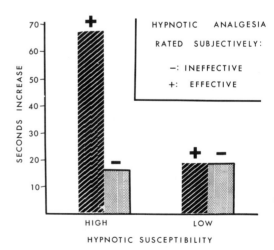

Figure 19.1.   Increased tolerance of ischemic pain in subjects of high and low hypnotizability (*N* = 12 each group) under conditions of hypnotic and placebo analgesia.

First, there was a dramatic increase in pain tolerance for deeply hypnotizable subjects during hypnotically induced analgesia. Hypnotic pain control in highly hypnotizable patients was unequivocally demonstrated. This is directly attributed to the dissociative aspects of the hypnotic conditions when it occurs in highly responsive hypnotic virtuoso subjects. This change only occurred in those highly hypnotizable subjects ($N = 6$) who subjectively experienced this relief.

Second, the much smaller but significant placebo-induced change in ischemic pain tolerance was equal in magnitude for both highly hypnotizable and unhypnotizable subjects. This shows that hypnosis is not related to placebo mechanisms per se. The later changes were due primarily to situationally induced anxiety (28).

Third, the most important finding is that the hypnotic analgesia suggestions significantly improved tolerance of ischemic pain even for unhypnotizable subjects who do not have the ability to enter hypnosis. This can be labeled as the "placebo" component of the hypnotic induction procedure. Indeed, for these hypnotically unresponsive subjects, the pain relief produced by the placebo component of the hypnotic context and the placebo component of ingesting a pill are about equal and highly correlated ($r = .76$, $N = 12$), and unrelated to the subjective ratings of relief. The expectation that hypnosis can be helpful in reducing pain produces significant reductions in pain similar to the expectation derived from taking a pain-killing pill, particularly in those individuals who otherwise have no special hypnotic skills. This somewhat manipulative and deceptive study indicated that hypnosis has both specific and nonspecific effects, just as the administration of medication has specific drug effects and nonspecific placebo effects.

In contrast to earlier studies in which attempts were made to minimize the nonspecific or placebo effects of the hypnotic context, they were maximized and allowed to run free in this study. Significant pain relief was achieved under both the placebo analgesia and placebo hypnosis conditions, even though this relief was not nearly as great as that obtained with hypnotic analgesia in hypnotizable subjects. In a similar fashion in drug research, it has been shown that for patients who respond to a placebo injection, over 90% also responded to a standard dose of morphine to reduce pain. However, in those patients who did not respond to the placebo trial, only about 50% responded to morphine (26). The expectation of relief and anxiety reduction that presumably mediates the placebo response produces

powerful therapeutic effects. Evans (28, 29) reviewed double-blind medication pain reduction studies and showed that the relative effectiveness of placebo compared to a standard dose of morphine is about 56%. The placebo is also from 50 to 60% as effective as other analgesics, including aspirin, codeine, Darvon, and Zomax, as well as nonpain procedures, including the pharmacologic and behavioral treatment of insomnia and the double-blind use of lithium in psychiatric patients. This is a remarkable finding, because it implies that the nonspecific factors arising from the treatment milieu are important clinical variables to the extent that the therapist communicates his/her enthusiasm and expectation of success to the suffering patient.

This study (27–30) documented that the mechanisms by which a placebo pill and hypnosis produced analgesia were different in subjects with high hypnotic capacity. Comparable findings have been obtained comparing hypnosis with other pain-reducing strategies (31–33). Results similar to those reported above for placebo versus hypnosis were reported for acupuncture versus hypnosis (31). The pain reduction with acupuncture was similar in high- and low-hypnotizable subjects, but the pain response of highly hypnotizable subjects was significantly greater with hypnosis than with acupuncture. It should be noted, parenthetically, that acupuncture is reversed by the morphine/endorphin antagonist naloxone, although hypnotic and analgesia is not (33). The independence of hypnotic analgesia from nonspecific pain reduction methods was also demonstrated in a recent study (32) that involved cold pressor pain in three groups, preselected for high and low hypnotizability, who were given: (a) Meichenbaum's (34) stress inoculation procedure; (b) the same procedure defined as a hypnotic intervention, without any hypnotic induction; or (c) hypnotic analgesia. Miller and Bowers argued that the two stress inoculation groups captured the essential features of interventions used by Spanos (18) and others from the social-contextual approach to hypnosis. Not surprisingly, the results were directly comparable to the hypnotic versus placebo (27) and acupuncture (31) studies. High- and low-hypnotizable subjects gained significant and equal pain relief from the stress inoculation procedures. However, the pain reduction of highly hypnotizable subjects with hypnotic analgesia surpassed the degree of relief obtained by all subjects where hypnosis was not involved.

In summary, then, these studies and others show that hypnosis can facilitate a number of cognitive strategies that can be helpful in alleviating pain. Specific interventions such as acupuncture, attention/distraction, placebo, relaxation, and stress inoculation all have a significant effect on pain, but these effects seem to be independent of individual differences in hypnotic capacity. The use of the label "hypnosis" produces a powerful, almost magical, connotation that *change* is expected. This expectation of therapeutic success may be strong in the therapist as well as in the patient, and is uncorrelated with the patient's hypnotizability. The communication of confidence and the message to the patient that help is on its way is a powerful therapeutic intervention that cannot be overlooked in treating chronic pain. The magical connotations of "hypnosis" and the ritual of the hypnotic induction process produce powerful nonspecific therapeutic effects that may lead to substantial pain control in many patients, even those with limited hypnotic capacity. In this sense, as many clinicians claim, hypnosis may work for everybody, except the treatment-resistant patient, even though for some the clinical effects are produced by the context of hypnosis rather than the hypnotic condition itself.

On the other hand, these studies show that for some highly selected individuals, hypnosis produces a means of controlling and mastering pain that is different from procedures such as placebo, acupuncture, stress inoculation, and naloxone-induced biochemical changes. Just as in the studies of the interaction between placebo response and morphine response, these interpersonal and individual trait aspects of hypnosis cannot easily be separated. However, only the trait components depend on measured hypnotic skill. The fact that there are two interacting mechanisms involved helps to explain why clinicians often see compelling pain relief in patients who otherwise seem unhypnotizable. The capacity to experience hypnosis may be at best a powerful bonus. Careful diagnosis of the nature of the pain will often suggest that the nonspecific components of the hypnotic situation may provide powerful therapeutic leverage. If hypnosis is useful with chronic pain cases where depression and secondary gain are the key therapeutic issues, it is likely to involve these nonspecific aspects of the hypnotic context rather than hypnotic capacity.

HYPNOSIS AND THE CLINICAL MANAGEMENT OF PAIN

It is important to make explicit the assumptions affecting the use of hypnotic techniques in pain management. Table 19.1 schematically differentiates the typical use of hypnosis in the treatment of several general kinds of pain, including acute and cancer pain, headache, and chronic pain of either known or unknown pathology. At least when hypnosis is involved low back pain is generally of the chronic type. This summary lists the typical way in which hypnosis is used in the particular pain type, the time course, and the goals of hypnotic intervention, as well as comments on anticipated additional benefits to the patient from the use of hypnosis. These summary statements will be expanded throughout the chapter.

Rational clinical applications of hypnosis for pain management must differentiate the typical sequence of events involved in acute versus chronic pain. The laboratory-confirmed assumption of a one-to-one correlation between the intensity of short-lasting, noxious stimulation and reported pain does not hold true for chronic pain. With most chronic pain patients, the intensity of the pain is not as significant as its psychological meaning, especially when a specific organic basis to the pain cannot be documented. A careful evaluation of the pain process itself must be made before hypnotic techniques can be employed as an adjunct in its management and control.

CANCER AND TERMINAL PAIN PATIENTS

Although an extended discussion of cancer pain is not relevant here, it should be noted that one of the most effective uses of hypnosis is in the management of the cancer patient. Hypnosis is often dramatic in helping the cancer patient control pain (although not usually in eliminating it completely), reducing medication, controlling nausea and vomiting and the side effects of chemotherapy, and helping (especially in children) minimize the threat of needles, bone marrow tests, and other invasive procedures. Cancer patients, especially those with excessive nausea and vomiting, are usually very responsive to hypnosis. Imagery techniques work very well. These patients can usually learn rapid self-hypnotic techniques that are then available to them whenever needed.

There are two important warnings for the therapist using hypnosis in this context. First, the improvement in the patient's functioning is easily misinterpreted as the remission of the cancer, and some family therapy is needed to assure all parties that hypnosis is being used to help the patient to suffer with dignity rather than to produce a cure. Second, the self-hypnosis procedures usually work— for a while. After days, or even weeks, self-hypnosis

Table 19.1
Generalized Overview of the Adjunctive Use of Hypnosis in the Treatment of Different Types of Pain[a]

TYPE OF PAIN	TYPICAL USE OF HYPNOSIS	TIME COURSE	TREATMENT GOALS	SECONDARY EFFECTS
Acute pain	Relaxation/anxiety reduction	Very short term, often crisis intervention	Reduce anxiety, provide support	Increase accessibility to appropriate treatment
Cancer pain	Self-hypnosis, often with relaxation and imagery	Very short term with "booster" sessions	Teach patient to suffer less with dignity	Reduction in nausea and other side effects of treatment, reduced medication
Chronic pain: clear organic pathology	Self-hypnosis usually directed at symptom, imagery and focused attention	Multiple sessions as needed	Teach self-control and mastery/ experiences	Reduction in suffering, improved ego strength due to self-control
Chronic pain: no clear organic basis	Self-hypnosis and dissociative skills	Short-term aggressive; long-term psychological and/or pharmacology therapy	Short term: control body functions (e.g., glove analgesia), learn self-control; long term: secondary gain, depression	Management of underlying depression
Headache	Varies based on type: relaxation, self-control, tension reduction, imagery	Variable, often with "booster" sessions	Symptom reduction, strategies for quality of life, as needed	Stress and tension reductions and self-control skills

[a]Assumes thorough medical psychological and diagnostic evaluation, and hypnosis used within the limits of professional training and competence.

often looses effectiveness. This may coincide with stressors, such as a new medical report, or a change in treatment, or a family dispute. Fortunately relatively rapid "booster" sessions with the hypnotist will usually recreate the effectiveness of self-hypnosis. If the technique is established well, these boosters can sometimes be conducted by telephone.

ACUTE PAIN AND HYPNOSIS

The management of acute pain primarily involves the management of anxiety. The growing anxiety about the short- and long-term consequences of the injury that accompanies the increasing intensity of the noxious stimulation is usually relieved by adequate treatment (e.g., pain medication, hypnosis, or other interventions to reduce anxiety). Many studies have shown an almost direct relationship between increases in anxiety and increases in pain intensity (22). It is clinically accepted (although there are virtually no studies documenting it) that the reverse will hold: reduction in anxiety will automatically be followed by reduction in reported pain. Hypnosis is a simple and effective method of

reducing anxiety either by direct suggestion or via any technique that helps the patient relax. Level of hypnotic responsivity is usually irrelevant, and the response is likely due to the nonspecific components of the hypnotic procedure. The mere soft, slow intonation of a hypnotic relaxation procedure is a dramatic contrast to the decibel level usually associated with emergency injury and resulting pain. If the sufferer has sufficient hypnotic talent, secondary effects (e.g., the control of bleeding, reduced medication, relaxation necessary for emergency medical intervention) are possible. It should be noted that patients with high levels of anxiety occasionally react counterexpectationally to relaxation methods. They may become even more anxious. These patients may respond well to imagery techniques, or may relax if they are allowed to leave their eyes open, or are positively assured that they will not loose self-control during hypnosis.

Even acute pain is not always a simple matter of stimulus intensity in the clinical situation. Wounded soldiers on the Anzio beachhead during World War II typically did not report pain as they waited to be removed from the battlefield, in spite of gunshot and shrapnel wounds that may eventually have needed major surgery, amputation, and long-term convalescence. Beecher (35) contrasted the wounded soldier's mild euphoria with similarly injured civilians in a hospital emergency setting, who typically writhed in agony and demanded immediate attention and medication. The soldier knew he was going home, and that he no longer had to fear being killed; for the civilian the pain has socioeconomic implications, fear of job loss, and so forth. Beecher's observations were not new, having been made during the Napoleonic Wars, and in China 2000 years ago (28). Beecher's (35) emphasis on the manner in which the psychological significance of the pain experience modulates wound severity has led to the delineation of learning factors and early experience in the development of long-term pain behavior (36). A young child, after falling, may survey the environs to establish whether a parent is nearby to provide tender loving care before deciding whether to cry or continue playing with his/her friends. Early learning experiences in handling transient pain may lead to an enduring developmental pattern in which pain and suffering can become instrumental in manipulating the environment (e.g., getting attention from Mommy, receiving the good-tasting cherry-flavored medicine, avoiding school). Learning and pain adaptation factors are prevalent in the psychological history of chronic pain patients.

FROM ACUTE TO CHRONIC PAIN: ANXIETY TO DEPRESSION

The management of acute pain primarily involves the management of anxiety. Partly because the pain is not relieved satisfactorily, a different set of dynamics arise as another pattern becomes established. Although pain intensity may have increased initially, it tends to abate gradually, but the fear of continued suffering remains. The anticipatory feelings of future fear give away from the initially vague feeling to the frightening awareness that a painful injury or lesion may have a more permanent effect. Despair and despondency gradually develop as the suffering remains partially unrelieved, and usual activities become restricted. Gradually a time-protracted pattern is established involving helplessness and depression that reinforces pain behavior (36). The seductiveness of seeking, demanding, and receiving help from significant others, the mildly pleasant and/or euphoric effects of medication, or the sedation by which sleep avoids the pain produces a reinforcement contingency for which the pain is a sufficient, and eventually a necessary,

experience. Feelings of helplessness lead to depression, guilt, and internalized anger concerning perceived loss of bodily parts or functions and diminished self-control.

Pain is sometimes positively reinforced by its pleasant consequences, and sometimes negative consequences are avoided by continued pain (37). Good things happen only when the patient has pain ("My low back pain allows me to watch the Sunday football game instead of mowing the lawn"); alternatively, pain prevents bad things from happening ("When I have my headache, I can avoid my spouse's advances and my impossible kids go outside and play"; "My poor spouse will not leave me while I am still suffering"). Hypnotic intervention based on anxiety reduction, relaxation, or symptom removal will only frustrate the patient and the therapist, and will usually be unsuccessful. The use of hypnosis in these patients may be helpful, but different strategies are needed. It is appropriate to consider that any chronic pain patient is depressed until proven otherwise, especially when there is no apparent somatic or organic basis to the pain. When using hypnosis for pain control it is necessary to address simultaneously the depression and secondary gain as psychotherapeutic issues.

CLINICAL ASSESSMENT OF CHRONIC PAIN

The typical chronic pain patient will have unsuccessfully experienced an average of five previous treatment modalities before coming to a therapist who uses hypnosis. These will often have included neurologists and neurosurgeons ("when in doubt, cut it out"), manipulative procedures by orthopedic and chiropractic specialists ("when in doubt, pound it out"), psychological interventions ("when in doubt, talk it out"), and extensive pharmacologic intervention ("when in doubt, medicate"). The typical chronic pain patient will be taking many different interacting medications. In addition, they will have been involved in psychological and psychiatric treatment, and have received input from other well-meaning sources, including spouses, lover, friends, and the local hairdresser. Partly because of the depression and internalized anger, the clinician is usually discouraged and the initial confrontation is often an adversarial one. The patient's demands to "help poor me, doc" (when the implicit meaning is "I know you can't"), "fix me up" ("you're probably another quack"), and "write me another prescription" ("I need to maintain my addiction") are not conducive to a meaningful therapeutic relationship (36). For many of these patients, the demand "hypnotize me and get rid of my pain" is often an invitation to failure. When the burden of cure is arrogated to an assumed magical technique, any initial attempt to use hypnosis will at best be unsuccessful and at worst precipitate an early termination of the therapeutic encounter.

The importance of the initial therapeutic contract must be emphasized when hypnosis is to be used with the chronic pain patient. This patient will usually require a confrontational style in order to evaluate the secondary gain issues quickly, because it will be these issues that will determine the focus of the treatment plan. Four direct questions are often helpful to achieve this:

1. *"What difference would it make to your life if suddenly you had no pain?"* The response to this question is often hedged with anger and impatience. It will quickly reveal hints about the psychic utility of the pain as a reinforcing system. For example, consider the implications of the response: "Oh, I would have to go back to my goddamned traveling salesman job and be away from my family most of the time."

2. *"Do you want to get better?"* Patients with chronic pain masking depression will rarely give an unequivocal "yes" to this question. An angry "What do you mean? Of course I want to get better!" is a typical response. This question should be repeated three times, giving the patient an opportunity to give a simple "yes" response. Failure to obtain a sincere "yes" usually indicates a poor prognosis. Depressed patients will quickly become more angry and frustrated with the repetition of this question.

3. *"Would you be satisfied if your pain could be reduced by about half?"* This is both a contractual and informational question exploring whether the patient has realistic expectations about pain relief. Patients who can accept partial relief as a goal have more realistic expectations about outcome.

4. *"Are you willing to work hard to get better?"* This question is useful to explain to the patient that the therapist has no magical cure, and that hypnosis does not guarantee dramatic results. The emphasis is on the ability of the patient to work at getting better rather than expecting the therapist to produce some effortless "quick fix." The importance of practicing self-hypnosis exercises can be stressed.

If the answers to the direct questions are unsatisfactory, it may be necessary to tell patients who cannot accept the basic therapeutic contract that this approach may not be right for them, and that

perhaps they should seek help elsewhere. The clinician then has to make a difficult decision: continue therapy with a patient with a poor prognostic outcome, or dismiss the patient, who may then seek help from another source that may be harmful.

These questions also provide a useful transition to discuss misconceptions about hypnosis and to emphasize that the responsibility for improvement rests with the patient rather than with the hypnotist. The hypnotist's role as a special and powerful teacher or facilitator must be emphasized. Finally, the way in which the patient is asked to describe his/her pain may be very useful later to help select appropriate imagery and cognitive strategies when it is time to use hypnotic interventions. Many patients find it difficult to describe their pain verbally, but can complete written instruments such as the McGill Pain Questionnaire (38). Techniques such as drawing the pain, asking about the color and shape of the pain, and exploring conditions under which it is more or less intense (heat, cold, sitting) may be relevant to help develop treatment strategies. Particularly in outpatient settings, chronic pain patients tend to resist extensive psychological testing. Elevations on the Somatic, Depression, and possibly Hysteria scales on the short Crown-Crisp Experiential Inventory (39) are as helpful as clinical indicators of somatic depression as are the elevated Hysteria, Depression, and Hypochondriasis scales of the much longer Minnesota Multiphasic Personality Inventory (MMPI) (36).

HYPNOTIC TECHNIQUES IN CHRONIC PAIN

The nature of the hypnotic intervention will largely depend on whether there are coexisting masked depression and secondary gain components to the pain, or whether the pain is primarily a residual of a clearly localized or carefully documented somatic process. The extreme clinical examples are low back pain injury in which the patient is involved in litigation versus terminal cancer pain. The patient involved in compensation or litigation cannot easily give up the pain until the legal proceedings are resolved. Although hypnosis will not be very successful initially, when gradually introduced with supportive psychotherapy, hypnosis may still be the adjunctive treatment of choice. Similarly, the low back pain patient who is masking depression will not easily relinquish his/her symptom with hypnotic intervention unless the depression is also treated. The symptom is too important to relinquish with simple hypnotic interventions such as direct symptom removal or posthypnotic suggestion. Where there is the possibility of unmasking depression as a result of too-rapid removal of the pain symptom, complications, including suicide risk, must be carefully considered. There have been clinical anecdotes of attempted suicide when low back pain has been abruptly removed by hypnotic suggestion, although the chances of successful direct, short-term symptom removal is low. The only exception to this guideline would be with cases in which the pain has suddenly stopped having secondary gain, such as when litigation is completed.

The Initial Hypnosis Session

After careful assessment, the initial work with hypnosis (in a first or later treatment session) will usually not involve the pain problem. This session should explore the patient's expectation about the nature of hypnosis, and provide opportunities for the patient to find out about his/her own hypnotic skills and to become familiar with the hypnotic procedures.

The initial hypnotic contact should build upon relatively easy suggestions that are based on subtle physical manifestations (e.g., eye fixation procedures based on eye strain and fatigue leading to suggestions of eye closure and relaxation). The aim is to provide opportunities for successful experiences that can be easily reinforced. These are typically suggestions for which an end point defining success is not obvious to the patient. For example, suggestions that the arm is light and floating up are appropriate as long as the patient does not find out how far up is "up." The therapist can easily reinforce partial responses. It is difficult for the suffering patient to recover from a clear-cut perception of failure if a hypnotic response cannot be positively reinforced.

Specific Hypnotic Procedures—Some Examples

The subsequent hypnosis experiences require a delicate balance between the initial authoritarian and manipulative approach by the hypnotist as he teaches the patient mastery experiences and the nondirective cognitive discovery of success and mastery in areas that the patient can see as related to pain control. At the same time, this progress must be sufficiently slow so that the patient can be drawn into the therapeutic alliance to handle the psychological issues that are more relevant than the pain experience (e.g., "What are the alternative career opportunities?"; "What if I don't win the compensation case?"; "How do I handle my spouse's sexual advances and the children's behavior?").

Suggested glove analgesia can be induced in almost all patients. Failure to induce a glove anal-

gesia, or at least a tingling sensations in the hand, is likely to involve resistance rather than lack of responsibility. Glove analgesia can be induced with a variety of suggestions directed at localized physical sensations, including those focusing on the sensations in the hand, any movement or twitching response, a breeze blowing on the hand, the sensation of pressure against clothing, or feelings of warmth or coolness. The novel experience of focusing on such limited physical events is usually surprising to the patient: most patients will attribute any changes to the therapeutic suggestions, rather than to the natural physiology of the event. It is sometimes helpful if the wrist is positioned over the sharp edge of the chair's armrest, or the therapist may hold the wrist between two fingers, applying mild pressure to an artery, and thereby inducing an ischemic numbness that can be tested by pinching the numb hand (somewhat less than the control hand). The patient gradually becomes impressed by the physiologic control experienced in part of the body. Repeated experience with this kind of analgesia can eventually be transferred to the pain-afflicted area. Hallucinated pain, which can then be taken away (e.g., with the analgesic hand), often impresses the patient.

Relaxation procedures are usually helpful to the patient, particularly when anxiety is also present. However, some patients, especially those with clear organic or cancer pain, are so involved in marshalling their own resources to help control their pain that relaxation experiences can sometimes intensify rather than reduce the pain. The use of relaxation techniques based on Jacobson's procedures, Benson's relaxation response, or modifications of Spiegel's eye roll method (40, 41) may increase the experience of self-mastery, and provide a method for teaching self-hypnotic procedures that the patient will eventually learn and use at home. Especially useful is a modification of Spiegel's procedure involving simultaneously rolling the eyes upward while taking in a deep breath, "feeling the relaxation surge down through your body as you breathe out and close your eyes and relax and let yourself float away to one of your very special places where you can enjoy the experience." The eye roll upgaze simultaneously performed with deep inhalation is a tension-inducing maneuver. It leads easily to deep relaxation as the eyes close with exhalation. Related strategies, including clenching and opening the fists with the breathing exercise, can heighten the tension/relaxation cycle, and later allow the transfer of pain (or anger) into the clenched fist, so that it can be crushed or "given away" as the first is released. Metaphors based on imagery are often helpful, including changing the color of the pain, for example, from intense red to a relatively mild pastel tone (blue, red, and purple are often associated with pain in depressed patients—changes to bright colors such as green or yellow are often helpful). Changes in pain intensity can be visualized as different sizes or shapes so that it can shrink away or be crushed as the pain dissipates. Many out-of-body dissociative floating experiences, and Sacerdote's magical mountain (2), can also be effective in learning self-control and mastery. Two outstanding books on hypnosis in children (42, 43) describe many creative techniques to control pain and most of them can be adapted to adults.

These techniques should be integrated with ego-strengthening suggestions, and with extensive use of imagery where relevant, including utilization of places or feelings or people that are exceptionally pleasurable and/or important to the patient. A suggested haven chosen by the patient (a special room, or garden, or beach) that can be "escaped to" under stress can be very important later when self-hypnosis procedures are introduced. The imagery need not be especially vivid, and sometimes nonvisual modalities are useful or preferred.

It is the melody rather than the lyrics that are important in hypnotic techniques. The procedures need to be a comfortable mix of the patient's abilities and the therapist's style. The goal is to learn mastery experiences, and to allow the patient to discover that he/she has the ability to gain mastery over the pain. However, it is especially important that the patient has permission *not* to use these mastery techniques in all situations. For example, in a litigation case a contract can be established that the pain can be controlled using hypnosis, but the patient will remain free to decide when and where to use these mastery techniques. Thus, the tactic of allowing the patient complete choice (usually while under hypnosis) as to when to control pain provides the patient an important way to handle the problems associated with possible exposure to psychological threat. The thrust of the hypnotic intervention is simply to teach the patient that he/she is capable of controlling pain, but not to become involved in the ethical and moral issues as to *when* the patient should use these techniques. Such contracts are often the key to success with this kind of patient. They allow the patient to manipulate pain when it is psychologically necessary, progress at his/her own pace, provide time to develop a therapeutic alliance, and treat the depression, either with antidepressant medication or psychotherapeutic

techniques. The use of large doses of L-tryptophan, combined with a high-carbohydrate, low-protein diet and vitamin B_6 supplement, is often helpful, especially when the pain is associated with depression and sleep difficulties (possibly due to common serotonergic mechanisms).

Finally, hypnosis may be the method of choice when, for whatever psychological reasons, the patient is ready to give up the pain (for example, at the end of litigation procedures). Hypnosis provides a face-saving way for the patient who needs an excuse to give up a long-lasting symptom when it no longer has any functional utility. If the patient is able to give up the pain, he/she may be confronted with a hostile family—"Why can you do it now, and not thousands of dollars ago with all of your therapists?" If the patient is allowed to capitalize on the magical label of hypnosis as a more powerful technique than other therapists have tried in the past, and if he/she can attribute the change to the hypnosis, the need for face-saving strategies for giving up a symptom is thereby successfully eliminated.

REPRESENTATIVE CASE STUDIES: HYPNOSIS IN CHRONIC PAIN

A case will be used to illustrate patient assessment and management, and typical clinical hypnosis techniques used in treating a chronic pain problem with no clear organic etiology. A second similar but unsuccessful case will be used to illustrate the importance of the careful evaluation of secondary gain and depression often masked by chronic pain. Responses to key diagnostic questions for both patients are summarized in Table 19.2.

SUCCESSFUL STUDY CASE
Ruby was a 59-year-old, slightly obese, middle-class white woman who had a series of major medical problems, including a renal infection, high blood pressure, electrolyte imbalance, and a history of headaches dating back many years. Ruby forgot many details of her headaches. Seven months after renal surgery she consulted a neurologist, and, as a result, a facial nerve was cut. Three weeks later the scalp was opened. She reported that the fascia was scarred and the occipital nerve was wrapped around an artery and literally blew up and was removed. The severe pain began 4 days after this surgery and has been almost constant since. She described the excruciating pain as a "hatchet" feeling, like something had pierced her head. Neuro-

Table 19.2

Management of Chronic Pain Summarized in Two Contrasting Cases of Functional Chronic Pain[a]

	JANET	RUBY
Diagnostic question		
1. What difference would it make to your life if your pain suddenly disappeared?	My poor husband. He would be able to stop cooking. He hates cooking so much. He would prefer to be out with his friends.	My poor husband worries so much. I try to hide the pain from my family so they can lead a normal existence. If it was less, I could carry out my activities (social groups, friends, and family).
2. Do you want to get better?	(Silence). What do you mean? (Angrily). Why do you think I am here. (Slamming fist on chair). (Stuttering). Of course, of course, why would you ask this. (Question repeated twice. Anger increased with similar responses. An unequivocal "yes" not obtained.)	Oh, yes, of course.
3. Would you be satisfied if your pain was reduced by about half its present intensity?	It is hopeless. It is so hard to survive this way. I want to be rid of my pain. All of it.	If I could reduce it some, I'm sure I could carry on a normal life again.
4. Will you work hard with me to learn how to control your pain?	I've done all I can. Doctor, please do something to take it away.	I will do whatever you want me to do.
Prognosis	Unsuccessful because of secondary gain.	Successful.
Result of hypnosis as an adjunctive treatment	Abruptly discharged herself from hospital.	Pain almost entirely eliminated except a mild discomfort during cold, damp weather.

[a] Illustrated by typical responses of a patient with (Janet) and a patient without (Ruby) underlying depression.

logic findings, including electroencephalogram and computed tomography scan, were negative. The pain was extremely pressure sensitive. She had reluctantly used different medications, including Dilantin, which was helpful but made her extremely nauseous so it was discontinued. The neurologist generally confirmed the above details, indicating that scar tissue could account for the pain, but that this was speculative. Her internist thought there may be secondary gain involved. A year after the onset of the head pain he suggested that hypnosis might be considered.

Her relationship with her husband and two married daughters seemed excellent. She preferred to be alone when the pain was at its worst. She often hid it from her family members so that they would not become "scared and concerned and overattentive" to her. This withdrawal reaction was very important to her. She did not seem to have much in the way of social interests except in her art, which she had not been able to continue easily with the headaches.

The pain often occurred during the course of the night, awakening her. She took Excedrin as soon as the pain seems likely to occur. She had noticed that the pain sometimes developed while she was reading a book, although her eyesight was normal. Her books grabbed her attention in the sense of losing track of time or becoming absorbed emotionally, but not as a distraction from the pain. She recently observed that her pain was associated with rain and excessive dampness. To help control the pain, she banged her head or squeezed her eyelid, which had led to a small growth. At the time of this treatment the pain occurred daily. Some days it did not reach intensity of greater than 4 or 5 on a 1–10 scale, but most days it would be around 8.

The MMPI produced no clinically significant scale elevations. The Melzack Pain Questionnaire (38) confirmed the pain descriptions but added no new information. Ruby scored 9 (out of a maximum of 12) in the high hypnotizability range on the *Stanford Hypnotic Susceptibility Scale: Form C* (SHSS:C) (44), administered by an independent trained clinician. Her answers to the diagnostic questions (summarized in Table 19.2) were clear, immediate, and compelling. No secondary gain was indicated in response to these questions. While there were psychological issues apparent in her relationship with her family (e.g., excessive attention), the pain was not an issue in the management of these problems. It seemed realistic that the problems would be in better balance if the pain was under control. The first session with her ended with some instruction and practice in self-hypnosis.

She arrived at the second session with a mounting pain of about 5. Most of the session was spent exploring hypnosis in various ways. She had practiced the self-hypnosis exercise a couple of times a day as requested, but not systematically, when she had pain. Hypnosis was reinduced with a standard right hand levitation–eye closure procedure. This was reinforced by allowing her time to relax and enjoy a pleasant scene. This was repeated with the left hand while she was still in trance, and this seemed to affect her visibly. When given the choice to come out of hypnosis when she wanted to, she took an extra few minutes to enjoy the experience. She did not want to come out of it. She felt no pain while she was in hypnosis, and found it very pleasant. The pain was rated 3 or 4 when she came out. Glove analgesia had been suggested, which she remembered as "working well." However, she remained amnesic for most of her hypnotic experiences.

Hypnosis was reinduced again and she was given ego-strengthening suggestions. This time the analgesia was reintroduced and transferred to her left hand. Whenever she talked about the facial pain, she lifted her hand up to her brow and let it rest there. It seemed reasonable to continue working with this natural movement as a dissociative experience coupled with an analgesic hand. She was taught to enter hypnosis with the left hand floating to her forehead, developing analgesia. The analgesia was then transferred automatically to her forehead using the natural movement, so that initially the glove analgesia and eventually the touch alone would allow her to gain control over pain. She remained amnesic for much of the hypnosis session.

Ruby arrived for the third session in an obviously good mood. She had been using hypnosis and had practiced the self-hypnosis procedure throughout the week, which had been mostly successful, particularly when she could anticipate the severe pain. It did not work once when the pain was severe on a night when it rained. She could use the technique when the pain awakened her at night, but it was more difficult during daily activities. She expressed impatience about learning to utilize the technique more effectively. She also noticed an association between sneezing and the onset of pain, and this was discussed as a useful anticipatory signal. Her left hand levitation technique to her head was very effective and she reported she was fascinated by the fact that her hand wanted to remain touching her head when pain removal was successful. The effectiveness of this dissociative movement was reinforced.

Time was spent on ways to make the procedure more inocuous. Suggestions were given emphasizing that hypnosis allowed her body to take over and to give messages that were helpful. She was taught to use her left hand levitating more rapidly to her forehead, and that on a cute "a,b,c," instead of floating up, her hands would quickly move to her forehead in a casual and stereotyped manner. This was most successful and surprising to her. Next she was told that she would have imaginary pain in the right side of her head. This time her right hand would float up and take away the pain. She was intrigued by this. She said it felt like a toothache in her ear, and that the pain was not necessarily like that on the left side, but it was immediately relieved. This was a breakthrough to signal to her that her body could really take control. She accepted that if the brain can produce and relieve imaginary pain, then real pain could also be removed by similar strategies.

Hypnosis was again induced but this time she was asked to leave her eyes open. She found this a little difficult and unpleasant the first time, but practice made it easier. She was then told stand up and go through the exercise. This she was able to do easily with the "a,b,c" technique. Suggestions were given under hypnosis, and while she was imagining a pleasant scene. She was reassured that she had a choice of procedures. If at home and with privacy she might prefer the slower levitation method. In a social situation a self-suggestion of "a,b,c" would allow her hand to come up quickly to her forehead as a normal conversational mannerism. All of these techniques worked well.

She was reminded under hypnosis that pain was an important warning signal, and this mild pain might recur, although it was suggested that, because she had good success using these various strategies, her body would not need to send pain signals as often or as severely. Although this was an accelerated session, she seemed to have good mastery for all of these dissociative experiences.

She was asked to call in about 3 weeks to indicate

her progress, although if for any reason the procedure was not working well for her, she could call anytime. She was reminded that under extreme stress the procedure might not work for a while, and that there might be other times when she felt the special techniques were unnecessary, but that she should continue using them.

This patient did not require any additional sessions after the 3-week phone call indicated that the pain had almost gone. The stabilization of the home relationship and the resumption of social activities was already in progress. Follow-up at 6 months indicated that the patient was doing well. Mild pain did recur occasionally, particularly in damp and cold weather. However, the patient was almost always able to handle this with the self-hypnosis exercises. All aspects of Ruby's life seemed stabilized, and she was leading the kind of active social life that she had desired.

In terms of the broad issues relevant to the adjunctive use of hypnosis in chronic pain this case appears straightforward. The pain was likely due to (unproven) lesions. There were no signs of significant psychological problems associated with pain. Whether hypnosis provided dissociative control mechanisms or served as a powerful nonspecific support system cannot be determined other than the evidence provided by the high hypnotic capacity of the woman.

CONTRASTING UNSUCCESSFUL CASE STUDY

The previous case should be contrasted with another patient with a similar referral profile. Janet was a 44-year-old, obese woman from a similar middle-class socioeconomic background. As a psychiatric hospital inpatient for severe chronic abdominal pain she was referred by a staff psychiatrist for possible work with hypnosis. The constant pain had become severe following a gallbladder and sphincter operation. The patient had been to several outpatient clinics. Her records were replete with unusual diagnoses, indicating diagnostic and etiologic confusion. Medical examination did not find a specific reason for the pain except for the untested possibility of some residual scar tissue. Medication, psychotherapy, and biofeedback had been unsuccessful. Hypnosis was suggested and she scored 8 out of 12 on the SHSS:C. The MMPI produced an elevated Hysteria-Depression-Hypochondriasis profile typical of the depressed pain patient (36). A diagnosis of current depression, concomitant with chronic pain syndrome, was made, although she did not meet the *Diagnostic and Statistical Manual of Mental Disorders,* Third Edition, criteria for

depression. Her answers to the standard diagnostic questions evaluating secondary gain are contrasted with those of Ruby in Table 19.2. These responses, plus the MMPI profile, plus other evidence from pain drawings and ratings indicating that the suffering was not as severe as her complaining might have suggested, all indicated a poor prognosis for the patient with hypnosis because the secondary gain was so intense and the underlying depression would be exposed.

She experienced hypnosis satisfactorily and deeply when it was introduced so she could learn about hypnosis. It was then made clear to her that the next hypnosis session would begin to address her pain. At the outset of the hypnosis she had a sudden, incapacitating pain attack and could not continue the session. She had to be carried back to her room. She refused hypnosis the next day, and the following day signed herself out of the hospital against medical advice. At a six-month follow-up, her husband indicated that hospital treatment elsewhere had not been successful, and she subsequently had unsuccessful abdominal surgery. The patient would not come to the phone.

The two patients provide a similar background and somewhat similar chronic pain history. The differentiating feature was the secondary gain supported by the pain for Janet, but not for Ruby. Back pain requires similar differential evaluation in terms of psychodynamic issues and depression. The initial evaluation should be conducted in a confrontational style to quickly evaluate the special meaning pain has for the patient. Treatment will involve a delicate balance as the therapist initially takes control in leading the patient to discover he/she can develop mastery over the pain experience, then gradually relinquishes that control to the patient to use the mastery experience under his/her own terms. At that point treatment gradually takes over, addressing the psychological issues that the patient should then be willing to handle.

In contrast, in the case of Ruby, standard medical treatment had not been successful but there was little suggestion of secondary gain (as opposed to the psychological problems that come with the hopelessness attached to chronic pain). Under these conditions it was predicted that a direct approach to the symptom would be safe and effective. At that point it becomes a matter of the skill of the therapist to find an intervention based on the expectation that a powerful and successful treatment is being introduced, and to explore ways in which the patient can be taught that he/she can exert control over the pain process even though this seems diametrically opposed to his/her prior experience. Hypnosis is often the method of choice to build these expectations and to lead to the discovery of self-control. However, the best way to use hypnosis (imagery, relaxation, regressive procedures, analgesia, dissociation, self-hypnosis) will depend on the abilities of the patient. It is then necessary to transfer these skills to the specific symptom (pain control), and this is usually best achieved by the use of self-help, self-hypnotic procedures. It is not important that the self-help strategy induces a hypnotic state, although it is helpful when this occurs because of the dissociative capacities possessed by the more hypnotizable person.

TRAINING IN HYPNOSIS

Training in clinical hypnosis should be sought from organizations restricting workshops to physicians, psychologists, dentists, or psychiatric social workers. The two national professional societies in the United States are:

American Society of Clinical Hypnosis
Suite 336
2250 East Devon Avenue
Des Plaines, IL 60018 (312-297-3317)

Society for Clinical Experimental Hypnosis
129-A King Park Drive
Liverpool, NY 13090 (315-652-7299)

These two national organizations are constituent societies of the International Society of Hypnosis, of which this author is currently president.

At press both U.S. societies are considering extending training opportunities to nurses with special qualifications and other health care professionals with relevant terminal degrees. There are many hypnosis training programs available. Unfortunately these are often conducted by groups who have no professional training and who do not limit courses to qualified health professionals. These groups can sometimes be recognized by use of terms such as "hypnotechnician" or "ethical hypnosis" in their literature. Training with such groups, or referring patients to them (even under medical supervision), may be considered a breach of professional ethics in many states and professional organizations. Colleagues seeking training should check with either of the above societies, or should check that the organization is sponsored by one of these societies, a university, a medical school, or a professional organization.

SUMMARY

Some of the ways in which hypnosis is relevant and useful in the management of chronic pain have been discussed. Differences in the theoretical understanding of hypnosis were highlighted, particularly as they relate to pain control research and clinical practice. Research on hypnotic analgesia has contributed to existing knowledge about pain mechanisms, but has had relatively few implications for the management of chronic pain. For highly hypnotizable subjects, hypnosis can effectively reduce pain. In selected individuals such pain reduction differs from that produced by a variety of physiologic (acupuncture, naloxone reversal) and psychological (placebo, distraction, stress innoculation) methods of pain reduction. The dissociative advantages of deep hypnosis cannot be overlooked, but are not available to some patients. However, hypnosis occurs in a special context that maximizes nonspecific components of expectation, trust, and belief, similar to the placebo response that occurs with medication, even in less hypnotizable patients. The combination of the specific and nonspecific components of hypnosis provides a powerful clinical tool even though the nonspecific components are independent of hypnotic capacity.

The specific applications of hypnosis in pain management are different depending on the nature and history of the patient's pain. *Acute* pain is best managed by anxiety-reducing strategies, particularly those having to do with interpersonal interactions that maximize the importance of the pain. Relaxation procedures can be designed that are incompatible with anxiety, and therefore will be pain reducing. Most of these procedures will not be directly relevant to back pain problems.

Chronic pain requires strategies that deal with handling one's social and psychological environment effectively. In such cases the pain has no clear organic basis, even though from the patient's viewpoint "it hurts." The difficulties in using hypnosis with chronic pain patients whose pain masks depression and who use pain instrumentally to reinforce psychological processes and behaviors (secondary gain) were highlighted, particularly as they apply to the initial stages of treatment. The use of several hypnotic strategies—relaxation, imagery, dissociation, and self-hypnosis—was summarized.

When the patient's pain is due to a chronic or *terminal* condition, where there is clear evidence of organic pathology, hypnosis can be used effectively while avoiding issues related to reactive depression. For these patients, hypnosis may be the method of choice to teach the patient to control and manipulate pain levels, as well as to reduce medication and to minimize side effects of treatment, including chemotherapy.

Further research and controlled clinical trials will be necessary to evaluate which of these approaches will be most helpful to individual patients with both acute and chronic pain. Each patient suffers in his/her own private way. Clinical sensitivity must always take priority over general guidelines and prescriptions for difficult and often misunderstood pain patients.

REFERENCES

1. Crasilneck HB, Hall JA: *Clinical Hypnosis: Principles and Applications,* ed 2. Orlando, FL, Grune & Stratton, 1985.
2. Sacerdote P: Theory and practice of pain control in malignancy and other protracted or recurring painful illnesses. *Int J Clin Exp Hypn* 18:160–180, 1970.
3. Domangue BB, Margolis CG: Hypnosis and a multidisciplinary cancer pain management team: role and effects. *Int J Clin Exp Hypn* 31:206, 1983.
4. Turner JA, Chapman CR: Psychological intervention for chronic pain: a critical review. II. Operant conditioning, hypnosis, and cognitive-behavioral therapy. *Pain* 12:23–46, 1982.
5. Hilgard ER, Hilgard JR: *Hypnosis in the Relief of Pain.* Los Altos, CA, William Kaufman, Inc, 1975.
6. Barber J: Rapid induction analgesia: a clinical report. *Am J Clin Hypn* 19:138–147, 1977.
7. Crasilneck HB: Hypnosis in the control of chronic low back pain. *Am J Clin Hypn* 22:71–81, 1979.
8. McCauley JD, Thelen MH, Frank RG, Willard RR, Callen KE: Hypnosis compared to relaxation in the outpatient management of low back pain. *Arch Phys Med Rehabil* 64:548–552, 1983.
9. Elton D, Burrows GD, Stanley GV: Chronic pain and hypnosis. In Burrows GD, Dennerstein L (eds): *Handbook of Hypnosis and Psychosomatic Medicine.* Amsterdam, Elsevier/North Holland Biomedical Press, 1980.
10. Esdaile J: *Hypnosis in Medicine and Surgery.* New York, Julian Press, 1957. (Originally titled *Mesmerism in India,* 1850.)
11. Dubin LL, Shapiro S: The use of hypnosis to facilitate a dental extraction and hemostasis in a classic hemophiliac with a high antibody titre to Factor 8. *Am J Clin Hypn* 17:79–83, 1974.
12. Evans FJ: The hypnotizable patient. Invited address, IVth European Congress of Hypnosis and Psychosomatic Medicine, Oxford, England, 1987.
13. Evans FJ: Suggestibility in the normal waking state. *Psychol Bull* 67:114–129, 1967.

14. Hull CL: *Hypnosis and Suggestibility: An Experimental Approach.* New York, Appleton-Century-Crofts, 1933.
15. Weitzenhoffer AM: *Hypnotism: An Objective Study in Suggestibility.* New York, John Wiley & Sons, 1953.
16. Barber TX: *Hypnosis: A Scientific Approach.* New York, Van Nostrand, Reinholt, 1969.
17. Sarbin TR, Coe W: *Hypnosis: A Social Psychological Analysis of Influence Communication.* New York, Holt, Rinehart & Winston, 1972.
18. Spanos NP: Hypnotic behavior. A social psychological interpretation of amnesia, analgesia, and "trance logic." *Behav Brain Sci* 9:449–502, 1986.
19. Wagstaff GF: *Hypnosis, Compliance and Belief.* New York, St. Martin's Press, 1981.
20. Bowers KS: *Hypnosis for the Seriously Curious.* New York, WW Norton, 1976.
21. Hilgard ER: *Hypnotic Susceptibility.* New York, Harcourt Brace Jovanovich, 1965.
22. Hilgard ER: *Divided Consciousness: Multiple Controls in Human Thought and Action.* New York, John Wiley & Sons, 1977.
23. Shor RE: Physiological effects of painful stimulation during hypnotic analgesia under conditions designed to minimize anxiety. *Int J Clin Exp Hypn* 10:183–202, 1962.
24. Sutcliffe JP: "Credulous" and "skeptical" views of hypnotic phenomena: experiments in esthesia, hallucination, delusion. *J Abnorm Soc Psychol* 62:189–200, 1961.
25. Frankel FH, Apfel RJ, Kelly SF, Benson H, Quinn T, Newark J, Malmaud R: The use of hypnotizability scales in the clinic: a review after six years. *Int J Clin Exp Hypn* 27:63–73, 1979.
26. Lasagna L, Mosteller F, von Felsinger JM, Beecher H: A study of the placebo response. *Am J Med* 16:770–779, 1954.
27. McGlashan TH, Evans FJ, Orne MT: The nature of hypnotic analgesia and the placebo response to experimental pain. *Psychosom Med* 31:227–246, 1969.
28. Evans FJ: Expectancy, therapeutic instructions, and the placebo response. In White L, Tursky B, Schwarts G (eds): *Placebo: Clinical Phenomena and New Insights.* New York, Guilford Press, 1985.
29. Evans FJ: Hypnosis and chronic pain. In Burrows GD, Elton D, Stanley R (eds): *Handbook of Chronic Pain Management* Amsterdam, Elsevier, 1987.
30. Orne MT: Pain suppression by hypnosis and related phenomena. In Bonica JJ (ed): *Pain.* New York, Raven Press, 1974.
31. Knox VJ, Gekoski WL, Shum K, McLaughlin DM: Analgesia for experimentally induced pain: multiple sessions of acupuncture compared to hypnosis in high- and low-susceptible subjects. *J Abnorm Psychol* 90:28–34, 1981.
32. Miller ME, Bowers KS: Hypnotic analgesia and stress inoculation in the reduction of pain. *J Abnorm Psychol* 95:6–14, 1986.
33. Goldstein E, Hilgard E: Failure to opiate antagonist

naloxone to modify hypnotic analgesia. *Proc Natl Acad Sci (USA)* 72:2041–2043, 1975.

34. Meichenbaum DH: *Cognitive-Behavior Modification: An Integrative Approach.* New York, Plenum Press, 1977.

35. Beecher HK: *Measurement of Subjective Responses: Quantitative Effects of Drugs.* New York, Oxford University Press, 1959.

36. Sternbach RA: *Pain Patients: Traits and Treatment.* New York, Academic Press, 1974.

37. Fordyce WE: *Behavioral Methods for Chronic Pain and Illness.* St. Louis, CV Mosby, 1976.

38. Melzack R: The McGill Pain Questionnaire: major properties and scoring methods. *Pain* 1:277–299, 1975.

39. Crown 3, Crisp AH. *Manual of the Crown-Crisp Experiential Index.* London, Hoddard Stoughton, 1979.

40. Benson H: *The Relaxation Response.* New York, William Morrow, 1975.

41. Spiegel H, Spiegel D: *Trance and Treatment: Clinical Uses of Hypnosis.* New York, Basic Books, 1978.

42. Gardner GG, Olness K: *Hypnosis and Hypnotherapy with Children.* New York, Grune & Stratton, 1981.

43. Hilgard JR, LeBaron S: *Hypnotherapy of Pain in Children with Cancer.* Los Altos, CA, William Kaufman, Inc, 1984.

44. Weitzenhoffer AM, Hilgard ER: *Stanford Hypnotic Susceptibility Scale, Form C.* Palo Alto, CA, Consulting Psychologists Press, 1962.

SECTION 6
SELECTED THERAPIES

Chapter 20

MULTIDISCIPLINARY PAIN CLINICS, CENTERS, AND PROGRAMS

HAROLD J. GOTTLIEB, PhD

While modern practitioners are comfortable with the view of acute pain as a symptom of a disease, they are deeply troubled by pain that refuses to disappear. This is especially frustrating when every tool in the physician's treatment arsenal has been tried and still the patient remains chronically in pain and disabled. This indeed represents a dilemma in modern medicine; however, it is out of the dilemma that we are today witnessing the increasing emergence of the multimodal multidisciplinary pain clinic.

What follows is the author's attempt to trace the origins and influences that have given rise to the multidisciplinary pain clinic. Discussion is focused on chronic low back pain patients as a patient population for whom the pain clinic has proven particularly efficacious. In addition, a review of empirical findings on the influence of cognition on pain perception is presented, and their particular influence on the development and implementation of a cognitive social learning–based pain clinic is discussed. An operant conditioning–based treatment model for chronic pain will also be presented. Based on the author's 15 years of experience setting up, developing, and implementing pain clinics, attention is given to the many issues and practical concerns involved in the implementation of a successful pain clinic, followed by some final comments on where this writer believes "we need to go from here."

Low back pain is one of the most common types of pain, yet it is one of the most poorly understood. Although not always found in patients with low back pain, the only definite causes of low back pain are herniation of disks and arthritis of vertebral joints (1). Yet, as pointed out by Loeser (1), as many as 60–78% of patients who suffer low back pain have no apparent physical signs. That is, despite x-rays and thorough orthopaedic examination, there is no evidence of disk disease, arthritis, or any other symptoms that can be considered the cause of pain. Notwithstanding, a sizeable number of these patients undergo one or more invasive surgical procedures anyway. Waddell et al. (2) reported that among a group of compensation patients who underwent back surgery, 97% had at least some complaint of persistent pain. Seventy-seven percent of these complained of impairments in functioning. Of the original group 15% underwent a second surgery, and of these 40% underwent a third and 23% a fourth operation.

Persistent pain, connected to failed intervention, decreases the livelihood of the patient returning to work. In this regard, the literature on return to work supports a general rule: the length of time out of work is inversely related to the likelihood of eventual return to work. McGill (3) reported that back-injured patients out of work more than 6 months have a 50% probability of returning, and those out more than 1 year only a 25% probability of returning to work. Pain-disabled patients out 2 years or more have about a 2% likelihood of returning to work (4).

Recent medical history has shown that pain has been attacked with every weapon available to the physician treatment arsenal. Furthermore, almost every site along the nervous system, from the periphery (sympthectomies and rhizotomies), along the spinal cord (percutaneous cordotomies), to the brain (thalamotomies and prefrontal lobotomies), has been surgically attacked without yielding long-term benefits for a sizeable number of patients (5). While standard medical and surgical interventions have proven reasonably effective with acute pain, it is estimated that approximately 60% of chronic pain patients have adequate reduction of pain as a function of purely somatic treatments (1). Moreover, only cursory attention is paid to the iatrogenic contribution to the chronic pain syndrome of multiple surgeries and polypharmacologic efforts to correct it. For example, one pain clinic, the University of Washington Pain Clinic, reports that while 86% of patients at the clinic had no pathologic diagnosis, 40% had undergone one or more surgical operations in an attempt to relieve their pain and 80% were taking one or more analgesic drugs on a physician prescription (6). These findings are also consistent with the findings reported by the Casa Colina Comprehensive Pain Program (7).

While the above illustrates the course taken by patients for whom objective signs are unclear, the results associated with surgical procedures for patients emitting clear-cut physical and neurologic signs of disk herniation are just as dismal. A review of the literature on this issue generates ranges of success of surgical procedures from 50 to 90% (1). Notwithstanding, somatic therapies for chronic pain are still regarded as the treatment(s) of choice for the restoration of low back pain disorders.

Analgesic medications as a treatment for the restoration of the chronic back pain patient provide yet another example of the failure of traditional medicine as a primary intervention for the alleviation of chronic back pain. Polypharmacy constitutes one of the most frequent companion treatments for patients with spinal pain problems. Drugs have been used for their sedating, anti-inflammatory, and analgesic effects. While a consensus exists among physicians as to the usefulness of nonsteroidal anti-inflammatory drugs and muscle relaxants during the acute phase, their utility in the chronic phase has not been clearly established. Analgesics (e.g., aspirin and acetaminophen derivatives) have generally been validated scientifically and have been found to be useful. Similarly, to the extent that depression is indeed a major element in the chronic back pain syndrome, antidepressants have been reported to be useful (8). However, as interventions for the alleviation of pain, that is, for the treatment of chronic pain, such efforts are surrounded by controversy. Equally discouraging as a primary intervention for the alleviation of chronic pain are the many single-modality treatments that have been applied as interventions for chronic pain, for example, bed rest, cryotherapy, manipulation, exercises in specialized centers, electroanalgesia, functional training, autotraction, biofeedback, and acupuncture. While these single-modality treatments for acute pain appear to produce symptomatic relief, their role outside of the multidisciplinary pain clinic raises grave doubt about their restorative efficacy for chronic pain (8).

To summarize, the persistence of low back pain occurs despite orthopaedic surgery, conservative management interventions, neurosurgery, and polypharmacy efforts to correct it.

ECONOMIC COST OF LOW BACK PAIN

The costs of chronic pain to industry and health care are prohibitive. Bonica (9) estimated that in the United States chronic pain may annually account for 700 million lost workdays and $65 billion in health care costs, compensation, and litigation. Low back pain alone, the most common pain complaint, has disabled an estimated 7 million Americans and accounts for more than 8 million physician office visits yearly in the United States (9). Approximately $14 billion is spent each year for treatment or compensation for low back pain (10). In summary, while the costs related to those injured who became chronic back patients are staggering, it should be noted that Spangler et al. (11) reported that 10% of all claims on back injuries accounted for 79% of costs for a back injury and 32% of total compensatory costs. More important, the costs analysis is in line with the fact that 7.4% of chronic back pain patients absent from work 6 months or more accounted for 75.6% of the total compensation costs (8).

CHRONIC BACK PAIN IN RESPONSE TO MISMANAGEMENT

Chronic back pain patients are not "accidents," they are created; that is, they are created by persistent attempts to apply standard medical knowledge and practices familiar to most physicians in the treatment of acute pain disorders to chronic low back pain. While most primary care physicians are familiar with acute pain disorders, they are less familiar with the diagnosis and treatment of chronic pain.

Typically, acute pain is viewed as a result of a sensation arising from the stimulation of nociceptive inputs generally due to tissue damage. Such inputs are seen as useful warning signs. They are often brief in duration (i.e., self-limiting), lasting less than 6 months in duration, well defined, and yield no permanent disability. Acute pain is often successfully treated by traditional medical means. In contrast, chronic pain has no apparent warning significance, is more than 6 months in duration, has questionable nociceptive inputs, is present most of the time with intensity varying, involves complications from layers of psychosocial problems, promotes suffering, and often leads to a disability.

The difference, while receiving token recognition, is mostly ignored by the primary treating physician, as evident in the myriad of treatments offered for acute pain that persists long after such treatments are justified. In short, the refractory low back pain patient is a creation of the 20th-century preoccupation with acute pain solutions to chronic pain problems.

EVOLUTION OF THE PAIN CLINIC

The history of ideas relative to the introduction of pain centers for the treatment of chronic low back pain can be traced to a number of notions about pain, its origins, and its cure. Historically, pain was viewed as having many sources. Either it originated from within the body or its origins were regarded as external. Within the body meant mind and/or body according to the dualistic distinctions associated with ideas originating from Rene Descartes. External causes for pain were often charged to "evil" forces, punishment from the gods, or spiritual magical entities. Pain was also viewed as being due to disturbances in mind and body (i.e., diseases). Bodily disturbances were viewed as diseases and mind disturbances were relegated to spiritual-magical psychological and/or theological (i.e., moral) issues. In a word, mind and body explanations for pain became split, and pain was either organic or functional.

In the 20th century, with attention focused on the medicalization of the emotions and the belief that emotions can be reduced to neurologic substrates, mental events, as diseases, were delegated to "cures" by medical means; hence terms like "mental disease," "mental illness," and psychiatric psychological "disorders" were applied to pain disabilities for which no organic evidence could be found.

The 20th century also witnessed major advances in medical technology: x-rays, laboratory test procedures, surgery, and analgesics. Such tools became increasingly popular adjuncts to the physician's ability to isolate and treat the specific causes of acute pain. With increased technology came increased confidence in finding a psychophysiologic or biomedical cause of all pain. When such a cause was not forthcoming, traditional medicine increasingly resorted to the application of psychiatric diagnosis (conversion hysteria, psychogenic pain, depressive equivalent, and compensation neurosis) as a replacement explanation for pain disorders without clear, objective clinical findings. However, such disorders were also subject to organic treatments and were therefore made the responsibility of the physician. It was soon realized that some pain disorders with or without clear organic findings were equally refractory to treatments within the medical model, and a growing uneasiness began to emerge as a number of pain disorders (phantom limb, tic douloureux, chronic pain), including those designated as psychogenic pain, began to appear equally unexplainable and resistant to regimens within traditional medicine. Thus, a climate was created within which alternative, nonsurgical approaches as treatments for chronic low back pain slowly began to emerge.

New discoveries identifying the role of important neurotransmitters (e.g., serotonin, norepinephrine, endorphins) in pain and the fact that emotions play a major role in sustaining "sick role behavior" also gave impetus to the gradual recognition and acceptance of the need for alternative, nonsurgical interventions such as pain clinics. It was not until the introduction of Melzack and Wall's gate control theory in 1965 that a medical scientific basis, and hence a climate of tolerance, for nonsurgical approaches began to clearly appear. The central tenant of Melzack and Wall's gate control theory gave support to the view that emotions play a significant role in the experience of pain. The gate control theory essentially argues that cognitive factors (i.e., thought, ideation, and feelings) can produce physiologic changes that actually modify physician sensations; that cognitive expectations regarding pain may affect the experience of pain by opening or closing the "spinal gate" mechanisms; and that pain that persists without an immediate organic source is not merely a matter of "suggestion" but an activity in the nervous system that affects the opening and closing of gates located in the dorsal horns of the spinal cord.

The net effect of the gate theory was to destroy

the prevailing ideas that pain is a simple sensation en route by direct transmission line to a pain center, that cognitive factors can have a direct effect on pain, and that cognitive-based treatment regimens can constitute treatments for the restoration of patients disabled by chronic low back pain. As stated by Melzack and Wall:

> The search for new approaches to pain therapy has been profited by directing thinking towards the contributions of motivational and cognitive processes. Pain can be treated not only by trying to manipulate the sensory inputs, but also by influencing motivational and cognitive factors as well . . . psychological methods, we know now, may decrease some kinds of pain from unbearable to bearable levels, an achievement which is gaining increasing recognition. (5)

ROLE OF PSYCHOLOGICAL PARADIGMS IN LOW BACK PAIN TREATMENT

Within the last two decades psychological theory and research have contributed an increasing influence to the growth and development of pain clinics. In fact, two major psychological pain centers owe their origins in conceptualization (i.e., treatment philosophy, techniques of treatment, and treatment modalities) to cognitive social learning theory and the operant conditioning paradigm (7, 12).

The Casa Colina Chronic Low Back Pain Treatment Center in Pomona, California (13) provides an excellent example of the application of a cognitive social learning–based treatment model. Central to the Casa Colina approach is the importance assigned to the role a "sense of personal control" has in the restoration of patients with chronic low back pain.

A number of empirical findings have had a direct impact on the development of the Casa Colina Comprehensive Pain Clinic. The work of Seligman on the role played by a loss of personal control in stress, tension, and pain provides interesting empirical support (14). Simply stated, Seligman's work demonstrated that when an organism cannot make an adaptive response or is unable to control a stressful outcome, the outcome can be said to be uncontrollable and unpredictable. Both uncontrollability and unpredictability, although hard to separate, have been found to be instrumentally related to anxiety, stress, tension, and pain. In another study with college students, Pervin varied both controllability and predictability of shock (15). When he asked the subjects which conditions they would choose to go through again, they significantly preferred predictability to unpredictability and control

to no control. Subjects who had control tended to report less anxiety. Most significant, subjects who self-administered their own control over shock were found to experience more pain relief benefits than subjects whose control over shock depended on actions performed by either an intermediary or an experimenter. The work of Davison and Valins (16) further supports the view they found that subjects who believed that they themselves were responsible for their improvement took significantly more shock than did those who were led to believe that the source of their pain relief was a drug (a placebo pill).

Having control over an aversive event can play a critical role in the effects morphine plays in pain reduction. Hill et al. demonstrated that morphine diminished pain reactions more when the anxiety level of the subject was initially high and when subjects were allowed to control pain-creating stimuli (17). Also, several workers pointed out that merely the attribution of self-control, that is, the belief that one has control over the stimulus or shock, regardless of whether one has control in fact, is sufficient to induce pain relief (11, 15, 16, 18).

The role of perceived control as an aid to the reduction of anxiety and pain gains further support from work derived from attribution theory. Attribution theory assumes that people are generally motivated to predict and control their environment and that in the service of this need, they attempt to establish causal connections between environmental events. In the realm of personal perception, observers tend to ascribe their actions, or the actions of others, to either internal or external forces. Attribution theory could predict that people are more likely to experience a sense of personal control when stress and pain are perceived to be under the internal control of cognitive coping strategies that are under one's predictable control (11, 19). In this regard, Davison and Valins (16) found that subjects who attributed their behavior changes to themselves—that is, believed they had ingested a placebo—subsequently perceived the shock as less painful and tolerated significantly more shock than subjects who attributed their behavior change to the drug.

FROM THE LABORATORY TO THE PAIN CLINIC

Based on the empirical evidence, a number of important treatment assumptions emerge:

1. Patients can be taught skills that enable them to control key cognitive and psychophysiologic parameters in stress and reactive pain.

2. Skill induction for pain control (and hence personal control) can be facilitated by imparting to the patient a great deal of preparatory information, including a precise description of expected reactions, medical procedures, and other medical information (20).

3. Patient self-control skills can promote self-reliance, independence, and patient independence and can reduce patient requests for help from physicians, nursing staff, and other medical and paramedical personnel.

4. Patient self-control attributions can be enhanced by experiences that attribute "power to the patient." Training in self-assertion, cognitive coping techniques, biofeedback training, and self-medication control procedures provide excellent examples of skill-based experiences that can impart to patients a sense of personal control (self-regulation) (5, 19).

5. Patients' self-control pain relief measures can draw them away from dependency on external pain-solving strategies such as (often toxic) medications and high-risk surgical procedures.

6. Self-regulated patients are less likely to over-utilize the traditional health care delivery system (21).

7. The attribution of "self-control" can replace depression, resignation, and pessimism with optimism, and despair with hope (19).

THE CASA COLINA COMPREHENSIVE BACK PROGRAM—A COGNITIVE SOCIAL LEARNING MODEL

The training program developed by Gottlieb et al. included the following elements:

1. Biofeedback training
   a. To eliminate the patient's belief in the classic mind-body dichotomy (biofeedback experience can provide the patient with experiential links among ideation, thought, images, increases or decreases in physiologic arousal, and increases or decreases in pain experience).
   b. To teach patients how to manage upper-body and lower-body physiologic indicators of pain.
   c. To teach patients how important they are in their own recovery.
   d. To implement a method of achieving patient self-responsibility.

   e. To teach the patient reduction techniques that can be used at home.

2. Individual and group counseling sessions aimed at teaching patients constructive cognitive control techniques for managing intra- and interpersonal sources of stress effecting pain.

3. A patient self-administered medication reduction program.

4. Patient participant case conferences.

5. Disability resolution conference—attended by key persons (attorney, third party payor, case manager, key family members, and employer)—for the purpose of establishing a comprehensive treatment plan designed to remove all barriers that prevent the patient from reentry into the work force.

6. Family therapy sessions to reduce the impact of family stress and styles of interaction that often reinforce the patient's pain, pain behavior, and suffering.

7. Vocational counseling program, including work hardening, functional capacity evaluation and work simulation training, assistance in work placement, and ergonomic on-job-site evaluation.

8. Assertion training program designed to enhance interpersonal skills, reduce the victim role, reduce passivity, and reduce a number of interpersonal stressors that mediate pain.

9. A lecture series covering the relationship between stress and anxiety and pain, nutrition, body mechanics, medication, and the role a sense of personal control plays in pain.

10. Physical therapy program including exercises that patients can easily acquire, that can be easily transferred to their postdischarge home environment. The physical therapy program is designed to increase sitting time, flexibility, endurance, strength, pain tolerance, and endorphin activity. Such exercises are designed to prepare the patient to utilize all gains toward achieving full vocational restoration.

11. A therapeutic milieu designed for maximum relaxation, recreation, and socialization.

12. A work hardening–work tolerance program, including work simulation, in vivo work training experiences, ergonomic assessment, job placement, and employment counseling.

PATIENT POPULATION SERVED

A common characteristic of treated pain patients is the diagnosis of chronic pain syndrome. Central elements in this disorder are: (a) severe and prolonged pain that is anatomically inconsistent or lacks a known organic explanation, (b) pain that is disproportionate to pathology discovered, and (c) pain that shows evidence of psychological overlay. Features typically associated with this syndrome include: analgesic abuse, "doctor shopping," request for surgery, invalidism, symbolic significance of the pain, anxiety, depression, bodily preoccupation, conviction of illness, and an unwillingness to allow that psychological factors play a central role in the maintenance of the pain. Many of these patients exhibit affective disorders, reveal early childhood abuses, describe a family member role model for pain, and exhibit histories of multiple surgeries without receiving benefit. These patients are typically out of work and are less likely to return to work. They are typically embroiled in litigation, are often angry at their physician and the health care system in general, and present major sexual and family problems for which pain foci becomes a defensive replacement. They typically present a premorbid picture of a passive-dependent narcissistic personality orientation, demonstrate disabling depression, and view their family members as need-fulfilling objects. Such patients typically focus on their pain and rely heavily on the health care system. Physically these patients exhibit sensitive trigger points, are deconditioned, and exhibit decreased or variable motion and/or bizarre movements or gaits. These patients are generally overreactive and exhibit exaggerated tenderness, groans, grimacing, and excessive guarding.

All of the above features contribute to rendering these patients poor candidates for traditional conservative and/or invasive procedures (22–24). Most of these patients display overt anger, often targeted at the insurance carrier and employer, who are often accused of being insensitive and advocating cost saving at the expense of the patient. Because most pain patients enter the program in litigation, an applicant attorney is usually involved. The applicant attorney is interested in an advantageous settlement for the client. To the patient this means he/she must amplify pain behavior and not return to work, lest he/she jeopardize the (often exaggerated) expected settlement. Most patients further recruit their families into their disability, often externalizing blame and exhibiting self-pity, victimhood, helplessness, and dependence. Key family members very often provide powerful reinforcement for continued pain behaviors. Fear of suffering and immobility result in a resistance to painful movement and consequent deconditioning. Many of the patients exhibit myofascial pain disorders with sensitive trigger points, and many patients become drug dependent and/or addicted. With time, these patients become increasingly depressed, and drink alcohol and/or take barbiturates, psychotropics, muscle relaxants, and often street drugs. By the time these patients come to the pain clinic they exhibit a full-scale emotional disability.

PROGRAM AND ADMISSION CRITERIA

The Casa Colina Low Back Pain Program is designed as both an inpatient and an outpatient program. The inpatient program is designed for patients with severe medical complications that require closer monitoring, and for patients whose home environments and/or medication abuse issues require a less stressful, more contained (inpatient) environment. Outpatient services (half-day, full-day, and single modality) offer acute, subacute, and chronic pain patients clinical services for a variety of pain-related disorders (particularly low back disorders) for patients already employed and/or living at home within a 30-mile radius of the clinic.

Programmatically, both inpatients and outpatients are screened for candidacy. Medical records are obtained by an intake liaison coordinator who obtains preauthorization from the insurance carrier. Medical records are then reviewed by the medical director, followed by a medical evaluation, a comprehensive psychological evaluation, and a comprehensive biomechanical and physical therapy assessment. A team conference evaluating all pertinent data is conducted (which includes the medical director) at which time—by admission triage criteria—a decision is made regarding which program the patient will enter. Patients who exhibit psychosis, sociopathy, and other severe affective and psychiatric states, including ancillary complicated medical management problems, are typically excluded from the program. Patients are also typically excluded who cannot speak English or whose intellectual level limits comprehension and prohibits full programmatic participation.

Treatment modalities are monitored for progress on all treatment goals and all patient progress reports are presented to the patient at bimonthly patient conferences.

ASSESSMENT AND TREATMENT PLAN

Patients are evaluated medically and psychologically (Minnesota Multiphasic Personality Inventory, Self-Efficacy Scale, Health Locus of Control, McGill Pain Questionnaire, Daily Activity Check List, Beck Inventory for Depression). Patients are evaluated for strength, flexibility, endurance, sitting tolerance, bending, stooping, lifting, and range of motion. A full battery of vocational assessments are administered that include an assessment of avocational hobbies the patient once enjoyed. Medication history and issues of dependence and/or addiction are assessed. Family financial and legal issues are also explored.

All pertinent data are evaluated and presented at staff conferences to determine the treatment plan, intervention strategy, and aftercare goals for every patient. A disability resolution conference is held and conclusions relative to the treatment plan, treatment goals, and expected outcomes are presented to the patient, his/her family, attorney, employer, case manager, and third party representative. Treatment goals are quantified and progress feedback reports are provided to the patient, staff, and relevant others. Staff progress reports are provided to the patient verbally on a daily basis and formally at patient conferences. Patients are given a treatment schedule and are reinforced for compliance. Family members are counseled and are made an integral part of the treatment program. Discharge plans are stated early in treatment and patients with vocational goals are ultimately expected to return to work.

PHYSICIAN–MEDICAL DIRECTOR'S ROLE

The physician–medical doctor is an essential member of the clinical team. By tradition, the physician is a powerful reinforcer. Traditionally, the physician role, albeit unwittingly, often reinforced dependency, the belief in "magical cures," and the physician's responsibility to the patient, rather than the patient's responsibility in his/her own recovery. The physician's role in the pain clinic is unique and clearly nontraditional. For example, the medical director, rather than dispense analgesic medication, reinforces decreased use of medication; rather than promote surgical cures, he/she promotes nonsurgical solutions. The medical director is expected to reinforce patient's responsibility in their own health care, reinforce the proper utilization of the health care system, and disabuse patients of their belief in "magical cares." Rather than a treater, the medical director is an educator who is expected to impart valuable health-promoting information to all patients.

MEDICATION REDUCTION

Pain programs embrace many treatment goals— vocational restoration, pain reduction, increased activity, better flexibility, strength, endurance, effective cognitive coping skills, medication reduction, and stress management skills. However, medication reduction and/or its total elimination

constitutes a major and uniquely exercised goal. In most acute pain settings, analgesic medication is given contingent on patient pain behavior. In most chronic back pain centers clinic treatment staff reinforce medication reduction. One approach to medication reduction recommended by Fordyce et al. (12) is referred to as the "pain cocktail." In this approach analgesic medication is administered in a liquid medium in which there is the systematic reduction of the proportion of active ingredients over time, under the control of the treatment manager (unusually a decrease of 20–25% per week). The pain cocktail is given at specific times instead of as needed. These arrangements are discussed with the patient but he/she is not told exactly when the dosage will be reduced. (Fordyce et al. suggested quantifying medication use by intake, expressed in terms of unit potency, based on average effective dosages of morphine.)

Consistent with the self-control theme outlined in Gottlieb et al.'s pain program, the Casa Colina Pain Program embraces an alternative approach to medication reduction: the patient, with proper training and detailed documentation, is assigned control over the amount, pace, and ultimate outcome of his/her medication reduction goal (25). In this approach, patients are provided their initial admission level of medication and a locker and key to store it in. Through a lecture series devoted to the presentation and discussion of a variety of medication issues (e.g., its side effects, chemical ingredients, and the role it plays in sustaining the patient's pain disability), patients and staff, monitored by the nurse, will review each patient's charting activity and objective pill count each morning with each patient. Discrepancies in pill count and the failure to demonstrate a quantified reduction of analgesic medication within 2 weeks of the beginning of the program invites counseling from staff and the possibility of discharge if abuse is demonstrated.

While reduction in analgesic medication is expected for all patients, those who resist this expectation do so out of fear of losing analgesic relief from pain, and myths about withdrawal symptomology. To combat resistance, emphasis (in lecture/counseling format) is provided to help patients understand the role that relaxation, biofeedback, and physical exercise play in the production of endorphins (natural body pain killers), and how their skill-based experiences, once acquired, can provide a substitute alternative to "mind-fogging medication."

In some carefully monitored situations, psychotropic medication may be used. Since the administration of such medications can reinforce an ternal/non-patient-based attribution for pain reduction, their efficacy is restricted to a time-limited application to facilitate mood changes to restore sleep, reduce high anxiety levels disruptive in task performance, and eliminate fatigue associated with sleep disturbance. The expectation for expediently administered (opiates, synthetic opiates, hypnotics, sedatives, tranquilizers, and analgesics) medication is that the patient will ultimately discontinue it/them as part of his/her overall medication reduction treatment goal.

Several points about medication reduction should be noted. First, the pain cocktail was not utilized. Instead, patients were pressed to engage in a self-control procedure. This appears to achieve good results (25). Second, these good results may have been enhanced only for patients living within the controlled environment of the hospital. Third, a self-control procedure was chosen over the pain cocktail in order to promote long-term maintenance. Patients who, at the suggestion of physicians, direct their own drug withdrawal rather than having withdrawal imposed upon them (as occurs with the pain cocktail) may feel a great sense of personal control over pain behavior. A large body of literature demonstrates that such a sense of self-control over pain (i.e., internal locus of control, self-efficacy) is associated with a tendency to engage in positive health behaviors (26–28).

FAMILY THERAPY

Many pain patients demonstrate a variety of family issues. Family therapy, therefore, provides an integral part of the pain treatment model. In many instances the patient's family suffers almost as much as the patient. Patients will often play "pain games" that result in reinforcing their disability. In some cases, the family member(s) are reinforced by the patient, especially when the patient's disability may fulfill`a latent family need.

Family involvement is an essential part of the treatment model. The failure to participate in treatment is cited as one of the major bases for failure of the patient to maintain continued health after discharge (29).

BIOFEEDBACK TREATMENT MODALITY

Gottlieb et al.'s program also utilizes feedback treatment for chronic low back pain. This modality involves the monitoring of a target physiologic response, providing the patient with feedback on the response, and instructing the patient to alter the response. The most obvious rationale for biofeedback relies on the assumption that pain complaints are related either to excessive tension or specific muscle groups, or to a more generalized state of tension. Neither assumption is conclusive. First, whether pain reduction is a direct result of frontalis or paraspinal muscle feedback (as measured by electromyography) is moot. Second, the possibility that expensive feedback equipment can be substituted for by less expensive cognitive coping techniques, guided imagery, positive self-statements, and the like has been suggested (30). Nevertheless, as applied in Gottlieb et al.'s program, biofeedback produces experience that supports the central theme of the program, namely that pain control must occur from skills attributed to the patient's actions.

TREATMENT GOALS

Patients in Gottlieb et al.'s pain clinic are expected to give up the invalid role, reduce and/or eliminate dependence on addictive medication, reduce pain behavior and suffering, reduce cognitive stress mediators of pain, and reduce sources and expressions of tension, anxiety, and depression associated with enhanced pain levels. Patients are expected to gain in strength, physical endurance, and flexibility related to stooping, sitting, walking, standing, and bending, and to improve in areas of overall increased mobility. All patients with vocational goals are ultimately expected to return to gainful employment, and to decrease heavy reliance on health care utilization.

TREATMENT STAFF

Staff composition consists of: (a) liaison coordinator (to coordinate intake process), (b) program manager (pain clinic administrator), (c) physical therapist (responsible for reinstating total reconditioning of the patient), (d) psychologist (conducts cognitive social learning–based individual, family, and group therapy), (e) occupational therapist (responsible for work hardening, work tolerance, ergonomic assessments), (f) vocational specialist (does vocational assessment, job analysis, training, simulation, and placement), and (g) R.N. nurse coordinator (predominantly responsible for medication reduction program, and conducts lectures on health and stress and nutrition). Other pain clinics may assign a more central role to one of the following professionals: psychiatrist, orthopaedic surgeon, neurologist, and anesthesiologist. However, the Casa Colina program's medical director is a rheumatologist.

All Casa Colina staff are licensed, highly skilled specialists in pain management, and are clearly aware of the treatment model and its philosophical and empirical origins. In a word, all treatment staff receive extensive training in the cognitive social learning treatment model. Many staff persons have years of experience working with pain patients, their families, and third party payors. By training, all staff are adept in handling the many games pain patients play, such as pitting one staff member against another and attempting to manipulate the medical director to release more medication. Team work is imperative, and staff communication and coordinated mutual support is an essential element in this treatment model. By design, clinical staff provide role models for healthy behaviors for the patient to imitate. Because of the multidisciplinary nature of the staff, creative solutions involving clear communications are often applied to daily problems that may not have occurred in a single-modality, nonmultidisciplinary treatment context.

DISCHARGE PLANS

All treatment plans, goals, and discharge decisions are coordinated with the applicant attorney, case manager, third party payor, and referring physician where applicable. Discharge planning is introduced early in the patient's program to provide a smooth transition from treatment to home environment. In addition, treatment interventions are made by the staff to inoculate the patient against postdischarge relapse (31). In this regard, patients about to be discharged are returned to their family, employment, and other environments by graded in vivo home trial visits.

VOCATIONAL RESTORATION

A great emphasis is placed on the vocational restoration of the patient. Through vocational counseling, the patient works through some of the initial fears that staff members may be advocates of the insurance carrier. These fears are eventually replaced with the view that, by returning to work, one can earn more money and improve the quality of one's life more than by accepting the invalid role. A dominant message is that by learning proper pacing of activities and more efficient communication skills, one can create a much less stressful environment in which to work than was ever possible in previous employment. Finally, the view is communicated that work involving what one wants to do can be enjoyable.

A full program of vocational counseling, planning, work tolerance, functional capacity evaluation and training, work simulation, work hardening, ergonomic assessment, and referral counseling is offered. This phase of the program addresses the ultimate vocational restoration of the chronic back pain patient.

LONGITUDINAL OUTCOME RESULTS

Assessment of long-term benefits of Gottlieb et al.'s program have been reported (32–34). Utilizing return to work as a criterion for success, it was reported that at 6 months after discharge 62% of patients were gainfully employed. In a recent paper published in *Pain* (33), several outcome measures were reviewed at 5 years after discharge: return to work, litigation, pain rating, pain-preventing activity, using medication, and hospitalizations for pain. For example, with respect to return to work, across all occasions the return-to-work variables were highly correlated ($r = .95$); thus, once having secured employment, a participant was likely to continue employment 5 years later. In general, the results found for each of the six variables examined over a 5-year period of follow-up pointed to progressive improvement. Using correlational and probabilistic methods, favorable outcomes on all measures were observed and the proportion of respondents who appeared to be chronically suffering decreased steadily over time and across all observations (33).

SUMMARY

To summarize, an in-depth example of a chronic pain clinic was provided. The focus in Gottlieb's et al. cognitive social learning program is to maximize patient perception of attributions of a sense of personal control. Patient-acquired skills in self-control result in a reduction of patient reliance on the physician, nursing staff, and other medical and paramedical personnel. Such derived skills are also strengthened by procedures that facilitate patient-controlled experiences that promote the patients' responsibility in their ultimate recovery. The goal of this multidisciplinary approach is to reduce dependency on such external pain-solving strategies as (often toxic) medications, high-risk surgical procedures, and a heavy reliance on health care delivery systems. Moreover, patient-acquired skill in self-control is also assumed to reduce the patient's tendency to assign blame and responsibility to others for his/her health and wellness. Finally, the clinical benefits of promoting a sense of personal control are to ultimately replace feelings of resignation and pessimism with optimism, and feelings of despair and depression with hope.

OPERANT CONDITIONING MODEL

The second model presented offers an analysis of the application of an operant conditioning paradigm for the restoration of the chronic back pain patient. Applying many of the associated assumptions, research, and techniques from the Skinnerian operant paradigm, pain in this model is viewed as a learned behavior, an operant that has come under the lawful control of a number of environmental contingencies (35, 36). As stated by Fordyce, the identified originator of one of the earliest and still most popular pain clinics (12),

> . . . responses by others to overt pain behavior accompanying the subjective experience of pain may serve to reinforce or to extinguish aspects of that behavior. When the pain behavior occurs with some consistency over a protracted period of time, as in chronic pain problems, the environment may come to be shaped in such a way as to reinforce the pain behavior and thereby sustain it. (p. 105)

Learning theory models of treatment are not concerned with the underlying causes of pain. Such paradigms make no assumptions about whether or not there is evidence of organic difficulty nor about the inner emotional state of the person. For the application of the learning approach, what is required is that pain behavior, however manifested, and the spinoff behaviors associated with pain, such as not working, be sufficiently isolated so that they can be effectively targeted for alterations by modification strategies. Since the behavior modification approach presupposes nothing about the patient him/herself, demographic variables, inner psychodynamics, affect states, or the organic status of the patient are not a primary focus of concern. In this model, pain behavior is real even if nociceptive inputs are not identified. The central tenant in Fordyce's approach is that when the subjective experience of pain manifest in behavior (grimacing, groaning, etc.) is systematically reinforced by its consequences (sympathy from others, etc.) over a protracted period of time, the environment may come to control pain behavior and consequently sustain it, shape it, and ultimately turn such behavior into a chronic disability.

Medication reduction is a central outcome goal in the operant paradigm. When patients cry out in pain, medication soon will follow. This is not the case in Fordyce's model. Patients are quickly shifted from a pain-contingent schedule to a time-contingent schedule. In behavior modification terms, medication is dispensed at specific time intervals.

Medication is never given when the patient complains of pain unless the complaints coincide with a specific time interval. After the patient is solidly established in an activity regimen, the narcotic content of his/her medication is decreased.

In Fordyce's operant model a number of other rehabilitatively important target behaviors were identified as important operants to modify: walking, pain behavior, up-time, and participation in occupational therapy. This model provides an example of some of the behaviors that have been selected for modification. Pain patients are also trained to record and monitor their experience of pain.

All significant others involved with the patient, including the patient's spouse, are taught the basics of the program and are taught not to reinforce pain behavior if and when it occurs. Family members are trained to reinforce, or maintain, all gains that patients demonstrate in the program. All procedures are also adapted for application in the patient's home milieu by family on weekend visits and when the patient returns home.

The patient's activity level is also assessed. In behavior modification terms, patients are asked to self-report up-time—the time spent out of a reclining position—using an hourly diary format (36). Each day the patient's up-time is recorded on a graph place above the patient's bed, and praise is dispensed on days when up-time is increased.

While other devices and measures have been designed to measure up-time, the results of this approach seem effective (36). In general, the operant model demonstrates that any nonillness behavior (when isolated for reinforcement) can increase or decrease contingent upon the systematic application of reinforcing stimuli.

Many clinics rely exclusively on operant learning treatment approaches, and others on combinations of operant and cognitive social learning strategies as effective treatment models for the restoration of chronic back pain patients (37). However, a number of issues surround the application of operant treatment regimens for chronic pain. First, a variety of practical issues involve the day-to-day implementation of such regimens in a free-standing ongoing hospital milieu. Staff require training and constant reinforcement, which is difficult to provide in the day-to-day world of the pain clinic. Second, staff need to apply coordinated and consistent reinforcers for all agreed-upon targeted behaviors. In other words, even though staff members may see some categories of behavior as undesirable and worthy of negative attention (e.g., complaining behavior), staff may not always differentially ignore or punish such behavior on a consistent basis, and in fact may respond positively to all forms of behavior. Third, questions are raised about the long-term benefits of applying this model over others in the treatment repertoire. Several important questions concerning the long-term efficacy of behavioral approaches in the treatment of a number of important disease entities have been raised (38).

Behavioral-based medication reduction strategies (e.g., the pain cocktail) raise important ethical issues that are of prime importance to the therapist. For example, several writers have addressed the ethical issues raised by the practice of withdrawing patients from pain medications without their knowledge or consent and without the consent of their treatment staff (39, 40). Although it is clear that such deception has important healing benefits (of a placebo nature), the question is whether these benefits override the ethical issues associated with deception. Notwithstanding, the general consensus is that the operant framework has pioneered a useful intervention for the restoration of the refractory low back pain patient.

PAIN CLINICS

The late 1960s and early 1970s witnessed the increasing proliferation of pain clinics for the treatment of chronic low back pain. In 1978 there were an estimated 325 pain clinics worldwide; there were 800 in 1980 (30), and today I would estimate there are over 1200 pain clinics in the United States alone. Broadly stated, the impetus to the development of chronic pain programs comes from five major sources: (a) the evidence that the biomedical model was inadequate as a restorative approach for a sizeable number of chronic pain patients; (b) political agencies at the federal level initiating an increase and interest in new therapies for the treatment of pain (National Institute of Drug Abuse and the National Institutes of Health); (c) the formation of international, national, and regional associations for the study of pain; (d) the prompting by these associations to form committees for the creation of taxonomies for the classification of pain; and (e) the creation of a new journal, *Pain.*

Pain clinics have been categorized by the American Pain Society of Anesthesiologists as major comprehensive, comprehensive, syndrome oriented, and modality oriented. Major comprehensive pain clinics, both inpatient and outpatient, offer multidisciplinary medical evaluation, as well as an integrated, behaviorally oriented treatment plan, a cohesive pain team approach, and a broad range of multidisciplinary techniques and technology geared to the removal of all barriers that prevent the patient from total emotional and vocational restoration. Common to the concept of the pain clinic is that, in the main, pain clinics provide a framework in which to eliminate and/or teach the patient to manage his/her pain (pain reduction, and/or pain management) through such conservative modalities as physical therapy, traction, hot packs, ultrasound, and biofeedback, and psychological methods such as individual and group therapy, cognitive coping skills, psychometric evaluation, stress reduction skills and family therapy. Pain clinics focus on reduction and/or elimination of drug dependence, treat underlying depression, improve family and community support systems, provide access to vocational and occupational rehabilitation, return patients to gainful employment (work hardening, job analysis, work simulation, etc.), and help patients to attain goals in quality of life. Furthermore, pain clinics attempt to decrease the cost and overutilization of traditional medical care and attempt to reduce the patient's fruitless reliance on iaotrogenic (i.e., surgical and polypharmacy) solutions to chronic pain problems.

While the Casa Colina treatment model is oriented toward the restoration of low back pain patients, pain clinics offer services for a variety of syndromes and diagnostic disorders (headaches, cancer pain, temporomandibular joint syndrome, etc.)—that is, for a variety of psychophysiologic disorders. Many syndrome-oriented programs offer services for dealing with specific types of pain disorders (e.g., headaches, cancer pain, temporomandibular joint syndrome, hand and neck disorders), and modality-oriented programs may stress one or another set of particular modalities (e.g., physical therapy, hot packs, ultrasound) as a primary programmatic focus.

Pain programs differ in length of stay. Some pain clinics offer 3-week programs, others require 4–6 weeks (37). Some programs are outpatient only, others inpatient in focus (37). Because all pain patients do not require 4–6 weeks of an inpatient program, many are referred to a less costly outpatient program. Some pain clinics utilize a motel residential component for patients requiring isolation from family and work stressors while receiving full-day inpatient treatment, and others, because of the patient's medical status, require a full inpatient program. However, many patients are treated in outpatient programs when their medical status justifies it, their insurance carrier authorizes it, and the impact of long-term hospitalization on the patient and his/her family is deemed harmful to the patient's overall compliance and ultimate success. Pain clinics also differ in their costs. A survey of California-based pain clinics conducted by Casa Colina Hospital revealed that the range of cost for an inpatient program can be from $12,000 on the low end to $34,000 on the high end for a 6–8-week major comprehensive pain service. For an outpatient program (half-day, full-day, and single-modality combinations) the cost can range from $2500 on the low end to $12,500 on the high end.

Typically, patients who exhibit pain for 3–6 months or more; who are unresponsive to everything the conventional medical model had to offer; whose life (including that of their family) is totally disrupted by pain, depression, and drug-seeking behavior; and who are employment candidates by virtue of the fact that they can benefit from a comprehensive work hardening and full-service vocational restoration program are patients for whom a major comprehensive inpatient residential pain program is typically recommended.

CHARACTERISTIC PROFILES OF CHRONIC BACK PAIN PATIENTS

Even before the establishment of pain clinics, the literature hypothesized that chronic back pain patients exhibited characteristic personality profiles, and that such profiles played a major role in rendering this patient population resistant to treatment by traditional medical means. Whether such profiles are antecedent (as suggested by engel's use of the term "pain-prone patient") (41) or the consequence of long periods of pain disability and suffering is moot. Nevertheless, a list of model personality and demographic characteristics of chronic back pain patients has emerged (42, 43). Typical of patients treated in Gottlieb et al.'s pain clinic, the literature supports the following profile: patients are typically hyperactive, emit extreme fatigue, exhibit suicidal depression, have somatic complaints, exaggerate or amplify their pain behavior, emit narcissistic borderline and/or hysterical personality characteristics, are likely to emit symptoms incongruent with physical pathology, exhibit poor coping skills, and display a variety of family problems. They typically come from families with significant role models for pain behavior; reveal having been abused as children; exhibit an enhanced sensitivity or decreased tolerance for pain; exhibit low stamina as a result of deconditioning, exhibit drug dependency and addiction; are more reactive, angry, stressed, and anxious; engage in

catastrophic thinking; demonstrate unfulfilled dependency needs; display helplessness, hopelessness, and suffering; stay in the hospital longer; remain out of work longer; and are less likely to return to work.

Evidence obtained from the Minnesota Multiphasic Personality Inventory (MMPI) points to an MMPI profile of elevated scores most associated with patients likely to fail surgical interventions (42, 44). High scale scores (T scale scores above 70) on Scales 1, 2, and 3, which represent hypochondriasis, depression, and hysteria, respectively, are not uncommon. Scale 1 translates into bodily focused complaints, while Scale 2 (depression) and Scale 3 (hysteria) point to a decreased mobility, depression, and decreases in the patient's pain threshold. Significant elevation in these scales point to the likelihood of these patients attributing stressors and pain to somatic complaints.

In general, elevations on Scales 1, 2, and 3 are descriptive of a variety of psychophysiologic disorders (43). Nevertheless, elevations on these scales have been shown to predict poor surgical outcomes: in one study, the MMPI scale scores of T values above 70 demonstrated a clear relationship between elevations on Scales 1, 2, and 3, and surgical failures from a chemonucleolysis procedure (45).

Several reviews of psychologically based multidisciplinary pain clinics have been published (46–50). One of the earliest reviews of multidisciplinary pain clinics was sponsored by the Department of Health and Human Services (National Institute of Drug Abuse) in collaboration with the interagency committee on New Therapies for Pain and Discomfort (37). In this monograph, a number of pain clinics and centers reported on their staffing and organization, structure, the problems for which patients are treated, drugs taken by entering patients, therapeutic approaches used, costs of treatment, and methods for long-term evaluation of treatment effectiveness (37).

OUTCOME RESEARCH OF PAIN CLINICS

Turk et al. have provided a comprehensive summary of the techniques employed, criteria for inclusion of patients, length of treatment, and number of patients who applied, received and completed treatment, and were included in follow-up studies conducted on the efficacy of comprehensive pain treatment programs (30). Their review included an analysis of programs that have made outcome research a priority. Their review is quite revealing; while many of the pain clinics reviewed may provide quality services, long-term follow-up studies are few and, when conducted, are of such poor quality that sound conclusions are hard to draw. Nevertheless, some studies are worth mentioning.

One of the earliest follow-up studies was conducted by Fordyce and his colleagues (35). This study gathered data from a mailed questionnaire sent to the patient 22 months after discharge. In the questionnaire, the patients were asked to remember their status on certain variables from before admission to the present time. Fordyce studied level of pain, activities interfered with because of pain, number of hours reclining, and medications subjects were taking. Results showed that there was a significant reduction in pain (35). However, patients still reported considerable levels of pain. They did improve in areas of up-time and in the degree to which pain did not interfere with necessary activities of daily living. Painter et al. (51) conducted a similar study with patients from the Northwest Pain Center. These workers found that 77% of patients felt improvement as a result of their experience at the pain center, with an average pain reduction of 35%. Further improvement following discharge was noted by 27% of the sample, with a further average reduction in pain of 21%. Deterioration was reported by 27% of the sample. A reduction in injury-related compensation from 70% at admission to 45% after discharge was also noted. A 90% admission rate of unemployment was reduced to 48% at follow-up. Sixty-one percent of patients reported they had had no further medical care for their pain and 17% stated they were seeking other medical solutions. Twenty percent reported having returned to use of narcotic medications, which had been eliminated by the pain unit program.

In another study, Roberts and Reinhardt (49) reported that 77% of patients in one clinic were leading normal lives 1–8 years after treatment. Cinciripini and Floren (52) found that at 12 months' follow-up 55% of patients in a behavior program were medication free, and 61% had avoided pain-related physician contacts.

Relying on data obtained from the Casa Colina Rehabilitation Hospital Program in Pomona, California, in two separate papers published in the journal *Pain,* McArthur et al. (32, 33) reviewed data from 710 participants covering a time span from 6 months to 5 years following treatment. Over the short term, outcomes appear to have been quite favorable on average across multiple measures from both physical and psychological realms. Evidence gathered at 12 months following treatment for a sample of 78 showed that 45% had returned to work and that a relationship existed between return to work and pain ratings, medication use, and utilization of physician services for pain during the intervening year.

This writer's intention is not to conduct an exhaustive review of the literature on the efficacy of multidisciplinary pain clinics; the literature so reviewed would support the fact that overall, pain clinics provide an effective, nonsurgical alternative to restoration of chronic low back pain patients.

Notwithstanding, the above impression must be somewhat cautiously embraced. The findings of research on long-term follow-up results point to many methodologic issues. For instance, most research fails to address the fact that chronic pain patients, on admission, differ in many ways: in organic pathology, disability, and psychological makeup and on a number of demographic variables. Despite earlier-cited efforts to find common characteristic profiles of chronic low back pain patients, chronic back pain patients are not homogeneous. The important task is to identify the kinds of chronic back pain patients (patient characteristics) that can most benefit from differing treatment models and modalities, under differing combination(s) of treatment(s), conditions, and outcome measures. Pain clinics utilize different treatment goals. Treatment goals for some patients (e.g., increase in activity, medication reduction, employability, changes in psychometric measures) may be irrelevant or unnecessary goals of treatment for other patients. Treatment goals are not standardized even though pressure exists to make efforts to do so.

Pain clinics employ a wide range of treatment modalities; however, most are unidimensional models, that is, they may rely on one or another psychological model. They may focus on physical therapy modalities or emphasize invasive procedures or stress biomechanical approaches. Sometimes pain clinics utilize a combination of modalities and treatment models.

Pain clinics differ in outcome measures employed. Reduction of pain may be a primary goal in one clinic, while the alteration of maladaptive sick role behavior may be a treatment goal in another. Other pain clinics focus on teaching patients cognitive coping techniques and/or reducing stress, and still others stress vocational outcomes.

Besides those pain clinics that demonstrate a purely operant or cognitive social learning paradigm, only some small number of pain clinics adopt a consistent empirically based treatment paradigm. One result is that few pain clinics select treatment modalities that reflect a theoretical paradigm; the array of treatment modalities they employ may be from a menu of paradigmically generated and/or scientifically proven treatments.

Pain clinics generate much data, but very few develop assessment batteries that integrate medical and physical findings with psychological and behavioral data, let alone employ prescriptive interventions from the data generated to prescribe combinations of treatments, conditions, and so forth that may best maximize optimal patient outcomes.

ORGANIZATIONAL STRUCTURE FOR PAIN CLINICS

Pain clinics differ in organization infrastructure. Some pain clinics retain a physical therapist or psychologist as program manager. The clinical staff may differ in training, in specialty, and in quality. Medical directors differ in specialty as well, and they may differ in the degree of influence they exert over their treatment team and in the treatment delivery system as a whole.

Pain clinics may be affiliated with a medical school, a hospital, an acute care facility, a rehabilitative medical unit, an industrial free-standing clinic, or a free-standing investor-owned outpatient unit. Pain clinics can be inpatient or outpatient in design. They can differ in staff composition and cohesion of staff. They may be wedded to a continuum of services (e.g., prevention programs, a back school, work hardening, and postdischarge service). In one pain clinic the physical therapist may administer biofeedback, whereas in another the psychologist provides this modality. Some pain clinics contract for services, others provide an in-house compliment of multidisciplinary specialists. Quality assurance concerns may be differentially addressed. In some clinics services may be integrated, sequenced, and consistently connected to all treatment goals, and in others they are fragmented and not reflective of an agreed-upon treatment plan. Some pain clinics are Commission on Accreditation of Rehabilitation Facilities (CARF)–accredited; others, by virtue of their standards of practice, are not. Policy and procedure manuals may or may not be in place. Such manuals may differ in scope, depth, clarity, and accuracy of program description, treatment goal, triage criteria, patients to be served, discharge criteria, range of modalities included, and program evaluation standards and strategies.

All pain clinics reflect the medical director's specialty. If a neurologist is the administrator, emphasis is typically placed on nerve blocks, the neurosurgeon may emphasize manipulation or ablation of pain pathways, the orthopaedist may focus on the removal of a herniated disk or "spine fusion" procedure, the internist may focus on rotation of pain medications, and the psychiatrist may rely on pharmacologic therapy. Finally, while mandatory under CARF regulations, many pain clinics do not have a comprehensive program evaluation system while others make program evaluation a priority.

As pain clinics become increasingly popular clinically, they have become increasingly popular financially as business ventures. This has proved both a bane and a benefit. The influx of capital support for outpatient hospitals or free-standing pain clinics has meant more clinics, but more clinics has not meant sustained or better quality.

ISSUES ATTENDANT ON THE IMPLEMENTATION AND MANAGEMENT OF A PAIN CLINIC

A number of factors have become increasingly important to the successful "business" of a pain clinic. Of primary significance to sound physical management is the quality, training, and business administrative skills of the pain clinic administrator. Most pain clinic administrators are responsible for: (a) assisting in the development of the business plan, (b) year-to-year budgets and operational pro forma, (c) the development of a short- and long-range marketing plan, (d) the management of day-to-day operations, (e) the anticipation of equipment needs, (f) the maintenance of referral patterns, (g) the maintenance of consumer third-party satisfaction, (h) staffing needs, (i) the maintenance of staff morale, (j) the continuing quality of all personnel, (k) the development an up-to-date maintenance of pain clinic policy and procedure guidelines (manual), and (l) the monitoring and continued maintenance of the pain clinic computerized program evaluation system.

Responsibility for coordinating all physical, clinical, vocational, and medical decisions (typically involving the third-party payor, patient's family, attorney, insurance carriers, industry, discharge coordinator, rehabilitation nurse, and referring physician) rests with the program manager and/or case manager. In this regard, pain clinic administrators (program managers) must be ever mindful of the clinical and marketing implications of the many extremely delicate decisions they make and their impact on consumer satisfaction. The alienation of attorneys, third-party payors, trade union officials, industry, referring physicians, and other community-based referring sources can have a severe impact on present and future referral patterns to the clinic.

Finally, but far from inclusive, pain clinic administrators must be knowledgeable about reimbursement issues, regulations, and prospective changes in reimbursement schedules. This includes state and federal reimbursement issues, federal licensing regulations, the workers' compensation laws, Medicare regulations, the Comprehensive Outpatient Rehabilitation Facility (CORF) regulations and guidelines, and Medicare reimbursement schedules. They must understand the insurance industry, their needs and concerns, and their perceptions of pain clinics. They must be prepared to respond promptly with clinical reports to referring physicians, attorneys, and third-party payors, and equally promptly to the many administrative demands exacted by hospital chief administrators and/or joint venture partners if there are any.

While the above list of concerns was not meant to be exhaustive, it does point to some of the many increasing concerns to which pain clinic administrators must attend in order to be successful fiscally as well as clinically.

PROGRAM EVALUATION

A well thought out program evaluation system is becoming an increasingly high priority for all pain clinics. Notwithstanding, the development and maintenance of a computerized program evaluation system has received slow priority. Hospital administrators and/or venture capitalists often view it as unnecessary and costly and therefore few hospital-based and/or free-standing or privately owned pain clinics allocate funds for this line item in their budget.

It must be stressed that although costly, the installation of a research program evaluation system is cost effective in the long run. A data-base program evaluation system can yield many benefits. It can generate data for research, marketing, billing, referral updates, referring patterns, and rates of referral as well as dates, frequency, and type of referral. It can facilitate the prompt implementation of reports, and empirically yield data for a variety of in-house (i.e., pain clinic) decisions. It can produce monthly consumer-oriented management reports and, most important, it can generate programmatic outcome studies as well as yield research commensurate with academic medical journal standards. To summarize, the major benefits of a program evaluation system are:

1. To increase the benefits to persons the program serves
2. To increase program productivity
3. To improve market position
4. To assess use of health care resources
5. To assess program costs
6. To assess programatic goals
7. To measure programs' longitudinal outcomes (programmatic success)
8. To record progress on all program (pain clinic) measures by medical findings, pain ratings, psychological adjustment, and so forth
9. To record medical referrals, reimbursement sources, diagnoses treated, and services provided
10. To conduct scientific research

Program (data-base) evaluation systems must be designed to address the issue of how well pain clinics do what they claim to do. The response to this issue not only serves the scientific and academic community, but is becoming increasingly important for the cost-conscious insurance industry as well. Third-party payors, although peripherally concerned with such clinical outcomes as pain relief, medication reduction, and improved quality of life, are pressing for hard scientific data regarding the costs-benefits and clinical efficiency of pain clinics. While third-party payors are interested in seeing their cases "closed" as well as returned to work, outcomes in pain reduction in their overall liability, and a reduction in patient health care utilization, pain clinics typically focus on the clinical restoration of the patient without salient regard for the concerns of the third-party payor.

Regional and national pain societies are also pressing for a standardized program evaluation system, and CARF is making program evaluation mandatory. Careful planning must go into the development of a program evaluation system. First and most important, planning for such a system must occur early, preferably at the very inception of the pain clinic proper. The purpose and scope of the program evaluation must be considered and computer needs must be determined. These tasks necessitate the staff inclusion of a half-time researcher. While pressure for standardization of key pain clinic data elements may be fixed, data reflecting other variables that are meaningful and indiginous to regionally different needs of pain clinics are not. Variables must be selected for inclusion or exclusion that reflect all relevant aspects of the pain clinics operation. Treatment outcome measures must be operationalized and quantified. All psychometric measures must be identified early on for inclusion, and all targeted hypotheses must be prospectively identified for investigation. While it is beyond the scope of this chapter to describe the many issues attendant on the important matter of program evaluation, the initiated reader would be wise to review the more technical issues involved in Gottlieb and Alperson's treatment of this topic (53).

COST-BENEFIT OF PAIN CLINICS

Are pain programs cost effective? Considering the degree of importance of this question, surprisingly few studies are available (54–56). Although we know medical costs are high as a rule, it is most difficult to gather definitive data on cost incurred by the average chronic low back pain patient prior to their pain clinic intervention. Nevertheless, Steig and Turk's (56) findings in this regard do support the view that pain clinic(s) can contribute to substantial cost savings. They compared the average cost of treatment of $8160 for a 3-week pain management program to the total cost (provided by the insurance carrier) of medical and disability payments for 1 year prior to and 1 year after pain treatment. The savings cited pointed to an average potential savings of $238,515 per patient (56).

Psychological interventions that prevent future high cost overutilization of medical resources are recommended and investigation (57), and more scientific and specific focus needs to address the question of costs-benefits of pain clinics.

WHERE DO WE NEED TO GO?

While pain clinics have been steadily gaining acceptance as viable alternatives to invasive medical procedures, a number of issues remain outstanding. Considering the incidence and prevalence of low back pain disorders, considerably little time is devoted in the curriculum of the physician to the many issues (i.e., theories, concepts, and research) that differentiate acute back pain from chronic (low back) pain. Efforts to repair this condition are underway. Medical schools are increasingly infusing their curriculum with courses devoted to topics in behavioral medicine, and they are also including psychologists trained in health psychology and behavioral medicine as integral members of their teaching staff. Similarly, third-party payors, the general public, attorneys, health care professionals, and a variety of relevant governmental agencies have differing impressions of pain clinics, some good and some bad. These bodies need to know much more about pain clinics, what they do, and how well they do it.

Pain clinics need to monitor their quality and produce outcome studies that validate what they do and how well they do it. CARF has begun to require program evaluation as a prerequisite to accreditation. However, this agency is not able to monitor the quality of treatment per se. Treatment quality is left to the integrity of the program administrator and his/her staff. In this regard, peer review procedures are becoming an increasingly viable component in many hospital-based pain clinics. Such procedures are needed in all pain clinics, free standing or otherwise.

Research needs to be directed at identifying the combination of treatments that work best with different subpopulations of low back pain patients. There is a need for treatment strategies to prevent and alter noncompliant behavior. Treatment strategies are needed for subpopulations of pain patients for whom pain clinics have not proven efficacious. Also, more attention needs to be paid to long-term follow-up research.

Waiting list control group studies are needed, and long-term follow-up protocol and supportive staff need to be committed to the arduous task of validation of pain clinic interventions. There needs to be a closer alliance between tertiary intervention (pain clinics) and primary care intervention (patient's physician).

Pain clinics need to address aftercare issues earlier and provide more coordinated services that facilitate smoother transition from discharge to family to work. Pain clinics need to support, if not create, more aftercare, community-based relapse prevention programs. They must provide more direct and effective consultation services for the community-based physician, and such services need to be systematically introduced to assist the community-based practitioner in the arduous task of "behavioral management" of the chronic low back pain patient. Since a large number of high-risk factors predictive of chronicity are psychosocial, the resources and expertise available for the early detection and management of high-risk acute and subacute low back pain patients renders the pain clinic an excellent adjunct to the community-based practitioner.

Medical criteria are given disproportionate notoriety as the basis for presuming or establishing the patient's inability to work. Other factors (i.e., pain behavior, emotional problems, illness behavior, and suffering) must be included as legitimate barriers, equal in significance to the role medical findings have in disability ratings. Pain clinics need to be closely identified with a continuum of efforts—from back injury prevention at the work site to chronicity prevention (related to improper case management and/or the administration of ineffective treatment(s)) during the early phase of the acute injury.

Pain clinics also must consider contributing their consultative expertise to a broader community base than they have to this point. They should include employee assistance programs and injury prevention and risk management programs. Moreover, pain clinics need to pay more attention to a number of concerns that have an impact on industry, one of which is the increasing cost to industry, the patient, and the patient's family of employee absenteeism due to on-job-site–related low back injuries and workers' compensations costs.

It is mainly through more effective community involvement with physicians, attorneys, employers, insurance carriers, patients, their families, and industry that pain clinics can obtain the respect they indeed deserve.

REFERENCES

1. Loeser JD: Low back pain. In Bonica JJ (ed): *Pain.* New York, Raven Press, 1980.
2. Waddell G, Kummel EG, Lotto WN: Failed lumbar disc surgery and repeat surgery following industrial injuries. *J Bone Joint Surg [Am]* 61:201–207, 1979.
3. McGill CM: Industrial back problems: a control program. *J Occup Med* 10:174–178, 1984.
4. Gordon E: Rehabilitating of chronic low back patients. *Indust Med Surg* 28:26–33, 1959.
5. Melzack R, Wall PD: *The Challenge of Pain.* New York, Basic Books, 1982.
6. Chapman CR: A behavioral perspective on chronic pain. Paper presented at the annual convention of the American Psychological Association, Montreal, Canada, August 1973.
7. Gottlieb H, Strite L, Koller R, Madorsky D, Hockensmith V, Kleeman M, Wagner J: Comprehensive rehabilitation of patients having chronic low back pain.
8. *Spine, European Edition Supplement,* Vol 16, No 7. New York, Harper & Row, 1987, 155N, pp 362–436.
9. Bonica J: Editorial. *Triangle* 20:1–6, 1981.
10. Social Security Administration: *Report to the Commission of Evaluation of Pain.* Washington, DC, Department of Health and Human Services, 1986.
11. Spengler DM, Bigos SJ, Martem MA, et al: Back injuries in industry: a retrospective study: I. Overview and cost analysis. *Spine* 11:241–245, 1986.
12. Fordyce WE, Fowler RS, DeLateur B: An application of behavior modification technique to a problem of chronic pain. *Behav Res Ther* 6:105–107, 1968.
13. Gottlieb HJ, Alperson BL, Koller R, Hockensmith V: Comprehensive rehabilitation of patients having chronic

low back pain. *J Am Phys Ther Assoc* 59.996–999, 1979.
14. Seligman ME: *Helplessness.* San Francisco, WH Freeman, 1975.
15. Pervin LA: The need to predict and control under conditions of threat. *J Pers* 31:570–587, 1963.
16. Davison GC, Valins S: Maintenance of self-attributed and drug-attributed behavior change. *J Pers Soc Psychol* 11:25–33, 1969.
17. Hill HR, Kornetsky CH, Flanary HG, Wikler A: Studies on anxiety associated with anticipation of pain: I. Effects of morphine. *Arch Neurol Psychiatry* 67:612–619, 1952.
18. Stotland E, Blumenthal A: The reduction of anxiety as a result of the expectation of making a choice. *Can J Psychol* 18:139–145, 1964.
19. Ross L, Rodin J, Zimbardo PG: Toward an attribution therapy: the reduction of fear through induced cognitive-emotional misattribution. *J Pers Soc Psychol* 12:N279–N288, 1969.
20. Nisbett RE, Schacter S: Cognitive manipulation of pain. *J Exp Soc Pyschol* 2:227–236, 1966.
21. Pranulis M, Dabbs J, Johnson J: General anesthesia and the patient's attempts at control *Soc Behav Pers* 3:N49–N54.
22. Beals RK, Hackman N: Industrial injuries of the back and extremities. *J Bone Joint Surg* 54:1593–1611, 1972.
23. Krusen FM, Ford DF: Compensation factor in low back injuries. 166:1128–1133, 1958.
24. Wilfling FJ, Klonoff H, Kokan P: Psychological, demographic, and orthopedic factors associated with prediction of outcome of spinal fusion. *Clin Orthop* 90:153–160, 1973.
25. Gottlieb HJ, Alperson BL, Schwartz HH, Beck G, Kee S: Self management for medication reduction in chronic low back pain. *Arch Phys Med Rehabil* 69:105–110, 1988.
26. Olbrish ME: Psychotherapeutic interventions in physical health. Effectiveness and economic efficiency. *Am Psychol* 32:761–777, 1977.
27. Rotter JB, Chance JE, Phares EJ: *Application of a Social Learning Theory of Personality.* New York, Holt, Rinehart & Winston, 1972.
28. Shofield W: The psychologist as a health care professional. *Intellect,* January, pp. 255–258, 1975.
29. Baranowski T, Nader PR: Family involvement in health behavior change programs. In Turk DC, Kernes RD (eds): *Health, Illness, and Families.* New York, John Wiley & Sons, 1985, pp. 81–107.
30. Turk DC, Meichenbaum D, Genst M: *Pain and Behavioral Medicine; A Cognitive Behavioral Perspective.* New York, Guilford Press, 1983.
31. Marlatt GA, Gordon JR: Determinants of relapse: implications for the maintenance of behavior change. In Davidson PO, Davidson SM (eds): *Behavioral Medicine: Changing Health Life Styles.* New York, Brunner/Mazel, 1980.
32. McArthur DL, Cohen MJ, Gottlieb HJ, Naliboff BD,

Schandler SL: Treating chronic low back pain: I. Admissions to follow-up. *Pain* 29:1–22, 1987.

33. McArthur DL, Cohen MJ, Gottlieb HJ, Naliboff BD, Schandler SL: Treating chronic low back pain: II. Admissions to follow-up. *Pain* 29:23–38, 1987.

34. Gottlieb HJ, Alperson BL: Low back pain comprehensive rehabilitation program: a follow-up study. *Arch Phys Med Rehabil* 63:458–461, 1982.

35. Fordyce WB, Fowler RS Jr, Lehmann JF, DeLateur BJ, Sond PL, Trieschmann RB: Operant conditioning in the treatment of chronic pain. *Arch Phys Med Rehabil* 54:399–408, 1973.

36. Fordyce WB, Steger JC: Chronic pain. In Pomerleau OF, Brady JP (eds): *Behavioral Medicine: Theory and Practice.* Baltimore, Williams & Wilkins, 1979.

37. Ng LK (ed): New approaches to treatment of chronic pain: a review of multidisciplinary pain clinics and pain centers. *NIDA Monograph 36.* Rockville, MD, National Institute of Drug Abuse, 1981, pp. 137–168.

38. Russel EW: The power of behavior control: a critique of behavior modification methods. *J Clin Psychol* 30:111–136, 1974.

39. Levundusky P, Pankratz L: Self-control techniques as an alternative to pain medication. *J Abnorm Psychol* 84:165–168, 1975.

40. Kelman HC: Was deception justified—and was it necessary? Comments on self-control techniques as an alternative to pain medication. *J Abnorm Psychol* 84:172–174, 1975.

41. Engle GL: *Psychological Development in Health and Disease.* Philadelphia, WB Saunders, 1962.

42. Philips EL: Some psychological characteristics associated with orthopedic complaints. In Adams JP (ed): *Current Practice of Orthopedic Surgery.* St. Louis, CV Mosby, 1964.

43. Sternback RA, Wolf SR, Murphy RW, Akenson WH: Traits of pain patients: the low back loser. Paper presented at the 19th Annual Meeting of the Academy of Psychosomatic Medicine, San Diego, California, 1972.

44. Hanvik LJ: MMPI profiles in patients with low-back pain. *J Consult Psychol* 15:350–353, 1951.

45. Witse LL: Psychological testing in predicting success of low back surgery. *Orthop Clin North Am* 6:317–318, 1975.

46. Turner JA, Chapman CR: Psychological interventions for chronic pain: a critical view: I. Relaxation and biofeedback. *Pain* 12:1–22, 1982.

47. Turner JA, Romano J: Evaluating psychologic interventions for chronic pain: issues and recent developments. In Benedetti C, Chapman CR, Moricca G (eds): *Recent Advances in the Management of Pain.* New York, Raven Press, 1984, vol 6.

48. Main CJ: Psychological approaches to management and treatment of back pain, ed 3. In Jayson MIV (Ed): *The Lumbar Spine and Back Pain.* Tunbridge Wells, UK, Pitman Medical, 1983.

49. Roberts AH, Reinhardt L: The behavioral management of chronic pain long term follow-up with comparison groups. *Pain* 8:151–162, 1980.

50. Arnoff GM, Evans WO, Enders PL: A review of follow-up studies of multidisciplinary pain units. *Pain* 16:1–12, 1983.

51. Painter JR, Senes JL, Newman RI: Assessing benefits of the pain center: why some patients regress. *Pain* 8:101–113, 1980.

52. Cinciripini PM, Floren A: An evaluation of an inpatient behavioral program for chronic pain. Paper presented at the 15th Annual Convention of the Association for Advancement in Behavior Therapy, New York, November 1980.

53. Gottlieb HJ, Alperson BL: Psychophysiological approaches to chronic low back pain. In Golden JC, Alcaparnas S, Studier F, Graber B (eds): *Applied Techniques in Behavioral Medicine.* New York, Grune & Stratton, 1981.

54. Steele RI: Are pain programs cost effective? *Pain* 2:438, 1985.

55. Steig RL, Williams RC, Timingmans-Williams G, Tafuno F, Gallagher L: Cost benefits of interdisciplinary chronic pain treatment. *Pain Manage* 1:189–193, 1988.

56. Steig RL, Turk DC: Chronic pain syndrome, demonstrating the cost-benefit of treatment. *Pain Manage* 1(2), 1988.

57. Gottlieb HJ, Strite LG, Koller R, Hockensmith V, Madorsky A, Stanley J: Symposium: Psychologically oriented treatment programs for the chronic pain patient. Presented at the American Psychological Association, Washington, DC, September, 1976.

Chapter 21

WORK HARDENING

BARBARA L. KORNBLAU, JD, OTR

Work plays an integral part in the development of an individual's self-esteem and in his/her own identification as a contributing member of our society (1, 2). Work fulfills numerous individual needs, including the needs for economic security, socialization, "belonging," status, creativity, and self-expression. As the individual develops his/her "work personality," he/she acquires work attitudes, the need for motivation or incentives, physical and psychological abilities to work, a value system, and specific work behavior patterns (2).

The ability to work derives from several prerequisite skills. One must possess adequate motor skills and abilities, such as coordination and the ability to lift, bend, and so forth. Social behaviors, such as the ability to cooperate and to relate to authority, are also required of the working individual. An individual must also develop appropriate work habits, such as the abilities to concentrate and to work in a structured environment. Another prerequisite to work is the ability to appropriately and independently address one's self-care needs. Work also requires that an individual develop work attitudes, self-concept, and the ability to make an appropriate vocational choice. Intervention becomes necessary when a person displays a defect or problem in his/her work personality or an inability to work because of an absence of one of the necessary prerequisite skills to work.

Low back pain interferes with an individual's ability to meet self-esteem needs and frustrates his/her "work personality." Individuals with low back pain may find themselves experiencing difficulty returning to the work force because of problems with one or more of the necessary prerequisite work skills. Often, the person with chronic pain has given up the role of a worker along with his/her role in other spheres of life (family, social, and community), leaving him/herself little sense of responsibility or control of his/her life (3). Rehabilitation attempts to address these inadequacies.

As a result, "return to work" almost always emerges as a pivotal goal to interdisciplinary rehabilitation of the person with low back pain. However, the road to "return to work" often detours short of its destination. A typical scenario often shows a low back pain patient who, following an injury, either before or after surgery, ends up spending perhaps an hour or two per day in physical therapy. After several months of this limited routine, the physician releases the patient to return to work. Miraculously, with the stroke of a pen, the system expects the patient to progress from an hour a day of "sheltered" physical therapy to a full, 8-hour workday. Miracles aside, most low back pain patients find themselves unable to physically, psychologically, and emotionally make this transition. Consequently, attempts to return to work often fail because the person with low back pain cannot bridge the gap from the medical portion of rehabilitation (the physical therapy, etc.) to the work force.

Work hardening bridges this gap. Work hardening is a structured, individualized, productivity-oriented program that provides the participant with simulated or actual work tasks that are structured and graded progressively to increase psychological, physical, and emotional tolerance and improve endurance and general productivity (4–8). Through work hardening, the person affected by low back pain may improve his/her "employability' and occupational performance so that he/she may function effectively in some type of employment.

HISTORICAL PERSPECTIVE

Although the term "work hardening" may be new, as a concept the therapeutic use of work in one form or another has played a significant role in rehabilitation efforts since before the turn of the century. The earlier therapeutic work programs limited themselves to the psychiatric setting, specifically to the psychiatric institution (8, 9). The advent of the therapeutic use of work with the physically injured population came with World War I.

During World War I, the government trained women as occupational and physical reconstruction aides to serve alongside soldiers in the battlefields of Europe (10). The reconstruction aides, precursors to occupational and physical therapists, used work activities to restore the wounded soldier to military duty as soon as possible. If return to military duty was not possible, the reconstruction aides employed work tasks to return the wounded soldier to civilian life in a physical condition that would enable him to function to the highest degree possible consistent with his injury (10, 11).

World War II again beckoned occupational therapists to rehabilitate injured servicemen. As the injured servicemen were discharged, federal funding for rehabilitating these disabled veterans increased. This led to an increase in the development of therapeutic work programs designed to evaluate and rehabilitate the physically disabled veterans returning with war injuries.

The late 1940s and 1950s brought various federal legislation to foster the continuing development and proliferation of vocational and prevocational programs for physically and mentally handicapped persons (5, 9, 12). These prevocational programs, run by occupational therapists, taught basic work skills to physically and mentally handicapped individuals seeking entry into the work force for the first time. Work programs for psychiatric patients continued to dominate the literature. Most of these work therapy programs were hospital based. Patients would be assigned various "work therapy tasks" in the hospital such as working in the laundry or the kitchen. Most of these programs fell victim to federal regulations because they were found to violate federal minimum wage laws since the patients were not paid for their "work."

In the 1960s, the occupational therapy profession shifted back to a stricter medical model, away from the vocational model. The passage of Medicare, the increase of therapy programs in the public schools, and the improvement of surgical and medical technologies all promoted this shift in the profession. The common usage of psychotropic drugs and the change in emphasis to deinstitutionalization of both psychiatric patients and the physically handicapped

pediatric population further affected the practice of occupational therapy. The former "prevocational" role held by the occupational therapist was assumed by the vocational rehabilitation counselor and the newly emerging vocational evaluator. Sheltered workshops, with their nonmedical focus, replaced the occupational therapist's domain. The sheltered workshop focused on habilitation of those new to the competitive work force, such as mentally retarded and severely physically disabled persons, rather than on rehabilitation of those reentering the work force following an injury.

The late 1970s and early 1980s brought a trend that returned the occupational therapist to work programs. These new work programs, called "work hardening," generally focused on community-based settings, emphasizing actual work tasks in a simulated "workplace-like" structured environment.

Work hardening programs guide the client back to work both physically and mentally. The clinic participates in a schedule of work activities specifically designed for him/her. The schedule of work activities derives from the activities that the worker is expected to perform upon return to employment—either to his/her former job or, if physical restrictions and limitations necessitate a change, to a new job. For example, a carpenter referred to a work hardening program will spend part of his day carrying wood, climbing a ladder, carrying his tool box up and down a ladder, and hammering items located overhead. An injured grocery store stock clerk/bag boy, as part of his work hardening regimen, will "bag" groceries, put filled grocery bags in a shopping cart, lift boxes of various sizes and shapes and load them onto a hand truck, maneuver the hand truck, and put the boxes on shelves.

This structured work activities program, based upon the specific activities of a particular job, helps put clients in a "work" frame of mind. Participants also punch timeclocks, take lunch breaks, and follow all of the other formalities of the work place. This gives the injured worker a nonthreatening job trial of realistic, functional, work activities.

Thus, work hardening is not a few fancy machines, some "standardized" boxes, and one or two expensive, state-of-the-art weight machines. Work hardening is not an extended regimen of exercise. While some of these may be components of a work hardening program, the core of work hardening is its work activities—the activities that remind the client, both physically and mentally, that he/she is on the road to returning to work. The work hardening program looks and acts more like an actual worksite or a sheltered workshop than a health club. Consequently, functional activities and functional restoration, rather than exercise, are the key to the work hardening program.

WORK HARDENING PROGRAM DEVELOPMENT

Work hardening programs focus on the whole individual rather than merely a part of the individual. The individual's relationship to the environment becomes the pivotal focus of his/her planned return to work. The work hardening model determines whether the individual can be adapted to the environment or whether the environment must be adapted to the individual. For example, can a person suffering from low back pain learn to perform job tasks in a new manner, with proper body mechanics, or must one change the job, its tools, or its physical layout in order to enable the worker to perform the job in a pain-free manner or at a lowered pain level?

Back pain patients make up the largest group of clients in work hardening programs, although work hardening effectively services other populations as well. Work hardening successfully assists the return-to-work process for persons with burns, hand injuries, head injuries, knee problems, cardiac conditions, and other physically challenging conditions. The low back pain patient will likely find him/herself in a work hardening program among an "injury-mixed" client population.

Often the injured worker spends months and in some cases years out of work, "recuperating" from his/her injury. This "recuperation" phase may include one or more hospitalizations, one or more surgical procedures, a possible pain clinic admission, and various courses of in- and/or outpatient physical and/or occupational therapy. This typical scenario usually ends with an extended "weaning period" of physical therapy. By this point, the injured worker's daily routine has become fixed around lying on the couch and watching soap operas, or perhaps babysitting for a child who previously spent time in day care when parents or relatives were working. Perhaps this injured worker performs a few household chores in between television and physical therapy appointments. For the most part, however, he/she has become fixed in a world of work distractors, which give little motivation to return to work. Work hardening eliminates work distractors and puts the injured worker on a return-to-work path. For those with work-interfering conditions, work hardening bridges the gap between the medical model, with its hospitals, therapy sessions, and doctor visits, and the work force.

Work hardening advances an injured worker from a hour or two per day of physical therapy to a full 8-hour workday. Once out of work for several months, a worker with a back injury, for example, will find it difficult to impossible to make the transition from the limited activity of 1 hour/day of physical therapy to 8 hours of heavy labor. Work hardening assists the injured worker in making this transition by teaching him/her to pace work activities while increasing the amount of work from 2 hours/day to 4 hours, then to 6 hours, and finally to an 8 hours/day of simulated or actual work tasks.

This transition includes not only the physical transitions from therapy to work but more importantly, the psychological transitions from sick person to well person, from symptom-directed behavior to productive behavior, from patient to worker and from dependent person to independent worker. Research shows us that early intervention with low back pain patients results in a faster and more frequent return to work (13, 14). For low back pain patients and others with pain, this transition takes place at a more rapid pace if intervention begins before the patient gives in to the "work distractor" routine with its soap operas and extensive naps. Work hardening can begin as soon after the injury as the patient/client is allowed to perform some work, however light in duty or limited in time the work may be.

In order to properly accomplish work hardening, one must be competent in several areas of knowledge. First, one must be versed in a client's neuromuscular abilities and limitations, including strength, range of motion, and endurance (4). One must possess knowledge of injury and illness and the functional limitations that accompany various illnesses and injuries (15, 16). Work hardening also requires the ability to perform a complex task analysis of a work setting to determine, for example, whether a task must be performed in a bilateral or unilateral manner (4). Work hardening requires knowledge of the psychosocial aspects of work and of disability (4, 15, 16). Finally, work hardening requires an understanding of the rehabilitation system and its players (15, 16).

THE WORK HARDENING TEAM

Work hardening programs employ various players from several related fields in order to design and implement these programs. The occupational therapist is trained to integrate the major areas of knowledge required to develop work hardening plans for clients. In 1954, Ayres wrote that occupational therapy could uniquely contribute to vocational programs two types of information: "the physical capacity of the patient to engage in work activities and an on-the-spot evaluation of behavior in a work situation" (17). Physical therapists also contribute to the knowledge base that work hardening requires. The physical therapist's knowledge of and experience with various back disorders can provide insight into the functional neuromuscular limitations of the back patient. Occupational therapy and physical therapy assistants may be employed to assist the clients with their work hardening tasks, monitor body mechanics, and assist with the on-site job analysis. The author's experience shows that a ratio of one staff member to every five clients works effectively with most clients.

Some work hardening programs employ vocational evaluators to assist with assessment. Psychologists, as members of the work hardening program's interdisciplinary team, can help to motivate the client by working to alleviate the fears and depression that often accompany chronic pain (18, 19). Vocational counselors and rehabilitation nurses may also be employed to meet placement needs for clients during and upon completion of the work hardening program. A "handyman" may be involved in the work hardening program that is geared toward the blue collar or construction/labor trades. Engineers may be employed to assist in developing new equipment.

In a well-organized work hardening program, the roles and functions of the various staff members will often overlap and intertwine. This blending of roles and functions in the work hardening program often obviates the distinction between the physical therapist and the occupational therapist. Other staff members will also share the various roles.

Ultimately, the work hardening staff must work together to foster a "holistic" approach to the client. Work hardening requires that the staff view the individual client's total needs in order to successfully rehabilitate the client. These needs reach beyond the mere physical to psychosocial needs, medical needs, and emotional needs as well. For example, a low back pain patient in a work hardening clinic may also have a heart condition. The heart condition has an impact upon the extent of the client's participation in the work hardening program and must be considered in planning an appropriate, individualized work hardening program. Staff members may have to take the client's blood pressure and consequently pay special attention to how the client paces him/herself.

Other medical factors become obvious in a population of clients who have been injured in accidents or suffered disabling illnesses. In light of the medical complications that tend to plague this population, the work hardening program must employ staff members who have a medical background and are prepared to act in a medical emergency. For example, someone on the staff of the work hardening program should be able to read and decipher medical records in order to determine the proper precautions to take in establishing a work hardening plan. It is wise to have a staff person who can perform cardiopulmonary resuscitation in an emergency. The work hardening client is often already involved in some sort of litigation and it is best to take precautions to avoid becoming the target of litigious clients.

The work hardening staff must incorporate new terminology into their practice. The former "patient" becomes a "client" when conversing with other staff members or with attorneys. He/she may still be referred to as a "patient" in communications with physicians. Communications with the insurance adjuster refer to the client as the "claimant," a term new to many health professions.

LOCATION

Work hardening can take place anywhere that people can work, and the more closely the program is linked to an actual work location the better for the client. Ideally, in choosing a site for work hardening, one should consider five factors: the number of clients the program accommodates, the types of workers, the location of the client population, the size of the facility, and the type of physical facility.

The number of clients that the program accommodates has an impact on the size of the space that is required. The type of workers who will use the program also affects the amount of space required. For example, if the program will gear toward blue collar, construction-type workers, then more space will be needed for constructing things and for large equipment such as scaffolds and wheelbarrows. If the work hardening program limits itself to clerical and computer personnel, then a smaller amount of space is required to house desks and computer terminals. Generally, an acceptable starting size for a work hardening program location is 1500 square feet.

New programs, however, especially those located

in hospitals or rehabilitation facilities, often find space at a premium and rarely have an extra 1500 square feet lying vacant. In these situations, practicality dictates location. This author worked in a rehabilitation hospital that planned to raize a building. A client in the facility's work hardening program whose goal was to become a locksmith removed all of the locks from the doors in the final days before the building's demise. Another work hardening participant, a painter, removed wallpaper and painted the walls. Other clients with outdoor jobs worked outside on the hospital's grounds.

In planning the program's location, one should consider the proximity of the population that the program will serve. For example, a work hardening program geared for factory workers should be located in an area surrounded by factories so that the transition to work is subliminally planted in the participant's mind. Further, access to public transportation, if available, should also be considered so that clients may independently get to the work hardening facility, the same way they independently get to work.

Work hardening planners have a choice of two types of physical facilities—the "medical or clinic" setting or the "warehouse." The medical or clinic-type facility usually emerges from a hospital or doctor's office. If a hospital decides to develop a work hardening program, it will undoubtedly use whatever available space it has at its disposal rather than rent alternative, perhaps more appropriate, physical facilities. Hospitals and rehabilitation centers tend to establish work hardening programs based upon the medical model that they know so well. Located in the hospital environment, these facilities look clean and sterile, like a typical institution.

Traditionally, the medical setting creates a place for the sick, emphasizing the "patient." This sick model encourages its patients to complain, creating confusion of purpose for the "well" work hardening participant who, through work hardening, works toward getting "weller." Further, the medical model often takes place as an adjunct to physical or occupational therapy. Thus, the client loses the opportunity to feel real progress, now that he/she has made it to the work hardening phase, which, in the medical-type facility, doesn't feel any different from the therapy phase.

The warehouse-type facility represents to the client a real worksite. In the warehouse, the clients are not sick and are not called patients. This attitude fosters wellness rather than "sickness." The facility is not sterile, but dirty—like a real worksite. The warehouse provides adequate space for performing various types of work. The high ceilings give the clients an opportunity to climb ladders, build large objects, and simulate various work tasks that require overhead space, such as hoisting.

The purpose of locating the program in a warehouse is obvious—to work. It represents a step further away from the medical system toward the workforce. Redkey suggested the nonmedical environment for work programs in 1957: "The atmosphere is different. It should emphasize to the patient that his being there . . . marks for him a long forward step toward his goal of employment. The atmosphere should reflect this—being more like a factory than a clinic. . . . [t]here should be noise and dust and dirt in moderation" (20). The change to such a facility shows the client that he has progressed from the medical setting with its doctors, nurses, and white uniforms to the road to work and self-respect.

REIMBURSEMENT

In considering placing a client in a work hardening program, reimbursement emerges as an important issue. Who pays for work hardening? The majority of work hardening's clients come from the injured worker population. Reimbursement for these clients comes from workers' compensation insurance carriers, self-insured employers, and self-insurance funds.

Another possible source of reimbursement is the disability insurance carrier. Many disability policies offer rehabilitation as a benefit under the disability plan. If the client's injury stems from a car accident, reimbursement may come from the automobile insurance carrier depending upon the type of coverage. Reimbursement for other accident-related injuries may come from other liability insurance carriers or settlement proceeds from personal injury lawsuits. State-level vocational rehabilitation funds will also reimburse work hardening programs for services provided to its clients. Further, an attorney may pay for work hardening if the program will help his/her client.

Sometimes, if work hardening is a function of physical or occupational therapists, certain health insurance carriers will reimburse the program depending on the contents of the program. If the work hardening program focuses on increasing physical capacities, that may be interpreted as physical or occupational therapy. However, many health insurance policies have disclaimers for work-related injuries and what they consider to be "vocational programs."

Neither Medicare nor Medicaid will pay for work hardening. Further, this author's experience has been that health maintenance organizations will not pay for work hardening.

Some reimbursement sources, such as state vocational rehabilitation, may only authorize reimbursement for their clients if the program is accredited. The Commission on Accreditation of Rehabilitation Facilities (CARF) has established accreditation criteria for work hardening programs. CARF considers work hardening to be a function of work adjustment and uses the work adjustment standards as the standards for accreditation for work hardening (21).

INTAKE ASSESSMENT

The work hardening program begins with an intake evaluation or assessment. Most work hardening programs use an intake assessment that measures the participant's physical ability to perform specific job task demands. This type of assessment may be referred to as a physical capacity, functional capacity, or work capacity assessment. Most commonly called the work capacity evaluation, this type of assessment gives one baseline data from which to develop a work hardening plan in order to meet the individuals' specific physical needs. The work capacity assessment is discussed at length in Chapter 24.

Other areas in addition to physical abilities require thorough examination in order to completely assess the starting point of the work hardening client. Often, work hardening programs videotape parts of the assessment to use as baseline data and/or instruction for the client. The following areas must be addressed as part of the intake procedure: activities of daily living, body mechanics, cardiopulmonary status, cognitive abilities, coordination, ergonomics of the job site, job analysis, perceptual abilities, psychosocial skills, symptom control, and work behaviors. These areas all have an impact upon the injured worker's ability to work.

Activities of Daily Living

This area involves the individual's ability to complete his/her own self-care activities, such as bathing, dressing, grooming, driving, and grocery shopping. Assessment in this area gives the therapist important information as to the impact the client's physical condition has on self-care abilities, and whether this may affect ability to work. For example, an activity of daily living assessment re-

vealed that a client who complained of low back pain accompanied by fear of lifting more than 10 pounds was actually lifting up to 25 pounds when he carried in the family's groceries each week. Another low back pain patient was able to return to work after his work shoes were adapted to enable him to put them on without bending over.

Body Mechanics

Assessment in this area looks specifically at how the person uses his/her body to perform various physical tasks. Physical tasks may be performed in specific manners calculated to protect the body from further damage and/or pain. The body can be used in many ways to perform lifting, for example. Lifting while bending one's knees puts less stress on the low back. An evaluation that shows improper lifting techniques will lead to teaching the client proper body mechanics, which will not only help to prevent reinjury but may make the difference between return to work and "disability."

Videotaping the body mechanics evaluations gives the clinician baseline data to show the client as he/she improves and learns to employ proper body mechanics during job tasks. In fact, viewing the videotaped material shows the client his/her mistakes and tells him/her precisely what not to do.

Cardiopulmonary Status

As a safety precaution, especially where programs include physical labor activities, program entrants should get cardiopulmonary clearance from their physicians before participating in work hardening. As previously discussed, often the prospective work hardening client develops a routine that involves sometimes months or years of inactivity. Although used to heavy work in the past, the return from inactivity to heavy- or even medium-duty labor may adversely affect the cardiopulmonary system.

Cognitive Abilities

A screening of the cognitive abilities of the work hardening applicant assists in determining placement options. For example, a laborer who previously performed heavy work and is now restricted to lighter work may make a change to different work, if he shows a level of cognitive abilities that allow him to be trained for or to perform a different job. Additionally, many employers require possession of a high school diploma as a prerequisite to employment. A cognitive assessment may help to predict whether the client has the skills necessary to obtain a high school diploma.

Coordination

Coordination provides the individual with the ability to functionally use his/her physical abilities, such as strength. Assessment of strength without coordination gives an incomplete picture of one's abilities. Both fine motor and gross motor coordination should be assessed. In some situations, certain medications taken by the client may adversely affect coordination.

Ergonomics of the Job Site

Ergonomics, the science of fitting the environment to man, has a significant impact upon the injured worker's relationship to his/her return to work. Assessment of the work site often leads to simple changes that make it possible for the patient with low back pain to return to work. For example, an airline customer service agent with back pain returned to work after the files she used were moved to a higher shelf in the file cabinet, the computer was moved to the other side of her desk, and a head set was attached to her telephone instead of a shoulder rest device.

Job Analysis

Perhaps the most significant component of the work hardening intake assessment process, the job analysis evaluates and assesses the job in the same way that the clinician evaluates and assesses the person. Job analysis is the process of collecting, organizing, evaluating, and analyzing information about a job in order to identify and accurately define the job, identify the tasks required by the job, and identify the physical and psychosocial demands the job makes upon the worker and the working conditions (22).

The job analysis helps predict "workability" and return to work by providing information about the job requirements that then can be compared and/or matched to the worker's abilities. While the worker is evaluated for his/her physical or work capacities, the job is evaluated for its physical demands or requirements (23). The individual's work hardening program goals come from the gap between the job's requirements and the worker's abilities. Since the training goals must be realistic and achievable, a large gap between the worker's abilities and the job's requirements will probably indicate the worker's inability to perform that job.

For example, if a carpenter is released to work permanently restricted by his physician to carrying no more than 20 pounds and not perform any bending or squatting, a job analysis indicating that the particular job requires lifting 50 pounds with frequent bending and squatting will eliminate the worker from returning to that job. A job analysis of another carpentry work site may be more compatable with this worker and allow him to return to carpentry. The job analysis also gives the clinician baseline data to determine the need for job modification.

The information gathered from the job analysis helps in setting up work samples, job simulations, and work hardening tasks. A work sample is a close simulation of an actual industrial task, or a component of a job. Work samples are designed to measure traits inherent in one or more jobs or job groups. This allows the worker to closely approximate actual performance of a job while receiving direct feedback relative to his performance in a given area. The University of Wisconsin–Stout, a national leader in the development of vocational materials, maintains a clearinghouse catalog of manuals for work samples that can easily be constructed from the instructions in the manuals (24). These work samples make excellent work hardening tasks. For example, the plumbing work sample requires the individual to install a toilet and a sink.

Six component parts make up the job analysis. First, one must define the principle tasks. For example, a glazier installs and removes windows. Second, the job's terms must be defined. To perform a useful job analysis of an insulator who performs "tear-outs and abatement," one must include a definition of these terms. The third component involves describing the tools, equipment, and work aides that the job requires and how the client uses them. Analyzing a sheet metal worker's job would include a description of the sheet metal shear and a description of its operation as well as other tools of the trade.

The fourth component is the performance standards inherent in the job. For example, a seamstress in a dress factory may be required to complete 250 sleeves per day. The final two components are the physical and the environmental demands. Physical demands would include, for example, that the butcher must carry 50-pound slabs of meat over a distance of 20 feet 28 times per day. An example of environmental demands is the dust that the mason creates when mixing cement. Each of the six components contributes information to the clinician to help determine if the injured worker can perform a given job. Information from any one of the of the six component areas may be enough to eliminate the job as a future goal. For example, if a client has asbestosis and the proposed new, light-duty job requires that he spend 8 hours per day surrounded by cotton dust, the environmental demands would probably eliminate him from this job.

The job analysis process begins by reading the *Dictionary of Occupational Titles'* (DOT) description of the job (25). The DOT gives a general description of a given job, including various physical, educational, and environmental demands of the job. In situations in which clinicians are ignorant of a particular job by title, or of its demands, the DOT gives a general, brief overview of what abilities the worker must have to perform the job. The information in the DOT is a good starting point. However, more information is needed to perform a complete job analysis.

Next, one must conduct a verbal interview during which the interviewer asks very specific questions about the job. For example, "How do you hold the instrument? Show me"; "How many times per minute do you perform that part of the task?"; "Show me how you sit"; or "How high is the shelf?" An important step is the on-site visit, during which the clinician actually performs the client's job where possible, in order to properly understand what the client does and analyze it.

For example, this author worked with a client who was a pile driver. Not knowing exactly what he did as a pile driver, it was necessary to visit a sewage treatment plant under construction, put on a hardhat, workgloves, and a raincoat, and jump into a pit to drive piles. Only after that experience could the author attempt to try to simulate the pile driver's job requirements.

The on-site visit gives the clinician the most complete picture of the job, allowing him/her the opportunity to develop worksite modifications that may enable the client to return to work. For example, from analyzing the specific job of a trash collector with a bad right knee, it was possible to determine that if he switched to the opposite side of the back of the garbage truck, he would jump off the truck leading with his good left foot thus, enabling him to return to work.

A tape measure is an essential element of the on-site job analysis. Specific measurements are taken of all relevant items. A client who reports that he is a truck driver gives the clinician little information. Trucks come in different shapes and sizes. A soft drink delivery truck, a semi-tractor trailer, and a milk truck all have different heights from the ground to the cab, and from the back of the truck where the delivery items are kept to the ground. Only through the on-site job analysis can the clinician determine the specific heights of the significant portions of the truck. A few inches here and

there can make the difference between working and not working. This author has measured the backs of numerous garbage trucks and discovered at least five different styles of truck. Each one is designed with different heights from the ground to the ledge on the back of the truck where the trash collectors stand. Further, in the county bus system where the author lives, the county uses over four different models of buses, each requiring different amounts of pressure to apply the brake and close the doors.

Finally, the on-site job analysis gives the clinician the opportunity to adapt the job to prevent further injuries or to make suggestions to the employer of ways the job could be performed in a safer manner.

Lytel and Botterbush have developed a physical demands job analysis checklist form that is a good starting point for the job analysis process (22). Their job analysis form looks at environmental conditions, common postures for work performed, visual demands, speech and hearing demands, and various physical demands such as weight that one must carry, and the amount that one must walk, stand, and sit.

Following the completion of the job analysis, the clinician develops the work hardening plan and the activities inherent to the plan. An example of the results is shown in Table 21.1.

Table 21.1
Counter Attendant, Cafeteria
(DOT Code 311.677-014)

JOB ANALYSIS TASKS	WORK HARDENING TASKS
Stands for 2½-hour periods without breaks while reaching and scooping food onto plates, and moving plates from table level to 72 inches from the floor (70%)	Activities in standing working up to a 2½-hour tolerance, scooping activities using plates, and moving 5-pound objects from table level to 72 inches from the floor
Lifts stacks of plates weighing up to 20 pounds and carries them a distance of 10 feet from table height to table height (20%)	Lifting tasks, using proper body mechanics, increasing to 20 pounds' tolerance, while carrying a distance of 10 feet
Cleans serving area (floor level to table height, 36 inches in depth) in bent and crouched positions (10%)	Simulated cleaning tasks from floor level to table height, cleaning tasks in bent and crouched positions (22)
Works 8 hours/day	To increase to 8-hour work day

Perceptual Abilities

Perceptual ability is the individual's ability to properly interpret information obtained through the five senses. An impairment in visual perception, for example, might render an individual incapable of discriminating right from left. Even a person able to lift 60 pounds might never be able to load a truck with 50-pound bags of manure if unable to visually determine how to properly load the truck.

Psychosocial Skills

Psychosocial status alone can thwart the work hardening programs efforts, and eliminate the goal of return to work. The evaluation process should include observations for depression, low self-esteem, and lack of motivation. Work hardening is a participatory program that requires the client to take an active role in his/her own rehabilitation. A depressed client with no motivation may not readily thrive in the work hardening environment or succeed at returning to work. Some clients may require some form of psychotherapy as an adjunct to the work hardening program to promote their progress.

Symptom Control

The method by which one deals with pain is also an important factor in the evaluation of return to work. A person with chronic low back pain who displays inappropriate pain behaviors will have difficulty getting and keeping a job, especially if the job involves contact with members of the public who are not sympathetic to the person's plight. Various pain medications often leave a person drowsy and lethargic and not able to concentrate on work. A client who is able to control his pain with a transcutaneous electrical nerve stimulation unit, for example, may have an easier time returning to work as a bank teller than one who relies on medications that tend to make her groggy and unable to concentrate on counting money.

Work Behaviors

As part of the intake process, clinicians evaluate work behaviors by observing the client's behaviors while he/she participates in the various evaluation tasks. The clinician looks at the worker's attention to task, and his ability to follow directions, complete tasks, concentrate, and work in a structured environment. Pain can interfere with these necessary work behaviors. Work hardening can give the injured worker a medium for developing appropriate work behaviors in spite of pain.

Since the evaluation process is so comprehensive, it is a rather lengthy process. The physical and mental condition in which one finds the prospective work hardening participant contributes to the length of the evaluation process. The client's levels of pain, activity, and motivation often force the clinician to evaluate the client in several sessions. The client may only tolerate a few hours per day of the evaluation's tasks. The necessary behavioral observations require that the client participate in the evaluation over several sessions so the clinician can note changes.

DETERMINATION OF CLIENT APPROPRIATENESS

After the evaluation phase, the work hardening team must decide whether the client, based upon his/her intake assessment, is an appropriate candidate for work hardening. Several factors determine whether an individual is an appropriate candidate for work hardening. Work hardening is a participatory program; it requires that the client take an active role in his/her own rehabilitation. Work hardening is unlike surgery, in which someone does something to the patient to make him/her "better." In the work hardening program, the participant must take an active role to work to make him/herself better. An individual who lacks the motivation to participate will not succeed in work hardening.

Another factor to consider in determining whether an individual is an appropriate candidate for work hardening is the purpose behind the referral—exactly why is this person being considered for work hardening? Insurance adjusters, attorneys, physicians, vocational counselors, rehabilitation nurses, psychologists, and other professionals refer clients to work hardening for a variety of reasons. The most obvious reason is to improve physical performance to meet the demands of the client's job within an 8-hour work day.

Other situations point to referral to the work hardening program. An injured worker with low back pain who is returning to work shortly after the accident may be referred to work hardening for a brief time to learn how to perform his/her job using proper body mechanics to prevent reinjury. A painter who fell off a scaffold and fears falling again is referred to work hardening to try to get back on a scaffold in a nonthreatening environment. A worker released to light-duty work with the goal to build up to heavier work goes to work hardening to begin light-duty work and gradually increase to heavier work since his company has no light-duty work available.

An insurance adjuster may send a client to work

hardening to end an addiction to soap operas, get him/her out of the house, structure his/her time, and develop a normal workday routine. An attorney may refer a client to work hardening to determine the client's specific limitations; this information may help the attorney negotiate a settlement. A rehabilitation nurse and an adjuster may send a client to work hardening as an alternative to surveillance to help ascertain whether the client is malingering.

A low back pain patient may return to work on a part-time basis while attending work hardening part-time to further increase his/her physical tolerances. An injured worker may be referred to work hardening for the sole purpose of adapting the job to accommodate his/her physical limitations so that he/she may return to work.

The work hardening team must decide, based upon the intake assessment, whether, working in concert with the client, it can accomplish both the client's and the referring party's goals. Most importantly, before the prospective work hardening candidate enters a work hardening program it is essential that he/she have a goal or purpose for attending the program. The purpose for attending must be clearly defined. For example, if the purpose for attending the program is to improve physical performance to meet the demands of the client's job within an 8-hour work day, then the client must have a vocational goal that specifies the job that he/she will do.

If the client attends the work hardening program merely to improve physical performance without a specific job goal upon completion at the outcome of the program, many problems will ensue. First, the client will lack the motivation that comes from working toward a set, measureable goal. Here, the specific goal would be employment in a specific job or specific type of work. Second, the client has no guarantee that anyone will give him/her a job and will have no idea what kind of job awaits. Further, the clinician and the client cannot set work hardening goals if they do not know what job-specific abilities the client must have at the end of the work hardening program. Finally, without a specific job to go to at the end of the program, the client is susceptible to falling into the same routine of watching soap operas, sleeping, and basically doing nothing when the program comes to an end.

PROGRAM LENGTH

Once the client is accepted into the work hardening program, and the vocational and program goals are established, the client is ready to begin the work hardening regimen. Work hardening programs generally aim toward an 8 hour/day, program by starting out with a few hours per day and gradually increasing as the client's tolerance for more work and more time increases. A typical program starts with a 2–3-hour day for the first week or two, increasing to 4 hours, then to 6 hours, and finally to a full 8-hour program. The work hardening program lasts from 4 to 8 weeks. This limitation in length is significant for several reasons.

First, the sources that refer the client to work hardening do not want the work hardening program to last forever. In this author's experience many insurance adjusters complain that they are tired of paying for "months and months" of therapy with no results. They want work hardening to be different. Adjusters—the holders of the purse strings—want to know the cost of the program, the success rate of the program, and the length of the program.

Further, it is important to the client to have a set program length, with a gradually increasing number of hours per day, so that the client can see him/herself progressing. Each time the number of hours per day is increased, the client sees progress. Progress acts as a motivating force.

As another motivating force, a definitive program length gives the client a set goal to work toward—the day of graduation from the program. Often the work hardening participant has taken on the role of the chronically ill person. He/she may have already been through months of therapy, pain clinics, and the like without any clue as to when and if it will all end, or if he/she will ever return to work. Previous experiences with therapy did not seem at all related to work. One client told the author about a pain program that had him climbing up and down five flights of steps on a repetitive basis. As a bus driver, this task was not relevant to his job at all. Once in the work hardening program, however, the tasks are calculated to be work related and there is a definite expectation that the client will return to work. If the work hardening participant knows when the program will end, this helps motivate him/her in that return to work.

A DAY IN THE LIFE

Work hardening is "client specific"; programs are specifically set for an individual based upon the individual's assessment. Some general principles exist within the work hardening philosophy that allow the author to describe a typical day of work hardening for the low back pain client.

The typical work hardening day begins with stretching exercises in a group. Since work hardening does not profess to cure low back pain but rather to teach the low back pain client to work within or around his/her physical limitations, the morning stretching is an important part of the program. It helps the client develop a personal routine to prevent increased pain while working. These stretching exercises become part of the client's daily routine after he/she returns to work. The work hardening program seeks to make stretching a habit for the client. Stretching should be taught by a team member who is acquired with the anatomy of the body, body mechanics principles, and all of the physical precautions and risks inherent in stretching.

Some programs promote walking as one of the first daily activities. First, walking helps the client increase his/her general physical activity level. Second, walking may be an integral part of the client's job. Further, walking serves the client as an excellent exercise after returning to work. Once again, walking in the program helps to promote walking as a habit for the return-to-work phase. Although exercise plays a role in the work hardening program, its use decreases as the program progresses so that the client performs the stretching and walking exercises on his/her own time.

Depending upon the client's individual goals, the balance of the day consists of a variety of activities designed to improve the client's functioning in the various areas in which he/she is required to perform in order to work at a preselected vocational goal. These areas include lifting, bending, stooping, reaching, sitting tolerance, standing tolerance, stair climbing, ladder climbing, jumping, pushing, pulling, crawling, hoisting, and fine motor coordination. Clinicians design activities that require the client to use these physical abilities. The activities are graded so that the client can easily perform them. As the client develops more tolerance, the task becomes progressively more difficult.

For example, a baggage handler whose job goal requires that he lift 70 pounds one time per minute for 2-hour periods, will begin by lifting suitcases weighing 10 pounds every 2 min. He will also learn to perform this task using proper body mechanics. As he becomes more comfortable and more proficient with this task, the clinician will add weight to the luggage so that he lifts 15 pounds every 2

min and then 20 pounds and so on until the client lifts 70-pound suitcases one time per minute. This whole progression may take the client 4 weeks.

Like all work hardening tasks, lifting must be client specific. In the example above, the client lifted luggage because his job requires him to lift luggage. A plumber would lift pipes and toolboxes and a television repairperson would lift televisions of various shapes and sizes. Lifting "standardized" boxes would be of little value to a department store stock clerk who lifts boxes of all different sizes and shapes all day or to a day care worker who lifts different sizes and shapes of children. The idea of work hardening is to simulate the tasks as closely as possible to the actual work task. Obviously, one would not expect a work hardening program to keep various sizes and shapes of children on hand. The alternative is for the work hardening program to "stock" boxes, bags, and sacks of various shapes filled with varying amounts of weight that can closely simulate the lifting that the worker's job requires.

Other work hardening equipment will vary among programs depending upon the characteristics of the client population—specifically, the occupations of the participants. Programs with an emphasis on the white-collar worker tend to use computers, drafting tasks, and other less physical work tasks. On the other hand, programs geared to the blue-collar worker typically use equipment such as ladders, scaffolds, tool boxes, truck cabs, shovels, wheelbarrows, and various tools. The Liberty Mutual Research Center in Boston, Massachusetts, for example, constructed an 8 foot square by 11 foot high multiwork station that simulates carpentry, plumbing, and electrical wiring. The work station also provides clients an opportunity to climb on and work on ladders as well as use a pulley system (26).

The equipment used by a work hardening program can be almost anything—a working conveyer belt, a telephone pole, a sheet metal sheer, or a sink and toilet, for example. Equipment is geared to the closest reproduction or simulation of the clients' job tasks. Wherever possible, clients should use their own tools since these are the tools with which they will return to work. The electrician needs to be able to physically manage his/her own toolbox, not a "standardized" toolbox located in some therapy clinic or work hardening program.

In situations in which the worker's own tools cannot be used in work hardening, the program's loaned tools should closely replicate the worker's tools. For example, the shovel should have dirt on it and the jack should be greased. These small touches put the injured worker closer to the work frame of mind and further away from the disability frame of reference.

Commercial equipment is also available that supplements—not replaces—the "real" thing. The BTE Work Simulator (Baltimore Therapeutics Equipment, Baltimore, MD), a popular, computerized, state-of-the-art device, can with a few attachments, simulate numerous activities from driving a truck to driving a golf ball to driving a vacuum cleaner. The clinician can change the tension on the BTE to simulate digging various weights of dirt, for example. Other companies manufacture various equipment used in work hardening for lifting, assembling, pushing, and pulling (e.g., Work Evaluation System Technology, Hunting Beach, CA; Valpar, Tucson, AZ; American Therapeutics, Macon, GA).

CASE STUDY 1

JR, a 35-year-old power company lineman, suffered a fall that left him with chronic low back pain accompanied by muscle spasms. He entered the work hardening program with this goal: to return to work at his former job with the power company.

The intake evaluation shows a motivated lineman with an employer who is willing to take him back in his former position. The job analysis shows two critical components of the client's job. First, the client's job required him to climb telephone poles. Second, the client must be able to lift 30 pounds.

The on-site job analysis showed that in order to climb a telephone pole, one must wear heavy work boots with spike-like attachments. The actual pole climbing is accomplished by placing one's feet on the pole so that the spikes dig into the wood. Then the climber takes steps up the pole in a circular fashion, digging the spikes into the wood as he goes. The climbers' weight rests on the spikes. Once at the top of the pole, he has a safety belt to help hold him up.

As the client climbs the pole, he is required to wear a tool belt with approximately 30 pounds of tools in place. Once he reaches his destination on the pole, his job requires him to lift the 30 pounds of tools, usually in one hand. His work requires that he stay on the pole for an average of up to 3 hours. The job analysis also revealed that the client performed his job outdoors.

Further evaluation showed that JR could lift 15 pounds 10 times with each arm. He used proper body mechanics during lifting tasks. JR dealt with pain by changing his position frequently and performing stretching exercises. He was not on any medication at the time of his initial evaluation. Further, JR spent most of his day watching television and fishing. He had been out of work for 18 months.

For the first 2 weeks, JR's daily work hardening program started with a regimen of stretching exercises followed by a 2-mile walk, gradually building up to a 5-miles-per-hour pace. Following the stretching and walking, JR practiced climbing an actual power company telephone pole located outdoors. He brought his own boots, spikes, tool belt, and tools. This was the first time JR had climbed a telephone pole since his accident.

JR would change to a "fresh" pole every few days because the climbing spikes would leave holes in the pole. He began climbing with an empty tool belt and gradually increased the amount of tools he carried.

The next step was to build up his tolerance for staying up on the pole. JR started by staying on the pole for 15-minute periods. As he reached ½ hour tolerance, he began lifting 10-pound weights with each arm while on the pole. The first 2 weeks JR participated in the work hardening program 4 hours/day. The third week he increased his time to 6 hours/day, and he reached 8 hours/day of work hardening by the fourth week. After 4 weeks, JR increased his tolerance to carrying 30 pounds on his tool belt, lifting 30 pounds with each arm, and remaining up on the pole for 3 hours.

CASE STUDY 2

A 33-year-old United Parcel Service (UPS) delivery person, LT suffered a back injury similar to JR's. His goal was to return to his work with UPS. LT worked outside near JR, serving to motivate both of them. LT's work hardening program also started out with stretching and walking.

Following the stretching and walking, LT used a hand truck similar to his UPS hand truck to deliver packages to a nearby apartment building. He was given boxes of various shapes and sizes, starting at 10 pounds and gradually increasing to 75 pounds, his job's requirement. LT walked, gradually increasing distances, and climbed up and down steps with the boxes as if he was actually performing his job. After 4 weeks, he too achieved his vocational goal of returning to his job with UPS.

ETHICAL CONSIDERATIONS

Work hardening presents an uncomfortable ethical dilemma for its staff members. The question arises: Who is the client? Is the client the injured worker who, on a daily basis, attends the work hardening program, or is the client the insurance company that pays the bill? Or, is the client the attorney who referred the injured worker to the work hardening program?

These questions surface, for example, when the work hardening program is asked to help determine whether the client is malingering. At times like this, the work hardening professional must choose between the wishes of the insurance carrier and the client's best interest. The ethics of the various professions involved in the work hardening team demand patient confidentiality. However, fulfilling the insurance carrier's wishes may be in direct conflict with the client's wishes. The insurance carrier may pressure return to work for an injured worker who, fearing reinjury, seeks court intervention to be declared permanently and totally disabled rather than return to work. Hence, a conflict arises placing the work hardening professional in the middle.

The solution to this ethical dilemma is not easy. The work hardening program that consistently "sides" with the client will lose its credibility with insurance carriers and defense attorneys. The work hardening program with a reputation for continuously backing the insurance company's position will similarly lose credibility with the clients and the clients' attorneys. Further, the work hardening program that repeatedly takes a "one-sided" position acquires a bad reputation in the community and loses its credibility among the local judges, before whom work hardening testimony would be presented, as well as the work hardening program's other referral sources.

LEGAL CONSIDERATIONS

The work hardening program also raises several legal concerns. First, since the work hardening program encourages its clients to become productive workers, there may be a temptation to have the clients actually produce something. For example, if carpenters fall among the program's participants, why not have them build some new equipment for other clients to use?

Unfortunately, this violates federal minimum wage laws. The Fair Labor Standards Act requires that all covered employees be paid minimum wage. There are certain exceptions under this law for handicapped persons but these exceptions apply to sheltered workshops, not work hardening. Under the law, if the work hardening participant does anything that is of economic benefit to the institution, he must be paid at least minimum wage.

One must be cognizant of these regulations in developing work program tasks. A painter can paint a room only if another painter repaints the room at a later time. A paperhanger can wallpaper a wall only if another client removes the paper. Essentially, things can be put together as long as they are taken apart.

Another legal concern surrounds staffing. Since work hardening programs fill themselves with people recovering from complicated medical conditions and those involved in pending litigation, this creates liability for work hardening personnel. Work hardening takes a person already at risk medically and places him/her in a position that could cause further injury if not handled properly. For example, assigning inappropriate lifting tasks to a client recovering from a spinal fusion, slipped disk, or cardiac arrest can cause serious injury to the client if the staff person fails to observe proper precautions.

The training and education of both the vocational evaluator and the rehabilitation counselor usually limit course work in "medical aspects of disabilities" to six credit hours. This training is not sufficient to adequately acquaint the rehabilitation professional with the client's proper medical precautions. The work hardening program must include staff members who are acquainted with medical precautions lest the purely vocational professionals open themselves up to malpractice suits.

SUMMARY

Work hardening seeks to return the low back pain client to his/her maximum attainable function through the use of actual work activities in a nonthreatening environment. Work hardening examines the person and the environment and attempts to change one to meet the needs of the other wherever possible. Work hardening requires a multidisciplinary, holistic approach to client management in order to meet the goal of return to work.

ACKNOWLEDGMENTS

I would like to thank my husband, Larry Sherry, and my children, Logan Aaron Kornblau-Stevens, Allan Sherry, Paula Sherry, Mindy Sherry, and Stephanie Sherry, for their patience, support, and cooperation during the many hours I spent at the computer writing this chapter.

REFERENCES

1. Llorens LA, Levy R, Rubin EZ: Work adjustment program: a prevocational experience. *Am J Occup Ther* 18:1, 1964.
2. Maurer P: Antecedents of work behavior. *Am J Occup Ther* 25:295, 1971.
3. Johnson JA: Occupational therapy and the patient with pain. *OT in Health Care* 1:7, 14, 1984.
4. American Occupational Therapy Association, Commission on Practice: Work hardening guidelines. *Am J Occup Ther* 40:841, 1986.
5. Smith PC, McFarlane B: Work hardening model for the 80's. In Smith C, Fry R (eds): *Proceedings of the National Forum on Issues in Vocational Assessment.* Menomonie, WI, Materials Development Center, University of Wisconsin–Stout, 1984.
6. Wegg L: The role of the occupational therapist in vocational rehabilitation. *Am J Occup Ther* 11:252, 1957.
7. Matheson LM, Ogden LD, Violette K: Work hardening: Occupational therapy in industrial rehabilitation. *Am J Occup Ther* 39:314, 1985.
8. Bockoven JS: Occupational therapy—a historical perspective: legacy of moral treatment—1800s to 1910. *Am J Occup Ther* 25:223, 1971.
9. Cromwell FS: Work-related programming in occupational therapy: its roots, course and prognosis. *OT in Health Care* 2:9, 1985.
10. Craine AG: *Medical Department of the U.S. Army in the World War.* Washington, DC, US Government Printing Office, 1927, Vol XII, part 1, p 57.
11. Office of the Surgeon General: *Army Medical Specialist Corp.* Washington, DC, US Government Printing Office, 1968, p 1.
12. Jacobs K: *Occupational Therapy: Work Related Programs and Assessments.* Boston, Little, Brown & Co, 1985, pp 1–10.
13. Murphy KA, Cornish RD: Prediction of chronicity in acute low back pain. *Arch Phys Med Rehabil* 65:334–337, 1984.
14. Pedersen PA: Prognostic indicators in low back pain. *J R Coll Gen Pract* 31:209–216, 1981.
15. Cromwell FS: Work-related programming in occupational therapy: Its roots, course and prognosis. *OT in Health Care* 2:9, 1985.
16. Ellexson MT: The unique role of occupational therapy in industry. *OT in Health Care* 2:36, 1985.
17. Ayres AJ: A form used to evaluate the work behavior of patients. *Am J Occup Ther* 8:73, 1954.
18. Keeie FJ, Block AR, Williams RB Jr, Surwit RS: Behavioral treatment of chronic low back pain: clinical outcome and individual differences in pain relief. *Pain* 11:221–231, 1981.
19. Sternbach RA: Psychological aspects of chronic pain. *Clin Orthop* 129:150–155, 1977.
20. Redkey H: The function and value of a pre-vocational unit in a rehabilitation center. *Am J Occup Ther* 11:22, 1957.
21. Commission on Accreditation of Rehabilitation Facilities: *Standards Manual for Organizations Serving People with Disabilities.* Tucson, AZ, Commission on Accreditation of Rehabilitation Facilities, 1987.
22. Lytel X, Botterbush K: *Physical Demands Job Analysis.* Menomonie, WI, Materials Development Center, University of Wisconsin–Stout, 1981.
23. Cranfield HV: Assessment of the working capacity of the physically disabled person. *Occup Ther* 26:128, 1947.
24. McCray X: *Work Sample Manual Clearinghouse Catalog.* Menomonie, WI, Materials Development Center, University of Wisconsin–Stout, 1980.
25. U.S. Department of Labor, Bureau of Employment Security: *Dictionary of Occupational Titles,* ed 4. Washington, DC, US Department of Labor, 1977.
26. Bettencourt CM, Carlstrom P, Brown SH, Lindau K, Long C: Using work simulation to treat adults with back injuries. *Am J Occup Ther* 1:12, 1986.

Chapter 22

THE BACK SCHOOL

HAMILTON HALL, MD, FRCSC

In spite of recent advances in investigative techniques, the diagnosis of mechanical back pain remains, in many ways, a mystery. Although myelograms, computed tomography scans, and magnetic resonance imaging have improved our understanding, they have raised more questions than they have answered, leaving the source of most common backache still a matter of conjecture and dispute. To compare our approach to back problems with the medical management of respiratory illness, we often postulate diagnoses with an accuracy comparable to that of "chronic chest disease." Our routine treatment of mechanical back pain possesses the scientific specificity that sunshine and a healthy diet did in the management of pulmonary tuberculosis. In short, we treat back pain empirically with an approach dictated by experience and our patients' acceptance and response.

Misconceptions abound. In the absence of clearly defined diagnoses with the resulting codified therapeutic regimens, the treatment of common backache has become the domain of anyone who can produce a plausible theory and effect a period of pain relief. Patients live in fear of the slipping or disintegrating disk and worry that their backs may go out and never return. Manipulative therapists speak of unlocking or realigning the spinal joints and family physicians prescribe weeks of bed rest while presenting an alternative of major, generally unsuccessful surgery.

Ironically, the very fear that pervades the subject of back pain is in itself a primary cause of trouble. Recognizing the medical profession's lack of specific information, the public assumes that no knowledge exists and so falls prey to the specter of an unknown and uncontrollable disease. Minor discomfort becomes a major concern and the source of unnecessary disability. Patients accept treatment with no

scientific validity and become dependent on those who promise to ward off the demon of back disease and offer temporary freedom from pain. Few physicians realize the amount of fear that surrounds the diagnoses of disk degeneration or arthritis of the spine. Eliminating this needless apprehension is a primary goal of "back school."

At first, the idea of back school seems a simple enough concept. It is easily defined as the location and process where individuals learn about their backs. The back school is an educational facility correcting misinformation and teaching anatomy, pathophysiology, and body mechanics to anyone who is interested. However, education and practical advise have been a part of good back pain management for years and have failed to stem the tide of growing concern and misapprehension about the "bad back." As early as 1958, Fahrni in Vancouver, Canada had developed a structured office program for the education of his back patients in proper body mechanics and flexion exercises (1). Why, then, is back school so different from the simple training programs conducted by physicians and physical therapists for their own patients? These programs addressed the immediate and practical needs of the individual, a necessary and worthwhile objective; however, a school for back education implies far more (2). Although the ultimate goal remains the return of the individual to normal activity and the prevention of further attacks of low back pain, enlarging the concept creates a series of often unexpected ramifications.

Health education has long been recognized to improve patient compliance and reduce treatment costs (3, 4). For subjects in whom the problem is well defined and the goals are limited, documentation has been relatively easy (5, 6). The situation is different and more difficult in the area of low back pain. The natural history of most low back disorders is one of rapid, spontaneous remission (7–9). This widely recognized but strangely often overlooked fact is ignored by many medical practitioners while being exploited by those who claim lasting results from the short-term use of passive pain-relieving techniques. The evaluation of any form of treatment must be gauged against this typical pattern of recovery. For example, a few modalities, including manipulation, traction, and bed rest, appear to eliminate suffering but do little to speed recovery or promote healing (10–12). They have never been shown to significantly affect the long-term outcome (13–18). When back school is seen as another separate form of management, its potential benefits and lasting effect must be justified and rendered cost effective (19). As an informal adjunct to other treatments, a simple spontaneous course of education required little effort or expense and its value could be casually gauged on purely subjective terms. The formal institution of back school demands a more precise assessment.

The rise in popularity of back schools reflects both a growing awareness and increasing frustration over the inadequate management of nonsurgical back pain patients. Because of our empiric approach to the management of low back pain and our inability to measure accurately the results of our own efforts, a wide range of approaches has emerged without good scientific assessment (20). Treatments as diverse as craniosacral therapy, which suggests that manual adjustments of the bones in the skull can relieve back pain, or the activator gun, which is supposed to produce minor adjustments of the spinal facet joints through impact on the skin by a spring-loaded rubber plunger, are part of the current spectrum of back pain management in North America. The problem is complicated further by the large amount of iatrogenic disease that exists in patients with low back disorders (21–23). Physical deconditioning from excessive bed rest or brace use, and emotional decompensation in a pattern of learned disability behavior, can be the results of inappropriate medical management.

In the absence of a specific diagnosis, the key elements for successful conservative treatment are the elimination of unnecessary fear, an improved basic understanding of back function, practical strategies to minimize attacks of back pain, and reduced dependence on all external sources of pain relief.

The demographics of the problem have been well documented. Back pain and spinal impairment are the most frequent causes of limited activity due to

a chronic condition in patients younger than 45 years of age (24–26). The incidence of back pain is about the same in men and women, although men undergo more spinal surgery (27). The cost to industry in lost time and medical and compensation payments is enormous (28–31). Clearly there is a role for effective authoritative education, both for the victim and for the public at large. The question is, can back school in its present form do the job?

HISTORICAL DEVELOPMENT OF BACK SCHOOLS

Twenty years ago, there were few if any organized back schools. in Sweden, the program originating at Danderyd Hospital in 1970 became the basis for several hundred similar back schools throughout the country (32, 33). The program, conducted by a physical therapist, consisted of four 45-min lessons over a 2-week period. Classes contained six to eight people. To encourage good back care, patients reclined in a semi-Fowler position on specially constructed couches while listening to the lectures. The instructors emphasized elimination of mechanical stress on the back and used prepared teaching aids to describe spinal anatomy. The last two classes were practical sessions designed to improve back care techniques and encourage the students to increase their level of physical activity. The formal structure of the program and the regular use of teaching materials set it apart from the informal back education courses that had previously existed. Although the content was largely the same as that offered by many physical therapists in one-to-one teaching situations, the school seemed to have a greater impact (34).

My own experience in organizing a back education program in Toronto, Canada is typical of many of the early attempts (35). In 1974, I assembled a small group of my patients with chronic low back pain for a two-lecture series on the cause and physical treatment of their problem. The classes were organized simply to eliminate the need for repetitive education in my private office. The second lecture was given by a physical therapist to broaden the information base. The original idea was simply to provide the patients, on a one-time basis, with as much knowledge as possible about their back problems. I hoped this would reduce their number of future office visits and expedite additional treatment. The emphasis in the classes was primarily on simple anatomy, the current theories of back pain production, and the fundamentals of safe lifting and good back care. The issues of fear and chronic pain behavior were not addressed.

The effect of the school approach was greater than I had anticipated. Patients rapidly developed patterns of group interaction that amplified and reinforced the information given. Questions were asked and topics discussed that had never arisen with these patients in my private practice. The classroom setting reduced the inhibition present in the doctor's office, and patients were anxious to express views and concerns they had previously suppressed. At the same time, the presence of two authority figures with different backgrounds, but with a similar viewpoint, strengthened the validity of the message contained in the lectures. Although not originally intended, a monthly program was rapidly developed and, within a year, had expanded to a regular series of four 60-min lectures. The inclusion of one session with a psychiatrist underlined our growing awareness of the psychological aspects of back pain. Gradually we shifted our emphasis from the traditional ergonomic approach typical of most physical therapy training programs to a more motivational style focusing on the elimination of fear and promoting confidence in the back's natural capacity for recovery. For our program, we found that a class of between 10 and 15 students encouraged active participation and made cost-efficient use of the instructor's time but avoided the patient's anxiety about speaking in front of a larger group.

In 1976, White and Mattmiller formed the California Back School (36). Their approach was directed at physical training and ergonomic assessment. Their facility also employed more invasive forms of conservative management such as epidural steroid injections and facet blocks. Students were treated individually in three weekly 90-min sessions and were observed going over an obstacle course and in work simulation techniques. A review session 1 month later tested both physical capacities and cognitive knowledge. This "hands-on" approach produced a back school similar in many respects to a conventional physical therapy back class yet possessing the perceived benefits of a structured educational program.

These early schools were rapidly copied. Within a decade, there were over 2000 patient education programs in North America designated as "back school" (37). The trend has continued to the present. Many programs influenced by the early success of the Canadian Back Institute in Toronto and the California Back School in San Francisco were patterned along similar lines. Other groups began to

develop in different ways from hospital-based clinics involving extended inpatient treatment to self-taught home study programs designed for use without a professional instructor.

EVALUATION OF EFFICACY

The proliferation of "back schools" in recent years should cause some concern. The wide range of formats and differences in approach make a valid comparison almost impossible. Even the generic title "back school" has come to hold little meaning. While patient education as a general principle is hard to refute, the specifics are open to far more criticism. As the cost of back education increases, there is a greater need to accurately ascertain its value. The assessment of any educational approach to the management of low back pain must be considered in terms of several defined parameters to measure the impact of comparable programs on comparable patient populations.

PATIENT SELECTION

Age

Back pain is most prevalent in the middle decades. The pattern is typically one of exacerbations and remissions with a decreasing frequency and severity of attacks over the age of 70 (38, 39). Educational programs must be tailored to the age of the students. Back care programs have been attempted in the public school system with limited success. Inadequate time within the curriculum, a shortage of teachers comfortable with the subject matter, and a lack of motivation in a young student population who have no fear of or interest in back pain are given as reasons for a poor response. Classes for the elderly in hospitals and nursing homes confront a student population with a greater percentage of specific, nonmechanical back problems, who will be poorly served by routine lectures on safe lifting or abdominal exercise. The most likely diagnoses and the most appropriate types of treatment both change with advancing years.

Sex

The incidence of back pain is approximately the same for men and women. The back education presentation must, however, have regard for the sex of the audience. Pictures depicting the proper way to stand at an ironing board will have little impact on a group of hard rock miners. A prepackaged back school program may be viewed as inappropriate or of little direct value to many members of the audience. One of the difficulties for an approach that focuses on modification of specific physical activity to protect the back is to obtain teaching aids that fit the particular circumstance. Many back schools of this type use pictures taken at the work place or employ simulation of the actual work environment (40). Increasing equality of the sexes may help resolve one aspect of this problem.

Workers' Compensation

Dissatisfaction concerning occupation, place of employment, and the monotony of the work performed have all been associated with an increased incidence of low back pain (41–43). Most studies record a lower success rate from all forms of treatment for patients still receiving compensation (44, 45). One method of dealing with this problem is to mix compensation and noncompensation patients together in the same class. Groups comprised entirely of workers' compensation patients can generate disruptive amounts of hostility. If the back education process is seen as a tool of the Compensation Board or of the employer, there will be immediate resentment and suspicion of any message that advocates a rapid return to work regardless of the validity of the advice on medical grounds. The inclusion of noncompensation patients in the student group introduces an element of peer pressure to improve performance, which may be the only positive motivation the class provides. These issues must be addressed both in planning a back school course and in evaluating its result.

Litigation and Insurance Claims

The possible role of secondary gain and the increased focus on nonsomatic complaints are factors to be considered in this group of patients (46, 47). A direct and open discussion of these topics in a small group setting can sometimes convey a message to the individual that is impossible to deliver in direct confrontation during an office visit. Patients suspected of malingering are often reacting more out of fear and misunderstanding than out of a conscious desire to defraud. One of the common features of chronic pain syndrome is a preoccupation with pain leading to visible changes in behavior. Attempts to alter this pattern of functional disability usually meet resistance from the patient, who remains convinced of the physical nature of the problem. Information about chronic pain and its real effect on performance can be delivered in a

back school lecture without arousing the defense mechanisms of an individual patient, who may, for the first time, actually understand the message. The time spent on the problem will depend upon the proportion of litigation and chronic pain patients within the general student population.

PAIN TYPE

No Pain

Preventative back education is a goal that has been sought by industry for many years, but the use of work site education through posters and the compilation of safety records have had little effect (48). Such passive measures have not influenced the increasing incidence of industrial low back injuries nor altered the workers' attitudes toward the problem. Most uninjured workers view back pain as something that only affects someone else. While there has been a general acceptance of increasing safety standards, there has been little change in the approach to the back. Industrial studies suggest that motivation to learn is low. Because so many back-sparing techniques rely on adapting unnatural postures and making increased use of the legs, most workers are reluctant to follow this advice. Because these alternate methods often require more energy than the conventional movements, workers tend to remain with the "easy" way. When an active education program is introduced, changes may occur but with a lowering of the interest level, it is generally noted that the effect on the behavior pattern is transient.

Minor, Acute, Intermittent Back Pain

Formal back education is not appropriate during an acute episode of low back pain. Following a single, short-duration attack, patients are rarely motivated to participate in an extensive training program. The need to prevent further episodes of pain becomes apparent only with time and additional attacks. The majority of these patients do well with almost all forms of treatment (49). In a study of patients attending the Canadian Back Institute, a pain pattern of short-duration attacks separated by periods of relief was found to be common and to respond to a number of different treatments. Because of their rapid spontaneous remissions, these patients probably form most of the group that responds so dramatically to the available fringe therapies. For some reason, it is difficult to assess the true value of back school in patients with this pain pattern.

Chronic Back Pain

Back school probably has its greatest role in improving the results of chronic back pain management. Patients with long-standing back pain tend to be motivated and willing to learn. They are often the victims of unnecessary fear that can be overcome when they discover how to modify and control their pain (50). Back schools working with these patients tend to stress the benign nature of back pain and attempt to make the individual more involved and self-reliant in the rehabilitation process. Because extended periods of back pain are often associated with long periods of physical inactivity, back education is usually combined with a progressive exercise and reconditioning routine. The increased activity is inevitably painful during the early phases, and a concurrent educational component is essential to reassure patients that in this instance, hurt does not equal harm, and that more, not less, activity is the way to recovery.

Chronic Pain Syndrome

The chronic pain syndrome requires intensive management. This syndrome is separated from chronic back pain by a predominance of the accompanying behavioral disorder. Patients exhibit a marked preoccupation with their pain, which comes to dominate their lives. They describe a widening array of symptoms and may actually worsen on conventional treatment. Many back schools use some psychological techniques, but the operant conditioning found in a chronic pain program lies outside the scope of most back education courses (51). Back school may be viewed as a first-line treatment to prevent the development of a complete syndrome or, alternatively, may be used as part of a more comprehensive program. Treating an established chronic pain syndrome with back school alone is an inappropriate use of the technique.

CLASS SIZE

Individual

Individual patient education in an office or clinic using pamphlets, blackboard drawings, or practical demonstrations was the forerunner of most back schools. This form of education obviously continues, although usually without a clearly defined format. As a method of conducting back school, it is rarely, if ever, cost effective. Where education is combined with physical training or the use of direct investigative or pain-relieving procedures, the one-on-one approach may still be considered a type of back school. Because this method is labor intensive, the cost per patient is generally high and the technique is almost always limited to those with third-party funding.

Small Group

The small group format allows patients to share their feelings, fears, and experiences with others in a supportive atmosphere. Groups of 10 to 20 people permit an informal approach. Lectures become conversations, albeit with clearly defined guidelines. Individual questions can be discussed and the answers used to advance the general knowledge of the class. Problem patients can be isolated and their disruptive influence minimized more easily than in a larger group. Group dynamics often reinforce the cognitive message while requiring patients to exhibit a degree of internal control and an expectation of positive outcome (52).

Large Group

Although apparently more efficient, significantly increasing the size of the back school class may interfere with the exchange of information. Patients are reluctant to speak out in front of a larger body. A greater number of students requires a higher degree of expertise in the lecturer and greater sophistication in the instructional aids. Points of detail, interesting in a small group, appear out of place in the large class. The air of informality disappears and the physician or physical therapist is once again viewed as an authority figure, not as a knowledgeable participant in an open discussion. Groups of more than 30 people lose the dynamics present in a smaller class. The sense of peer pressure, competition, and feedback are diminished.

Didactic Lecture

The purpose of didactic lectures is to provide information and to motivate the audience. There is limited opportunity for interplay between the instructor and the students. Patients who attend receive no individual attention and the result is therefore that of watching a prepackaged program. Because of the strange sense of isolation about their problem that affects so many chronic back pain patients, the majority of the audience may view the performance as something that applies to situations other than their own. The same criticism can be made, of course, about video or tape/slide presentations given without the opportunity for follow-up discussion. These types of presentation will serve to educate the public but have little or no place in the regular schedule of a conventional back school.

PRIMARY EMPHASIS

Ergonomic

Evidence supports a strong relationship between mechanical stress and low back pain (53–56). As the natural outgrowth of physical therapy programs, most early back schools stressed body mechanics and proper body movement. Considerable emphasis was placed on proper standing and sitting postures as well as on the correct techniques for lifting or carrying. Although the educational scope has expanded, many instructors still consider disseminating this ergonomic information their principle objective. Unfortunately, the biomechanical evidence supporting the various "correct" techniques is constantly changing. The rigid maintenance of a pelvic tilt, once considered essential for good posture, is now being questioned, and many therapists have begun to advocate the preservation of a neutral lordosis instead. As a major source of patient information, back school has an obligation to constantly upgrade its material and keep its message in line with the current state of knowledge. When ergonomic information is the primary emphasis, this may prove particularly difficult both logistically in the provision of new teaching aids and psychologically in the reeducation of staff firmly convinced of the value of the established methods.

Psychological

Information about the benign nature of mechanical back pain helps dispel myths, allay fears, and minimize the patient's natural preoccupation with his/her symptoms. The principal goal for this type of program is to change attitudes, modify personal interaction, and increase independence and self-reliance. Because emphasis is placed on a basic understanding of spinal anatomy and the recognized sources of back pain, there is less demand with this approach to constantly revise the information. Rather than attempt to provide absolute answers to specific questions, this variety of back school promotes a philosophy of self-help and experimentation as a method of coping with the changing rules of proper physical movement.

Back Exercise

It has long been accepted that weak muscles contribute to back pain. Current knowledge indicates that the strength of the trunk extensors is often reduced in patients with chronic back complaints, that decreased muscle endurance is a contributing factor, and that balanced strength in all the trunk muscles is necessary for full functional recovery (57–62). As with ergonomic training, the biomechanical theories used to advocate one approach to exercise rather than another are changing. Abdominal strengthening, long the fundamental objective of back exercise, has been supplanted in many clinics by an emphasis on back extension programs. Maintaining a balance while providing the best available therapeutic routine is the goal of this type of education. The term "back school" may be used to denote a course of remedial exercise comparable to the standard physical therapy "mat class," but in such cases the title is poorly employed. An exercise-oriented back school is not merely the extension of a physical therapy exercise session nor is it a fitness club for back patients. Neither of these alternatives provides the continuing educational input and psychological support that set the back school apart.

General Fitness

The current enthusiasm for aerobic exercise and overall physical conditioning has led to the incorporation of general exercise and fitness routines into many back schools. As the proportion of specific back exercise is reduced and the educational content diminishes, it becomes difficult to justify the title "back school," and even more difficult to compare the results of treatment.

FREQUENCY OF TREATMENT

Single Session

There is no justification for labeling a single instructional session as a back school. The industrial application of back education often demands time constraints dictated by production quotas or shift schedules. Convincing management of the value of an educational program for their employees can be difficult. The financial returns of good back care are slow to materialize and may not be reflected in the year-end financial statement. Spending prevention dollars today in expectation of injury cost savings tomorrow is not always an accepted strategy. When an industrial back school is established, it must conform to the demands of the work place and function with a minimum of disruption to plant operation. But since the goal of any valid educational effort is a change in observed behavior, compression of the format into a single session is ineffective.

Multiple Sessions

The amount of instruction necessary for the individual back school student has yet to be determined. Estimates range from as little as 3 to more than 12 hours (63). The longer courses tend to focus on the more difficult chronic pain patients or combine education with ergonomic and exercise training. Most back schools run between two and four classes for each patient. These may be held on consecutive days as part of an intensive, sometimes residential, program or spaced over days or weeks to allow gradual assimilation of the information. Individual sessions are from 30 to 90 min in length. Prolonged sitting can be painful for someone with a bad back.

TREATMENT TYPE AND INTENSITY

Education Only

The teaching, learning, and retention of information about spinal anatomy, the causes of back pain, the psychological implications of a bad back, proper back care, and remedial exercise is generally the basis for the designation "back school." It is hoped that patient education will lead to a willingness to accept responsibility and to active participation in the recovery process. Implicit in this approach is the belief that greater understanding by the patient will lead to greater control of the problem (64). This seemingly self-evident proposition has, in fact, rarely been tested. Its acceptance lies in the broader acceptance in our society of education as a means of improving performance. Because back school is generally based on a medical model and because formal education in medicine is viewed as the only way to obtain the knowledge necessary to practice effectively, it is little wonder that the concept of back education has gained wide medical support. Only in recent years has the purely educational approach been questioned.

Treatment Only

The hospital-based back school has been regarded by some critics as primarily a means of directing patients to other, more invasive forms of conservative back pain management (65). In this version, individual assessment is most important and the "school" aspect may be little more than the cursory dissemination of back care instruction. This substantial shift in direction under the same designation "back school" poses a major concern for the future. In the absence of any binding regulation or even accepted guidelines, a back school can become whatever its organizers wish it to be. The name may bear little relevance to the program it is supposed to describe.

Outpatient Education, Assessment, Treatment, and Training

In light of concerns over the value of a purely educational program, many back schools have expanded to include patient management. Others have developed in association with established rehabilitation medicine clinics. The combination of an educational approach with specific patient treatment and long-term training addresses one of the major requirements for back school in a work environment. The same expertise used to deal with more financially pressing short-term case management can provide long-term prevention through training and education. Promoting back education as a means of providing an overall reduction in back injury claims is far more difficult than offering a treatment program for currently disabled workers with back problems. Often it is the assessment and treatment of the individual that creates receptiveness to the education and training of the remaining work force.

Inpatient Education, Assessment, and Treatment

Chronic back pain patients require a thorough assessment and lengthy management routines. A hurried approach and rapid disposition may only reinforce the patient's hostility and promote further disability (66). Here the back school becomes part of an interdisciplinary clinic employing a battery of investigative procedures and an extensive inpatient routine of operant conditioning. Cognitive input as well as psychomotor training are both required, and a formal educational program is an efficient means of providing the first part of the combination. Group sessions not only impart knowledge, they create a pattern of positive reinforcement, reduce the sense of isolation, and generate an atmosphere in which back pain can be understood and controlled. Because of the significant expense and the amount of professional time required, patients admitted to such programs should be those who are severely disabled (67, 68).

PAYMENT

Direct Patient Charge

Most back schools providing only education charge the students directly. By using small classes rather than individual instruction and by maximizing the time commitment of the involved professionals, the unit cost can be reduced to affordable levels. Lectures can be prepared and slides or teaching aids provided so that the physician or therapist requires a minimum of preparation time. Individual sessions can be structured so that most of the routine questions are answered in the formal presentation, reducing the need for extended discussion at the end of the class. If back school is to be a "front-line" management strategy, it must be accessible to all those who need it. If it is to remain an attractive idea to private clinics and practitioners, it cannot run at a financial loss. Keeping the price of a back education program within the means of the average back pain sufferer while retaining the potential for profit is the challenge of the back school business.

Third-Party Payment

The more extensive programs combining education with direct patient treatment are expensive and become cost efficient only against a background of inflated insurance and compensation benefits. An inpatient pain management clinic can expect a 25–70% return-to-work rate even when drawing from a carefully screened patient population (69, 70). Because of the enormous financial burden of a back-injured worker in lost productivity, medical expenses, and disability payments, cost effectiveness can be achieved if only 1 patient in 20 returns to regular employment.

Government Support

In some areas, the cost of back education is supported by government funding. The amount of money available from this source is usually sufficient to provide only cursory assessment, basic education, and limited follow-up. Socialized health care tends to move treatment toward the lowest common denominator, and back school is no exception. On the other hand, this method of payment greatly increases access and makes at least a rudimentary back school available to anyone who needs it. As a purely educational experience, this "ounce of prevention" may be worth "a pound of cure."

ISSUES INVOLVED IN BACK SCHOOL

If back school is to survive as an effective and scientifically valid form of treatment, several issues must be addressed. The very popularity of back school among its student population has made the approach suspect to some observers. Nothing in medicine can be so simple and so effective, and still be honest. Yet 94% of the people attending the California Back School were satisfied with the program, and 96% of the students at the Canadian Back Institute found the lecture series worthwhile. The cause of this consistently high level of patient

acceptance has never been fully explained. It must be pointed out, however, that patient satisfaction does not necessarily equate with functional recovery. These same programs report a 70% success in the elimination of disabling back pain or the return to full employment and normal daily activity. Still, it seems clear that back school answers a need and corrects a deficiency in our routine regimen of back care.

PATIENT GAINS IN INFORMATION

The usual goals of back school, including the development of a positive attitude, reduced reliance on external forms of therapy, a willingness to actively participate in rehabilitation, and the acceptance of responsibility for the recovery process, may be accomplished primarily through the patient's exposure to concerned, knowledgeable authority figures. Contrary to popular opinion, not all back pain sufferers are malingering. Many, in fact, are prevented from returning to normal living by overcautious medical management and unnecessary fear of the dire consequences of working with back pain. A change in the physician's approach to a problem can alter patients' expectations (71). There is, however, little scientific evidence that learning actually occurs. One of the most quoted early studies on the value of back school was carried out by Bergquist-Ullman and Larsson in Sweden (72). Automotive plant employees with back pain were randomly divided into three groups. The first group received the classic Danderyd Hospital Swedish Back School, consisting of four 45-min sessions over a 2-week period. The second group received manual therapy and manipulation as well as 5 min of instruction on lifting techniques and the importance of avoiding strenuous movements. The third group received placebo treatment consisting of an average of five treatments of short-wave diathermy at the lowest possible intensity. Seventy patients were treated by back school. Comparable numbers were treated with physical therapy and placebo. Excluded from the study were patients with back pain of more than 3 months' duration, any pain in the year preceding the current attack, previous back surgery, structural scoliosis, pregnancy, and osteoporosis. The results of the study showed that patients treated with back school or physiotherapy returned to work more rapidly than those treated by placebo. However, the study found no decrease in the long-term pattern of pain or the recurrence rate after back school compared to physical therapy, suggesting that the short-term improvement was due more to the interaction with the authority figures involved than to the cognitive information obtained and remembered by the workers.

Although the basic premise that increased knowledge leads to the patients' increased ability to control back pain is appealing, it is deceptively simplistic and difficult to prove. Some support for the proposition comes from the review of multiple-choice examinations carried out in a study of patients educated at the Canadian Back Institute. Ten multiple-choice questions were given before the start of the standard four-lecture series. A second test of 10 different questions was given immediately after the program and a review test of 10 additional questions was administered 6 months or more after the back school had been completed. To ensure the questions were of approximately equal difficulty, the three tests were regularly interchanged. When the score on the review test was compared with the score obtained on the pretest, a highly significant correlation was found between the gain in information retention and the patient's subjective assessment of his/her improvement. The percentage increase in the individual student's score between test 1 and test 3 appeared to be a valid indicator of the ability to control back pain. In at least one study of patient education, the more they knew the better they did.

ACCURACY AND COMPREHENSIVENESS

If information is retained and remembered, and if this information has an effect on performance, it is obviously important to ensure that the correct knowledge is being disseminated. Low back treatment is empiric and full of contradiction. Nonsurgical management includes bed rest, traction and massage, exercise, passive mobilization, hydrotherapy, electrotherapy, acupuncture, and postural training (73). Medication includes muscle relaxants, analgesics, antidepressants, and sedatives. Injections into trigger points, nerve root canals, the epidural space, and the intervertebral disk are all accepted by various practitioners as legitimate treatment methods. Therapies as diverse and questionable as palpating the rhythm of movement in the suture lines of the skull or injecting hypertonic sugar solutions to toughen the ligaments of the spine have their adherents. Can a back school be expected to arbitrate and choose, or should it present all the available information without bias or comment? Also, the information changes. The abdominal strengthening Williams exercises and pelvic tilt that were the mainstay of physical therapy instruction 30 years ago have been challenged by the concept of a neutral lumbar lordosis and exten-

sion exercising (74–76). The traditional role of intra-abdominal pressure as a source of low back support has been disputed by more recent studies of abdominal pressure while lifting. Prolonged bed rest and long-term bracing are no longer fashionable.

If the educational process is used to support only one point of view or, worse, one form of treatment, its ability to resolve the apparent confusion is reduced and much of its value is lost. The role of back school should be to provide the patient with as complete an understanding as possible while explaining and clarifying the origins of current trends in treatment. Confusion and uncertainty in the mind of the first contact physician can easily lead to doubt and fear in the mind of the patient. Unless back school can address these issues with clear, factual information, it is not fulfilling its intended role (77).

ADDRESSING PATIENTS' EDUCATIONAL NEEDS

The degree of sophistication in the knowledge of the average back pain patient about the spine and its function is surprisingly low. To be effective, the level of education should be far more basic than most practitioners realize. Simply explaining the basic structure of the spine and identifying the common sources of pain removes much of the mystery. Emphasizing that most back pain disappears with time and does not produce paralysis seems so obvious that it hardly requires teaching, and yet many patients live in fear for lack of such basic knowledge. Back school need never enter the controversy about the benefits of specific types of spinal treatment; it is enough to explain what the various modalities attempt to do and to discuss the alternatives.

A great deal of unnecessary fear results from prevalent and frightening misconceptions. To explain to the typical back pain sufferer that disks do not slip out from their positions between the bones of the spine is often of greater value than a discussion on the modern thinking about the role of raised intra-abdominal pressure while lifting. Maintaining the educational input at a level that is both useful and noncontroversial can be difficult and requires a surprising amount of preparation. The message must not appear patronizing. Technical information should be available in detail for those with the necessary educational background, but must be understood by all. The program should address the concerns of the class and so must be tailored to the particular age, sex, or occupational needs involved. There must be a free exchange of ideas so that every member of the group feels that his/her problems are being discussed. Yet, the average back school is not the place for private consultation, and the demands of a vocal minority cannot be allowed to overshadow the fundamental message or the needs of the other participants. Developing a teaching style that accomplishes these objectives takes practice. No matter how simple the message is made to appear, there is much more to conducting a successful back education program than knowing spinal anatomy (78).

Implicit in an effective back school is a strong element of pragmatism and common sense. By eliminating fear and misunderstanding, patients can be encouraged to experiment with approaches to their own problems. The ideal class, for example, does not teach by rote one correct lifting technique. It offers alternative methods and invites the students to choose for themselves the maneuver that is appropriate for their own circumstances. It stresses that for most back pain sufferers, hurt and harm are not synonymous, and therefore an unsuccessful and uncomfortable experiment in lifting does not mean further damage to the spine. To perform in this fashion, a back school must communicate its message clearly. Educational objectives should be carefully developed and clearly stated so that both the instructor and the student know what is expected. As with all good educational objectives, those prepared for a back school should include a visible and measurable outcome to allow proper evaluation.

EVALUATION STANDARDS

At present, there is little scientific validation for the concept of back school as an independent treatment modality. Many of its components, however, have long been recognized as useful. Early attempts at behavioral modification such as those conducted at Rancho Los Amigos in the 1960s demonstrated the value of reinforcing healthy behavior (79). The reward structure was based on group activities, peer pressure, competition, and positive feedback. A similar approach exists today in successful back education courses.

Fordyce and his colleagues at the University of Washington Clinical Pain Center have developed behavioral techniques to return patients to a satisfied life situation (80). Their emphasis is to eliminate the patient's inappropriate dependency on physicians, hospitals, and other health care providers, and to decrease verbal and nonverbal pain behavior. The principles developed in this type of

comprehensive program can be readily adapted to a less sophisticated back school.

Many popular educational programs with comparable strategies have proven and validated records of success. Using award systems and peer pressure, groups such as Alcoholics Anonymous and Weight Watchers have demonstrated their ability to modify behavior. Medical acceptance of this approach has been guarded. These programs, with their obvious appeal to the emotions and direct marketing techniques, are contrary to many doctors' perception of the traditional medical model. Their reliance on group support and psychological motivation is foreign to the conventional medical approach of patient dependence and frequent medication. Partly because of the public perception of back pain as a particularly threatening occurrence, partly because of the overwhelming prevalence of the problem, and partly because of the high level of medical involvement, evaluation standards found acceptable for other self-help groups are often judged inadequate for back school. Although the need exists for controlled prospective studies to provide objective information, well controlled subjective assessments may, in fact, be equally valid (81, 82).

BACK SCHOOL AND INDUSTRY

Industry is well aware of the value of safety education. Goals including the prevention of recurrent injuries, a reduction in the number of days lost from work, and a decrease in the financial burden of back pain to industry are all meaningful and measurable outcomes. Changes in the workplace and a greatly increased safety consciousness on the part of the workers have combined to reduce work-related accidents in many areas (83). Unfortunately this has not yet occurred with back injury and back pain. Conventional approaches such as posters depicting the proper techniques of material handling have been available for decades but have had little impact. The cost of lost time due to back pain continues to increase.

The industrial back school is perceived by some as a possible solution (84). Schools involving employer, employee, union, and insurance carrier would provide better understanding of the problem and eliminate many of the potential difficulties that arise through a lack of knowledge (85). Back education programs could improve the employer's understanding of an ergonomically correct work place and lead to better working conditions for back pain sufferers. Programs could convince the employees to take responsibility for their own back care and lead to greater participation in exercise and fitness activities. They could show unions that a rapid return to work is in the best interest of their membership and lead to selected rule changes in seniority and job classification. Finally, back education programs could induce insurance companies to put more time and money into rehabilitation and lead to increased funding for retraining and alternate employment schemes rather than for long-term disability.

There are, however, dangers in this approach. A typical educational program designed to instruct the work force may be relatively inexpensive, but it is not necessarily cost effective. If there is no management involvement, there will be no meaningful commitment within the company. Short-term modifications can produce only short-term benefits with no positive financial implications. In addition, employees require the opportunity to work safely and to keep fit. Ergonomic modifications and the provision of a fitness facility may be required. Both will necessitate a considerably larger commitment of funds than the provision of education alone and may be ignored. Both workers and their unions may view the back school solely as a means of levering greater concessions out of management while missing completely the messages of self-help and responsibility. Insurance companies may regard the funding of a back school as an inexpensive alternative to the more difficult responsibilities of developing active rehabilitation programs. Even if it is effective and fully supported by all concerned, the back care message must be continually reinforced. A single series of back school lectures cannot be expected to produce lasting change. If back education is seen by each group involved merely as a means of avoiding a more substantial commitment, it will certainly fail. As part of an integrated program with the support of management and labor, it is indispensable.

FINANCIAL ASPECTS OF BACK SCHOOL

By its very nature, as an uncontrolled educational establishment back school is open to abuse. Currently there is no regulatory body nor even a widely held consensus of what constitutes proper back education. Because most back pain improves within a few weeks or months, the effectiveness of any treatment is difficult to determine, and when a particular treatment is promoted aggressively, the apparent benefit may come more from merchandising than from medicine. Back school is no exception. The rapid proliferation of back education programs has inevitably allowed the development of some programs run by professionals with ques-

tionable qualifications. Recognizing the vast number of back pain sufferers and the obvious confusion over the most effective forms of treatment, a school may be seen as a potentially lucrative endeavor. There is certainly nothing inherently wrong in "doing well by doing good." The difficulties arise when the quality or content of the program begins to suffer to support the profit margin. Larger classes or unskilled lecturers are two obvious ways to cut costs. Both reduce the beneficial impact of the primary message or, in the case of a poor lecturer, may change the message completely.

Back school can also be subverted to a particular therapeutic approach (86). A course can easily be developed placing unwarranted emphasis on a particular piece of equipment or therapeutic modality. Students can be encouraged to purchase, without proof of their value, specific items in which the back school has a financial interest. Students may be advised to obtain additional therapy that will require a commitment of time and money far beyond that advertised as part of the original educational package. Subtler methods of increasing the back school's financial return may blur the margin between medical caution and unnecessary investigation. Special x-ray procedures, serial nerve conduction studies, or thermography may have more impact on the "bottom line" than on measuring the patient's response to back education.

The potential for abuse exists in many areas of medicine and is not unique to back school. Greater involvement by concerned and knowledgeable professionals, a more concise definition of the process and its limitations, broader public understanding of the basic concept, and valid comparisons of the results are all required.

CONCLUSIONS

In the final analysis, the success of back school will be determined by its potential to reduce low back disability. Does it really work? Industrial back schools such as that conducted for the Southern Pacific Transport Company produced a 22% decrease in back injuries and a 43% decrease in lost time from back pain in the year following the educational program. A controlled study of industrial back education with the Federal Cartridge Corporation in Anoka, Minnesota produced a 50% reduction in compensation costs over a 3-year period (87). Eighty-nine percent of the participants at the California Back School did not feel the need to seek further treatment. Many people, patients and professionals alike, believe that back school is effective. Its success, however, awaits validation.

Perhaps more importantly, the reasons for its apparent benefit have yet to be clearly defined. According to Robinson, one important factor is a consistency of approach (88). In an effective back school, every member of the staff presents the same attitude and basic information. Patients obtain a clear consensus without conflicting opinion and are presented with an overriding sense of optimism. Equally significant is the feeling of confidence that rapidly pervades the program. Patients, accustomed to the cautious and often uncomfortable response back pain engenders in many doctors, are impressed with the positive approach and lack of confusion inherent in this technique. Within this aura of understanding, patients lose the intimidation that is so often part of the doctor-patient relationship. They are willing to try and are even hesitantly confident of success. Recognizing the widespread pessimism that permeates the common perception of back pain, the back school approach may be almost as important as the back school message.

Regardless of the style or content, there is no doubt that the timing of back education is important. Most patients stricken by acute low back pain recover quickly. Nachemson estimates that within 6 weeks 80% will have returned to regular employment. It is the remainder who require immediate attention, including a program to reduce apprehension and promote active rehabilitation. These patients must be reminded repeatedly that a graduated early return to work will not worsen their condition or lead to future complications. At the same time, however, they must accept and cope with the possibility of a temporary increase in their pain during the early stages of recovery. Symptoms recur in about 50% of patients during the first 24–36 months after an acute episode of back pain, but no evidence has been found to suggest that these recurrences are related to a controlled return to work. The destructive effects of chronic pain and the creation of disability behavior develop over several months. Too often this time is spent in programs dominated by short-term, passive pain-relieving modalities. Patients encouraged to remain passive become dependent and accept the need for extrinsic methods of pain control. Getting the message of active participation to the patient in time for it to have a beneficial effect is something back school can do very well.

McGill (89) and Kelsey (90), reporting on separate studies, found that employees with back problems who are absent from work for longer than 6 months have only a 50% chance of reachieving productive employment in the same capacity. The chance is reduced to 25% after 1 year and becomes negligible after 2 years. Back school can be an effective means of early intervention. Back education, however, does not compensate for poor physical evaluation or inappropriate treatment methods. Neither is it a substitute for good medical care and the judicious use of medication. Back school is a resource with the potential to help a wide range of patients regardless of the nature of their physical problems. An effective back education program will alter the patient's perception of him/herself from that of a passive observer to one of an active participant in an understandable and goal-oriented treatment and rehabilitation routine.

REFERENCES

1. Fahrni WH, Orth M: Conservative treatment of lumbar disc degeneration; our primary responsibility. *Orthop Clin North Am* 6:1, 1975.
2. Pawlicki RE, Gil KM, Joplins CA, et al: The low back school: a new palliative approach to low back pain. *W Va Med J* 78(10):249, 1982.
3. Egbert LD: Reduction of postoperative pain by encouragement and instruction of patients. *N Engl J Med* 270:825, 1964.
4. Healy KM: Does preoperative instruction make a difference? *Am J Nurs* 68:62, 1968.
5. Levine PH, Britten AF: Supervised patient-management of haemophilia. A study of 45 patients with haemophilia A and B. *Ann Intern Med* 78:195, 1973.
6. Miller LV, Goldstein J: More efficient care of diabetic patients in a county-hospital setting. *N Engl J Med* 286:1388, 1972.
7. Lidström A, Zachrisson M: Physical therapy on low back pain and sciatica; an attempt at evaluation. *Scand J Rehabil Med* 2:37, 1970.
8. Nachemson AL: Work for all. For those with low back pain as well. *Clin Orthop* 179:77, 1983.
9. Reisbord LS, Greenland S: Factors associated with self-reported back-pain prevalence: a population-based study. *J Chronic Dis* 38(8):691, 1985.
10. Haldeman S: Spinal manipulative therapy. *Clin Orthop* 179:62, 1983.
11. Kirkaldy-Willis WH, Cassidy JD: Spinal manipulation in the treatment of low back pain. *Can Fam Physician* 31:535, 1985.
12. Saunders HD: Use of spinal traction in the treatment of neck and back conditions. *Clin Orthop* 179:31, 1983.
13. Christy B: Discussion on the treatment of backache by traction. *Proc R Soc Med* 48:811, 1955.
14. Farrell JP, Twomey LT: Acute low back pain. Comparison of two conservative treatment approaches. *Med J Aust* 1:160, 1982.

15. Glover JR, Morris JG, Chosla T: Back pain; a randomized clinical trial of rotational manipulation of the trunk. *Br J Ind Med* 31:59, 1974.

16. Lawson G, Godfrey C: A report on studies of spinal traction. *Med Serv J Can* 12:762, 1958.

17. Mathews J, Heckling J: Lumbar traction: a double blind control study for sciatica. *Rheumatol Rehabil* 14:222, 1975.

18. Sims-Williams H, Jayson MV, Young SMS, et al: Control trial of mobilization and manipulation for patients with low back pain in general practice. *Br Med J* 2:1338, 1978.

19. White AH: A model for conservative care of low back pain: back school, epidural blocks, mobilization, AAOS Instructional Course Lectures. St. Louis, CV Mosby, 1985, vol. 34, pp 78–84.

20. Wiesel SW, Cuckler JM, De Luca F, et al: Acute low back pain: an objective analysis of conservative therapy. *Spine* 5:324, 1980.

21. Brown MD, Jackson C: Editorial comment. *Clin Orthop* 179:2, 1983.

22. Hall H, Iceton JA: Back school; an overview with specific reference to the Canadian Back Education Units. *Clin Orthop* 179:10, 1983.

23. Tarsh MJ, Royston C: A follow-up study of accident neurosis. *Br J Psychiatry* 146:18, 1985.

24. Fisk JR, DiMonte P, Courington S: Back schools, past, present and future. *Clin Orthop* 179:18, 1983.

25. Kelsey JL, Pastides H, Bisbee G: Musculoskeletal disorders; their frequency of occurrence and their impact on the population of the United States. New York, Prodist, 1978.

26. National Center for Health Statistics: *Limitation of Activity due to Chronic Conditions, United States, 1969 and 1970*. Washington, DC, U.S. Government Printing Office, 1973, series 10, no 80.

27. Frymoyer JW, Pope MH, Costanza MC, et al: Epidemiologic studies of low back pain. *Spine* 5:419, 1980.

28. Bonica JJ (ed): Symposium on pain (Parts 1 and 2). *Arch Surg* 112:783, 1977.

29. Nagi SZ, Riley LE, Newby LG: A social epidemiology of back pain in a general population. *J Chronic Dis* 26:796, 1973.

30. Rowe ML: Low back disability in industry: updated position. *J Occup Med* 13:476, 1971.

31. Taugher NJ: *Incidence of Industrial Back Injuries and the Significance to our Community. Workmen's Compensation Data*. Madison, State of Wisconsin, Department of Industrial Labor and Human Relations, 1973.

32. Zachrisson-Forsell M: The Swedish Back School. *Physiotherapy* 66(4):112, 1980.

33. Zachrisson-Forsell M: The back school. *Spine* 6:104, 1981.

34. Lankhorst GJ, Van de Stadt RJ, Voselaar TW, et al: The effect of the Swedish Back School in chronic idiopathic low back pain. A prospective controlled study. *Scand J Rehabil Med* 15(3):141, 1983.

35. Attix EA, Nichols J: Establishing a low back school. *South Med J* 74(3):327, 1981.

36. Mattmiller AW: The California Back School. *Physiotherapy* 66(4):118, 1980.

37. White LA: Community resource back school (abstract). The Challenge of the Lumbar Spine 7th Annual Meeting, Minneapolis, Minnesota, September 1985.

38. Nachemson AL: The lumbar spine. An orthopaedic challenge. *Spine* 1:59, 1976.

39. Nachemson AL: The natural course of low back pain. In White AA, Gordon SL (eds): *Symposium on Idiopathic Low Back Pain*. St. Louis, CV Mosby, 1982, p 46.

40. Bettencourt CM, Carlstrom P, Brown SH, et al: Using work simulation to treat adults with back injuries. *Am J Occup Ther* 40(1):12–18, 1986.

41. Magora A: Investigation of the relations between low back pain and occupation. Physiological aspects. *Scand J Rehabil Med* 5:191, 1973.

42. Svensson H, Andersson GBJ: Low back pain in 40 to 47 year old men: work history and work environment factors. *Spine* 8:272, 1983.

43. Caruso LA, Chan DE, Chan A: The management of work-related back pain. *Am J Occup Ther* 41(2):112–117, 1987.

44. Taylor PJ: Personal factors associated with sickness absence. *Br J Ind Med* 25:106, 1981.

45. White AWM: Low back pain in men receiving Workmen's Compensation, a follow-up study. *Can Med Assoc J* 101:61, 1969.

46. Fordyce WE, Fowler RS, Lehmann JF, et al: Some implications of learning in problems of chronic pain. *J Chronic Dis* 21:179, 1968.

47. Mendelson G: Not "cured by a verdict"—effect of legal settlement on compensation claimants. *Med J Aust* 11:132, 1982.

48. Bigos SJ, Battie MC: Acute care to prevent back disability. Ten years of progress. *Clin Orthop* 221:121–130, 1987.

49. Sikorski JM: A rationalized approach to physiotherapy for low back pain. *Spine* 10(6):571–579, 1985.

50. Black RG: The chronic pain syndrome. *Surg Clin North Am* 55:999, 1975.

51. Tollison CD, Kriegel ML, Downie GR: Chronic low back pain: results of treatment at the Pain Therapy Center. *South Med J* 78(11):1291–1295, 1985.

52. White AH: Back school. AAOS Instructional Course Lecture St. Louis, CV Mosby, 1979, p 184.

53. Andersson JAD: Back pain and occupation. In Jayson M (ed): *The Lumbar Spine and Back Pain*. London, Pitman Medical, 1980, pp 57–82.

54. Chaffin DB: Human strength capability and low back pain. *J Occup Med* 16:248, 1974.

55. Pope M, Wilder D, Matteri R, et al: Experimental measurements of vertebral motions under load. *Orthop Clin North Am* 8(1):163, 1977.

56. Troup JDG: Dynamic factors in the analysis of stoop and crouch lifting methods: a methodological ap-

proach to the development of safe material handling standards. *Orthop Clin North Am* 8(1):201, 1977.

57. Cady LD, Buschoff DP, O'Connell GR, et al: Strength and fitness and subsequent back injuries in fire-fighters. *J Occup Med* 21:269, 1979.

58. Caldwell LS: Relative muscle loading and endurance. *J Eng Psychol* 2:155, 1963.

59. Jackson CP, Brown MD: Is there a role for exercise in the treatment of patients with low back pain? *Clin Orthop* 179:39, 1983.

60. Nachemson AL, Lindh M: Measurement of abdominal and back muscle strength with and without low back pain. *Scand J Rehabil Med* 1:60, 1969.

61. Soderberg GL, Barr JO: Muscular function in chronic low back dysfunction. *Spine* 8:79, 1983.

62. Suzuki N, Endo S: A quantitative study of the trunk muscle strength and fatiguability in the low-back-pain syndrome. *Spine* 8:69, 1983.

63. Selby N: Industrial back school (abstract). The Challenge of the Lumbar Spine 7th Annual Meeting, Minneapolis, Minnesota, September 1985.

64. Klaber Moffett JA, Chase SM, Portek I, et al: A controlled, prospective study to evaluate the effectiveness of a back school in the relief of chronic low back pain. *Spine* 11(2):120–122, 1986.

65. White AH: *Back School and Other Conservative Approaches to Low Back Pain.* St. Louis, CV Mosby, 1983.

66. Spengler DM: Chronic low back pain: the team approach. *Clin Orthop* 179:71, 1983.

67. Anderson TP, Cole TM, Gullickson G, et al: Behaviour modification of chronic pain. *Clin Orthop* 129:96, 1977.

68. Gottlieb HJ, Koller R, Alperson BL: Low back pain comprehensive rehabilitation programme: a follow-up study. *Arch Phys Med Rehabil* 63(10):458, 1982.

69. Rosomoff HL, Green C, Silbert M, et al: Pain and low back rehabilitation program at the University of Miami School of Medicine. *Natl Inst Drug Abuse Res Monogr Ser* 36:92, 1981.

70. Seres JL, Newman RI: Results of treatment of chronic low back pain at the Portland Pain Center. *J Neurosurg* 45:32, 1976.

71. Deyo RA, Diehl AK, Rosenthal M: Reducing roentgenography use. Can patient expectations be altered? *Arch Intern Med* 147(1):141–145, 1987.

72. Bergquist-Ullman M, Larsson U: Acute low back pain in industry: a controlled propective study with special reference to therapy and confounding factors. *Acta Orthop Scand [Suppl]* 170, 1977.

73. Lehmann TR, Russell DW, Spratt KF, et al: Efficacy of electroacupuncture and TENS in the rehabilitation of chronic low back pain patients. *Pain* 26(3):277–290, 1986.

74. McKenzie RA: *The Lumbar Spine: Mechanical Diagnosis and Therapy.* Waikanae, NZ, Spinal Publications, 1981.

75. Williams PC: Lesions of the lumbosacral spine, Part 1. *J Bone Joint Surg* 19:343, 1937.

76. Williams PC: Lesions of the lumbosacral spine, Part 2. *J Bone Joint Surg* 19:690, 1937.

77. Hall H: The Canadian Back Education Units. *Physiotherapy* 66(4):115, 1980.

78. Hall H, Hunt M, Tennant H: *Talking Back in Class.* Toronto, The Canadian Back Institute, 1983.

79. Mooney V: Alternative approaches for patients beyond the help of surgery. *Orthop Clin North Am* 6:331, 1975.

80. Fordyce WE: *Behavioral Methods for Chronic Back Pain and Illness.* St. Louis, CV Mosby, 1976.

81. Roland M, Morris R: A study of the natural history of low back pain: Part 1: Development of a reliable and sensitive measure of disability in low back pain. *Spine* 2:141, 1983.

82. Roland M, Morris R: A study of the natural history of low back pain: Part 2: Development of guidelines for trials of treatment in primary care. *Spine* 2:145, 1983.

83. Litster R: Foot injuries in North America. Paper presented at the COPE Conference, Toronto, 1984.

84. Snook SH: Approaches to the control of back pain in industry: job design, job placement and education/training. *State Art Rev Occup Med* 3(1):45–59, 1988.

85. Morris A: Program compliance key to preventing low back injuries. *Occup Health Safety*, March, p 44, 1984.

86. Brill MN, Whiffen JR: Application of a 24-hour burst TENS in a back school. *Phys Ther* 65(9):1355, 1985.

87. Hall H: A successful industrial back education programme; its design and outcome (abstract). The International Society for the Study of the Lumbar Spine 12th Annual Meeting, Sydney, Australia, April 1985.

88. Robinson GE: A combined approach to a medical problem—the Canadian Back Education Units. *Can J Psychiatry* 24:138, 1980.

89. McGill CM: Industrial back problems, a control program. *J Occup Med* 10:174, 1968.

90. Kelsey JL: An epidemiological study of acute herniated lumbar intervertebral discs. *Rheumatol Rehabil* 14:144, 1975.

Chapter 23

LUMBAR TRACTION

GARY D. GOLDISH, MD

Traction is taken from the Latin *tractio,* meaning to draw or apply force in order to pull on an object. Lumbar traction has been in use in one form or another since the beginning of recorded history. Egyptian priests treated deformities and painful local conditions of the spine with traction (1). Hippocrates (460–357 BC) used traction tables in the fifth century BC for the treatment of dislocations, fractures, and spinal deformities (2). Avicenna (980–1037) and Ambroise Paré (1510–1590) applied traction along with manipulation to treat scoliosis (2). Traction resurfaced in modern medical literature during the early 19th century when leg traction was used to stabilize and decompress femur fractures. During the Civil War, Dr. Gurdon Buck attached tape to the skin of the leg in order to suspended a traction rope over a pulley at the end of the bed. This form of traction is often called Buck's extension, skin traction, or leg traction. Sometime around the turn of the century, leg traction was applied bilaterally in an attempt to treat low back pain and sciatica. In 1954 Dr. Samuel Vargo described the use of a pelvic belt for the attachment of the traction rope (3). This pelvic traction became a popular treatment for low back pain and sciatica. Over the ensuing years a flurry of literature has appeared, describing numerous methods for applying traction to the lumbar spine. Clinical trials of these various methods have produced conflicting results. This chapter reviews the literature on lumbar traction and tries to develop a rational approach for its use.

BIOMECHANICAL AND PHYSIOLOGICAL PRINCIPLES OF LUMBAR TRACTION

STABILIZATION/IMMOBILIZATION

It has often been stated that traction's main therapeutic effect is to keep the patient immobilized at strict bed rest. Outpatient traction would not have any true stabilizing or immobilizing effect, since between treatments the patient is ambulatory. Even when traction is applied continuously (i.e., 24 hours/day) to the lumbar spine, the patient is not actually immobilized, because the applied force is not strong enough to prevent the powerful trunk muscle from moving the spinal segments. Stronger forces, if applied continuously, would cause skin discomfort and breakdown. If traction does not actually produce true immobilization, is it any better than just bed rest alone? Traction would tend to improve compliance by enforcing bed rest, but this alone hardly justifies the added expense and personnel time.

Later in this chapter it will be noted that appropriately applied lumbar traction can decompress traumatized tissue, thus leading to a reduction in muscle spasm, pain, and inflammation. Pain therefore acts as a constant reminder not to move. An example of this concept is Buck's traction for the treatment of femoral fractures. Although the patient could easily overcome the relatively small force of traction, it is quickly apparent that if he/she does not try to resist the traction, his/her muscle spasm relaxes and the fracture remains in good alignment. Even the infant with a femoral fracture quickly learns to play in bed without resisting the traction. Thus, if the patient is more comfortable with lumbar traction then he/she is more likely to comply with the prescription of bed rest. In fact, comfort can be a guide to the adequacy of decompression. If the patient is still uncomfortable with traction then he/she may not be adequately decompressed. Conversely, if the patient is perfectly comfortable with bed rest alone then the addition of traction is probably unnecessary.

If we assume that some degree of stabilization is possible with traction and/or bed rest, then under what conditions and for how long should a back injury be stabilized? After an injury, initially a fibrin clot is laid down between damaged tissue. By the fourth day scar tissue begins to form in the fibrin clot. It is often unclear, for any given injury, how long the immature scar tissue has to be protected from motion. Too much motion risks disruption of the scar but no motion at all results in delayed healing and a shortened, irregular scar. Side effects of bed rest include generalized deconditioning, loss of bone mass, and significant adverse psychological effects. Very few low back injuries do better with any more than a few days of bed rest (4). One must therefore balance the need to protect the patient from further injury with the side effects of bed rest.

Bed rest and continuous lumbar traction should both be reserved for the more acute patient with an unstable fracture, unstable ligamentous disruption, herniated disk with acute neurologic signs, or severe incapacitating exacerbation of low back pain. Remobilization should be started as soon as the wound can tolerate it. This decision is usually based on radiographic appearance, as well as on individual tolerance to a gradually advanced and appropriately guided rehabilitation program.

If stabilization is considered to be essential to the healing process, then continuous lumbar traction may be a legitimate means of increasing the efficacy of bed rest. When we consider the cost of taking time off from work to stay in bed as well as the consequences of deconditioning, it may be justified to try to maximize the yield and shorten the recovery period by using lumbar traction in selected cases of acute lumbar pathology.

DISTRACTION

Distraction is the separation of surfaces by the application of tractional force. It is generally accepted that it is possible to distract the vertebral bodies of the cervical spine because the force required to overcome the weight of the head and the cervical musculature is relatively small. There has been more controversy as to whether the lumbar vertebrae can be distracted because of the greater weight of the trunk, the more powerful trunk muscles, and the more dense ligaments of the lumbar spine.

Coste et al. (5) studied two lumbar segments of a cadaver spine with the muscle removed but ligaments intact. They observed an average of 1–1.5 mm of distraction with 9 kg of axial traction. DeSeze and Levernieux (6) used segments T9–L5 from a cadaver and observed that 9 kg of traction produced 9.5 mm of elongation, 15 kg produced 11 mm of elongation, and 40 kg produced 16 mm of elongation. When the traction was removed 4 mm of elongation persisted, but when traction was reapplied no further gains in elongation were recorded. Twomey (7) applied 9 kg of traction to L1–S2 cadaver spines and measured an overall average increase in length of 8.7 mm. It would seem from these cadaver studies that a small but significant amount of distraction is allowed by the lumbar vertebral ligaments.

When assessing studies that measure lumbar distraction on live subjects one must keep in mind that the methods of measurement, methods of delivering traction, and amount of force all vary considerably from one study to the next. An example is the study by Rothenberg et al. (8) in which distraction was measured in six patients with ruptured intervertebral disks during posterior laminectomy. Bony landmarks were drilled into adjacent vertebral bodies and calipers were used to measure distraction. No measurable distraction occurred with 25 lb of traction applied to each leg while the patient was in the prone position. As will be seen later, this amount of tractional force would not be expected to produce any distraction since it did not overcome the inherent frictional force between the table and the lower half of the body. In addition, traction in the prone position would tend to produce less disk space widening at the posterior endplates compared to the anterior endplates. DeSeze and Levernieux (6) produced an average of 8–10 mm of lengthening of the lumbar spine with tractional forces of up to 366 kg. Lehmann and Brunner (9) measured an average of 0.3 mm of distraction per disk space of 300 lb of traction. Colachis and Strohm (10) measured an average of 1.75 mm of increase in posterior vertebral body separation during 100 lb of split-table traction. No significant distraction was detected when only 50 lb of traction was applied.

It would appear from these studies that if appropriately high tractional forces are applied to the lumbar spine, the lumbar trunk muscle and the weight of the trunk can be overcome. The amount of distraction in live subjects is similar to that observed in the cadaver spine with the muscle removed. It can therefore be concluded that with sufficiently high tractional force, lumbar distraction is primarily limited by the spinous ligaments.

If we assume that traction can produce distraction then how does this distraction produce a physiologic effect on the various disease processes affecting the low back?

Herniated Nucleus Pulposus

Cyriax (11) has hypothesized that traction can produce negative intradiscal pressure, which if strong enough can actually suck the herniated disk back in. Mathews (12) studied patients with what he termed "dynamic discography" during traction. He injected contrast into the epidural space in three patients and found disk herniations. Traction was then applied at 115–120 lb. Two out of three patients showed actual indentation at the previous site of disk herniation during traction. Anderson et al. (13) placed a pressure transducer in the L3 disk in four healthy volunteers during autotraction and manual traction. They found that intradiscal pressure went up in direct proportion to the force of pull during autotraction. Mean intradiscal pressure in the supine position was 110 kPa and standing was 270 kPa. During autotraction, intradiscal pressure went up to 540 kPa and during manual traction intradiscal pressure averaged 280 kPa. It was hypothesized that contraction of trunk muscles was responsible for increased intradiscal pressure during these two forms of traction. Anderson et al. concluded that at no time was negative intradiscal pressure observed, and therefore the disk could not be sucked back in, as proposed by Cyriax. They went on to suggest that in order to produce a relative reduction in disk pressure (i.e., below that obtained in the supine position but not actually negative), traction must be administered in such a way as to allow trunk muscle relaxation. Unfortunately, this study looked only at two types of traction, and neither method provides the type of steady tractional force that would be most conducive to trunk muscle relaxation.

Since herniated disks and degenerative disk disease are both associated with a decrease in disk space height, several studies have focused attention on the potential of traction to increase disk space height (5–7, 9, 10, 14). It is generally well accepted that bed rest results in an increase in disk height because intradiscal pressure goes down in the supine position. This allows more fluid to be imbibed into the disk, and the volume or height of the disk is increased. If the intradiscal pressure during traction could be lowered beyond that obtained with bed rest alone, then more fluid would be imbibed into the disk and the disk height or volume would be even more increased. To our knowledge, no one has compared the increase in disk height obtained with traction to that obtained with bed rest alone. An increase in disk height has been documented radiographically during traction but return to baseline was noted shortly after returning to a standing position (6, 9, 14).

Is a temporary increase in disk height actually beneficial? It may be helpful to increase disk height if the disk is merely degenerated but this may not necessarily be the case with a herniated disk. Patients with herniated disks frequently complain that they feel fine while receiving traction but when they subsequently stand up again, the pain may initially be worse. The intradiscal pressure is relatively decreased during traction and therefore the nerve root is temporarily decompressed. Fluid is imbibed into the disk, and the volume of the nucleus pulposus increases and makes it a larger space-occupying lesion. When the patient stands, the extra volume takes the path of least resistance and, rather than the height of the disk being increased, the size of the herniation increases. This may be especially troublesome if the nucleus is extruded. Thus, traction could in fact exacerbate a nerve root compression by a herniated disk if the patient is simply allowed to stand up without other intervention. This adverse effect can be avoided by appropriate instruction in posture, body mechanics, and rest between treatment sessions. Even if traction only produces a relative decrease in pressure on a herniated disk during traction, this may be all that is needed to decompress the nerve root and prevent progressive neurologic deterioration long enough to avoid the need for surgery. Eventually, as inflammation subsides, the nerve root may accommodate to the new narrow confines created by the disk hernia or the disk may degenerate enough to resolve the nerve root compression. If the disk is still contained, the hernia may be reduced and the ligamentous defect may eventually heal.

If the herniated nucleus pulposus is still contained by the annulus fibrosus or the posterior longitudinal ligament, pulling these ligaments taut may be another potential mechanism for decompression of the nerve root. Raney (15) demonstrated that during flexion, the posterior longitudinal ligament and annulus fibrosus are pulled taut, which flattens the myelographic defect of the herniated nucleus pulposus. He noted that patients with disk protrusion often say that flexion is more comfortable because of this effect. McKenzie's theory (16) would argue that lumbar flexion provides only temporary relief but cannot be expected to push the deformed nucleus back toward midline, because of the increased pressure at the anterior vertebral endplates. The flexed position actually may aggravate the situation by stretching out the posterior longitudinal ligament and annulus fibrosus so that it is even less able to contain the disk. With traction in a neutral axial plane, the pressure at both anterior and posterior rims would theoretically be the same. The force exerted on the nucleus by the taut ligaments would be equal around the entire perimeter of the disk and therefore would tend to push the nucleus back toward the center of the disk. This would depend on the integrity of the annulus fibrosus or the posterior longitudinal ligament and therefore would not be expected to be beneficial for an extruded nucleus.

Degenerative Disk Disease

Twomey (7) classified cadaver spine specimens according to age and degree of disk degeneration. There was no significant difference in overall distraction length according to age; however, there was significantly less distraction in those spines that had even one degenerated disk. One may conclude that traction does not have a significant effect on degenerative disk disease. On the other hand, the degenerated disk may have more to gain by traction, since *living* connective tissue conforms to the conditions that are imposed on it. One may also speculate that lowering intradiscal pressure by distraction may have an effect on the nutritional state of the nucleus pulposus because nutrients must diffuse across the vertebral endplate to get to the nucleus.

With a severely degenerated nucleus pulposus, there may not be enough nucleus to herniate (17); however, the annulus fibrosus and the posterior longitudinal ligament may cause nerve root compressive symptoms secondary to hypertrophy and redundancy. Traction thus would be able to pull these ligaments taught and thereby decompress the spinal nerve root long enough to allow inflammation to subside and to allow the nerve root to accommodate.

Lumbar Vertebral Fractures

Vertebral fractures are often managed by axial traction. The main effect is stabilization of the fracture in a decompressed and aligned position. This position is obtained by placing distracting force on the supporting ligaments. If the ligaments are intact then, just as with the nucleus fragment, the fracture fragment may be drawn back into alignment and away from the spinal cord and roots.

Lumbar Scoliosis

Lumbar traction has been used as a treatment of scoliosis and kyphosis. Traction is still used in Europe for the treatment of structural scoliosis (18). The proposed mechanism of action is neutralization of the deforming force by applying a distracting force in a neutral position.

COMBINATION OF DISTRACTION AND POSITIONAL STRETCH

Cailliet (19) believes that traction does not normally distract vertebrae but rather decreases lordosis, thereby separating the facets, opening the foramen, and decreasing muscle spasm. Twomey (7) found that flexing a cadaver spine consisting of segments L1–S2 produced a 3-mm increase in overall length. Adding 9 kg of traction to the already flexed spine produced an additional 8.7-mm increase in overall spine length. Thus, forward flexion combined with axial traction produced more distraction of the posterior vertebral element than either one alone. This tends to contradict Cailleit's assumption that lumbar traction primarily produces a decrease in lordosis.

Colachis and Strohm (10) found a greater degree of anterior compression of the vertebral endplates than posterior separation when patients flexed in a Thomas curl position. When lumbar traction was applied at 18° from the horizontal, posterior distraction was much greater than anterior compression. In other words, while simple flexion exercises may separate the posterior elements, at the same time they also compress the anterior endplates. This can be detrimental when disk disease is present. Traction combined with flexion can be used to produce an increase in the separation of posterior elements without compromise of the anterior elements.

Foraminal Stenosis

Traction combined with flexion can be effective for the decompression of certain types of stenosis. Spinal stenosis has been subclassified into central, subarticular, lateral (foraminal), or extraforaminal ("far-out") (20). It is foraminal stenosis that sometimes responds to lumbar traction. The walls of the lumbar intervertebral foramen are formed by the facet processes posteriorly, vertebral body anteriorly, pedicle superiorly, and pedicle inferiorly. A stenotic intervertebral foramen may cause spinal nerve root compression or root sleeve irritation. Forward flexion opens the foramen by separation of the facet joints and the pedicle. The addition of traction would maximize this separation. Widening of the foreman even temporarily might be expected to relieve nerve root compression long enough to allow nerve root swelling to decrease.

Heitoff et al. (20) has described the following three types of foraminal stenosis:

1. *Up-down stenosis,* which is responsible for 92% of the cases of foraminal stenosis, most often at the L5–S1 level. Up-down stenosis is classically used to describe the foraminal stenosis caused by spondylolisthesis, but the majority of cases of up-down stenosis are caused by an osteophyte arising from the disk endplate or uncinate process of the L5 vertebral body. As the osteophyte enlarges it compresses the L5 nerve root up against the L5 pedicle. There is no potential motion between the osteophyte of L5 and the pedicle of L5; therefore traction would be unable to widen this type of stenosis. Up-down stenosis also occurs when an osteophyte arises from the superior margin of S1. As the osteophyte enlarges or as the L5–S1 disk space collapses, the L5 nerve root is compressed against the L5 pedicle. Since motion may still occur between the osteophyte of S1 and the pedicle of L5, traction could potentially widen this type of stenotic lesion.
2. *Front-back stenosis,* which is caused by hypertrophic encroachment on the foraminal space by the articular process of the facet joints. Nerve root compression is rare because the nerve root lies superiorly in the foreman just below the pedicle, whereas most of the hypertrophic changes occur more inferiorly. When the nerve root does get compressed it is usually between the upper ventral aspect of the superior articular process of the lower segment and the vertebral body of the higher segment. If the facet joint is not fused, traction combined with forward flexion would pull the superior articular process away from the vertebral body and, at least temporarily, decompress the nerve root.
3. *Pinhole stenosis,* which is a combination of the elements that cause up-down and front-back stenosis. It is usually difficult to determine radiographically if any of the bony confines are mobile; therefore a trial of traction is appropriate.

Lumbar traction can also be used in combination with lumbar extension, rotation, or lateral bend. This can be accomplished by changing the position of the patient during traction or by changing the direction of tractional pull (see below for details of techniques). Saunders (21) found in one healthy man that unilateral traction of 100 lb on a split table produced 10 mm of separation on the side of

pull and 2 mm of separation on the side opposite the pull. This was compared to side bending in the same individual, which was found to produce 7 mm of separation on the side he was bending away from, but 11 mm of *narrowing* on the side he was bending toward. Again it is apparent that traction can be used to prevent simultaneous compression on the side opposite where the stretching force is being applied.

Herniated Nucleus Pulposus
Saunders (21–23) noted that there is often a protective list away from a *lateral* disk protrusion or toward a *medial* disk protrusion. He believes that with unilateral traction he can maintain this protective scoliosis while intradiscal pressure is still minimized. He also believes that the mechanical shift of the nucleus pulposus can be corrected with proper positioning and angle of pull during traction. McKenzie extension exercises are occasionally not tolerated well because the disk becomes pinched off between the vertebral endplates. It is often helpful to start with traction in a flexed position and gradually progress to extension by positioning the patient prone on the traction table. When the patient is able to tolerate extension he/she can then be advanced to the standard extension program without traction.

Stretch of Contracted Connective Tissue
Scar tissue tends to heal in a disorganized, shortened fashion unless it is stretched. Even undamaged connective tissue has a natural tendency to contract with inactivity. Guarding of motion is a natural protective mechanism after an injury but leads to contractures of the involved joints. Chronic poor posture produces shortening of connective tissue in one direction, painful overstretch in the other direction, and a chronic deformation of the nucleus pulposus. This can lead to a vicious cycle of progressive poor posture, pain, and disk degeneration. Simple stretching exercises can be quite helpful for both prevention and treatment of these contractures. Concomitant disk herniation may make stretching exercises difficult because there are usually compressive forces in the opposite direction of the tissue being stretched.

It is also sometimes difficult to apply stretch to the specific lumbar segment that is contracted because there are multiple joints involved in the same motion. All but the involved segment may be stretched during a range-of-motion exercise. If one joint becomes hypomobile with respect to the others, then the more mobile joints may become relatively hypermobile in an attempt to compensate for the stiff joint. With manipulation, the slack in the more mobile segments is taken up or the mobile joints are manually fixed. Then the hypomobile segment is abruptly stretched or gradually mobilized.

With traction, slack can be taken up in the more mobile segments by proper positioning during traction. There is no need to immobilize the more mobile segments, because each segment theoretically gets the same amount of distracting force. Traction is actually a form of manipulation that is applied by mechanical means, thus enabling the force to be applied for longer periods of time (i.e., prolonged stretch). An abrupt stretch of connective tissue is more likely to cause microtrauma, which leads to inflammation and subsequent recurrence of the contracture. Prolonged stretch produces a longer lasting increase in connective tissue length because there is less microtrauma.

Breaking or Stretching Adhesions

Inflammation associated with injury can cause adhesions to form between any involved structures. These adhesions can restrict motion of segmental joints and the normal gliding motion between fascial plains. Adhesive scar tissue can also compress spinal nerve roots or restrict their normal excursion during spinal motion, thus resulting in a typical radicular pain pattern. Simple range-of-motion exercises may not be able to direct force specifically to the involved lumbar segment. Traction or manipulation can be used to direct a stretching force at specific adhesions. Manipulation may give a more rapid and dramatic effect, with a typical pop that is believed by some to represent the breaking of adhesions. Often these adhesions recur because inflammation is produced by this microtrauma. Thus, repeated manipulations may be necessary. Traction probably acts more by stretching these adhesions so that they are less restricting and therefore less painful. This effect may be longer lasting, especially if maintained by range-of-motion exercises.

Release of Apophyseal Joint Impingement

The facet joints may become restricted in motion by impingement of the meniscus, capsule, synovial membrane, or free bodies (17). Manipulation is often used to isolate the involved joint in order to release the entrapped tissue. Traction is another option for a lower, more controlled release of the impinged facet joint.

Relief of Muscle Spasm

A rapid stretch of skeletal muscle causes reflex excitation but a more prolonged stretch will produce relaxation. Both traction and range-of-motion exercises have the ability to relieve muscle spasm. Traction has the advantage of also being able to decompress painful structures at the same time. If painful impulses are relieved by decompressing injured or inflamed structures, then muscle spasm will be relieved as a result of relaxation of nociceptive reflexes. In healthy volunteers, erector spinae muscle electromyogram (EMG) activity decreased back to baseline within a few minutes of initiating lumbar table traction (24, 25) and tended to be lower than baseline with gravity inversion traction (26). Since these studies were done on healthy volunteers, there was no lesion that needed decompression; therefore resting EMG would be expected to be nearly silent. Therefore traction would not be expected to decrease EMG activity below this normal baseline.

Miscellaneous

It has also been suggested that traction exerts its beneficial effects on some patients by stretching the mechanoreceptors of the disk, ligaments, and apophyseal joints (17).

TYPES OF LUMBAR TRACTION

BED TRACTION

Bilateral leg traction (Fig. 23.1) and pelvic traction (Fig. 23.2) are methods still used for delivering traction while in bed. The traction rope is pulled over a pulley at the foot of the bed and free weights are attached. The patient may be positioned in Trendelenburg to provide countertraction for the upper half of the body. Very low forces are tolerated when traction is used continuously in this fashion.

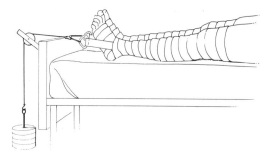

Figure 23.1. Bilateral leg traction while at bed rest.

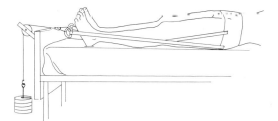

Figure 23.2. Pelvic traction while at bed rest.

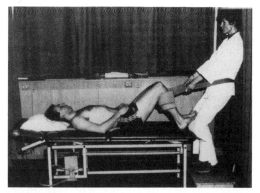

Figure 23.3. Manual traction. (From Ljunggren AE, Weber H, Larsen S: Auto-traction versus manual traction in patients with prolapsed lumbar intervertebral discs. *Scand J Rehabil Med* 16(3):117–124, 1984.)

A frequently cited study by Pal et al. (27) involved a blinded approach in which half the patients were treated with 3–4 lb of continuous bed traction while the other half were treated with 12–18 lb of continuous bed traction. No statistically significant difference in clinical response was seen between these two groups. However, in neither group was tractional force sufficient to overcome the frictional force between the bed and the lower half of the body; therefore neither group was actually receiving any traction to the lumbar spine. It was concluded from this study that any benefit from continuous traction devices is due to enforced immobilization rather than actual traction forces on the lumbar spine. This study is often cited as proof that all forms of lumbar traction do nothing more than enforce bed rest.

MANUAL TRACTION

Cyriax (11) uses a form of manual traction in which the therapist pulls on the legs to deliver the tractional force (Fig. 23.3). He noted that the therapist has a better feel for the patient's response to the treatment. Problems with this technique are similar to those with manipulation in that a sudden thrust of an uncertain amount of force is applied and can result in further damage. Furthermore, the patient may be unable to relax because the amount of tractional force cannot be anticipated, and a steady prolonged stretch is also more difficult to maintain since the therapist eventually fatigues. It has been estimated that slightly more than half of the therapist's body weight is applied as tractional force (28, 29). Comparison trials between manual traction and autotraction (28) and between manual traction and isometric exercises (29) failed to show any significant difference in improvement. Manual traction did provide greater temporary relief than the isometric exercise. It was therefore recommended that manual traction be used in the more acute phase, especially since force and angle of pull

are easily controlled by the therapist and the equipment is inexpensive.

Manual traction can also be used as a quick clinical test to assess if a more prolonged mechanical form of traction may be helpful. The examiner may pull on the legs while the patient is supine to see if table traction might be effective, or the patient can be lifted by the elbows while sitting to see if gravity traction might be beneficial. Cottrell (30) tested for the effectiveness of 90/90 traction by flexing the patient's hips and knees to 90° while lifting the pelvis off the examining table.

TABLE TRACTION

Table traction differs from bed traction in that traction is applied periodically on a therapist's table, rather than continuously in bed. Since table traction is not continuous, much higher tractional forces can be tolerated without risking skin breakdown. The simplest tables use free weights and a pelvic harness similar to that used with bed traction. With higher forces, a chest harness is usually used to provide countertraction to prevent the patient's entire body from slipping down the table. Mechanical gear systems have also been used (2, 11, 31), but have the disadvantage of being unable to automatically take up slack as the patient relaxes and the pelvic harness slips. Free weights, on the other hand, automatically and continuously take up slack as long as the weights remain above the ground. Unfortunately free weights can be quite cumbersome to deal with, especially in the amounts used with table traction.

Several uncontrolled studies have reported excellent results with mechanical forms of table traction (2, 31, 32). Mathews and Hickling (33) used a double-blind crossover technique to compare table traction to simulated traction. Twenty-seven patients with "clear sciatica" by history and physical examination were selected. The treatment group received table traction at forces of 80–135 lb while the control group received 20 lb ("an amount insufficient to overcome the inherent friction in the system"). Mathews and Hickling noted no statistically significant difference because of the small size of the group, but a trend toward better results was noted with the higher tractional force. This trend was also noted when the control group crossed over.

Home units with the same basic concept as table traction are available, but the patient usually lies on the floor rather than a table. Free weights, mechanical gears, or hydraulics can be connected to a door or a free-standing frame.

SPLIT-TABLE TRACTION

Judovich (34–36) studied the frictional forces involved with table and bed traction by making serial cuts at progressively lower levels of a cadaver and measured the force required to move the body part across the table. He demonstrated that the horizontal force required to move a body part across a mat was always about 54% of the weight of that body part. The surface resistance would be less with a firm, slippery mat than with a soft bed. He found that the weight of the lower half of the body below L3 was 49% of the total body weight. Therefore the force required just to overcome the surface resistance of the lower half of the body was 49% × 54%, or 26% of the total body weight. For a 150-lb male 39 lb of tractional force is needed just to overcome the surface of the lower half of the body, and any smaller force would not be transmitted to the lumbar spine.

Judovich (35, 36) proposed split-table traction to eliminate surface resistance (Fig. 23.4). As the name implies, a table is split into cephalad and caudal halves. The lower half of the table is freely mobile on wheels. In this way the lower half of the body moves freely with the lower half of the table and surface resistance of the lower half of the body is said to be eliminated. Mechanical testing of this principle has shown split-table traction to be 96.6% efficient with a load of 75 lb on the lower half of the table and a tractional force of 100 lb (37). Several versions of split-table traction are on the market today, and the more expensive tables have

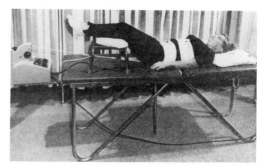

Figure 23.4. Split table traction. (From Hood LB, Chrisman D: Intermittent pelvic traction in the treatment of the ruptured intervertebral disc. *Phys Ther* 48:21–30, 1968.)

a computerized motor with automatic tension adjustment.

Hood and Chrisman (38) did an uncontrolled trial of split-table traction and reported slightly better than 50% excellent to good results. Christie (39) compared split-table traction to a placebo pill and reported significantly better results with traction than placebo. This study can be faulted in that any "hands-on" treatment is likely to have a higher placebo effect. Weber (40) compared patients treated with split-table traction at one-third body weight to a control group with simulated traction ("only enough force to tighten the straps"). The study group consisted of 72 patients with disk herniation as diagnosed by myelogram. There was no significant difference between the two groups as far as pain ratings, spine mobility, or neurologic signs after treatment. However, it should be noted that one-third body weight on a split table is usually the minimum or initial force used for lumbar traction.

AUTOTRACTION

Lind (41) first described autotraction in her 1974 thesis as consisting of a table that is split and hinged to allow lumbar motion in three planes during simultaneous traction (Fig. 23.5). The pelvis is secured by a harness and the patient provides the tractional force by pulling on arm bars at the head of the table. The patient is usually able to maintain a pull of 400–800 Newtons from a few seconds to at the most a couple of minutes. Treatment sessions usually last about 1 hour, or until the patient is exhausted. Lumbar rotation and lordosis are gradually normalized as treatment progresses.

Autotraction as originally described by Lind includes strict bed rest, a corset, a lumbar roll belt, equalization of leg lengths, and back ergonomic

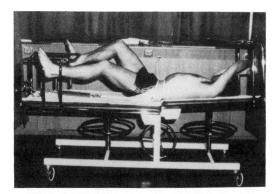

Figure 23.5. Autotraction. (From Ljunggren AE, Weber H, Larsen S: Auto-traction versus manual traction in patients with prolapsed lumbar intervertebral discs. *Scand J Rehabil Med* 16(3):117–124, 1984.)

education. In her original thesis, Lind claimed 100% excellent results in a controlled study. In an uncontrolled study, she treated 20 patients, with myelogram-documented disk herniation, and reported that 15 recovered so dramatically that no surgery was needed. She also reported a 30% increase in disk height during autotraction, but only at the posterior vertebral endplates. Not surprisingly, this posterior distraction was most marked when hips and lumbar spine were flexed.

Autotraction has become very popular in Europe and is starting to receive considerable attention in the United States. Variations along the same theme have been reported elsewhere (42, 43). Considerable recent European literature has further explored the clinical application of autotraction. For example, Ljunggren et al. (28) compared autotraction to manual traction in 52 patients with disk prolapse. Approximately 25% in both groups avoided surgery, so the authors concluded that manual traction was as effective as autotraction. Larson et al. (44) treated 41 patients with a 1-week course of autotraction as described by Lind, and 42 controls with corset, lumbar roll, ergonomic education, and 1 week of bed rest. All patients had "sciatica" of 2–14 weeks' duration, and with or without neurologic deficits. At 1 week, 15% of the traction group and none of the control group had resolved completely. At 3 weeks 17% of the traction group and 7% of the control group had resolved. At 3 months there was no statistical difference between the two groups.

Gillstrom and Ehrnberg (45) applied autotraction to 45 patients with "sciatica" present for greater than 6 weeks, resulting in improvement in 79%. Gillstrom et al. (46, 47) performed two similar

studies with myelography computed tomography (CT) scan–documented disk herniations. Follow-up myelograms and CT scans failed to reveal any change in appearance of the disk despite favorable clinical results. In four patients CT scans were obtained during autotraction and again no radiographic change in appearance of the disk was seen. In another study, Ljunggren and Eldevik (48) reported 47% clinical improvement with autotraction, but again no change in CT scan appearance of the disk herniation was noted even after 3 months of sustained symptom improvement. Natchev and Valentino (49) also looked at CT scans before and after autotraction in 17 patients with disk herniations. Eleven cases demonstrated no radiographic change in appearance, two had decreased in size, two had increased in size, and two had a change in shape. At the very least, autotraction seems to be adding to the controversy over the correlation between symptoms and radiographic appearance of disk herniations.

COTTRELL 90/90 BACKTRAC

Cottrell (30, 50) introduced a system of traction that involves positioning the patient with the knees and hips bent at 90° while the pelvis is tilted to decrease lumbar lordosis (Fig. 23.6). A rope attached to a pelvic belt is draped over the top of a triangular frame, and the patient pulls on the rope to lift the pelvis off the floor. Cottrell traction can also be initiated in a hospital bed by attaching it to the bed frame. Cottrell traction is usually well tolerated and easy to apply and can be sent home with the patient. In an uncontrolled study, Cottrell (30) reported 97% complete relief in acute low back pain and 94% improvement in chronic low back pain. In another uncontrolled study, Hanai et al. (51) reported 87% subjective improvement. They also compared lateral radiographs supine and while

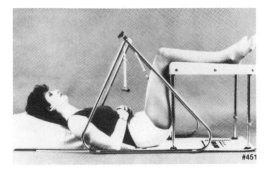

Figure 23.6. Cottrell 90/90 traction. (From Backtrac 1987 brochure, photo #451. Lossing Orthopedic, Minneapolis, MN.)

in Cottrell traction, and measured greater posterior disk distraction than anterior disk compression. It should be noted that flexing the hips to 90° without traction also produces posterior distraction; therefore radiographic comparison between this position with and without 90/90 traction applied needs to be evaluated. Dimaggio and Mooney (52) compared Cottrell traction, the McKenzie program, and back school in 136 patients with low back and/or leg pain. They found that 97% improved with the McKenzie program, while only 50% improved with Cottrell traction and 38% with back school.

At the Institute for Low Back Care in Minneapolis, Cottrell traction is frequently used for distraction of the posterior elements. It is gentle, patient controlled, well tolerated, and therefore especially effective for the older individual who is often troubled by foraminal stenosis.

INVERSION TRACTION

Sheffield (53) was one of the first to report the use of inversion traction in 1964. He adapted a tilt table so that the patient is suspended upside down by the lower extremities; thus the upper half of the body provides tractional force to the lumbar spine. Today several inversion devices are on the market (Fig. 23.7) (54), but the limiting factor in all of these devices is the intolerance of most people to hang in an inverted position. Reported side effects include headache, hypertension, nasal congestion, nausea, dizzyness, petechial hemorrhages, increased intraocular pressure, and reversible visual field defects (55–58). Equipment failure has re-

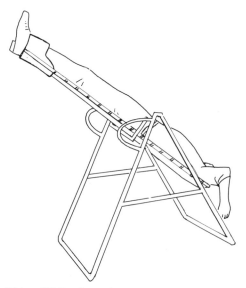

Figure 23.7. Inversion traction.

sulted in quadriplegia (54). The only clinical trial of the results of inversion traction (55) found 13 out of 16 patients were subjectively improved while inverted, and distraction averaged 1.7 mm/disk space.

GRAVITY TRACTION

Using the body's own weight as the source of tractional force is not a new idea. Hippocrates attached patients to a ladder, head up or down, and then dropped the ladder from a second story roof to the ground (2). In 1954 Fazer (59) described a technique of suspending the patient from a chest corset with upper arm gutters. Counterforce was supplied by a pelvic band attached to the floor and a crank was used to increase the force of traction. Since friction from a table is eliminated, the entire weight of the lower half of the body provides additional tractional force. Lehmann and Brunner (9) used a similar vest, but up to 300 lb of intermittent traction was delivered by a hydraulic machine. Complications included "uncomfortable stretch and tendency for fainting." There is also potential for radical nerve compression by the upper arm gutters. Masturzo in 1955 (60) and Gray in 1963 (61) both published reports on the use of an inclined plane with the upper half of the body secured by a chest corset. The lower half of the body was allowed to slip down the incline and thus provide tractional force to the lumbar spine.

Burton and Nida (62) introduced Gravity Lumbar Reduction (GLR) at Sister Kenney Institute back in 1974 (Fig. 23.8). GLR consists of an adjustable incline table with the upper half of the body secured to the caudal end of the table by a soft foam-rubber chest harness. The lower half of the body provides tractional force to the lumbar spine as it slides down the incline. Tractional force is increased by increasing the angle of the incline. With gradual increases, most patients can tolerate incline angles of 60–90°. At an angle of 90°, an estimated 40% of total body weight is providing tractional force. At lower angles the force drops off as a result of friction between the lower half of the body and the table, as well as loss of vertical vector force. The attractiveness of GLR is heightened by the fact that it can be continued at home.

In a retrospective analysis, Salib (63) reported 78% good to excellent response in private-pay patients and 70% in compensation or litigation patients when the disk herniation was acute (within 6 weeks of onset). Response dropped to 47% and 21%, respectively, in chronic cases. Oudenhoven (64) reported similar good results in patients with noncompensible unoperated low back pain, but re-

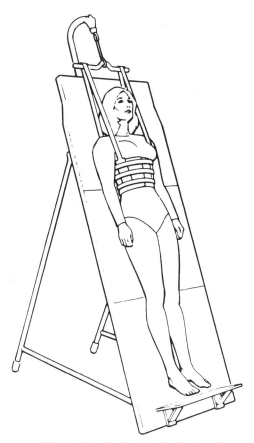

Figure 23.8. Gravity Lumbar Reduction therapy. (From Burton C, Nida G: *Gravity Lumbar Reduction Therapy.* Rehabilitation Publication no 731. Minneapolis, Sister Kenny Institute, 1976.)

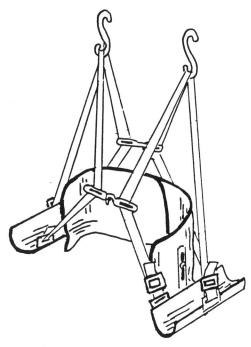

Figure 23.9. Prototype of a new gravity traction vest.

sults dropped off sharply with compensation cases and previous surgeries.

The greatest limiting factor to the use of GLR has been chest pain caused by chest compression (55). Several investigators (65–71) have documented the adverse respiratory effects associated with any type of chest compression; therefore pulmonary disease may be a relative contraindication to all forms of traction that use the chest for securing the upper half of the body. In addition, chest pain could lead to muscle guarding, which would counteract the force of traction.

Goldish (72) presented a prototype of a new gravity traction vest developed at the University of Minnesota, which improves comfort by distributing body weight over forearm gutters (Fig. 23.9). A new suspension system allows the vest to be open in the front, allowing free anterior and posterior chest expansion. The patient is able to tolerate a full

vertical position and therefore a simple doorway chin-up bar can be used. Traction is initiated by simply lifting the toes off the ground, and can be done intermittently by lifting and lowering the toes; therefore the patient remains in control of the traction treatment. Using data from the cadaver study by Judovich (34), 49% of body weight is below the third lumbar vertebra, and since there is no loss to friction this full force is producing traction to the lumbar spine. Higher force can be obtained by the use of ankle weights or a pelvic weight belt. Without a table behind the patient, the therapist can manipulate the back and pelvis during traction (Fig. 23.10). Modalities such as superficial heat, ultrasound, ice, or vapocoolant sprays can also easily be applied during traction to improve relaxation. For a prolonged positional stretch combined with traction, the patient can be placed in flexion, extension, lateral flexion, or rotation (Fig. 23.11). This new form of Interactive GLR requires a skilled therapist to utilize all of its dimensions. If maintenance traction is needed the patient can be sent home with a vest and a simple chin-up bar. Charles Burton, MD, and the author are presently combining efforts to develop this vest for clinical use.

Thery et al. (73) looked at spinal distraction while patients hung from a chin-up bar by holding on

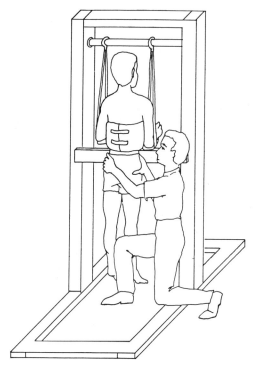

Figure 23.10. Interactive GLR—combined gravity traction and manipulation.

with their hands. Even though relaxation would be suboptimal in this position, Thery et al. found that 70% of their subjects showed an average of 2 mm of distraction per lumbar disk space. Sallade (74) described a modification of the McKenzie program in which the patient hung from a chin-up bar while

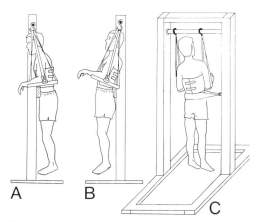

Figure 23.11. Interactive GLR—combined gravity traction and positional stretch. *Left,* Flexion. *Center,* Extension. *Right,* Lateral bend and/or rotation.

the therapist manipulated the patient's lumbosacral spine to correct lateralization. By combining distraction with manipulation, he was able to obtain a more rapid reduction with less guarding. Hanging from a chin-up bar can be used as a quick clinical test to see if more prolonged traction such as gravity traction might be effective. Sometimes patients volunteer that hanging from a chin-up bar or pushing up on the armrests of a chair relieves their pain.

OTHER TECHNIQUES

Numerous other techniques for delivering lumbar traction may be found in the literature, but those most commonly used have been discussed.

VARIABLES TO CONSIDER WHEN USING LUMBAR TRACTION

FORCE

Reported forces have varied anywhere from 50 to 810 lb, but the efficiencies of the different systems have also varied considerably. Most studies using split-table traction applied forces of between 50 and 120 lb, but this of course needs to be determined by individual tolerance and response. At these weights there does seem to be a high margin of safety since forces of 800 lb are required to rupture a lumbar disk (75).

TIME VARIABLES

Continuous traction is used 24 hours/day to decompress and stabilize acute back injuries. *Sustained* or static traction is the application of steady tractional force anywhere from a few minutes to about one-half hour. *Intermittent* traction involves a cycling on and off of tractional force during the treatment session, with cycles varying anywhere from a few seconds to a couple of minutes. The distinction between sustained and intermittent becomes somewhat gray when using over 2 min on/off cycles.

The advantage of intermittent traction is that higher forces can be used because there are no sustained areas of high pressure between the harness and skin causing discomfort. However, it is often argued that intermittent traction does not produce as much stretch as sustained traction. With cadaver spines, Twomey (7) found that 85% of distraction occurred immediately, and the other 15% occurred gradually over the next 30 min. Colachis and Strohm (10) found no difference between the posterior separation of lumbar vertebrae with 100 lb of sustained traction for 5 min versus

100 lb of intermittent traction for 15 min. Cyriax believes that traction must be sustained because it takes 2–3 min for paravertebral muscle relaxation (11). Hood and Chrisman (38) compared quantitative lumbar paravertebral EMG activity during 80 lb of both intermittent and sustained traction on a split table. Intermittent cycles were 7.5 sec on and 7.5 sec off. They found no significant difference in the EMG activity between the two methods. EMG activity fell to resting level within a few minutes with both methods. They concluded that Cyriax was correct in assuming that 2–3 min of traction is required for relaxation, but it does not have to be a sustained pull. However, if the goal of traction is to relieve an inflamed nerve root, then sustained traction would give a longer period of decompression. Intermittent or sustained traction could both be useful for stretching soft tissue.

Length of treatment session is another time variable to consider. Saunders (22) believes that traction for treatment of a herniated disk need not be carried out for longer than 10 min if traction is intermittent or 8 min if it is sustained. He believes that longer periods are not beneficial because intradiscal pressure equalizes with the surrounding tissue and the "suction" effect is lost. Weatherell (25) showed that lumbar paravertebral EMG activity decreased after a few minutes of traction but began to increase again after 10 min. In each individual case, a gradual increase in the length of treatment, with close monitoring of the clinical response, is the best method for determining the most effective length of the session.

Frequency of treatment sessions varies from twice a day to an as-needed basis with home units. The need for more frequent treatment in the therapy department should be determined by the results of treatment with early attempts at tapering to avoid dependency. *Duration of treatment* can best be minimized by close follow-up. If no improvement is seen after even a few sessions or improvement reaches a plateau, consider changing one of the traction variables or the type of traction, or discontinue traction altogether. If improvement lasts no longer than a few hours it may be worth considering a form of traction that can be used at home for maintenance.

POSITIONAL TRACTION

Positional stretch with autotraction and Interactive GLR have been discussed above. Lumbar flexion, extension, rotation, and lateral bend can also be obtained during split-table traction by changing the direction of pull or by changing the position of the patient during traction. Flexing the hips during traction provides some degree of increase in lumbar flexion (76) (Fig. 23.8). Lumbar flexion can also be increased by raising the angle of the traction rope above the table to increase lumbar flexion. However, as the traction rope angle is raised, true axial traction in the horizontal plane decreases because traction force is lost by lifting the pelvis off the table (37). This loss of force can be avoided by simply prepositioning the patient in lumbar flexion by raising up the head of the table or propping the patient up on pillows. Also, with this method, traction force need not be expended on fighting the erector spinae muscles. Moreover, most tables do not allow traction rope angles greater than 30°; therefore a greater range of lumbar flexion can be obtained by raising the head of the table.

Katz et al. (77) believe that by applying traction with the rope 15° above the horizontal the pelvis can be lifted off the table and thus surface resistance can be reduced enough to obviate the need for a split table. This hypothesis was tested (37) on a standard traction table at a traction rope angle of 15°. The split table was still 23% more efficient than the standard table.

The patient can also be positioned prone on the table to increase lumbar lordosis during traction. The head of the table can also be raised up while the patient is prone, to accentuate this effect.

Saunders (21) advocated the use of *unilateral traction* to maintain "protective scoliosis" while simultaneously allowing distraction. The method involves the use of a split table with a pelvic harness that is attached to the traction rope on only one side. He recommended attaching the rope on the same side as the pain, if the list is away from the painful side. He recommended attaching the rope to the side opposite the pain if the list is toward the painful side. A similar effect can be obtained by positioning the patient in side-lying on a pillow during split-table traction. Rotation can be obtained by appropriately wedging pillows under the patient during traction.

MODIFICATIONS TO INCREASE RELAXATION

The more relaxed the patient is the less the paravertebral muscles will be guarding against distraction. Narcotics and muscle relaxants have been used with traction but are usually reserved for very acute problems. Saunders (22) noted that modalities such as ice, heat, ultrasound, or massage before or during traction can be very helpful in evoking relaxation. Patient position also has an effect on muscle relaxation. Erector spinae EMG activity was slightly higher with supine table traction than with prone table traction (25). EMG returned to baseline within 6 min in the prone position and 8 min in the supine position.

CONTRAINDICATIONS

Contraindications that have previously been noted in the literature include spinal infection (osteomyelitis and discitis), spinal malignancy, cord compression from a central disk herniation, vascular disease, acute inflammatory arthritis, pregnancy, hiatal hernia, other abdominal hernias, severe hemorrhoids, aortic aneurysm, Paget's disease, severe osteoporosis, severe respiratory disease, uncontrolled hypertension, and claustrophobia (2, 22, 53, 78). Contraindications vary depending on the method and force to be used. Traction in patients with acute ligamentous disruption, dislocations, and fractures is contraindicated unless the traction is intentionally and specifically used for decompression or stabilization.

SUMMARY

After review of the literature it becomes apparent that a meaningful comparison of studies that evaluated the effectiveness of lumbar traction is difficult because there are so many different types of traction that have been used. It is rare to find a controlled trial of lumbar traction. In addition, most of the clinical trials have concentrated on the use of lumbar traction in the treatment of the herniated disk and all but ignore any other causes of low back pain that may be benefited by traction. Many studies have attempted to show radiographic changes such as increased disk space or a change in the appearance of the disk protrusion, but there is no clear correlation between these radiographic changes and clinical status.

Dimaggio and Mooney (79) have rightfully observed that the failure of most therapeutic modalities has largely been because they "supply only one mode of treatment to all patients—regardless of the underlying problem." However, it should be pointed out that this is mostly an artifactual problem induced by the study protocols, which attempt to minimize variables by comparing one modality to another. In clinical practice modalities are usually skillfully combined by the experienced therapist to enhance overall effectiveness. Using heat by itself does little more than produce temporary mild an-

algesia and relaxation. Combining heat with a stretching exercise often produces a greater increase in range of motion because the patient is more relaxed and connective tissue is more distensible when heated. Traction also need not be applied so one dimensionally. Combining lumbar traction with stretch, manipulation, and other modalities increases its potential therapeutic range, especially if applied with an understanding of the variables of technique and underlying pathology.

The effectiveness of lumbar traction is probably only limited by our understanding of the different causes of low back pain and by our understanding of the many traction variables that can be manipulated to provide a more specific treatment.

REFERENCES

1. Natchev E: *A Manual on Auto-Traction Treatment for Low Back Pain.* Emil Nathev, Tryckenibolaget i Sun dvall AB, 1984.
2. Neuwirth E: Management of sciatica by vertebral traction by means of mechanical table. *Rheumatism* 10:12–17, 1954.
3. Varco S: New method of pelvic traction for relief of low back pain. *Surg Gynecol Obstet* 98:760–761, 1954.
4. Deyo RA, Diehl AK, Rosenthal M: How many days of bedrest for acute low back pain? A randomized clinical trial. *N Engl J Med* 315:1064–1070, 1986.
5. Coste F, Gamiche P, Pajault L: Apropos du traitement des lombosciatiques par les methodes de traction. *Rev Rhum* 17:298, 1950.
6. DeSeze S, Levernieux J: Les tractions vertebrales; premieres etudes experimentales et resultats therapeutiques apres d'une experience de quatre annees. *Sem Hop Paris* 27:2085–2104, 1951.
7. Twomey LT: Sustained lumbar traction. An experimental study of long spine segments. *Spine* 10(2):146–149, 1985.
8. Rothenberg, SF, Mendelsohn HA, Putname TL: The effect of leg traction on ruptured intervertebral discs. *Surg Gynecol Obstet* 96:564–566, 1953.
9. Lehmann JF, Brunner GD: A device for application of heavy lumbar traction: its mechanical effects. *Arch Phys Med Rehabil* 39:696–700, 1958.
10. Colachis SC, Strohm BP: Effect of intermittent traction on separation of lumbar vertebrae. *Arch Phys Med Rehabil* 50:251–258, 1969.
11. Cyriax, E: *Textbook of Orthopedic Medicine, Vol II, Treatment by Manipulation and Massage,* ed 9. Baltimore, Williams & Wilkins, 1977.
12. Mathews JA: Dynamic discography: study of lumbar traction. *Ann Phys Med* 9:275–279, 1968.
13. Anderson G, Schultz A, Nachemson A: Intervertebral disc pressures during traction. *Scand J Rehabil Med [Suppl]* 9:88–91, 1983.

14. Lawson GA, Dofrey CM: A report on studies of spinal traction. *Med Serv J Can* 14:762–771, 1958.

15. Raney FL: The effects of flexion, extension, valsalva maneuver and abdominal compression of the large volume myelographic column. Paper presented at the International Society for the Study of the Lumbar Spine, San Francisco Meeting, June 5–8, 1978.

16. McKenzie R: *The Lumbar Spine.* Waiknae, NZ, Spinal Publications, 1981.

17. Tasuma T, Makina E, Saito S, Michio I: Histological development of intervertebral disc herniation. *J Bone Joint Surg [Am]* 68:1066–1072, 1986.

18. Calliet R: Spine: disorders and deformities. In Kottke RJ, Stillwell GK, Lehman JF (eds): *Krusen's Handbook of Physical Medicine and Rehabilitation,* ed 3. Philadelphia, WB Saunders, 1982, pp 720–722.

19. Calliet R: *Low Back Pain Syndrome,* ed 3. Philadelphia, FA Davis, 1981.

20. Heitoff KB, Ray CD, Schellhas KP, Fritts HM: CT and MRI of entrapment syndromes. in Genant HK (ed): *Spine Update 1987.* San Francisco, Radiology Research and Education Foundation, 1987, pp 203–236.

21. Saunders HD: Unilateral lumbar traction. *Phys Ther* 61:221–225, 1981.

22. Saunders HD: Use of spinal traction in the treatment of neck and back conditions. *Clin Orthop* 179(Oct):31–38, 1983.

23. Saunders HD: *Evaluation and Treatment of Musculosketal Disorders.* Minneapolis, H Duane Saunders, 1982, pp 143–150.

24. Hood CJ, et al: Comparison of electromyographic activities in normal lumbar sacrospinalis musculature during continuous and intermittent pelvic traction. *J Orthop Sports Phys Ther* 2(3):137–141, 1981.

25. Weatherell VF: Comparison of electromyographic activity in normal lumbar sacrospinalis musculature during static pelvic traction in two different positions. *J Orthop Sports Phys Ther* 8(8):382–390, 1987.

26. Nosse LJ: Inverted spinal traction. *Arch Phys Med Rehabil* 59:367–370, 1978.

27. Pal B, Mangion P, Hossain MA, Diffey BL: A controlled trial of continuous lumbar traction in back pain and sciatica. *Br J Rheumatol* 25:181–183, 1986.

28. Ljunggren AE, Weber H, Larsen S: Auto-traction versus manual traction in patients with prolapsed lumbar intervertebral discs. *Scand J Rehabil Med* 16(3):117–124, 1984.

29. Weber H, Ljunggren AE, Walker L: Traction therapy in patients with herniated lumbar intervertebral discs. *J Oslo City Hosp* 34:61–70, 1984.

30. Cottrell GW: New, conservative, and exceptionally effective treatment for low back pain. *Comp Ther* 11(11):59–65, 1985.

31. Neuwirth E, Hilde W, Campbell R: Tables of vertebral elongation in the treatment of sciatica. *Arch Phys Med* 33:455–460, 1952.

32. Parsons WB, Cummings JDA: Mechanical traction in lumbar disc syndrome. *Can Med Assoc J* 77:7–11, 1957.

33. Mathews JA, Hickling J: Lumbar traction: a double-blind controlled study for sciatica. *Rheumatol Rehabil* 14:222–225, 1975.

34. Judovich BD: Lumbar traction therapy and dissipated force factors. *J Lancet (Minneapolis)* 74:411–414, 1954.

35. Judovich BD: Lumbar traction therapy: elimination of physical factors that prevent lumbar stretch. *JAMA* 159:549, 1955.

36. Judovich BD, Nobel GR: Traction therapy: a study of resistance factors, preliminary report on a new method of lumbar traction. *Am J Surg* 93:108–114, 1957.

37. Goldish GD: A study of the mechanical efficiency of split table traction. *Spine* 1989 (in press).

38. Hood LB, Chrisman D: Intermittent pelvic traction in the treatment of the ruptured intervertebral disc. *Phys Ther* 48:21–30, 1968.

39. Christie BGB: Discussion on the treatment of backache by traction. *Proc R Soc Med* 48(2):811, 1955.

40. Weber H: Traction therapy in sciatica due to disc prolapse. *J Oslo City Hosp* 23:167–176, 1973.

41. Lind GAM: Auto-traction-treatment of low back pain and sciatica. *Scand J Rehabil Med* 2:37–42, 1974.

42. Bihaung O: Autotraksjon for ischialgipasienter. En kontrollert sammenlikning mellon effekten av Auto-traksjon-B og isometriske ad modum Hume Kendell og Jenkins. *Fysioterapeuten* 45:377–379, 1978.

43. Myrin SO: *Bedomning av Ryggpatienter.* Stockholm, LIC Rehab, 1978.

44. Larson U, et al: Auto-traction for treatment of lumbago-sciatica. A multicentre controlled investigation. *Acta Orthop Scand* 51:791–798, 1980.

45. Gillstrom P, Ehrnberg A: Long-term results of auto-traction in treatment of lumbago and sciatica. An attempt to correlate clinical results with objective parameters. *Arch Orthop Trauma Surg* 104:244–298, 1985.

46. Gillstrom P, Ericson K, Hindmarsh T: Computed tomography examination of the influence of auto-traction on herniation of the lumbar disc. *Arch Orthop Trauma Surg* 104:289–293, 1985.

47. Gillstrom P, Ericson K, Hindmarsh T: Auto-traction in lumbar disc herniation. A myelographic study before and after treatment. *Arch Orthop Trauma Surg* 104:207–210, 1985.

48. Ljunggren AE, Eldevik P: Auto-traction in lumbar disc herniation with CT examination before and after treatment, showing no change in appearance of the herniated tissue. *J Oslo City Hosp* 36:87–91, 1986.

49. Natchev E, Valentino V: Low back pain and disc hernia observation during autotraction treatment. *Manual Med* 1:39–42, 1984.

50. Cottrell GW: 90/90 traction in the treatment of low back pain. *Orthop Trans J Bone Joint Surg* 4(1):80, 1981.

51. Hanai K, Kamei K, Nojiri H: 90/90 traction for lumbar disc herniation. *Contemp Orthop* 16(6):1–7, 1988.

52. Dimaggio A, Mooney V: The McKenzie program: ex-

ercise effective against back pain. *J Musculoskel Med* 4(12):63–74, 1987.

53. Sheffield FJ: Adaptation of tilt table for lumbar traction. *Arch Phys Med Rehabil* 4:469–472, 1964.

54. Lancourt JE: Traction technique for low back pain. *J Musculoskel Med* 3(4):44–50, 1986.

55. Gianakopoulos G, Waylonis GW, Grant PA, Tottle DO, Blazek JV: Inversion devices: their role in producing lumbar distraction. *Arch Phys Med Rehabil* 66:100–102, 1985.

56. Plocher DW: Inversion petechia (letter). *N Engl J Med* 307:22, 1982.

57. Sanborn GE, Friberg TE, Allen R: Optic nerve dysfunction during gravity inversion. Visual field abnormalities. *Arch Ophthalmol* 105:774–776, 1987.

58. Friberg RR, Weinreb RN: Ocular manifestation of gravity inversion. *JAMA* 253:1755–1757, 1985.

59. Frazer EH: Use of traction in backache. *Med J Aust* 2:694–697, 1954.

60. Masturzo A: Vertebral traction for treatment of sciatica. *Rheumatism* 11:62–67, 1955.

61. Gray RJ: The lumbar disc syndrome: a preliminary report on a method of treatment combining body weight traction on a inclined plane and manipulation. *Med J Aust* 50–441, 1963.

62. Burton C, Nida G: *Gravity Lumbar Reduction Therapy.* Rehabilitation Publication no 731. Minneapolis, Sister Kenny Institute, 1976.

63. Salib R: Use of Gravity Lumbar Reduction in acute and chronic disk herniation documented by CT scan. Paper presented at the North American Spine Society meeting, 1984.

64. Oudenhoven R: Gravitational lumbar traction. *Arch Phys Med Rehabil* 59:510–512, 1978.

65. Caro CG, Butler J, DuBois AB: Some effects of restriction of chest cage expansion on pulmonary function in man. An experimental study. *J Clin Invest* 39:573–583, 1960.

66. DiMarco AF, Kelson SG, Chemiack NS, Hough WH, Gothe B: Effects on breathing of selective restriction of movement of the rib cage and abdomen. *J Appl Physiol* 50:412–420, 1981.

67. Klinberg PIL, Rehder K, Hyatt RE: Pulmonary mechanics and gas exchange in seated normal men with chest restriction. *J Appl Physiol* 50:412–420, 1981.

68. McIlroy MB, Butler J, Finley T: Effects of chest compression on reflex ventilatory drive and pulmonary function. *J Appl Physiol* 17:701–705, 1962.

69. Quain MB, Tecklin JS: Lumbar traction: its effect on respiration. *Phys Ther* 65:1343–1346, 1985.

70. Scheidt M, Hyatt RE, Rehder K: Effects of rib cage or abdominal restriction on lung mechanics. *J Appl Physiol* 51:1115–1121, 1981.

71. Sybrecht GW, Garnett L, Anthonisen NR: Effect of chest strapping on regional lung function. *J Appl Physiol* 39:707–713, 1975.

72. Goldish GD: Presentation of a new gravity traction device. Scientific Meeting of the Minnesota Physiatric Society, February 1987.

73. Thery Y, Bonjean P, Calen S, Roques JC: Anatomical and roetgenological basis for the study of the lumbar spine with the body in suspended position. *Anat Clin* 7(3):161–169, 1985.

74. Sallade J: Variation on Robin McKenzie's technique for correction of lateral shift. *J Orthop Sports Phys Ther* 8:417–420, 1987.

75. Harris R: *Massage, Manipulation and Traction.* New Haven, CT, E Licht, 1960.

76. Reilly JP, Gersten JW, Clinkingbeard JR: Effect of pelvic femoral position on vertebral separation produced by lumbar traction. *Phys Ther* 59:282–286, 1979.

77. Katz K, Mizrahi J, Ross S, Seelenfreund M, Maor P: Constant inclined pelvic traction for treatment of low back pain. *Orthop Rev* 15:540–545, 1986.

78. Yates D: Indications and contraindications for lumbar spinal traction. *Physiotherapy* 58:55–57, 1972.

79. Dimaggio A, Mooney V: Conservative care for low back pain: what works? *J Musculoskel Med* 4(9):27–34, 1987.

SUGGESTED READINGS

Barbor R: Spinal traction. *Lancet* 1:437–439, 1954.

Bettman EH: Therapeutic advantages of intermittent traction in musculoskeletal disorders. *GP* 26:605–608, 1963.

Biaco AJ Jr: Low back pain and sciatica: Diagnosis and indications for treatment. *J Bone Joint Surg [Am]* 50:170–181, 1968.

Boone T, Hammett J: Postinversion responses to inversion in normal subjects. *Arch Phys Med Rehabil* 69:502–505, 1988.

Boysen G: Sciatica, especially the prognosis by conservative treatment. *Acta Med Scand* 128:473–485, 1947.

Burton CV: Conservative management of low back pain. *Postgrad Med* 70(5):168–171, 174–183, 1981.

Chrisman OD, Mittnacht A, Snook G: A study of the results following rotatory manipulation in the lumbar intervertebral disc syndrome. *J Bone Joint Surg* 46:517–524, 1964.

Colonna PC, Friedenberg ZD: Disc syndrome: results of conservative care of patient with positive myelograms. *J Bone Joint Surg [Am]* 31:614–618, 1949.

Crisp EJ: Discussion on the treatment of backache by traction. *Proc R Soc Med* 48:805–808, 1955.

Durbin FC: The conservative treatment of sciatic pain by immobilization in a plaster jacket. *J Bone Joint Surg [Br]* 30:487–489, 1948.

Eie N, Kristiansen K: Complications and hazards associated with traction therapy in patients with ruptured lumbar intervertebral disc. *Tidsskr Nor Laegeforen* 81:1517–1520, 1526, 1961.

Gartland GJ: A survey of spinal traction. *Br J Phys Med* 20:253–258, 1957.

Gray FJ: An assessment of body weight traction on a

polished inclined plane in treatment of discogenic sciatica. *Med J Aust* 2:545–549, 1969.

Grechko VE, Rezkov GI, Puzin MN: Device for treating vertebrogenic lumbosacral radiculitis by the spinal traction method. *Zh Nevropatol Psikhiatr* 3:1158–1160, 1983.

Gupta R, Ramanao S: Epidurography in reduction of lumbar disc prolapse by traction. *Arch Phys Med Rehabil* 59:322–327, 1978.

Henderson RS: The treatment of lumbar intervertebral disc protrusion. An assessment of conservative measures. *Br Med J* 2:597–598, 1952.

Hickling J: Spinal traction technique. *Physiotherapy* 58:58–63, 1978.

Keega J: Alternations of lumbar curve related to posture and seating. *J Bone Joint Surg [Am]* 35:589–603, 1953.

Kekosc VN, et al: Cervical and lumbopelvic traction: to stretch or not to stretch. *Postgrad Med* 80(8):187–194, 1986.

Li YF, Fei JX, Luo ZL, Lu ZO: Traction and manipulative reduction for the treatment of protrusion of lumbar intervertebral disc—an analysis of 1455 cases. *J Tradit Chin Med* 6(1):31–33, 1986.

Lidstrom A, Zachrisson M: Physical therapy on low back pain and sciatica. Dissertation, Linköping University, Linköping, Sweden, 1974.

Mathews JA: The effects of spinal traction. *Physiotherapy* 58:64–66, 1972.

McKee GK: Traction manipulation and plastic corsets. In: The Treatment of Disc Lesions of the Lumbar Spine. *Lancet* 1:472–475, 1956.

Neagoe C: (Vertebral traction with Tru-Trac electronic device, a modern method of functional rehabilitation in cervical and lumbar spondylosis). *Vista Med (Medii Sanit)* 30(2):29–34, 1982.

Politer LP: A brief history of traction. *J Bone Joint Surg [Am]* 50(8):1603–1607, 1968.

Scott BO: A universal traction frame and lumbar harness. *Ann Phys Med* 2:258–260, 1955.

Siebens AA, Hohf JP, Engel WE, Scribner N: Suspension of certain patients from their ribs. *John Hopkins Med J* 130(1):26–36, 1972.

Stauffer TS: Gravity traction reduction. *J Neurosurg Nurs* 13(6):299–302, 1981.

Street DM: Roller board traction. *JAMA* 169:1876–1877, 1959.

Vanharanta H, Videman T, Mooney V: McKenzie exercise, back traction, and back school in lumbar syndrome. *Orthop Trans* 10:533, 1986.

Worden RE: A new spinal traction table. *Arch Phys Med Rehabil* 44:605–608, 1963.

Worden RE, Humphrey TL: Effect of spinal traction on the length of the body. *Arch Phys Med Rehabil* 45:318–320, 1964.

Yefu L, Jixiang F, Zuliang L, Zhengian L: Traction and manipulation reduction for treatment of protrusion of lumbar intervertebral disc—an analysis of 1,455 cases. *J Tradit Clin Med* 6(1):31–33, 1986.

Chapter 24

WORK CAPACITY EVALUATION

LEONARD N. MATHESON, PhD

This chapter presents the conceptual and philosophical background of work capacity evaluation and highlights some of the major evaluation and treatment approaches in the rehabilitation of individuals who suffer from low back pain. It is important to note that, while most of the work capacity evaluation services will apply without distinction between injured workers who suffer from low back soft tissue injuries and injured workers who suffer from intervertebral disk injuries, in certain occasions distinctions will exist. In each of these instances, the distinction is noted.

BACKGROUND AND DEFINITION

Combining elements of physical therapy, occupational therapy, vocational evaluation, ergonomics, kinesiology, and industrial psychology, work capacity evaluation can be conceptually described as occurring at the interface between medical rehabilitation and vocational rehabilitation. The rehabilitation professionals in each of these areas work together to assist the low back–injured worker to resume his/her preinjury roles. More formally, work capacity evaluation is defined as:

A systematic process of measuring and developing an individual's capacity to dependably sustain performance in response to broadly defined work demands. (1)

It is often incorrectly assumed that work capacity evaluation is primarily a measurement process. Actually, work capacity evaluation combines measurement with developments as dual aspects of the process. That this is so becomes apparent when one carefully considers the definition presented above and reflects that the force of the process is on "capacity," which connotes potential that is not yet

achieved. Just as the physicist must recognize that measurement involves interaction with the object being measured and, hence, requires a posture of uncertainty with regard to the true properties of the object, the work capacity evaluator assumes that measurement of the low back–injured worker not only marks current status but will precipitate further development.

WORK CAPACITY EVALUATION AND LOW BACK INJURIES

It is important to distinguish between low back injury, impairment, a "low back disability" (sic), and any vocational handicap that is the result of low back impairment. In concordance with Waddell's "biopsychosocial" concept of low back illness (2), the implementation of any approach to the treatment of low back injury, including the choice between a surgical or a nonsurgical approach, should often rest with the vocational significance of treatment. If any treatment provides a reasonable advantage over another in terms of returning the low back–injured worker to his/her usual and customary employment, it should be recommended to the injured worker. Work capacity evaluation is used to assist the injured worker and the treatment team to determine which treatment will provide sufficient functional return so that the probability of a return to work is maximized. As treatment is undertaken, it is necessary to determine when and whether the low back–injured worker can return to his/her usual and customary employment. Work capacity evaluation is used to determine if the injured worker has made sufficient functional gains to safely return to work. If a return to usual and customary employment is not possible, work ca-

Table 24.1
Stage Model of Industrial Rehabilitation[a]

STAGE	AREA ASSESSED	MEASURED BY OR IN TERMS OF . . .
One	Pathology	Studies of tissue and bone
Two	Impairment	Anatomy, physiology, psyche
Three	Functional Limitation	Symptoms and limitations
Four	Occupational Disability	Social consequences of functional limitations
Five	Vocational Feasibility	Acceptability of the patient as an employee in the most general sense
Six	Employability	Ability to become employed
Seven	Vocational Handicap	Ability to perform a particular job
Eight	Earning Capacity	Income measured over expected worklife

From Matheson LN: Work Capacity Evaluation. Trabuco Canyon, CA, Rehabilitation Institute of Southern California, 1982.

pacity evaluation is used to identify alternate occupations that the low back–injured worker may consider. If return to work is substantially delayed, work capacity evaluation is used in the identification and treatment of the psychological and social factors that impede return to work.

CONTEXT OF PRACTICE

Work capacity evaluation is most easily understood within the context of the "stage model of industrial rehabilitation" (3), which provides an organized framework within which to consider the issues that are addressed. The stage model encompasses eight stages, beginning at the point at which pathology is identified and extending to the point at which earning capacity is determined (Table 24.1). Each stage has one unique area that is assessed. Each area is assessed or measured in terms of particular types of information collected by different professionals. The stages of Functional Limitation, Occupational Disability, Vocational Feasibility, Employability, and Vocational Handicap are integral to work capacity evaluation and define its focus. These stages apply to low back–injured workers and, indeed, to all workers at all levels of employment.

FUNCTIONAL LIMITATION

The measurement of functional limitation is based on the evaluation of impairment[a] provided at a

[a] The American Medical Association, in its *Guides to the Evaluation of Permanent Impairment* (1984), draws a clear and firm distinction between disability and impairment. The AMA has taken the position that, while disability ratings are based on impairment, physicians must "refrain from speculating about non-medical consequences of an impairment." In addition, "it is not possible for a physician, using medical information alone, to make reliable predictions about the ability of an individual to perform tasks or meet functional demands."

prior stage by the physician, psychiatrist, or psychologist. While all functional limitations are of interest to the clinician, the focus of measurement of those functional limitations that are manifestations of the low back–injured worker's presenting impairment is encouraged by most compensation systems. That this is so short-sighted as to lead to substantial difficulties in rehabilitation is attested to by the author's experience with low back–injured workers who had completed rehabilitation programs but were unable to return to work. In a series of 227 cases, 23% of these "rehab failures" were found to have measurable memory deficits and 15% were found to have measurable visual acuity deficits that were uncorrected. While the impact on ability to return to work varied from substantial to negligible, it is important to note that none of these so-called secondary impairments were considered in these injured workers' disability ratings. Given this institutional bias, the usual approach to the measurement of functional limitations in modern work capacity evaluation is based on the dynamic function of the spine (4).

This artificial narrowing of focus is important to keep in mind because it leads to much of the disparity between degree of impairment and subsequent ability to work, especially with older workers and workers who are at lower socioeconomic levels. That this is actually an artificial narrowing of focus can be seen when one considers compensation systems that are based on the stage model, such as those found in the personal injury tort system and, indeed, found to be underlying even a schedule-based disability rating system such as that in California. The California State Supreme Court has held on several cases that the California Disability Rating Schedule (1972) should be only taken as a guide and should be set aside if substantial evidence exists that the economic consequences of an individual's impairment differ from what the

Schedule provides. While the burden of proof is on the injured worker in the workers' compensation system and on the plaintiff in personal injury tort actions, the author's experience with several hundred cases of these types leads to the conclusion that the current bureaucratic "disability rating" conventions will gradually be replaced with systems for evaluating the consequences of pathology that reflect the injured person's occupational disability separate from the pathology's economic consequences (5). These emerging systems follow the stage model presented earlier.

OCCUPATIONAL DISABILITY

Occupational disability is defined as *the vocational consequence of the patient's functional limitations.* Disability is a question of the manner in which these functional limitations affect the patient's customary work role. The determination of occupational disability is based on a comparison between the injured worker's residual functional limitations and the demands of his/her usual and customary job as presented in a job analysis that follows the U.S. Department of Labor system (6). This evaluation varies somewhat between individuals who have sustained low back soft tissue injuries and individuals who have sustained low back intervertebral disk injuries. For the worker who has suffered a low back soft tissue injury, the occupational disability is usually a biomechanical problem based on a mismatch between the injured worker's functional limitations and one or more of the following job demands, presented in order of usual importance:

1. Frequent submaximal lifting and lowering
2. Sustained off-center postural holding
3. Repetitive horizontal reaching
4. Vertical reaching below knuckle level
5. Infrequent maximal lifting and lowering

In slight but significant contrast, for the low back–injured worker who has suffered an intervertebral disk injury, the usual causes of occupational disability are:

1. Infrequent maximal lifting and lowering
2. Vertical reaching below knuckle level
3. Sustained off-center postural holding
4. Repetitive horizontal reaching
5. Frequent submaximal lifting and lowering

VOCATIONAL FEASIBILITY

Feasibility for competitive employment is defined as the *acceptability of the patient (as an employee)*

to an employer. We are concerned here with the work behavior of the employee-to-be. This is a transitional stage in that the low back–injured worker is no longer considered a "patient" and is now identified as a "worker." This is the first stage in which the injured worker is formally assessed in terms that are used by potential employers. The evaluee's work behavior is considered in general terms, with issues of productivity, safety, and interpersonal behavior of primary importance. Feasibility is the injured worker's acceptability as an employee in the most general sense based on those factors that any employer in the competitive labor market has of any employee. Some of the questions that are asked here are:

1. Will he/she be safe in the workplace?
2. Can he/she get to work every day?
3. Can he/she put in a full workday?
4. Can he/she get along with supervisors?

Employers consistently require acceptable responses to these issues, whether they are considering hiring a clerical worker, a laborer, or a physical therapist. These issues pertain to all employers and employees in the competitive labor market.

EMPLOYABILITY

Employability is defined as the low back–injured worker's *ability to become employed within a particular labor market.* This is distinct from the Feasibility stage in that the latter is concerned with the general acceptability of the injured worker as an employee in any occupation, whereas Employability is concerned with the ability of a person to become employed within a particular labor market. An injured worker may be feasible for competitive employment and may not be employable because no occupations exist in the particular labor market for which he/she qualifies. This happens with individuals who live in rural areas. This also happens with older workers in all employment settings, a rapidly growing problem for older females. As American society ages, females have remained in the workforce longer while males continue to demonstrate a stable retirement age. An increase in the number of older females competing with each other in the labor force, coupled with technological changes that are displacing unskilled and semiskilled workers at a disproportionate rate, has placed older low back–injured females who are attempting to return to work after a serious injury in a very difficult predicament.

Employability assumes that the injured worker is feasible for competitive employment. Employability considers the evaluee's work tolerances, general educational development, aptitudes, temperament, interests, and geographic location. It can be statistically calculated as the proportion of jobs in a particular labor market that are accessible to the low back–injured worker given the constellation of these factors that the injured worker presents to the labor market. In this sense, employability can be thought of as the probability that an injured worker will become employed.

VOCATIONAL HANDICAP

Vocational handicap has to do with the *ability of the low back–injured worker to become employed in a particular job,* and addresses the residual mismatch between a worker's capabilities and the demands of a particular job. The nature and severity of the handicap is wholly determined by the interface between the worker and the job. "How well does the low back–injured worker match this particular job?" is the issue here. It assumes that the injured worker is feasible for competitive employment and can find employment in a particular labor market. Within that labor market, there will be several occupations and, within each occupation, several jobs. Each job will be more or less demanding on the injured worker. Some of the job demands will be within the injured worker's work tolerances and some will be beyond these work tolerances, thus imposing a vocational handicap. The degree of vocational handicap imposed on the injured worker by each of the job demands must be considered. Unless the degree of vocational handicap is minimal or can be overcome through work hardening, training, or job and tool modification, the job will not be acceptable.

DOMAINS OF FUNCTION

Work capacity evaluation considers each injured worker in terms of three coincident domains of function. Additionally, the work capacity evaluator recognizes that each performance measure reflects the injured worker's most limiting domain. The three domains of function are:

1. *Biomechanical*—the demands placed on the worker by the work task that challenge the injured worker's anatomic and musculoskeletal levers and fulcrums. For the low back–injured worker, the biomechanical domain will be especially important in tasks that demand high strength and occur infrequently, or occasionally on a frequent basis (more often than

once every 2 min). Skeletal muscles produce torque at the various biomechanical linkages in the body. In the biomechanical model (7–13), the stresses on the musculoskeletal system during lifting are evaluated by combining isometric maximal strength tests with application of newtonian mechanics. Researchers using this model estimate the reactive forces and torque at various joints, including compressive and shear forces in the L4–L5 and L5–S1 disks. Recently, isokinetic techniques have been developed to determine lifting capacity through assessment of dynamic muscle strength (14–16).

2. *Psychophysical*—the demands placed on the worker by the work task that challenge the injured worker's self-perceptions, fears, and built-in work function themes (17). For the low back–injured worker, the psychophysical domain will be especially important in tasks that are similar to the task in which a traumatic injury took place. More to the point, it is tautologically the most limiting domain for most low back–injured workers who suffer pain disorders. The psychophysical model (18–26) predicts lifting capacities for several lifting ranges and sizes of objects with a degree of reliability that exceeds the biomechanical model.

3. *Cardiovascular/Metabolic*—the demands placed on the worker by the work task that challenge the injured worker's cardiac, respiratory, and metabolic systems. This domain will limit the worker in tasks that require prolonged, sustained work. For the low back–injured worker who has remained off work for more than 3 months and has not maintained a level of activity that approximates his/her previous work demands, the cardiovascular/metabolic domain will present significant limitations. Similarly, the injured worker who has become depressed will present problems that exist within this domain and exhibit themselves as malaise and fatigue. Research on cardiovascular/metabolic capacity for manual materials handling has its roots in exercise physiology. Physiologic models of endurance and the metabolic energy expenditure limits of the individual, often based on measurement of oxygen consumption during lifting tasks, have been offered by Bink (27), Bonjer (28), Erb (29), and Genaidy and Asfour (30).

It is important to note that these domains are pertinent in all work tasks for every injured worker, all of the time. The work capacity evaluator recognizes that every evaluee has one or another of these domains operating as the most limiting domain at all times. While the presenting issue may be clearly identified to exist in one domain, to perform work results in demands on the evaluee in all of the domains. Given the evaluee's particular strengths and weaknesses, the most limiting domain may or may not coincide with the domain that is the intended focus of study.

WORK CAPACITY EVALUATION GUIDELINES

Criteria for the selection of testing procedures developed by the American Psychological Association (31) and endorsed for use in industrial performance evaluation by the National Institute of Occupational Safety and Health (32) can be used as a guideline in the selection, administration, and interpretation of evaluation procedures. Every procedure used for the evaluation of a disabled worker or, for that matter, of any employee, must meet five criteria.

SAFETY

The evaluation equipment, procedures, and environment must not expose the injured worker to undue risk of reinjury. The evaluation of an already-disabled worker within the litigious medicolegal system requires more than the usual degree of care and professional acumen, and requires rigorous adherence to procedures that are accepted standards of community practice.

RELIABILITY

Reliability is the degree to which the evaluee's performance is consistent over time, between different raters, or across different parts of the same test. This is an especially troublesome factor in work capacity evaluation in that it is not possible to assume that the injured worker has "tried his/her best" or performed at a level that will be consistent, without regard to the previously demonstrated reliability of the evaluation equipment and procedures. Rehabilitation professionals have developed numerous measurement techniques and devices that are said to be reliable. The developers of those that are commercially available have demonstrated the reliability of their equipment in studies that assume that the evaluee is providing maximum voluntary effort in the evaluation task. This is not a safe assumption to make in industrial

rehabilitation. Given the litigious context within which the back-injured person is evaluated and treated, challenges to the reliability of the measure of performance are to be expected. Methods have been developed to confirm the reliability of the low back–injured worker's impairment (33–36), functional limitations (37), and disability (38–43).

VALIDITY

The third standard by which to judge evaluation measures is validity, the extent to which the measure of performance is related to some true criterion. That is, how closely does the evaluee's performance in the evaluation task approximate his/her performance when subsequently faced with the job demand? The Equal Employment Opportunity Act of 1974 requires that tests not unfairly discriminate against the evaluee. The focus is on the fairness of the discrimination. Obviously, tests must discriminate. In fact, a test that does not discriminate has no utility. Unfair discrimination is defined by the EEOC Guidelines as that which is found when individuals with equal probabilities of successful performance on the job have unequal probabilities of being placed on the job because of factors that are not relevant to the job, such as age, sex, race, ethnicity, or handicap.

The statistical determination of the validity of a performance measure is extremely difficult and, except in rare circumstances, will not be undertaken by the rehabilitation professional. The usual (and legally acceptable) alternative to the statistical validation of a measure is the use of content validation procedures that reflect the degree to which the measure of performance that is used to evaluate the individual samples the demands of the job for which the individual is being evaluated. The content validity of a measure is a professional judgment as to the degree to which the test measures the job's demands. The content validity process is based upon a thorough and systematic job analysis. Thus, a good job analysis is a necessary ingredient of the validation of any evaluation procedure. The value of the use of work simulation tasks in work capacity evaluation is that the relationship between the evaluation and the job can be easily demonstrated; work simulation has inherent content validity.

As the low back–injured worker participates in a work capacity evaluation program, he/she is evaluated in terms of current work tolerances. This information is used to develop inferences about his/her potential work capacity. It is important to keep in mind that work capacity is never directly measured; it is always inferred from the low back–

injured worker's performance. The distinction between work tolerance and work capacity noted above is coincident with the fact that there are barriers between the evaluee's demonstrated work tolerance and his/her inferred work capacity that cause the measurement of work tolerance in the laboratory to be different from the demonstration of work capacity at the work site. The evaluator must recognize that the validity of the evaluation requires a well-rounded and reasoned application of the evaluation's findings to the question at hand. It is not possible merely to assume that the results of a test will directly and unequivocally apply to the evaluee when he/she subsequently performs at the work site. Of special note here are the psychophysical issues present in the evaluation of every low back–injured worker. Such factors as motivation, fear, expectation of the outcome, and self-perception often strongly color the application of the finding and, hence, have an impact on its validity. Generally speaking, to the degree that the content of the evaluation varies from (does not simulate) the job's demands, the validity of the findings will be suspect.

PRACTICALITY

The task must be reasonably easy to administer and of reasonable expense. Equipment expense must be balanced against cost of administration. The evaluation must be accepted by the evaluee so that full participation is quickly achieved. Evaluation results must be quickly available, readily understood, and easily defendable.

UTILITY

Utility is the application of the findings to the problem at hand. It is often defined in industrial rehabilitation as "ability to predict future injury," but is more generally defined as "ability to predict future work performance."

DESCRIPTION OF SERVICES

It is important to note that work capacity evaluation is an "umbrella" term denoting a professional field of practice that includes work capacity evaluation and several specific services that may be offered separately, including work tolerance screening, work hardening, and specific vocational exploration. In a typical work capacity evaluation program, the low back–injured worker will receive all three services. However, each service is available separately and may be provided to the low back–

injured worker in place of full-scale work capacity evaluation. Additionally, after a work capacity evaluation program has been concluded, there may be additional need for services such as work hardening, which would then be provided to the injured worker on a more intensive basis.

WORK TOLERANCE SCREENING

Work tolerance screening is the functional evaluation component within work capacity evaluation, and is defined as:

> . . . an intensive short-term evaluation that focuses on major physical tolerance abilities related to strength, endurance, speed, and flexibility. (1)

Work tolerance screening is a generic term used in the vocational rehabilitation community to denote a form of work evaluation that focuses on work tolerances. It is a systematized assessment that uses evaluation instruments available in the public domain. Work tolerance screening may be offered as a stand-alone evaluation program or may be integrated into a full-scale work capacity evaluation program. When used as part of a work capacity evaluation program, work tolerance screening is conducted early in the process and provides benchmark measures of the low back–injured worker's development to allow the rehabilitation team to pace the worker's progress.

The usefulness of graded work simulation in vocational rehabilitation stems from the fact that the collection of *work-relevant* physical capacity information provides a context within which the evaluator can consider other factors such as the low back–injured worker's skills, aptitudes, interests, and temperament. An adult who has been injured after several years of experience in the workforce tends to have developed a constellation of these factors that center around a particular work capacity level. Physical work capacity is an *organizing factor* that is of central importance to the disabled worker. Additionally, without this work-relevant context, the validity of the evaluation findings is easily challenged.

Whether used as a stand-alone service or as part of a work capacity evaluation program, work tolerance screening measures the low back–injured worker's response to selected demands of work that are simulated and presented to the injured worker in a controlled setting. This work simulation allows the injured worker to demonstrate his/her own unique response to these work demands. The availability of this information can be of great benefit to the injured worker and to the treatment team.

WORK HARDENING

Work hardening is the primary developmental or theapeutic component within work capacity evaluation, and is defined as:

> . . . a highly structured, goal oriented, individualized treatment program designed to maximize the individual's ability to return to work. Work hardening programs, which are interdisciplinary in nature, use real or simulated work activities in conjunction with conditioning tasks that are graded to progressively improve the biomechanical, neuromuscular, cardiovascular/metabolic and psychosocial functions of the individual. Work hardening provides a transition between acute care and return to work while addressing the issues of productivity, safety, physical tolerances, and worker behaviors. (44)

Work hardening is effective for several reasons. The simplest (and not necessarily most important) reason is that the low back–injured worker becomes gradually conditioned to work through his/her involvement with work simulation tasks. Another reason for improvement is that the injured worker who has been afraid to perform job tasks begins, within the context of the work capacity evaluation center, to experiment with methods to improve his/her ability to respond to work demands and develops impromptu job and tool modifications in order to accomplish work.

An important part of the low back–injured worker's improvement in productivity has to do with the orientation to pain held by the injured worker. On admission, the injured worker is "disabled by pain" (a frequent self-description). Injured workers frequently report no change in symptoms over the course of the program while reporting a major improvement in productivity. Work hardening is effective in improving work performance because it teaches the low back–injured worker to maintain work productivity in spite of symptoms. "My symptoms are as bad as they were before but I can work now" is often heard as low back–injured workers complete work hardening. Work hardening is especially useful with individuals who have low back pain as the presenting cause of disability because the low back–injured worker is expected to take responsibility for his/her symptoms and experiment with different symptom control strategies. Experience has shown that each injured worker has a symptom control strategy that can be patterned to his/her own work behavior. Some people are effective in maintaining control of pain through pacing of the work. Others are able to maintain control of pain through the use of body mechanics or work

posturing. Each person has a unique strategy that must be discovered. This discovery is best accomplished in the laboratory environment of the work capacity evaluation center. While a pedagogic classroom approach to training in pain control techniques is useful to impart information, such instruction is minimally effective in bringing about the behavior changes (45) that will foster return to work. The opportunity to use the work hardening experience to experiment with these new behaviors under supervision leads to identification and subsequent adoption of enduring strategies.

As with work tolerance screening, work hardening may be offered as a stand-alone program or integrated into a full-scale work capacity evaluation program, often to learn whether or not subsequent involvement in a full-scale work hardening program would be likely to be of benefit. As a stand-alone service, work hardening usually requires 4 weeks of daily involvement, while the length of fully implemented programs ranges from 3 weeks to 8 weeks.

SPECIFIC VOCATIONAL EXPLORATION

The third component in work capacity evaluation is specific vocational exploration, defined as:

> . . . a systematic process of identification of appropriate vocational goals, including assessment of general educational development, vocational aptitudes, temperament, and vocational interests. (1)

In the specific vocational exploration process, the low back–injured worker's work history is combined for indicators of vocational direction through the use of a transferable skills analysis. With this information in hand, the evaluator is able to systematically develop a model of the low back–injured worker in terms of his/her general educational development, vocational aptitudes, temperament, and vocational interests. This information is supplemented with psychometric tests and work samples within the context of the injured worker's work tolerances to develop a model of the injured worker that can be used to interrogate one of several computerized data bases to identify occupations that subsequently can be explored more fully.

As with work tolerance screening, specific vocational exploration may be offered as a stand-alone program or integrated into a full-scale work capacity evaluation program. The low back–injured worker who enters a full-scale work capacity evaluation program will receive specific vocational exploration–type services as an integral part of the program.

SERVICES WITHIN A WORK ENVIRONMENT

The identification of the work demands that will be placed on the low back–injured worker begins with the physical environment within which the evaluation is conducted. Whenever possible, work capacity evaluation is conducted in a setting that simulates a real work setting. As an example, the Employment and Rehabilitation Institute of California presents two milieux, one that simulates an industrial setting and one that simulates an office setting. The industrial setting includes concrete floors, minimal temperature control, and substantial ambient noise. The office setting exposes the injured worker to professional-level office equipment, including computer keyboards and video display terminals used at work desks much like the desk one would find at a typical place of employment.

In addition, the temporal and rule structure of the work capacity evaluation program simulates the work environment. The low back–injured worker's day begins by selecting his/her time card from the time card rack, "punching in" on the time clock, and reviewing the clipboard on which his/her individual daily schedule is laid out in quarter-hour increments. The injured worker is involved in the work capacity evaluation program from Monday through Friday with regular hours that are set to meet his/her needs, progressing up to a full 40-hour work week. The following behavioral demands also must be met:

1. *Safety*—follow rules and instructions, do not exceed work restrictions, use proper body mechanics
2. *Interpersonal behavior*—accept supervisors' directions, get along with fellow workers
3. *Attendance*—daily, Monday through Friday
4. *Workplace Tolerance*—start each morning on time; take only scheduled breaks and return on time; remain in the workplace for a full work day
5. *Productivity*—work at the maximum pace that will allow:
   a. Next-day attendance
   b. Completion of the scheduled workday
   c. Sustained activity without an unscheduled break from work.

These demands are consistent with the expectations of employers in the competitive labor market. The subtle but very important prioritization of factors in this list is of central importance to the work capacity evaluation.

WORK CAPACITY EVALUATION PROCESS

The work capacity evaluation process can be presented in a series of flowcharts, the first of which is shown in Figure 24.1. The reader will discover that there are three contiguous "tracks" through the work capacity evaluation process. The process begins with a look at the low back–injured worker's job demands, against which are compared his/her job-relevant functional limitations in order to determine his/her occupational disability.

JOB ANALYSIS AND DATA COLLECTION

The work capacity evaluation process begins with collection of information about the demands of the

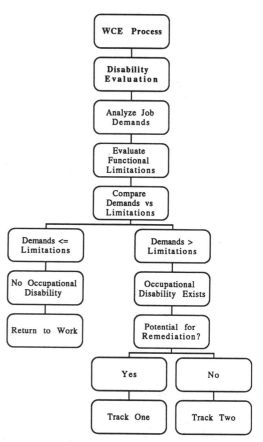

Figure 24.1. Overview of the work capacity evaluation process.

low back–injured worker's job. Using systems such as that of the U.S. Department of Labor (6) or the Lifting Risk Analysis (3), the clinician gathers information about the demands of the injured worker's usual and customary job in such a way that the job demand data will "dovetail" with the subsequent evaluation of the injured worker.

The job analysis system of the Department of Labor defines work factors in gross functional terms. While this approach complements the evaluator's subsequent use of work simulation tasks, it falls short of providing the degree of specificity required, especially with regard to the strength demands of work. This factor is measured by involvement of the worker with standing, walking, sitting, lifting, carrying, pushing, and pulling. Standing, walking, and sitting are expressed in terms of duration while lifting, carrying, pushing, and pulling are expressed in terms of both intensity and duration. Intensity involves consideration of the weight handled, position of the worker's body or part of the worker's body used in handling weights, range of motion under load, and aid given by helpers or by mechanical equipment. Duration is the time spent by the worker in carrying out each task. Carrying most often is expressed in terms of duration, weight carried, and distance carried. The five degrees of strength [*Dictionary of Occupational Titles* (46)], supplemented with ratings of typical energy expenditure based on metabolic equivalencies (METs) of work metabolic rate over basal metabolic rate [defined as the rate of energy expenditure requiring an oxygen consumption rate of 3.5 ml oxygen/kg body weight/min (3, 29)] are:

Sedentary Work—exerting up to 10 lb of force occasionally and/or a negligible amount of force frequently or constantly to lift, carry, push, pull, or otherwise move objects, including the human body. Sedentary work involves sitting most of the time, but may involve walking or standing for brief periods of time. Jobs are sedentary if walking and standing are required only occasionally and all other sedentary criteria are met. typical energy expenditure of 1.5–2.1 METs.

Light Work—exerting up to 20 lb of force occasionally, and/or up to 10 lb of force frequently, and/or a negligible amount of force constantly to move objects. Physical demand requirements are in excess of those for sedentary work. Light work usually requires walking or standing to a significant degree. However, if the use of arm and/or leg controls requires exertion of forces greater than that for sedentary work and the worker sits most of the time, the job is rated for light work. Typical energy expenditure of 2.2–3.5 METs.

Medium Work—exerting up to 50 lb of force occasionally and/or up to 20 lb of force frequently, and/or up to 10 lb of force constantly to move objects. Typical energy expenditure of 3.6–6.3 METs.

Heavy Work—exerting up to 100 lb of force occasionally, and/or 50 lb of force frequently, and/or up to 20lb of force constantly to move objects. Typical energy expenditure of 6.3–7.5 METs.

Very Heavy Work—exerting in excess of 100 lb of force occasionally, and/or in excess of 50 lb of force frequently, and/or in excess of 20 lb of force constantly to move objects. Typical energy expenditure of greater than 7.5 MET.

In this system, "occasionally," "frequently," and "constantly" describe activities or conditions that exist up to one-third of the time, from one-third to two-thirds of the time, and for two-thirds or more of the time, respectively. The author's experience in the use of this system in work capacity evaluation led to the development of the Physical Demand Characteristics (PDC) of Work chart (3). An updated version of this chart is presented in Table 24.2. The "PDC Chart" is in use throughout the world as a simple and straightforward means of summarizing the physical demands of a job and, correspondingly, the general physical capacity of a worker. As is readily apparent, however, this approach to the strength demands of work is not very specific.

In order to improve the specificity of the Department of Labor system and the subsequent validity and utility of evaluation procedures based on this system, the author has developed the "Lifting Risk Analysis" (1) based on guidelines developed by the National Institute of Occupational Safety and Health (NIOSH) (32). In 1981, NIOSH published the *Work Practices Guide for Manual Lifting*. The *Guide* reviews the causes of overexertion injuries with a focus on injuries to the lower back and provides recommendations about methods that can be used to assess and modify the injury risk of particular job tasks. The risks associated with lifting can be considered from three general perspectives.

Table 24.2
Physical Demand Characteristics of Work

PHYSICAL DEMAND LEVEL	FORCE IN POUNDS			TYPICAL ENERGY REQUIRED (METS)
	OCCASIONAL (0–33% OF THE WORKDAY)	FREQUENT (34–66% OF THE WORKDAY)	CONSTANT (67–100% OF THE WORKDAY)	
Sedentary	10	Negligible	Negligible	1.5–2.1
Light	20	10 (and/or walk/stand/push/pull of arm/leg controls)	Negligible, and/or push/pull of arm/leg controls while seated	2.2–3.5
Medium	50	20	10	3.6–6.3
Heavy	100	50	20	6.4–7.5
Very heavy	Over 100	Over 50	Over 20	Over 7.5

Infrequent Lifting—The primary risk factors to be considered in lifting tasks that are carried out on an infrequent (less often than once per 2 min) basis exist within the biomechanical domain. Lifting produces biomechanical stresses throughout the body based on the relationship between the amount of weight lifted and the method of handling the load. The load that is grasped by the hands and moved vertically combines with the body weight of the worker to produce rotational movements at various joints of the body. These forces are counterbalanced by skeletal muscles and by changes in whole body position to maintain balance.

Occasional High-Frequency Lifting—The primary risks associated with occasional high-frequency lifting tasks stem from the worker's exceeding his/her psychophysical limits. In psychophysical terms, strength is defined as the maximum voluntary force a person is willing to exert in a single effort. Endurance is defined as the force a person is willing to exert repeatedly for an extended period of time.

Continuous High-Frequency Lifting—The primary source of risk for continuous high-frequency lifting tasks has to do with exceeding the cardiovascular and metabolic capacity of the worker. The body has a finite store of metabolic energy that, as it is depleted, brings about fatigue and eventual exhaustion. In a related manner, the body has a limited ability to utilize available oxygen. Tasks that, in the short run, can be sustained without biomechanical risk and are acceptable to the worker on a psychophysical basis may, in the long run, produce fatigue and exhaustion as the metabolic and oxygen consumption limits of the body are reached.

In the evaluation of the risk of injury associated with any lifting task, all three of the risk factor domains must be considered. In order to facilitate the accurate evaluation of risks due to lifting, NIOSH has developed a simple mathematical model that includes each domain's primary components, the action limit (AL) formula (Fig. 24.2). The action limit can be taken as a unifying concept that allows a "risk boundary" to be established, given certain information about the lifting task. By collecting this information and entering the values gathered into the action limit formula, a value (expressed in terms of pounds) can be achieved that is the load at or below which 99% of the American adult male population and 75% of the American adult female population should be able to perform without increased risk of injury from the lifting task itself. The four variables in the action limit formula presented are:

Horizontal Displacement (H)—has the most potential impact. Horizontal displacement is primarily a biomechanical factor that rapidly increases the force of the load at each of the body joints by multiplying the value of the load by the distance that the load is displaced from the fulcrum, taken to be the L5–S1 disk interspace. Within 6 inches from the spine there is no discernible decrease in work capacity but there is a rapid decrease thereafter. It should be noted that objects that are grasped bilaterally in the sagittal plane will not be held closer than 6 inches from the spine because this represents the minimum possible abdominal depth.

$$AL = 90\,lb \times [(6 \div H) \times (1 - .01\,|\,V - 30\,|\,) \times (.7 + (3 \div D)) \times (1 - (F \div F_{MAX}))]$$

H = Horizontal displacement of lift

V = Vertical location of hands at origin of lift

D = Vertical travel distance from origin to destination

F = Average number of lifts per minute

Figure 24.2.   Action limit (AL) formula developed by NIOSH.

Vertical Starting Height of the Lift (V)—represents the effect of the vertical location of the hands at the origin of the lift. Optimal starting height of a lift is 30 inches from the floor, roughly comparable to knuckle height. Less than 30 inches from the floor requires that the worker begin to stoop and flex the knees to retrieve the load, with an attendant decrease in metabolic and cardiovascular efficiency. Lifts that begin more than 30 inches from the floor require additional upper extremity involvement, with a similar though less pronounced decrease in efficiency.

Displacement of the Load (D)—represents the vertical travel distance from origin to destination of the worker's hands as they grasp the load. The vertical distance over which the load is lifted has a slight but significant impact on safe working capacity. Vertical displacement of a load that is less than 10 inches does not decrease safe work capacity. Beyond this lower limit, however, safe work capacity gradually decreases as the vertical displacement of the load increases.

Frequency (F)—the average frequency in terms of lifts per minute has a direct and inverse relationship on safe work capacity. The primary factor affecting the extent of the decrement due to frequency is the posture in which the worker is performing the lift.

Derived from the action limit is the maximum permissible load (MPL), the point at which only 25% of men and 1% of women will not experience an increased risk of injury as a result of the lifting task. Maximum permissible load is derived by simply multiplying the AL times three. Job tasks that exceed the MPL are recommended by NIOSH to require engineering controls, which usually means redesign of the job itself. The range between the AL and MPL is quite large and represents a load that, if it is present in a lifting task, requires that the lifting task be undertaken with administrative controls in place. Administrative controls usually refer to selection of the individual worker so that the job's demands do not exceed the worker's capacity.

This author has developed the Lifting Risk Analysis as a straightforward procedure that accurately describes lifting in terms of "range of motion under load" (3). Based on the action limit, the Lifting Risk Analysis describes the lifting demands of a job in graphic form. It provides sufficient specificity about the lifting and lowering demands of a job to allow the evaluator to compare job demands to the evaluee's functional limitations and, thus, determine occupational disability.

MEASUREMENT OF FUNCTIONAL LIMITATIONS

The second step in the work capacity evaluation process focuses on measurement of the injured worker's functional limitations and the comparison of these functional limitations with the demands of his/her usual and customary job. (It is important to note that functional limitations are not merely the complement of the injured worker's functional tolerances. Commonly, limitations include prophylactic restrictions that stem from the impairment in addition to the functional tolerances that the injured worker has demonstrated.) This author has developed procedures to measure the functional limitations of low back–injured workers in simulated manual materials handling tasks.

An early study (1) with healthy male workers demonstrated the realiability of this approach. Subjects were 28 employed males, none of whom reported any chronic disability. All had normotensive cardiovascular responses as measured by pretest sitting and standing resting blood pressure measurement. Age of the subjects ranged from 28 to 63 years, with a mean of 40 years. Each subject was required to participate in the full evaluation procedure and repeat a portion of the complete evaluation procedure two additional times. After the initial procedure (trial 1) was completed, the subject was given a 15-min rest period. He resumed testing (in both trial 2 and trial 3) at a load that was approximately equal to 50% of the maximum load that he had been able to lift from shoulder to eye level in trial 1. The subject was naive about the trial 2 and trial 3 starting load. The weight tray was designed so that the number of weights in the tray could be masked through the use of a light cardboard cutout placed upon the weights. Trial 2 proceeded in the same manner as trial 1. In this manner, maximum values were obtained for trial 2 and, after a 15-min rest period, trial 3. The maximum load that could be lifted from shoulder to eye level was selected as the reference upon which the coefficient of variation was to be calculated. The transition from shoulder to eye level appears to be a critical segment of the range of motion in a lifting task, in all likelihood due to a shift in the biomechanics that are required. Coefficient of variation is an elegant means to compare the variability of measures that occur in a ratio scale, such as force, load, or weight. It is frequently used in ergonomic studies of able-bodied performance, especially those in which strength is the variable under study (15, 47). The coefficient is calculated by dividing the standard deviation of a set of scores by the scores' mean and is expressed as a percentage. An average coefficient of variation of 5.73% was obtained when the able-bodied subjects' shoulder–to–eye level maximum load was considered. The coefficient of variation is within the range of results reported by Kroemer (15) and compares favorably with isometric measures of lifting capacity, which are usually less reliable, typically resulting in coefficients of variation on the order of 10–15% (32).

In a study of the safety and utility of this approach

with a sample of disabled workers, Matheson (1) studied 162 ambulatory disabled adults referred for vocational evaluation. Seventy-nine per cent of the subjects under study were male. The age of the sample ranged from 17 to 68 years (mean = 35 years). All of the subjects were previously screened for presence of cardiovascular or pulmonary disease and were excluded from the sample if any indication was noted. Sixty-six per cent of these subjects had diagnoses that involved injury to the lumbosacral spine and/or supporting tissue. Twenty-two per cent of this subset had diagnoses that indicated impairment of the L4–L5 or L5–S1 intervertebral disk. Twenty-eight per cent of the subjects with lumbosacral injuries of all types also had other impaired body parts. The most frequently encountered accompanying injury was to the knee. All subjects had been disabled from work for at least 3 months, with a median time off work at the date of evaluation of 27 months. Each was believed by his/her primary care physician to be unable to return to usual and customary employment and had been referred for vocational rehabilitation. Eighty-eight per cent of the subjects were evaluated as part of the vocational rehabilitation program provided under the worker's compensation laws of the State of California. Based on subjects' response to questions during the evaluation and in next-day telephone contact, there was not a single new injury reported nor any exacerbation of a previous injury as the result of these procedures. Maximum load attained by a disabled worker in this study was 80 pounds.

In addition to the measurement of the strength of the evaluee, the relative risk that is a consequence of the evaluee's lifting style should be evaluated. Through the use of the High Risk Work Style Measurement system (1), it is possible to reliably document styles of manual materials handling in a clinical setting. The use of these guidelines to set functional limitations should increase the likelihood that a subsequent return to work will be as safe as possible:

Conservation of Horizontal Displacement—the ability of the evaluee to maintain minimum distance between the center of gravity of the load and the center of his/her spine at the sacrum is measured during a manual materials handling test in which the evaluee lifts a load in six-inch increments from the starting point to the extent of his/her full upward range.

Control of Spinal Torque—the evaluee's ability to maintain the shoulder in alignment with the pelvis while retrieving a weight from the lowest point of his/her range. The degree to which the evaluee maintains his/her shoulders in alignment with the pelvis is observed. Measurement of this factor is greatly facilitated through the use of stop-action or slow-motion videotape photography.

Stance—as the evaluee lifts a weight during a manual materials handling test from the starting point to his/her full upward extension, the placement of his/her feet is observed. Good lateral and forward/rearward stability is required in order to achieve a "plus" rating on this factor.

Pace and Object Control—the degree to which the evaluee controls the lifting and lowering of a load during a manual materials handling test, breaking it up into segments so that rapid acceleration and deceleration of the load is avoided.

REMEDIATION OF OCCUPATIONAL DISABILITY

If the injured worker's limitations do not preclude the performance of any significant job demand, the injured worker returns to work. If the injured worker's limitations preclude the performance of any significant job demand, an occupational disability exists. If potential for remediation of the functional limitations to a level that will allow return to his/her usual and customary job exists, the injured worker will enter Track One (see Fig. 24.1). If there is insufficient potential for remediation, the injured worker will enter Track Two (Fig. 24.1). In work capacity evaluation Track One (Fig. 24.3), the low back injured worker participates in a Track One version of work hardening. This approach to work hardening utilizes an aggressive approach to functional restoration (48), including biomechanical and cardiovascular conditioning, combined with the simulation of job demands so that the injured worker is prepared to make an immediate return to his/her usual and customary job. The focus here is on remediation of the functional limitations sufficiently so that an occupational disability does not exist. Track 1 work hardening begins with a comprehensive evaluation of the current functional status of the patient by an interdisciplinary team that includes a physician, psychologist, physical therapist, and occupational therapist. Based on this evaluation, a therapeutic regimen is prescribed that simultaneously addresses the psychophysical, biomechanical, and cardiovascular/metabolic domains. Such programs are pro-

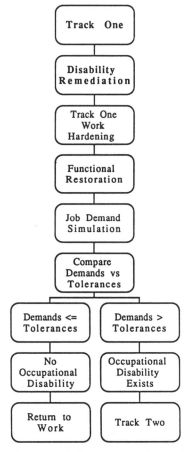

Figure 24.3. Track One of the work capacity evaluation process.

gressive in their treatment focus in a manner that is similar to a sports medicine approach to an athlete. Such a program is also time limited, with expectations and a time line for functional improvement clearly communicated to the patient prior to the program's inception. The early treatment focus is on remediation of functional limitations with a gradually increasing focus on functional restoration and improvement toward the patient's theoretical functional capacity.

This program continues until the patient's functional tolerances equal or exceed the functional demands of his/her usual and customary employment or until functional tolerances plateau and it is determined that further improvement is not probable. At this point, if the patient is unable to safely return to his/her usual and customary employment, contact with the employer to seek a modified job or alternate employment is undertaken. If either is possible, the individual will return

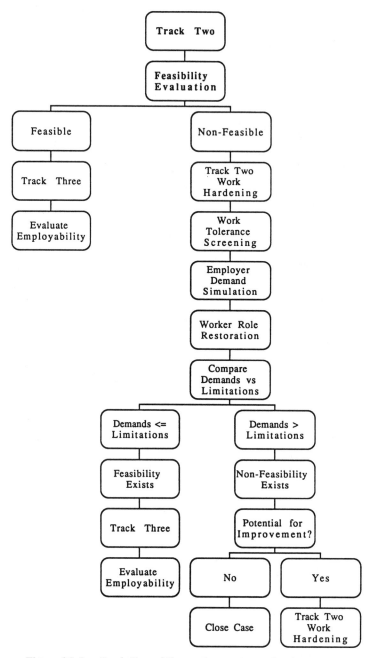

Figure 24.4. Track Two of the work capacity evaluation process.

to the previous employer in new job status. If neither is possible, the injured worker will enter Track Two, the first task of which is to evaluate vocational feasibility (Fig. 24.4).

EVALUATION OF VOCATIONAL FEASIBILITY

The feasibility issues are considered because experience has shown that, if the low back–injured worker is not able to return to work after Track One intervention, it is often because one or another of these behavioral issues continues to be unresolved. Feasibility for competitive employment is evaluated in terms of the injured worker's behaviors, which can be grouped into three major areas as found in the Feasibility Evaluation Checklist (3):

1. *General Productivity*—the evaluee's ability to perform work tasks with sufficient speed, endurance, quality, and consistency to allow the employer to profit from his/her employment.
2. *Safety in the Workplace*—the evaluee's ability to perform the job tasks within the work environment in a manner that is safe to the evaluee and his/her fellow workers.
3. *Interpersonal Behavior*—the evaluee's ability to get along with his/her fellow workers, accept direction from a supervisor, and adjust to different supervisory styles.

The evaluation of feasibility for competitive employment makes three important contributions to the rehabilitation process. First, it acts as a gatekeeper to triage injured workers as they enter the vocational rehabilitation process, helping to triage the evaluees in terms of three categories:

1. Individuals who are identified as being able to benefit from vocational rehabilitation services directed at competitive employment, who will receive those services.
2. Individuals who are identified as being unable to benefit from vocational rehabilitation services directed at competitive employment, who will be denied those services and will be identified as being "nonfeasible for competitive employment."
3. Individuals in this latter group who are identified as having the potential to benefit from vocational rehabilitation services, who will receive prevocational service that has feasibility for competitive employment as its eventual goal.

Second, the evaluation of feasibility is used to certify that the individual who is feasible for employment possesses those basic attributes that are necessary for employment at that level of competition somewhere in the labor market. Any subsequent unsuccessful attempts to secure employment are interpreted in this light and may reflect other important factors, such as the evaluee's work skills and knowledge, or important trends in the local labor market. Each of these factors is separate from the issue of feasibility and can be dealt with on that basis. Finally, the feasibility evaluation maintains safety in the work capacity evaluation program. Experience has shown that when work demands exceed work tolerances for an appreciable length of time, the worker will become nonfeasible. The work capacity evaluation process is conducted within the context of feasibility because this context ensures a safe evaluation that will result in valid recommendations.

The evaluation of feasibility can actually begin in the subacute hospital setting. A low back–injured worker who may eventually return to work can benefit by early adoption of feasibility as a framework for treatment. The concept of feasibility as an external touchstone allows the hospital staff to bring part of the reality of the injured worker's eventual context of living into the hospital environment to be used as part of the rehabilitation process. Vocational rehabilitation begins as soon as pathology is identified and should not be left to the vocational counselor to implement. The interpretation of the injured worker's behavior in terms of the acceptability of the injured worker as an employee can begin to orient the injured worker (and his/her family) toward eventual return to work as a goal. There may be no better opportunity to begin to learn appropriate employer-relevant behavior than in the supportive atmosphere of the hospital or rehabilitation center.

Feasibility can also be a very effective communications link between the injured worker and the treating professional, superior to the traditional communication link that is termed "symptoms." Typically, health care practitioners interpret the injured worker's behavior in terms of his/her symptoms. The injured worker communicates through the use of symptom reports. While the use of symptomatology as a communications link between injured worker and health care practitioner has stood the test of time, an alternative approach is to consider the injured worker's behavior in terms of feasibility. Feasibility can actually be superior to symptomatology as a communications link for four reasons. First, feasibility is the context of the employer. The factors that we consider within feasibility are those factors that are easily understood by any employer. Similarly, the injured worker who has been an employee understands very quickly the measures that are being used to conduct the evaluation. Second, feasibility is a multidimensional factor. Through the application of the concept of feasibility, it is possible to identify specific feasibility issues and develop specific strategies to remediate the feasibility problems. Third, feasibility is verifiable. Feasibility can be validated through cross-reference to observable behaviors. Whereas agreed-upon standards of feasibility have been developed, symptomatology is not verifiable.

Finally, feasibility has a positive orientation to results. As the injured worker is considered in terms of feasibility, he/she is assisted to achieve improved attendance, workplace tolerance, and productivity. By comparison, when the injured worker is considered in terms of symptomatology, the focus is on something to avoid, such as pain or dizziness. Rehabilitation professionals teach people that it is important to avoid these experiences when possible, even though many are not avoidable. Unfortunately, learned avoidance behavior is easily generalized and produces a conservatism that tends to limit the person in the exercise of his/her options which, in turn, limits his/her chances of success in rehabilitation. In direct contrast, a focus upon output and productivity are readily reinforced in the external environment and contribute to the growth of the person and his/her perception of his/her options. Additionally, while pain behavior and the injured worker's reports of symptomatology can be difficult to extinguish, competing behaviors that are productivity oriented can be strongly reinforced. This will result in a loss of the injured worker's focus on symptoms with a subsequent refocus on productivity. Feasibility, once it is established and carried through to employment, usually is strongly reinforced. This in large part explains the decreased medical recidivism among those patients who have been successfully placed in the labor market. Numerous studies have demonstrated that success in medical rehabilitation is often lost when placement is not achieved or when employment is not sustained beyond the short term. Much of this is attributable to an insufficient focus on feasibility early in the rehabilitation program.

EVALUATION OF EMPLOYABILITY

To be employable, the injured worker must be feasible. However, an injured worker may be feasible for employment without being employable. This is especially true with older workers. As an example, the older construction worker may be feasible in terms of productivity, safety, and interpersonal behavior but be unable to find employment because his transferable skills are not needed in the immediate labor market. The older worker's lack of employability may not be recognized for what it is. It may be mistaken for a lack of feasibility for employment, when, in fact, the problem is a lack of opportunity for employment. The older worker in this circumstance will often begin to develop a self-image that is consistent with lack of potential rather than focus on the personal factors that he/she can change (skills, knowledge, goals) or on the labor market–dependent factors that have frustrated his/her return to work. Such occurrences are, unfortunately, only too common. For this reason, it is important to remember that feasibility and employability are not synonymous.

If the low back–injured worker becomes feasible for competitive employment, evaluation of employability is undertaken. However, if the low back–injured worker is not feasible for competitive employment, Track Two work hardening will ensue. Utilizing an aggressive approach to restoration of worker behaviors combined with the simulation of general employer demands, the injured worker is prepared to return to the labor market. Once feasibility for competitive employment is achieved, the work capacity evaluation process continues to Track Three, the evaluation of employability (Fig. 24.5).

Employability combines information about the low back–injured worker's goals, transferable skills, aptitudes, and interests within the context of his/her already-established work tolerance profile to identify occupations that exist in the labor market that may be appropriate, often utilizing a computerized job-matching system. Goals are identified through the use of a structured interview (1) that assists the injured worker to develop an appropriate future orientation and to begin to take responsibility for the plans and actions that are required to achieve the envisioned future.

Transferable Skills

Transferable skills are the skills that remain after the effects of the chronic disability have been considered. Transferable skills are based upon the evaluee's work history, training, and education. Transferable skills may be identified through the use of the Vocational Factors Profile (1) procedure to analyze the evaluee's work history through the use of job analysis data that are supplied by the U.S. Department of Labor. This is a clerical and counseling procedure that should be conducted very early in the specific vocational exploration process and often forms the basis for subsequent skills testing. Another approach to the identification of transferable skills is the use of an activity sort technique, such as the WEST Tool Sort (43). This can be used for an in-depth review of the evaluee's experience with tools and work activities in addition to an analysis of his/her perception of residual transferable skills.

Intellect, Aptitudes, and Interests

While literally thousands of tests are available to evaluate general intellectual function, aptitudes, interests, and temperament, certain tests have been found to be more useful than others with the low back–injured worker.

General Reasoning

Raven's Standard Progressive Matrices (49) is a 60-item paper-and-pencil nonverbal test that measures abstract reasoning ability. In each problem,

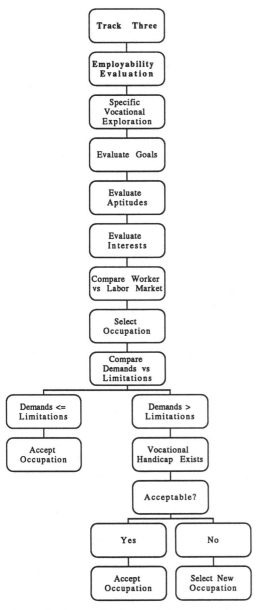

Figure 24.5. Track Three of the work capacity evaluation process.

the evaluee is presented with a pattern or figure design that has a part missing. The evaluee's task is to select one of six to eight possible parts to complete the pattern.

Intelligence

The Wechsler Adult Intelligence Scale–Revised (WAIS-R) (50) is the predominant test of general intelligence in use in the United States today. This individually administered test is composed of 11

subtests that are divided into two major divisions, Verbal and Performance. The WAIS-R is a revision of the original Wechsler Adult Intelligence Scale (51) with a standardization sample based on the 1970 census consisting of subjects who are grouped in terms of socioeconomic status, sex, and occupation in proportions similar to those found in the United States population as a whole. Norms are presented over nine age groups from 16 years through 74 years.

Language Skill

The Gates-McGinitie Reading Test (17) is a multiple-item paper-and-pencil test that measures reading achievement in the areas of vocabulary and reading comprehension, Six different levels of test difficulty allow appropriate evaluation of individuals in grades 1 through 12. Another excellent test in this area is the Adult Basic Learning Examination (52), a multiple-item paper-and-pencil measure of vocabulary, reading comprehension, spelling, arithmetic computation, and arithmetic problem solving.

Mathematics

In addition to the Adult Basic Learning Examination, the Employee Aptitude Survey (EAS) Test 2 (Numerical) is quite useful. The EAS 2 is a 75-item paper-and-pencil multiple-choice test arranged in three parts (integers, decimals and percentages, and fractions) of 25 items each. This test measures basic arithmetic skill. The Personnel Test For Industry–Numerical (53) is a multiple-item paper-and-pencil test of mathematical competence that evaluates the ability to solve "word problems" that are common in the industrial environment.

Secondary Aptitudes

Depending on the "expert" that you ask, the number of secondary aptitudes ranges from 10 to more than 100. There are several aptitude batteries that have been developed and are used with success that address the most vocationally relevant secondary aptitudes. Those that have been found to be most appropriate for use in industrial rehabilitation include the following.

Employee Aptitude Survey. Eleven subtests (Psychological Services) that cover verbal comprehension, numerical ability, visual pursuit, visual speed and accuracy, space visualization, numerical reasoning, verbal reasoning, word fluency, manual speed and accuracy, and symbolic reasoning. Normative data are provided for several occupational groups as well as for the general population.

Differential Aptitude Tests. A multiple-item paper-and-pencil test (The Psychological Corporation) of eight scholastic abilities that have direct application for industrial work. Abilities assessed include verbal reasoning, numerical ability, abstract reasoning, clerical speed and accuracy, mechanical reasoning, space relations, spelling, and language usage.

Temperament Factors. The Sixteen Personality Factors (16 PF) Questionnaire (Institute for Personality and Ability Testing) is a paper-and-pencil test of 105 to 187 items, depending on which of the five forms is used. This test measures 16 primary personality traits. Properly interpreted, the 16 PF can predict such items as probable length of employee tenure, tolerance for routine, and work efficiency. Occupational profile data based upon 11,000 cases are available.

Interest Patterns. The Career Assessment Inventory (NCS Interpretive Scoring Systems) is a 300-item paper-and-pencil test that measures Holland's six general occupational types, 22 basic occupational interest scales, and 91 specific occupational scales. The Self-Directed Search (Consulting Psychologists Press) is a multiple-item paper-and-pencil self-guided assessment of Holland's six general occupational types. The Strong Vocational Interest Inventory (Stanford University Press) is a 325-item paper-and-pencil multiple-choice test that measures occupational interest in a wide range of career areas requiring advanced technical or college training. As does the Career Assessment Inventory, the Strong yields scores on Holland's six general occupational types and 23 basic interest scales. The Strong offers 162 specific occupational scales.

Worker Profile–Job Demands Comparison

Once the worker's profile is developed, a comparison between the occupation's demands and the profile is made. Computerized job matching systems are widely available to assist with this task. Data collected in the specific vocational exploration process are used to present a profile of the evaluee that is matched against profiles of occupations maintained in one of several computerized data bases. The OASYS System (Vertek, Inc., 1986) is a highly sophisticated relational data base/expert system that can reside on an IBM XT. It contains and can rapidly access all of the occupational titles, descriptions, and statistical profiles for the U.S. Dictionary of Occupational Titles.

Once an occupation is identified, a close comparison between its demands and the low back–injured worker's goals and resources, with a special focus on functional tolerances, is made. If the

worker's goals and his/her resources provide an adequate match, a formal vocational rehabilitation program will follow. This may or may not involve formal or on-the-job training, but will usually involve rehabilitation counseling support, job search training, assistance with placement, and postplacement follow-up to ascertain job maintenance.

EVALUATION OF VOCATIONAL HANDICAPS

If the worker's functional profile is not adequate, a vocational handicap exists. The degree of this handicap and whether or not it is acceptable to the injured worker and may be acceptable to a potential employer is the focus of the last stage of the work capacity evaluation process (see Fig. 24.5). Vocational handicap has to do with the ability to become employed in a particular job and is evaluated in terms of the match between the injured worker's capabilities and the job's demands. The injured worker's ability to perform the specific work tasks of a targeted job is the focus of this stage of the evaluation.

Everybody has potential vocational handicaps. For each person, jobs exist that exceed one's capabilities. The task in work capacity evaluation is to develop a sufficiently clear picture of the match between the injured worker and the job so that vocational handicaps can be minimized or avoided altogether. The importance to the injured worker of evaluating his/her vocational handicaps comes from the relationship between the level of job demand and the level of remuneration. Generally speaking, the more demanding the job the more the remuneration, and the greater the risk of reinjury. A clear understanding of vocational handicap will assist the injured worker to avoid reinjury by learning to work around those aspects of the job that are most dangerous.

SUMMARY

This chapter has presented a brief overview of work capacity evaluation, including its philosophy and basic concepts. In addition, the use of work capacity evaluation in the rehabilitation of individuals who are disabled as a result of low back pain has been presented. It is clear that work capacity evaluation is a comprehensive approach that is effective with low back–injured workers because it addresses the broad constellation of issues that these individuals present to the treatment team. As a comprehensive process, it is effective in identifying secondary impairment issues and other factors that are often found to magnify the low back–injured worker's functional limitations. This provides a basis for subsequent treatment that can be more effective with the "problem patient" than traditional unitary intervention.

REFERENCES

1. Matheson LN: *Work Capacity Evaluation: Systematic Approach to Industrial Rehabilitation.* Anaheim, CA, Employment and Rehabilitation Institute of California, 1986.
2. Waddell G, Morris EW, Di Paola M, Bircher M, Finlayson D: A concept of illness tested as an improved basis for surgical decisions in low-back disorders. *Spine* 11:712–719, 1986.
3. Matheson LN: *Work Capacity Evaluation.* Trabuco Canyon, CA, Rehabilitation Institute of Southern California, 1982.
4. Mooney V: Impairment, disability, and handicap. *Clin Orthop Rel Res* Aug(221):14–25, 1987.
5. Clark WL, Haldeman S, Johnson P, Morris J, Schulenberger C, Trauner D, White A: Back impairment and disability determination. *Spine* 13:332–341, 1988.
6. US Department of Labor: *Handbook for Analyzing Jobs.* Washington, DC, US Government Printing Office, 1972.
7. Chaffin DB, Baker WH: A biomechanical model for analysis of symmetric sagittal plane lifting. *AIIE Trans* 2(1):16–27, 1970.
8. Chaffin DB, Herrin GD, Keyserling WM: Preemployment strength testing. An updated position. *J Occup Med* 20:403–408, 1978.
9. Chaffin DB: Ergonomics guide for the assessment of human static strength. *Am Ind Hyg Assoc J* 36:505–510, 1975.
10. Chaffin DB: Human strength capacity and low back pain. *J Occup Med* 6:248–254, 1974.
11. Harber P, SooHoo K: Static ergonomic strength testing in evaluating occupational back pain. *J Occup Med* 26:877–884, 1984.
12. Keyserling WM, Herrin GD, Chaffin DB: Isometric strength testing as a means of controlling medical incidents on strenuous jobs. *J Occup Med* 22:332–336, 1980.
13. Mital A, Ayoub MM: Modeling of isometric strength and lifting capacity. *Human Factors* 22:285–290, 1980.
14. Kishino ND, Mayer TG, Gatchel RJ, Parrish MM, Anderson C, Gustin L, Mooney V: Quantification of lumbar function. Part 4: Isometric and isokinetic lifting simulation in normal subjects and low-back dysfunctional patients. *Spine* 10:921–927, 1985.
15. Kroemer KHE: An isoinertial technique to assess individual lifting capability. *Human Factors* 25:493–506, 1983.
16. Pytell JL, Kamon E: Dynamic strength test as a predictor for maximal and acceptable lifting. *Ergonomics* 24:663–672, 1981.
17. MacGinitie G: *Gates-MacGinitie Reading Tests,* ed 2. Iowa City, The Riverside Publishing Company, 1900.
18. Ayoub MM, Mital A, Asfour SS, Bethea NJ: Review, evaluation, and comparison of models for predicting lifting capacity. *Human Factors* 22:257–269, 1980.
19. Ciriello VM, Snook SH: A study of size, distance, height, and frequency effects on manual handling tasks. *Human Factors* 25:473–483, 1983.
20. Jiang BC, Smith JL, Ayoub MM: Psychophysical modeling of manual materials-handling capacities using isoinertial strength variables. *Human Factors* 28:691–702, 1986.
21. Karwowski W: Reliability of the psychophysical approach to manual lifting of liquids by females. *Ergonomics* 29:237–248, 1986.
22. Mital A: The psychophysical approach in manual lifting—a verification study. *Human Factors* 25:485–491, 1983.
23. Mital A, Comprehensive maximum acceptable weight of lift database for regular 8-hour work shifts. *Ergonomics* 27:1127–1138, 1984.
24. Snook SH: A study of three preventive approaches to low back injury. *J Occup Med* 20:478–481, 1978.
25. Snook SH: Psychophysical considerations in permissible loads. *Ergonomics* 28:327–333, 1985.
26. Troup JDG, Foreman TK, Baxter CE, Brown D: The perception of back pain and the role of psychophysical tests of lifting capacity. *Spine* 12:645–657, 1987.
27. Bink B: The physical working capacity in relation to working time and age. *Ergonomics* 5(25), 1962.
28. Bonjer FH: Actual energy expenditure in relation to the physical working capacity. *Ergonomics* 5(29), 1962.
29. Erb BD: Applying work physiology to occupational medicine. *Occup Safety Health,* June, 1981.
30. Genaidy AM, Asfour SS: Review and evaluation of physiological cost prediction models for manual materials handling. *Human Factors* 29:465–476, 1987.
31. American Psychological Association: *Standards for Educational and Psychological Testing.* Washington, DC, American Psychological Association, 1985.
32. National Institute of Occupational Safety and Health: *Work Practices Guide for Manual Lifting.* Cincinnati, Ohio, US Department of Human Services, Division of Biomedical and Behavioral Science, 1981.
33. Ransford AO, Cairns D, Mooney V: The pain drawing as an aid to the psychologic evaluation of patients with low-back pain. *Spine* 1:127–134, 1976.
34. Waddell G, Bircher M, Finlayson D, Main CJ: Symptoms and signs: physical disease or illness behavior? *Br Med J* 289:739–741, 1984.
35. Waddell G, Main CJ, Morris EW, Di Paola M, Gray ICM: Chronic low-back pain, psychogenic distress, and illness behavior. *Spine* 9:209–213, 1984.
36. Waddell G, McCulloch JA, Kummel E, Venner RM: Nonorganic physical signs in low-back pain. *Spine* 5:117–125, 1980.
37. Mayer TG: Using physical measurements to assess low back pain. *J Musculoskel Med* 2(6):44–59, 1985.
38. Fairbank JCT, Davies JB, Couper J, O'Brien JP: The

Oswestry Low Back Pain Disability Questionnaire. *Physiotherapy* 66(8):271–273, 1980.

39. Feuerstein M, Greenwald M, Gamache MP, Papciak AS, Cook EW: The Pain Behavior Scale: modification and validation for outpatient use. *J Psychopathol Behav Assessment* 7:301–315, 1985.

40. Gatchel RJ, Mayer TG, Capra P, Diamond P, Barnett J: Quantification of lumbar function. Part 6: The use of psychological measures in guiding physical functional restoration. *Spine* 11:36–41, 1986.

41. Gatchel RJ, Mayer TG, Capra P, Barnett J, Diamond P: Millon Behavioral Health Inventory: its utility in predicting physical function in patients with low back pain. *Arch Phys Med Rehab* 67:878–882, 1986.

42. Keefe FJ, Crisson JE, Maltbee A, Bradley L, Gil KM: Illness behavior as a predictor of pain and overt behavior patterns in chronic low back pain patients. *J Pschosom Res* 30:543–551, 1986.

43. Matheson LN: Reliability crisis in industrial rehabilitation. *Ind Rehabil Q* 1(1):1, 8–10, 1988.

44. Commission on Accreditation of Rehabilitation Facilities: *Guidelines for Work Hardening Programs.* Tuscson, AZ, CARF, 1988.

45. Carlton RS: The effects of body mechanics instruction on work performance. *Am J Occup Ther* 41(1):16–20, 1987.

46. US Department of Labor: *Dictionary of Occupational Titles, 4th Edition Supplement.* Washington, DC, US Government Printing Office, 1986.

47. Chaffin DB: Biomechanics of manual material handling and low back pain. In *Occupational Medicine: Principles and Practical Applications.* Chicago, Year Book Medical Publishers, 1975, pp 443–467.

48. Mayer TG, Gatchel, Mayer H, Kishino ND, Keeley J, Mooney V: A prospective two-year study of functional restoration in industrial low back injury. *JAMA* 258:1763–1767, 1987.

49. Raven JC: *Standard Progressive Matrices.* London, HK Lewis & Co. Ltd, 1958. [New York, The Psychological Corporation (US distributor.)]

50. Wechsler D: *Wechsler Adult Intelligence Scale—Revised (WAIS-R).* Cleveland OH, The Psychological Corporation, 1981.

51. Wechsler D: *Wechsler Adult Intelligence Scale (WAIS).*

Cleveland, OH, The Psychological Corporation, 1955.

52. Karlsen B, Madden R, Gardner EF: *Adult Basic Learning Examination (ABLE).* Cleveland, OH, The Psychological Corporation, 1967.

53. Wesman AG, Joppelt JE: *Personnel Tests for Industry (PTI).* Cleveland, OH, The Psychological Corporation, 1980.

SUGGESTED READINGS

Ayoub MM, Mital A, Bakken GM, Asfour SS, Bethea NJ: Development of strength and capacity norms for manual materials handling activities: The state of the art. *Human Factors* 22:271–283, 1980.

Chaffin DB: Functional assessment for heavy physical labor. *Occup Health Safety* 26:24–27, 1981.

Chaffin DB, Andersson GBJ: *Occupational Biomechanics.* New York, John Wiley & Sons, 1984.

Matheson LN, Ogden LD, Vilette K, Schultz K: Work hardening: occupational therapy in industrial rehabilitation. *Am J Occup Ther* 39:314–321, 1985.

Mayer TG: *Assessment of Lumbar Function.* In Clinical Orthopaedics and Related Research, Dallas, 1986, pp 99–109.

Mayer TG, Tencer AF, Kristoferson S, Mooney V: Use of noninvasive techniques for quantification of spinal range-of-motion in normal subjects and chronic low-back dysfunction patients. *Spine* 9:588–595, 1984.

Mital A: Maximum weights of lift acceptable to male and female industrial workers for extended work shifts. *Ergonomics* 27:1115–1126, 1984.

Snook SH: The design of manual handling tasks. *Ergonomics* 21:963–985, 1978.

Snook SH, Webster BS: Cost per case of compensable back pain—1985. Hopkinton, MA, Liberty Mutual Insurance Company, 1987.

Snook SH, Webster BS: The cost of disability. *Clin Orthop* May, 77–84, 1986.

US Department of Labor: *Dictionary of Occupational Titles,* ed 4. Washington, DC, US Government Printing Office, 1977.

Waddell G, Main CJ: Assessment of severity in low-back disorders. *Spine* 9:204–208, 1984.

Chapter 25

FUNCTIONAL RESTORATION FOR CHRONIC LOW BACK PAIN

TOM G. MAYER, MD
ROBERT J. GATCHEL, PhD

Rehabilitation in low back pain implies that we are speaking about the *chronic* patient with low back pain. This assertion emerges from the recognition that the vast majority of low back pain episodes resolve spontaneously in a short period of time, with more than 50% improved in less than 2 weeks. More than 90% of back pain episodes resolve within 3 months, but about 40% of those with acute back pain episodes will have a recurrence. Spontaneous recovery results in two remaining groups of individuals: (a) chronically disabled low back pain patients, often involving unskilled or semiskilled and poorly educated workers whose back pain becomes an impediment to work return; and (b) individuals with chronic episodic back pain suffering from intermittent acute recurrences leading to brief periods of total disability and more frequent limitations of recreational activities.

It is safe to say that the interests of the general public are focused on only two issues: cost and human suffering. In the latter category, one would include two subissues: pain and disability. The staggering costs have been variously estimated, depending on which aspects are included (weekly benefits, permanent disability payments, Social Security, and long-term disability payments; loss of productivity; medical cost and vocational retraining; etc.) at from $20 to $60 billion annually in the United States. Comparable costs relative to population demographics are experienced in other industrialized countries, although cost declines in countries where life-and-death issues prevail over quality-of-life issues.

In terms of human suffering, pain perception has been one of the primary indices used in its documentation. Pain perception is a subjective phenomenon whose expression and secondary gain characteristics are discussed extensively in the literature (1, 2). Pain perception may be related to structural, functional capacity, or psychosocioeconomic issues and remains an unvariable element of performance. Consequently, it is also the most difficult problem to deal with. While several authors have created standardized measures of pain, they are only useful for intraindividual comparisons since similar lesions may produce such variable reporting between subjects (3–6).

The issue of disability, on the other hand, has received relatively scant attention in comparison to the above two issues. Yet, it probably represents the central problem from which all others spring. Lower productivity of individual labor certainly produces major losses for society. We have found it also produces the loss of self-confidence and self-esteem in most individuals, although a small percentage of patients may take advantage of an opportunity for "premature retirement." Disability itself may lead to mental and physical deconditioning, which perpetuates itself and produces a general decline in human performance. Yet, many of our treatments, if devoted solely to the alleviation of pain, fail to assure a simultaneous goal of alleviation of disability. As clinicians, we may sometimes go even further, ending up blaming the patient for therapeutic failures in the guise of recognition of "secondary gain" concomitants of their failure to get well.

The rate of rise of low back disability in the

United States has been accelerating dramatically over the past 20 years (7) with a staggering 14 times increase in disability in the United States in the decade of the 1970s (8). This increase can no longer be ignored, particularly in view of the declining work force. It is the recognition of disability as the central problem related to lumbar dysfunction that characterizes the functional restoration approach. In essence, functional restoration has, as its primary goal, the elimination of disability; once this has been accomplished, pain relief and cost control can be anticipated as secondary phenomena.

QUANTIFICATION OF PHYSICAL FUNCTION

Loss of the capacity to perform physical tasks may be associated both with structural lesions and decrements in physical capacity. An example of the first situation would be a tibial fracture, and an example of the second is the joint stiffness and muscle atrophy attendant upon prolonged cast immobilization and pain-induced neural inhibiting influences while primary healing occurs. This example delineates general principles of behavior of the organism following musculoskeletal injury. Soon after injury, effects of the trauma on structural factors predominate. Inflammation leads to repair of the tissue with the original mesothelial element, or (in the case of large defects) replacement with collagenous scar.

In more significant trauma, the period of immobilization/inactivity may be prolonged and lead to dysfunctional behaviors, abetted by a variety of psychosocial and cultural situations. These dysfunctional behaviors may be succeeded by loss of physical capacity measured by deterioration of a variety of *basic elements of performance (BEPs)* such as motion, strength, endurance, and agility (9, 10). The longer the period of inactivity, the greater the opportunity for disuse to create physical capacity deficits leading to decreased human performance, and ultimately to a variety of psychosocial and affective concomitants such as depression, medication abuse, and disability habituation. Pain may be a parallel factor, but its direct relationship to changes in muscles or other mesothelial structures remains elusive.

Of the two primary factors of *structural* and *functional* change following injury, the structural change is most dominant in the early stages following injury. Healing almost invariably occurs in a reasonable soft tissue repair time period (albeit with replacement of original tissue by suboptimal scar in severe cases). By contrast, physical capacity deficits are rarely a factor in human performance in the early posttraumatic stages, but become a gradually increasing factor accompanying inactivity and disuse. As time progresses, functional deficits become the dominant physical impairment disabling the chronic case. Clinically, the chronic patient is the most important in terms of financial cost to society and human suffering. Strength testing during the early posttraumatic time period will be hampered by invalid measurements due to pain-induced neuromuscular inhibition. There is also some limited concern that overaggressive attempts at performance might actually exacerbate the injury. Given usual soft tissue healing periods, such concerns should no longer be necessary 3–6 weeks after trauma, at the latest. While testing may be feasible from that point forward, deconditioning produced by inactivity is likely to make its appearance only after that acute time period. Epidemiologically, we would anticipate that about 75% of acute low back pain cases will have resolved spontaneously by then.

One way of viewing the human organism is as a set of biomechanical links (or functional units) in a chain. Transcending purely anatomic considerations, these "functional units" work together to provide the organism certain safety and efficiency advantages in maintaining homeostasis. There is probably no more important human factor in our industrialized society than our manual manipulation of the environment. In most postures, the lumbar spine is necessary for supporting the loads held in the hands, and transmitting them to ground contact. Through changes in posture, the lumbar spine may effect a variety of changes in hand reach and height placement capabilities, thus increasing performance efficiency. Following injury, the lumbopelvic functional unit may become a "weak link" in the biomechanical chain. Under these circumstances, it may be important to measure the strength of the isolated unit to evaluate its place in the pathologic process. In other cases, the compound activity of multiple functional units involved in performing whole body tasks may be most important to measure. The classical compound strength measurement is generally thought to involve lifting.

Extremity deficits are easily noted because they are susceptible to simple visual observation of atrophy through muscle circumference measures and comparison with the contralateral side. For this reason, sports medicine programs have focused considerable therapist effort on restoring strength/

endurance in the para-articular musculature as a natural part of any rehabilitation process. In the spine, because of lack of visual feedback and a comparison side, these connections have not generally been made. While certain neuromuscular conditions (polio, muscular dystrophy, spinal cord injury) have been recognized as causing lumbar dysfunction through muscle wasting, clinicians usually only accept the muscle relationship when spine deformity results from gross, asymmetrical loss of muscle bulk. More subtle forms of loss of trunk strength are generally not perceived, and therefore not taken into consideration as a cause of symptoms. While more research has been done relating trunk muscle strength to low back pain (11–15) than relating range of motion to low back pain, most clinicians tend to pay more attention to motion deficits that can be partially visualized as a reflection of lumbar spine dysfunction. The lack of visual feedback, and the consequent need for mechanical devices to supplement the senses for strength assessment, probably accounts for this finding.

We know that surgical treatment is performed on only 2–3% of patients with spinal disorders. Nevertheless, surgeons will search diligently for that small percentage with a wide variety of expensive and sophisticated diagnostic tools (computed tomography, magnetic resonance imaging, electromyography, myelography, etc.). A structural diagnosis, when made, may lead to the ability to "fix" an anatomic aberration such as a prolapsed disk. For the remaining 97% of the back-injured population, spontaneous recovery may account for many "cures." However, a substantial percentage of patients, perhaps as high as 30–40%, will show some evidence of disuse and deconditioning, making them candidates for physical retraining once the functional deficits are identified. Without quantification, the deficits are simply not recognizable, leading to inevitable over- or underutilization of therapeutic services. This observation is not merely true for spinal disorders, nor has it escaped the attention of health care planners. Medicare requires periodic testing to document progress in other areas of rehabilitation. It is likely that similar rules will ultimately apply to treatment of spinal problems, since their necessity becomes more generally perceived.

The term "deconditioning syndrome" has been applied to the cumulative disuse changes produced in the chronically disabled patient suffering from spinal dysfunction. The syndrome is initially produced by the immobilization and inactivity attendant upon injury. It is supplemented by disruption of spinal soft tissues and scarring resulting from a surgical approach or repetitive microtrauma. As pain perception is enhanced, learned protective mechanisms lead to a vicious cycle of inactivity and disuse. As physical capacity decreases, the likelihood of fresh sprains/strains to unprotected joints, muscles, ligaments, and disks increases. These inevitable alterations of pain and function are perceived by the patient as a "recurrence" or "reinjury."

There are now methods available to objectively quantify the degree of deconditioning. However, one must carefully select the appropriate type of test for such quantification. For example, isometric lifting tests have been used to "measure back strength" (16, 17). In fact, although engineering principles require that the force of an isometric test be transmitted through the body from hands to foot/floor contact, the spine can often be placed into such a position that virtually no spinal muscular strength is required to support the load (18)! This exemplifies the first criterion for any functional evaluation: the test must be *relevant* to the physiology being measured. If isolated spinal muscular strength is what one wishes to assess, then measures of trunk torques in flexion/extension, rotation, or lateral bend must be sought, not whole-body tasks such as lifting.

A second critical principle of measurement is the need to know the *validity* and *reproducibility* of the measurement. Validity refers to the accuracy of the test device itself, and reproducibility refers to the ability of the test (device *plus* subject) to give a repeatable and precise measure of a clinical variable. *A valid test is not necessarily reproducible and vice versa.* An invalid test is simply useless, but an irreproducible test may reflect actual clinical reality (such as comparing intersubject body weight or changes in spinal mobility before and after exercise in the same individual). As in the examples, reproducibility problems can often be corrected by restructuring the test protocol.

Once a functional test has been found to be valid, reproducible, and relevant, an *effort factor* must be defined. Without the ability to identify suboptimal effort, invalid low readings may be accepted as true physical deficits. Because suboptimal effort may reflect a clinical abnormality (such as low motivation or a personality disorder leading to conscious malingering), the clinician must be able to assess whether he/she is dealing with a true physical deficit or not.

Finally, once the appropriate device and test

protocol have been chosen, the hard work begins! A *normative data base* must be compiled on a large population sample to permit comparisons to be drawn to a patient grouping. Degree of deviation from "normal" may significantly affect treatment protocols. While much more should be said about measurement criteria, it is most important to select the optimal measurement device in the first place, to avoid the tedious task of collecting additional normative data (7, 17, 19–24).

RANGE OF MOTION TESTS

Trunk motion is a compound movement combining intersegmental and hip motion components. Thus, a patient with a completely fused spine can often bend forward to perform toe touches using hip motion alone. While we are not yet able to measure intersegmental motion noninvasively, biplanar radiography may confirm inclinometry in selected cases (25, 26). Inclinometers may be used to separate the hip motion component from the lumbar spine motion component and derive valuable information (19, 23). As in all functional capacity measurements, information obtained with range-of-motion techniques must be compared with a normative data base. In addition, an "effort factor" must be available to validate adequate motivation in performing the test. For range of motion, this effort factor is generally the repeatability of sequential measures. However, in the most important spine flexion measure, where ultimate range of motion is approximately the same in the hips and the six lumbar motion segments, the comparison of the hip motion component with the supine straight leg raising measurement creates an effective effort factor (4, 7, 19). In the sagittal plane, the inclinometers, which are available in mechanical or computerized forms from various manufacturers, may be positioned at two points or moved from one point to another (4).

Measurements are taken in both flexion and extension and validated through the effort factor of straight leg raising. There are many reasons for limitation of effort on any single test and thus the "effort factor" is not a test for malingering. Effort may be reduced by pain, fear of injury, physiologic perception of excessive load, and psychological factors of anxiety/depression, as well as conscious effort to mislead the examiner.

Many alternative techniques for spine mobility measurement have been described (27). However, many of them are relatively cumbersome to perform or require large and expensive pieces of equipment such as the three-dimensional digitizer. Probably the most commonly utilized technique is the Schober

method (28), which is essentially only useful for measuring true spine flexion isolated from the hip component. Unfortunately, there are several problems with this technique, including its variable number of segments measured and the absence of the "dimples of Venus" (a critical anatomic marker) in a significant percentage of subjects. Careful evaluation of all available spine motion techniques leads to the inescapable conclusion that inclinometry is the only technique combining simplicity, relevance, validity, and reproducibility. As noted above, these are the essential prerequisites for development of a normative data base using any functional capacity measurement.

As in all other physiologic measurements, there is some variation in the normal population. Interestingly, our normative data show that mean true lumbar motion is almost identical in males and females, even though females tend to have higher hip and straight leg raising mobility components. Patient values are expressed as a "percentage of normal" as related to mean scores of the asymptomatic subject population. These scores may be normalized for such factors as age, gender, and anthropometric factors (especially body weight) when applicable. The system allows the clinician to judge the significance of small variations from the anticipated value. More importantly, he/she may track the progress of the rehabilitation process and patient effort from one examination to the next.

ISOLATED TRUNK STRENGTH TESTS

While trunk strength measurement devices have nearly a 50-year history, it is only recently that the number of publications in this area has risen dramatically (11, 12, 14, 29–38). The most commonly utilized approach has been for individual investigators to use a strain gauge or modify a standard Cybex dynamometer (Lumex Corp., Ronkonkoma, NY) to construct a trunk testing unit for use in various positions. These include sagittal measurement devices in standing, sitting, sidelying, and prone/supine positioning, thus offering a variety of starting positions, physiologically induced motion restriction, and gravity effects (32–34, 36–39). While most of these publications concerned muscle strength testing in normal individuals, the link between trunk muscle strength deficits and deconditioned chronic back pain patients has recently been shown (20, 24). Thus, two critical points appear to be established:

1. Trunk muscle strength is one important factor in functional capacity assessment of the lumbar spine.

2. Because of lack of visual feedback, mechanical devices to indirectly measure trunk strength are essential. Because strength and endurance measures require subject motivation, and the clinician lacks a visual validity check, an objective "effort factor" to assure optimal subject compliance is also necessary.

This brief chapter does not allow detailed discussion of the various devices currently available commercially for research or clinical use in testing isolated trunk strength or lifting capacity. However, it is important to point out that the back presents an area where the tools of measurement themselves have gained a certain notoriety with an aura of commercial exploitation. It is clear that the various devices for measuring trunk strength will be ultimately recognized simply as measurement tools, as useful to the spine muscle researcher as a microscope is to an anatomist. However, at the present time, so little is generally understood about these tools in both the research and clinical communities that a certain level of misperception appears to surround the various machines. Unfortunately, measurement has never been a major part of spinal diagnosis, and thus neither the surgeon nor the therapist has taken a great interest in these devices in the past.

At present, several devices are commercially available for assessing isokinetic trunk strength. Selection of a device must not only take into consideration such commercial aspects as price, tolerance of abuse, repair record, and resale value, but also the critical factors of *validity, reproducibility, relevance, effort factor,* and *simplicity of operation.* While the University of Texas Southwestern Medical Center and the Productive Rehabilitation Institute of Dallas for Ergonomics (PRIDE) groups initially had the advantage of working with the prototype Cybex (the developers of isokinetics) devices, several other units are now commercially available. They include sitting and standing models, as well as those that are stand-alone versus "add-on" units combining extremity and spine measurement ability. The Cybex TEF unit (Lumex Corp., Ronkonkoma, NY) is the first sagittal strength testing unit restricting motion to the sagittal plane only. This manufacturer also has an axial (torsional) measurement device. Biodex, on the other hand, has a reclining unit that adds on to its all-purpose dynamometer (Biodex, Inc., Shirley, NY). The dynamometer may be disconnected from the sitting isokinetic sagittal plane unit for use on a variety of alternative fixtures used for isolated extremity joint measures. Lido (Loredan Corp., Davis,CA) and Kin-Com (Chatteck

Corp., Chattanooga, TN) also manufacture isokinetic trunk strength testing equipment. Lido permits both sitting and standing measurements on a dedicated isokinetic sagittal plane testing unit. Nonisokinetic devices are also available, utilizing isometric, isotonic, or isoinertial systems. Although these devices may have advantages for physical training, particularly when multiplanar motion capability is present, they lack the advantages of isokinetics that are critical for useful measurement: (a) isolation of a single independent variable (torque) rather than allowing changes in multiple independent variables; or (b) dynamic motion with greater safety ensured by "accommodating resistance."

Major differences in trunk strength in both sagittal and axial planes between a normal subject and a patient population have been demonstrated (24, 32, 40, 41). Moreover, through efforts at functional restoration with a "sports medicine" approach, trunk strength in the patient population can be markedly improved (20). Effort can generally be assessed by repeatability of curve production, and information on work performance, power consumption, and endurance can be delivered by the computerized assessment devices. It is interesting to note that trunk strength deficits may exist independently of symptoms, and act to produce recurrent injury risk.

LIFTING TESTS

The previously described tests of mobility and strength focus primarily on the alterations in the lumbar spine functional unit induced by injury or disuse. Measurement of whole body task performance represents the interaction of multiple functional unit links in the biomechanical chain. While the body may utilize substitution of higher performance of one body link for deficits in another (as in the case of squatting rather than bending after back injury), this is not the optimal biomechanical situation and requires frequent conscious compromises of function that predispose to recurrent injury. Optimum physical capacity involves the highest possible functioning of each functional unit involved in a task, and a relearning of coordination/agility dimensions linking the functional units to provide optimum safety and efficiency.

One approach taken at PRIDE is to perform multiple tests of varying complexity to examine a single task. A case in point is examination of lifting, which has been implicated in 60–70% of back injuries. Three separate tests of lifting, all performed along standardized protocols in the sagittal plane, are used. An *isometric* test sequence is performed according to the NIOSH guidelines produced by Chaffin and colleagues (16, 42). *Isokinetic* tests are performed utilizing the Cybex Liftask (Lumex Corp., Ronkonkoma, NY), currently the only available isokinetic lifting device (7, 17). Finally, a progressive *isoinertial* lifting evaluation (the PILE) is performed to simulate "real world" lifting while using a standardized protocol controlling vertical distance, weight, and duration of lift to produce comparable data (43, 44). Tests are normalized to age, gender, and a body weight variable.

OTHER TESTS

Aerobic capacity is an important factor in disability. Inactivity leads to loss of cardiovascular function, particularly in older individuals spending unusual amounts of time reclining in order to protect painful spinal segments. Aerobic capacity tests can be performed using a variety of protocols attached to treadmill or bicycle ergometers. Oxygen consumption and fitness levels may be obtained from standardized tables.

Positional and activity tolerance is another area of interest in functional task measurement directed toward return to productivity. Following spine surgery, patients often cannot tolerate the long static positioning (sitting/standing) and often complain of inability to perform various tasks such as squatting, kneeling, walking, carrying, or climbing. We have devised an obstacle course requiring use of multiple positions in an attempt to assess the patient's tolerance of a variety of positions and daily living activities. Observation of the patient through a testing or training session can give the therapist an idea of the patient's activity tolerance. Because of the lack of corroborative tests, the latter measures are somewhat less "objective" than the battery of lifting tests.

Quantification of physical function represents a new and important tool in assessing patients with chronic disabling low back pain. Although the measures are in a relatively early stage of development and standardization, experience with extremity rehabilitation suggests that these tests will, in time, become an important supplement to our sophisticated but expensive imaging devices in determining the full gamut of spine treatments. Quantification of physical functional capacity requires patient motivation, but since an "effort factor" can be identified with each functional capacity test, suboptimal effort can be recognized and utilized to validate the actual test scores. In general, the clinician will attempt to shorten and simplify the battery of testing in the desire to come up with a "single number" of use in making a decision. Unfortunately, from the point of view of this investigator involved in

research in this area for the past several years, the number of measures is likely to increase rather than decrease in the short run. Tests commonly recognized as being important in the extremities, such as stability, fatigue resistance, and coordination/balance, either are unavailable for the spine currently or are in laboratory development only. Considerably more clinical experience will be necessary before the usefulness of the various tests and their cost-benefit ratios can be assessed.

QUANTIFICATION OF PSYCHOSOCIAL FUNCTION

Chronic pain is now appropriately viewed as a complex and interactive psychophysiologic behavior pattern that cannot be broken down into distinct, independent psychological and physical components. In the functional restoration approach used at PRIDE, psychological assessment is not used to try to differentiate "organic" from "functional" cases. Rather, the assessment is directed at evaluating the important psychological characteristics of each individual patient in order to help *guide* the treatment process, as well as help predict therapeutic outcome. This psychological assessment evaluates not only the patient's self-reported pain, but also evaluates overall psychological functioning in order to help therapeutic team personnel to effectively integrate each patient into the intensive treatment program. Quantified changes in many of these measures are also used to document therapeutic improvement.

In past publications, we have provided an overview of the various psychological assessment devices used in our functional restoration treatment (3, 7, 45). These include the Minnesota Multiphasic Personality Inventory (MMPI), the Millon Behavioral Health Inventory (MBHI), the Beck Depression Inventory (BDI), Quantified Pain Drawings, and the Oswestry Scale, as well as a comprehensive clinical interview. Currently, this wide variety of diverse tests is used because there has not been a comprehensive instrument developed specifically for chronic low back pain. We are currently in the process of developing such a psychometrically sound test, which we hope will be available for use in the near future.

Such a comprehensive psychosocial assessment of each patient is essential to "guide" the patient effectively through the intensive treatment regimen, as well as to evaluate the patient's cognitive-psychologic resources that may affect response to treatment. It should be noted that, presently, no one psychological test can reliably be used for this psychosocial assessment process. Indeed, one of the major misapplications of psychological measures in the field of medicine has been the assumption that one psychological instrument can be used as a sole conclusive predictor or descriptor variable. As Gatchel and Mears (46) noted in their discussion of the field of personality psychology, such data should be viewed as just one source of information to be used with other types of information in helping to make a probability statement concerning the prediction of some behavior. It is extremely rare to make a totally accurate prediction of some behavior based upon a single psychological instrument.

Finally, it is obviously of extreme importance to integrate these psychosocial assessment data with the quantified physical data in order to maximize the treatment process. In general, in the functional restoration program as conducted at PRIDE, these assessment results are reviewed at a general staff meeting during the start of the treatment program, at which time any modifications of the basic program are formulated for each patient. Subsequent weekly staff meetings then evaluate progress of each patient and initiate any modification needed.

FUNCTIONAL RESTORATION: MULTIMODAL DISABILITY MANAGEMENT

We have labeled the psychologic approach developed and refined at PRIDE as the *Multimodal Disability Management Program* (MDMP). It is based upon a cognitive-behavioral approach to crisis intervention, and focuses on overcoming physical and psychosocial difficulties that interfere with returning to a productive, functional life-style. Treatment issues deal with events in the present or the recent past, and patients are helped in understanding how thoughts contribute to feelings and behaviors. Within this framework, therapists contribute to feelings and behaviors. Within this framework, therapists also maintain an awareness of early learning experiences and long-standing psychologic issues that can affect reactions to recent life experiences. For example, many patients come from family backgrounds where there was some significant emotional deprivation. As a result, many experience chronic feelings of anger, depression, and low self-esteem. Relatedly, they also have a sense of entitlement stemming from a frustrated search for an idealized caretaker. These issues, along with the cognitions and emotions accompanying them, are

rekindled quickly when the patients find themselves involved in a medical/compensation/disability system that fosters dependency.

It should be noted that this MDMP approach differs from many typical "pain clinics," of which there are now estimated to be some 2000 in the United States with a wide variety of treatment approaches. The early proliferation of pain clinics was stimulated primarily by a philosophy of focusing on "quality of life outcome criteria," rather than those having socioeconomic impact (1). However, not only did such clinics proliferate in a nonstandardized manner, but when the rare scrutiny of treatment effectiveness has taken place, results sometimes no better than placebo results have often been observed (1). Indeed, as Fordyce and colleagues indicated, the tendency of pain clinics to merely treat the experience of pain, and not the *disability* associated with pain behavior, has often led to unsuccessful treatment (1). Such overly narrow approaches were also frequently accompanied by the lack of recognition of physical capacity deficits such as the deconditioning syndrome, as well as the lack of technology to measure it. The lack of effectiveness has led to a general perception, particularly among third-party carriers, that rehabilitation for chronic back pain may be ineffective and, in fact, may be no better than placebo in attaining specific societal goals such as return to work (20). The MDMP approach is an alternative to many of these unsuccessful pain clinics, with the major focus being on the *disability* associated with the pain behavior, and not merely the experience of pain.

Again, in past publications, we have discussed aspects of MDMP in some detail (7, 20, 21). Basically, however, there are four major areas involved:

1. Individual and group counseling emphasizing a crisis-intervention model (e.g., coping with family problems, unemployment). Group counseling is conducted on a daily basis; the amount of individual counseling is dependent on the particular needs of the patient.

2. Family counseling, which is conducted on a weekly basis. During these sessions, family members are encouraged to take an active part in the rehabilitation process and are provided with information about the philosophy and specific details of MDMP.

3. Behavioral stress management training that involves initial training in muscle relaxation, followed by exercises in guided imagery in which patients practice relaxing while imag-

ining themselves in various stress situations. They also receive daily electromyography/temperature biofeedback sessions during which they refine their relaxation skills, with the understanding that these skills will help them copy more effectively with residual pain and discomfort.

4. Cognitive-behavioral skills training that includes instruction in assertiveness, rational versus irrational thinking, and the management of stress and time.

Besides involvement in the above four treatment components of MDMP, the maintenance by the psychological staff of a positive therapeutic environment is important. Part of this therapeutic environment maintenance is accomplished with each patient individually through counseling and educational interventions. Moreover, frequent and clear communication between the psychological staff and all members of the treatment team working with a particular patient is essential.

FUNCTIONAL RESTORATION: REACTIVATION AND OUTCOMES

The above disability management approach emphasizes the return of patients to their previous productive life-style as quickly as possible through aggressive functional restoration. Indeed, a major conceptual breakthrough has been the recognition of the relationship between fitness and back pain. While Cady's initial study was limited primarily by reliance on cardiovascular fitness measures, engineers and clinicians have added substantially to the body of knowledge in this area, leading ultimately to the quantification of function technology discussed previously (17, 19, 22, 24, 31, 42, 47–49). All that remained was the development of truly objective outcome criteria to assess the relationship of a treatment program to address *disability*, not merely subjective *pain* self-report. Nachemson summarized the interrelationship between cost and disability and set the stage for use of objective outcome criteria to assess *cost* and *disability* responses to rehabilitation programs (50).

In this way, the evolution to the functional restoration program occurred. There are nine critical elements to the program, as noted in Table 25.1. First of all, quantification of function is the key to the entire process. We have spent quite a bit of time discussing this previously. Patient self-report of pain, disability, and affective disorders is a nec-

Table 25.1
Characteristics of a Functional Restoration Program

1. Quantification of physical capacity.
2. Quantification of psychosocial function.
3. Reactivation for restoration of fitness.
4. Reconditioning of the injured functional unit.
5. Retraining in multiunit task performance.
6. Work stimulation.
7. Multimodal disability management approach.
8. Vocational/societal reintegration.
9. Formalized outcome tracking.

essary part of the process, and standardized self-report tests to permit intraindividual comparisons can be very helpful.

The reconditioning and work simulation aspects of the program involve physical and occupational therapists utilizing active, not passive, treatment modalities. This may be difficult to encourage in view of traditional reimbursement schedules in much of the industrialized world that encourage ancient passive treatments that produce temporary comfort and discourage exercise and education. Quantification is necessary for these aspects of the program, since they provide the initial levels of exercise from which a progressive resistive program emerges. The indirect assessments confirm functional deficits and psychosocial barriers to effort, leading to a combination of education and exercise training to resolve the deconditioning syndrome. Initial treatment is directed toward mobilizing and strengthening the "weak link" in the biomechanical chain, while whole-body work simulation integrates the performance of this link with other parts of the body deconditioned simply by inactivity.

Finally, just as the quantification of physical function and self-report provides feedback to the staff and patient on individual performance, so follow-up outcome measures provide objective statistical confirmation of success in achieving program goals. The Productive Rehabilitation Institute of Dallas for Ergonomics (PRIDE) comprehensive program performs 1- and 2-year structured follow-up telephone interviews as a routine part of its ongoing program at no additional cost. The interview includes information on working status, additional surgical/medical/chiropractic treatment, resolution of compensation issues (long-term disability, Social Security disability, permanent partial/total disability, etc.), and injury recurrence. At PRIDE, we have found that it may be difficult to entice workers back for 1- and 2-year physical evaluations to obtain quantified physical capacity and pain/disability self-report scores, although it may be possible to obtain this information in a higher percentage of patients elsewhere. However, with judicious attempts to maintain patient contact, a high percentage of success in performing follow-up interviews may be anticipated. The interviews must be performed in the context of possible remaining barriers to full disclosure by the patient, thus necessitating further investigation through contacts with employers, attorneys, family members, or third-party pairs in some cases. Combining the follow-up interview information with preprogram demographic data on the same subjects can provide valid statistical comparisons of the ability of a comprehensive functional restoration program to deal with disability and cost. Since the chronic low back pain patient ultimately accounts for 80% of the cost of low back pain problems through a combination of medical treatment, lost productivity, indemnity, and government support, program evaluation, including involvement of other members of the disability system, provides a major resource to clinicians, employers, health care planners, and legislators alike.

Functional restoration is a new conceptual framework combining both new and old methodology. Given the system developed for this specialized type of spinal rehabilitation, certain specific outcomes can be anticipated. These outcomes might vary according to the geographic area, percentage of chronically disabled patients, and factors within the disability system, including the laws of the area involved. Based on our research, however, outcomes can be anticipated as noted in Table 25.2 (7, 20, 21, 51).

SUMMARY

In summary, spinal rehabilitation is entering an important new era. Focus on disability rather than pain, new technology to quantify physical capacity, physical reactivation, and work simulation approaches oriented to specific goals and outcome tracking have provided exciting new options for the chronically disabled and chronic episodic patient with spinal disorders. Techniques of providing such care are truly multidisciplinary, with a treatment approach involving physicians and therapists who interact with an intensity rarely seen in rehabilitation programs. Staff communication and morale are the essence of providing effective care for this difficult, and previously refractory, group of pa-

Table 25.2
One-Year Follow-up Outcomes of Functional Restoration[a]

Return to work	>80%
Posttreatment surgeries	<10%
Percentage unsettled claims	<15%
Spine-related medical visits (except for functional restoration or referring physician visits)	<5 visits
Rate of recurrent injury (major lost time) in patients returned to working status	<6%

[a] Data from Mayer et al. (20) and Hazard et al. (52).

tients. With attention to treatment details, realistic outcomes can be obtained and maintained.

REFERENCES

1. Fordyce W, Roberts A, Sternbach R: The behavioral management of chronic pain: a response to critics. *Pain* 22:113–125, 1985.
2. Turk D, Meichenbaum D, Genest M: *Pain and Behavioral Medicine: A Cognitive-Behavioral Perspective.* New York, Guilford Press, 1983.
3. Gatchel R, Mayer T, Capra P, Diamond P, Barnett J: Quantification of lumbar function. Part 6: use of psychological measures in guiding physical functional restoration. *Spine* 10:36–42, 1986.
4. Mayer T: Using physical measurements to assess low back pain. *J Musculoskel Med* 2:44–59, 1985.
5. Million R, Haavik K, Jayson M, Baker R: Evaluation of low back pain and assessment of lumbar corsets with and without back supports. *Ann Rheum Dis* 40:414–449, 1981.
6. Mooney V, Cairns D, Robertson J: A system for evaluating and treating chronic back disability. *West J Med* 124:370–376, 1976.
7. Mayer T, Gatchel R: *Functional Restoration for Spinal Disorders: The Sports Medicine Approach to Low Back Pain.* Philadelphia, Lea & Febiger, 1988.
8. Frymoyer J, Mooney V: Current concepts review: occupational orthopedics. *J Bone Joint Surg [Am]* 68A:469–474, 1986.
9. Kondraske G: Human performance: measurement, science, concepts and computerized methodology. *Neurology* (in press).
10. Kondraske G: Towards a standard clinical measure of postural stability. In Kondraske G, Robinson C (eds): Proceedings of the 8th Annual Conference of the IEEE Engineering in Medicine and Biology Society. *IEEE Trans Biomed Eng* 3:1579–1582, 1986.
11. Flint M: Effect of increasing back and abdominal muscle strength on low back pain. *Res Q* 29:160–171, 1955.

12. Mayer L, Greenberg B: Measurements of the strength of trunk muscles. *J Bone Joint Surg* 24:842–856, 1942.

13. Nachemson A, Lindh M: Measurements of abdominal and back muscle strength with and without low back pain. *Scand J Rehab Med* 1:60–69, 1969.

14. Oneidi O, Pederson R, Staffeldt E: Back pain and isometric back muscle strength of workers in a Danish factory. *Scand J Rehabil Med* 7:125–128, 1975.

15. Pederson R, Staffeldt E: The relationship between four tests of back muscle strength in untrained subjects. *Scand J Rehabil Med* 4:175–181, 1972.

16. Chaffin D: Pre-employment strength testing: updated position. *J Occup Med* 10:105–110, 1978.

17. Kishino N, Mayer T, Gatchel R, Parrish M, Anderson C, Gustin L, Mooney V: Quantification of lumbar function. Part 4: isometric and isokinetic lifting simulation in normal subjects and low back dysfunction patients. *Spine* 10:921–927, 1985.

18. Gracovetsky S, Farfan H: The optimum spine. *Spine* 11:543–573, 1986.

19. Keeley J, Mayer T, Cox R, Gatchel R, Smith J, Mooney V: Quantification of lumbar function. Part 5: reliability of range of motion measures in the sagittal plane and an *in vivo* torso rotation measurement technique. *Spine* 11:31–35, 1985.

20. Mayer T, Gatchel R, Kishino N, Keeley J, Capra P, Mayer H, Barnett J, Mooney V: Objective assessment of spine function following industrial injury: a prospective study with comparison group and one-year follup-up. Volvo Award in Clinical Sciences. *Spine* 10:482–493, 1985.

21. Mayer T, Gatchel R, Mayer H, Kishino N, Keeley J, Mooney V: A prospective two-year study of functional restoration in industrial low back injury: an objective assessment procedure. *JAMA* 258:1763–1767, 1987.

22. Mayer T, Smith S, Kondraske G, Gatchel R, Carmichael T, Mooney V: Quantification of lumbar function. Part 3: preliminary data on isokinetic torso rotation testing with myoelectric spectral analysis in normal and low back pain subjects. *Spine* 10:912–920, 1985.

23. Mayer T, Tencer A, Kristoferson S, Mooney V: Use of noninvasive techniques for quantification of spinal range-of-motion in normal subjects and chronic low-back dysfunction patients. *Spine* 9:588–595, 1984.

24. Smith S, Mayer T, Gatchel R, Becker T: Quantification of lumbar function. Part 1: isometric and multi-speed isokinetic trunk strength measures in sagittal and axial planes in normal subject patients. *Spine* 10:757–764, 1985.

25. Pearcy M, Portek I, Sheperd J: The effect of low back pain on lumbar spinal movements measured by three-dimensional x-ray analysis. *Spine* 10:150–153, 1985.

26. Pearcy M, Shepard J: Is there instability in spondylolisthesis? *Spine* 10:175–177, 1985.

27. Moll J, Wright V: Measurement of spinal movement. In Jayson M (ed): *The Lumbar Spine and Back Pain.* New York, Grune & Stratton, 1976, pp 93–112.

28. Schober P: Lendenwirbelsaule und kreuzschcmerzen. *Munch Med Wochenschr* 84:336, 1937.

29. Alston W, Carlson K, Feldman D, et al: A quantitative study of muscle fatigue in the chronic low back syndrome. *J Am Geriatr Soc* 14:419–423, 1966.

30. Andersson G, Ortengren R, Herbert T: Quantitative electromyography studies of back muscle activity related to posture and loading. *Orthop Clin North Am* 8:85–96, 1977.

31. Cady L, Bischoff D, O'Connel E, Thomas P, Allan J: Strength and fitness and subsequent back injuries in firefighters. *J Occup Med* 21:269–272, 1979.

32. Davies G, Gould J: Trunk testing using a prototype Cybex II Isokinetic Stabilization System. *J Orthop Sports Phys Ther* 3:164–170, 1982.

33. Hasue M, Fuguwara M, Kikuchi S: A new method of quantitative measurement of abdominal and back muscle strength. *Spine* 5:143–148, 1980.

34. Langrana N, Lee C, Alexander H, Mayott C: Quantitative assessment of back strength using isokinetic testing. *Spine* 9:287–290, 1984.

35. McNeill, Warwick D, Andersson C, et al: Trunk strength in attempted flexion, extension, and lateral bending in healthy subjects and patients with low back disorders. *Spine* 5:529–538, 1980.

36. Smidt G, Herring T, Amundsen L, Rogers M, Russell A, Lehmann T: Assessment of abdominal and back extensor function: a quantitative approach and results for chronic low-back patients. *Spine* 8:211–219, 1983.

37. Thorstensson A, Arvidson A: Trunk muscle strength and low-back pain. *Scand J Rehab Med* 14:69–75, 1982.

38. Thorstensson A, Nilsson J: Trunk muscle strength during constant and velocity movement. *Scand J Rehab Med* 14:61–68, 1982.

39. Suzuki N, Endo S: A quantitative study of trunk muscle strength and fatigability in the low-back pain syndrome. *Spine* 8:69–74, 1983.

40. Mayer T, Smith S, Keeley J, Mooney V: Quantification of lumbar function. Part 2: sagittal plane trunk strength in chronic low back pain patients. *Spine* 10:765–772, 1985.

41. Thompson N, Gould J, Davies G, Ross D, Price S: Descriptive measures of isokinetic trunk testing. *J Orthop Sports Phys Ther* 7:43–49, 1985.

42. Chaffin D, Andersson G: *Occupational Biomechanics.* New York, Wiley Intersciences, 1984.

43. Mayer T, Barnes D, Kishino N, Nichols G, Gatchel R, Mayer H, Mooney V: Progressive isoinertial lifting evaluation, Part I: a standardized protocol and normative database. *Spine* 1988 (in press).

44. Mayer T, Barnes D, Nichols G, Kishino N, Coval K, Piel B, Hoshino D, Gatchel R: Progressive isoinertial lifting evaluation, Part II: a comparison with isokinetics in a disabled chronic low back pain industrial population. *Spine* 13:998–1002, 1988.

45. Capra P, Mayer T, Gatchel R: Using psychological

scales to assess back pain. *J Musculoskel Med* 2:41–52, 1985.

46. Gatchel R, Mears G: *Personality: Theory, Assessment and Research.* New York, St. Martin's Press, 1983.
47. Gould J, Davies G (eds): *Orthopedic and Sports Physical Therapy.* St. Louis, CV Mosby, 1985.
48. Langrana N, Lee C: Isokinetic evaluation of trunk muscles. *Spine* 9:171–175, 1984.

49. Pope M, Frymoyer J, Andersson G: *Occupational Low Back Pain.* New York, Praeger, 1984.
50. Nachemson A: Work for all. *Clin Orthop Rel Res* 179:77–82, 1983.
51. Hazard R, Reid S, Fenwick J, Reeves V: Isokinetic trunk and lifting strength measurements: variability as a predictor of effort. *Spine* 13:54–57, 1988.

Index

Page numbers in *italics* denote figures; those followed by "t" denote tables.